PARLIAMENT OF VICTORIA

DRUGS AND CRIME PREVENTION COMMITTEE

INQUIRY INTO AMPHETAMINE AND 'PARTY DRUG' USE IN VICTORIA
Final Report

Ordered to be printed

May 2004

by Authority
Government Printer for the State of Victoria

No. 66 Session 2003-2004

The Report was prepared by the Drugs and Crime Prevention Committee.

The Committee records its appreciation to Kate Hiller for permission to use images from her video *Rave Culture 2002* in the artwork of the Discussion Paper and this Report.

Drugs and Crime Prevention Committee

Inquiry into Amphetamine and 'Party Drug' Use in Victoria – Final Report

DCPC, Parliament of Victoria

ISBN: 0-9579188-3-6

Drugs and Crime Prevention Committee

Level 8
35 Spring Street
Melbourne Victoria 3000
Telephone: (03) 9651 3541
Facsimile: (03) 9651 3603
Email: sandy.cook@parliament.vic.gov.au
http://www.parliament.vic.gov.au/dcpc

Drugs and Crime Prevention Committee – 55th Parliament

Members

Ms Carolyn Hirsh, M.L.C.– **Chair**

The Hon. Robin Cooper, M.L.A. – **Deputy Chairman**

Ms Kirstie Marshall, M.L.A.

Mr Ian Maxfield, M.L.A.

Dr Bill Sykes, M.L.A.

The Hon. Sang Minh Nguyen, M.L.C.

Mr Kim Wells, M.L.A.

Drugs and Crime Prevention Committee – 54th Parliament

Members

The Hon. Cameron Boardman, M.L.C. – **Chair**

Mr. Bruce Mildenhall, M.L.A. – **Deputy Chair**

The Hon. Robin Cooper, M.L.A.

Mr. Kenneth Jasper, M.L.A.

Mr. Hurtle Lupton, M.L.A.

The Hon. Sang Minh Nguyen, M.L.C.

Mr. Richard Wynne, M.L.A.

Committee Staff

Ms Sandy Cook, *Executive Officer*

Mr Peter Johnston, *Senior Legal Research Officer*

Ms Michelle Summerhill, *Office Manager*

Ms Joyce Wong, *Acting Office Manager*

Functions of the Drugs and Crime Prevention Committee

The Victorian Drugs and Crime Prevention Committee is constituted under the *Parliamentary Committees Act 2003* (Vic)

Section 7

The functions of the Drugs and Crime Prevention Committee are, if so required or permitted under this Act, to inquire into, consider and report to the Parliament on any proposal, matter or thing concerned with:

a. the use of drugs including the manufacture, supply or distribution of drugs;

b. the level or causes of crime or violent behaviour.

Terms of Reference

The Governor in Council, under section 4F of the *Parliamentary Committees Act 1968*, requests that the Drugs and Crime Prevention Committee of Parliament inquire into, consider and report to Parliament on amphetamine and 'party drug' use in Victoria. In particular the Committee is required to:

a) examine the nature, extent and culture of amphetamine and 'party drug' use;

b) determine the demographic profile of users;

c) examine the short and long-term consequences of amphetamine and 'party drug' use;

d) examine the relationship of amphetamine and 'party drug' use to other forms of licit and illicit substance use;

e) review the adequacy of existing strategies for dealing with amphetamine and 'party drug' use;

f) consider best practice strategies to address the issue of amphetamine and 'party drug' use, including regulatory, law enforcement, education and treatment responses; and

g) examine national and international legislation, reports and materials relevant to the issue.

Chair's Foreword

The Inquiry into Amphetamine and 'Party Drug' Use in Victoria was commenced in 2002 by the Drugs and Crime Prevention Committee of the 54th Parliament, during which time a literature review was initiated. Following the 2002 election, the new Drugs and Crime Prevention Committee, established by the 55th Parliament, was asked to continue the work already underway. The same Terms of Reference were resubmitted to the Committee to enable the work to be completed. The Committee produced a discussion paper in September 2003, in which the questions developed from submissions and evidence to the Committee were posed.

The Inquiry was extremely complex, with the Terms of Reference encompassing two very distinct drug groups, and drug use by two discrete populations, those using amphetamines alone, and those ingesting drugs such as ecstasy and other drugs typically available or used in a 'party' environment. Moreover, within these two broad classifications many 'subtypes' of user can be identified.

The formulation of the recommendations contained in this Report was, as a result of the complexity of the Reference, quite difficult. The Recommendations are wide-ranging and all encompassing, reflecting the many and varied topics and issues reviewed throughout the Report. While some of the recommendations are applicable to all groups discussed in the Report, other groups require specifically tailored interventions.

The recommendations reflect the key concept of harm minimisation. This concept, which places equal emphasis on supply, demand and harm reduction as described in the National Drug Strategy, is endorsed by and underpins the work of this Committee.

During the Inquiry, the Committee made numerous of visits to rural and regional Victoria. Through consultation and evidence gathering, Members became aware of the specific issues which confront workers and drug users in those communities. As a result of this information the Committee has made a number of recommendations specifically targeted toward drug problems in rural and regional Victoria.

Another specific set of recommendations in the Report is directed toward the media. The Committee acknowledges, and indeed appreciates, the valuable role played by the media in their dissemination of information on important issues, and the contribution of the media to social policy debates. However the use of the term 'party drugs' to describe diverse drugs used in a 'party' environment could be problematic in that it glamourises these substances, some of which are very dangerous. The Committee has used the term throughout this report, as required by the Terms of Reference but hopes that the media will play a leading role with the community in discouraging the use of this term.

At the conclusion of this exhaustive and extensive Inquiry I am very pleased that the Committee has produced a Report with which all members agree unanimously.

The Committee and I wish to express our sincere thanks those who have assisted in the production of this major piece of work. In particular, the commitment of the Committee's staff needs to be acknowledged. The Report could not have been completed without the dedication of Sandy Cook, the Executive Officer, Pete Johnston, Senior Legal Researcher, who drafted the report, office staff Michelle Summerhill, Joyce Wong and Sandi Jensen and Sarah Kerwick, a student from the University of Melbourne who was responsible for researching and drafting much of the Chapter on rural and regional Victoria.

The Committee also wishes to express its gratitude to Debra Reeves and Jon Breukel from the Parliament of Victoria Library for their library assistance, Mignon Turpin for her contribution in editing the Report, Chris Watson from Zapwhizz.com.au who has designed and laid out the contents of the Report and Matt Clare for designing the cover. In particular the Committee records its appreciation to Kate Hiller for permission to use images from her video *Rave Culture 2002* for the covers of both the Discussion Paper and the Final Report. The assistance of Natalie Russell from RaveSafe, Ben Horan and all those members of the community who gave so generously of their time and knowledge is also most appreciated.

I would also like to thank the members of the Committee for their participation and contribution to the Inquiry.

The Committee hopes that this important Report will inform the Government and the Victorian community in policy and programme development on the growing problem of the use of amphetamine-type substances and other drugs used by people in a recreational environment.

Carolyn Hirsh M.L.C.

Chair

Executive Summary

The Drugs and Crime Prevention Committee was given Terms of Reference to investigate and report to Parliament on the use of amphetamines and 'party drugs' in Victoria. This included examining the nature and extent of use, the consequences of such use, and the strategies employed to restrict such use and provide treatment for users. A major concern identified through this Inquiry has been the dearth of information relating to the extent of amphetamine and 'party drug' use, the long-term effects of use and the lack of specific education, services and appropriate treatment for specific users of specific drugs. The need for further targeted research and partnerships between all groups working in areas related to the supply and use of these drugs was seen to be essential for effectively addressing these issues.

PART A – Introduction

The introductory chapters of this Report discuss the framework against which this Inquiry took place, the people and organisations consulted and the research process undertaken.

This Part also argues in Chapter 3 that a multi-faceted 'all of community' response is needed if the problems associated with the use of amphetamines and 'party drugs' are going to be effectively addressed. The importance of collaborative approaches is incorporated in the recommendations of the Committee.

PART B – The Nature and Extent of Amphetamine and 'Party Drug' Use

This Part contextualises the problem of amphetamine and 'party drug' use in Victoria. It is noted that amphetamines in particular are increasingly popular on an international level and the second most commonly used illicit drug in Australia.

Chapter 4 provides a detailed account of the nature of amphetamine and 'party drugs'. It notes that there are problems associated with coupling these drug groups together in an Inquiry such as this, given the diversity of drugs included under this rubric. It also notes the problematic nature of the language and nomenclature associated with these drugs. For example, does the use of the term 'party' trivialise or even render acceptable this form of drug misuse?

The second part of Chapter 4 discusses the nature of those drugs or groups of drugs that have been selected as the focus of this Report. This includes an examination inter alia of:

- the history of the use of the drug;
- the pharmacological and chemical properties of the drug;
- how such drugs are used;
- the mode of administration; and
- a brief account of why some drugs may be seen as 'desirable' by their users.

Chapter 5 examines prevalence rates for the use of amphetamines and 'party drugs'. The first part of this chapter examines briefly the extent of use of amphetamine and 'party drugs' from a global perspective, basing its analysis chiefly on United Nations data.

The second section of Chapter 5 is similarly an examination of the quantitative data, however this time from a local perspective. Prevalence data is examined from both national and Victorian sources. Much of this is based on population surveys, although disparate sources such as treatment and ambulance data are also used. The limitation of such surveys, and indeed the problems generally encountered in measuring drug activity, are discussed at length. The chapter and Part conclude with a call for further research that provides more accurate assessments of trends in the use of amphetamines and 'party drugs'.

PART C - Effects of Amphetamines and 'Party Drugs' – Physical, Psychological and Social Consequences

Chapter 6 of this Part examines the complex issues pertaining to the medical effects of amphetamines and 'party drugs'. It commences with a discussion of the physical and psychological consequences of taking amphetamines. Topics of discussion include the issue of 'speed psychosis', withdrawal and dependence, an examination of whether there is an amphetamine dependence syndrome, behavioural and co-morbidity problems associated with amphetamine use and issues pertaining to depression and cognitive functioning. A particular aspect of the chapter that requires separate consideration is a comparison of injecting versus non-injecting amphetamine use.

The second half of the chapter examines physical and psychological problems associated with the use of 'party drugs' such as MDMA (ecstasy), ketamine and GHB. In particular it examines such diverse issues as the effect of the 'comedown period' after the use of MDMA, MDMA and cognitive functioning and the vexed issue of whether there are any long-term effects from the use of MDMA (ecstasy).

Chapter 7 switches from a discussion of the medical effects of using amphetamines and 'party drugs' to the social consequences of using these drugs, examining the links between amphetamine use, violence, and crime. This is followed by a discussion on 'drink spiking through the use of 'party drugs' such as GHB, often for the purpose of 'date rape'. The chapter then looks at how amphetamine is used for functional reasons in the transport and other industries before examining the issue of road trauma and 'drug driving', particularly in the context of new Victorian legislation which will allow for the testing of drivers who may have been ingesting amphetamine. Finally, a discussion of the economic costs of amphetamine and 'party drug' use is undertaken with particular emphasis on the costs of absenteeism from work, school or college due to the after-effects of 'party drug' use.

The final chapter in this Part consists of a discussion of the issue of 'poly-drug' use. The chapter notes that rarely are either amphetamines or 'party drugs' such as MDMA used exclusively. Poly-drug use, including the use of cannabis and alcohol, is increasingly common among drug users, whether through the use of several drugs in succession over a period of time (for example, the use of marijuana to 'come down' from the effects of MDMA) or more worryingly the use of a wide 'repertoire' of drugs at the same time.

PART D – The Culture and Patterns of Use

Part D moves away from a medical appraisal of amphetamine and 'party drug' use to a more descriptive and qualitative based discussion of the patterns, profiles and cultures of this form of drug taking.

Chapter 9 examines the profiles and cultures of varied and discrete groups of drug user. It commences with a discussion of 'street use' of amphetamine, particularly among street workers and the homeless. This is followed by the related issue of amphetamine use among young people, particularly young people 'in crisis'. Amphetamine use as a 'functional' measure is then discussed, concentrating particularly on those who use it in the transport industry. Sections devoted to the use of amphetamines by women, Indigenous Victorians and people from culturally and linguistically diverse communities follow. A section on amphetamine, particularly methamphetamine, and 'party drug' use in the gay and lesbian community and a discussion of MDMA use among 'middle-class' 'party drug' users concludes the chapter. The disparate needs of various groups who use amphetamines and 'party drugs' are reflected in the accompanying recommendations.

Chapter 10 profiles the use of 'party drugs' by one particular subset of user – the 'clubber' or 'raver'. It examines the cultures and lifestyles of those who use the drugs in the context of dance parties and outdoor 'raves'. It notes that elements such as the choice of music, lighting, venue and fashion are an integral part of the dance party scene. While the use of 'party drugs' such as ecstasy is clearly part of this scene, it is true to state, as many academics have done, that dance parties cannot simply be viewed as 'drug supermarkets'.

The final chapter in this Part is a discussion of drug use in rural and regional areas of Victoria, an issue that is often overlooked. It examines the prevalence of amphetamine and 'party drug' use in non-metropolitan regions of Victoria noting that one cannot speak of either licit or illicit drug use in Victoria on the basis that all country areas are homogenous entities with the same extent and types of drug use and the same problems stemming from such use. The chapter also examines issues such as access to and availability of drug treatment services and programmes, the adequacy of staffing levels of drug and alcohol services, the lack of research and data with regard to patterns of amphetamine and 'party drug' use by people in non-metropolitan areas, and the disadvantages related to location and distance for those living and/or working in country regions. Finally, the chapter discusses whether drug policy and service delivery in Victoria can be viewed as 'Melbourne centric' and if so how this can be remedied.

PART E – Law, Law Enforcement, Policing and Supply Control

This Part examines a variety of issues that impact upon the way the legal and criminal justice systems deal with the issue of amphetamines and 'party drugs'.

The first chapter in the Part contains a brief discussion of the law, both domestic and international, as it applies to these drugs.

Chapter 14 examines the international and domestic supply control of amphetamines and 'party drugs' and Chapter 15 discusses the manufacture of amphetamines and 'party drugs' at both domestic and international levels. In particular it focusses on the investigation of clandestine laboratories and the dangers faced by the officers of Victoria Police who are part of the Illicit Laboratories Task Force.

Chapter 16 discusses a particular issue that encompasses both manufacture and supply issues, namely the difficulties associated with precursor control. In doing so, it examines both the importation of precursor chemicals, their wholesale supply and, at a domestic level, the role that pharmacies and retail chemists play in curtailing the use of precursors for the manufacture of illicit drugs.

Chapter 17 moves away from the supply or manufacture of amphetamines and 'party drugs' to the issues surrounding the distribution of the drugs once they are in Australia. In particular it concentrates on the macro distribution of amphetamines. The local level distribution of 'party drugs' is discussed in Chapter 18, which examines local level policing and law enforcement. The emphasis in this discussion is on the problems police face in policing amphetamines and 'party drugs' at a local level. In particular, it examines the issues surrounding the use of law enforcement in Victorian nightclubs.

PART F – Education, Information and Harm Reduction Issues Pertaining to Amphetamines and 'Party Drugs'

This Part discusses the separate but related issues of drug education, information provision and the concept of harm reduction as it applies to drug programmes and drug service delivery.

Chapter 18 commences with an examination of the debates pertaining to drug education generally, before canvassing education issues specific to amphetamines and 'party drugs'. It notes that for the most part education strategies should draw from young people's own experiences of their drug use. It also takes cognisance of the fact that 'negative' drug education campaigns rarely have success in stopping young people either taking up drugs or discontinuing use. A discussion of interventions such as outreach and peer education follows before examining the role of the media in disseminating and commenting upon issues pertaining to 'party drugs'.

The examination of 'party drugs' concludes with a discussion of the use of new technologies such as the Internet in providing both useful and possibly dangerous information with regard to these drugs. The chapter concludes with a brief examination of education and information provision with regard to amphetamine use.

Chapter 19 discusses the controversial and often misunderstood concept of harm reduction. It also examines some of the theoretical writing about harm minimisation and the related issue of the 'normalisation' of youth drug use.

The major part of the chapter is devoted to an examination of strategies, policies, services and programmes that aim to prevent or at least minimise the harms associated with amphetamine and 'party drug' use, particularly in the context of dance clubs, parties and 'rave events'.

The related recommendations recognise that the use of 'party drugs' does occur. They do not, however, condone such use. Instead, in accordance with harm minimisation principles, they seek to prevent adverse or dangerous reactions and consequences for the user or other affected party.

PART G – Treatment and Research Issues Pertaining to Amphetamine and 'Party Drug' Use

Part G examines the distinct but interrelated issues of treatment for and research into amphetamine and 'party drug use'.

Chapter 20 is a discussion of the treatment issues associated with these drugs. It notes that the concept of treatment is much more applicable to the use of amphetamines than to 'party drugs'. People who may suffer from the ill effects of 'party drugs' such as MDMA or GHB rarely present with chronic conditions. Rather they are more likely to attend casualty or emergency room departments after having ingested a contaminated pill or suffered from a condition such as hyperthermia. **[check]**

On the other hand, while there may be long-term and chronic conditions associated with the regular or long-term use of amphetamines, amphetamine users are often reluctant to seek treatment or attend medical services. The chapter discusses why this may be so and how services may become more 'user friendly' for those people who take amphetamines.

The most commonly accessed service for amphetamine users experiencing problems with their drug use is likely to be a general practitioner. This may be in part because there *are* few discrete specialist interventions available, particularly pharmacological interventions. The issue of substitution therapies for amphetamines, such as oral use of dexamphetamine, is contentious. The arguments for and against such therapies are canvassed in detail in this chapter, as is a range of other intervention methods.

Chapter 21 examines the need for comprehensive and targeted research into amphetamine and 'party drugs'. It argues that a wide range of research projects, and methodologies of both a quantitative and qualitative nature, need to be undertaken, noting that while a huge amount of research literature on amphetamines and 'party drugs' exists, there is still an enormous gap in our knowledge of the effect of these drugs and the patterns of their use.

PART H – The Way Forward: Concluding Remarks

The concluding part of this Report gives a summary of the issues pertaining to amphetamines and 'party drugs' as discussed and examined throughout this Inquiry. It notes that given the complexities of amphetamine and 'party drug' use and the differences between and within these classifications, it is quite clear that a 'one size fits all' approach will be inadequate to address this issue. For example, the strategies required to prevent MDMA use among party-goers will be very different to interventions needed for the chronic adult amphetamine abuser.

The Committee notes throughout this Report that addressing amphetamine and 'party drug' abuse requires a whole of community response. Local solutions, including local partnerships, are required for local communities. Drug misuse requires interventions that range across a number of areas – policy development, training and education, legal regulation, treatment, research, media reporting, employment and recreation and local community initiatives, to name a few.

Such programmes and initiatives will also require adequate and ongoing funding if they are to be successfully initiated and maintained. The Committee therefore makes a number of recommendations with regard to the funding of amphetamine and 'party drug' programmes, projects and services.

The remaining section of this concluding chapter contains brief summaries of the Committee's position on the key issues that have arisen from this Inquiry. It should be read in conjunction with the Inquiry recommendations. As the conclusion notes, reaching these positions has not been easy. It has involved balancing and reconciling a number of competing interests and positions, all of which have strong arguments to support them.

Recommendations

Statement of Principles underlying the Recommendations

The Committee's endeavours have been guided by a series of principles that have formed the bedrock of the Report and informed the recommendations that follow them. These Principles are as follows:

A. The Committee believes that there is no 'one size fits all' response to amphetamine and 'party drug' use. This is particularly the case given that these are two very distinct drug groups. It is an extremely complex problem that requires a co-ordinated multi-faceted 'all of community response'. Such a response requires commitment and participation at Commonwealth, state and local levels. It will involve input from and partnerships between the government, private and community sectors.

B. In formulating these recommendations the Committee acknowledges that amphetamine and 'party drug' use is a problem for a diverse range of users and groups. Many of the Committee's recommendations will be applicable to all profiled groups. Nonetheless, the Committee recognises that specific groups require tailored interventions. As such, many of the recommendations will be targeted accordingly.

C. The Committee endorses the importance of placing an equal emphasis on the three tiers of supply, demand and harm reduction as outlined in the National Drug Strategy.

D. The Committee believes that the laws and legislation pertaining to drug-related crime should reflect the seriousness of the harms associated with amphetamines and 'party drugs'.

E. The Committee believes that law enforcement agencies and personnel play a key role in supply reduction and control. It is essential that all branches of the law enforcement apparatus, local, state and federal authorities, work together collaboratively to reduce the supply and distribution of amphetamines and 'party drugs'.

F. Demand reduction for both illicit and licit drugs requires the development and dissemination of best practice education strategies and information provision. Such strategies need to be tailored and delivered to a diverse range of audiences.

G. Amphetamine and 'party drug' use is not solely a drug problem. In a complex society people experience a range of economic, social and personal problems and their drug use is a symptom of these problems. Strategies must therefore address the underlying causes of this drug use.

H. Similarly, the Committee believes that in addressing a person's use of amphetamines and 'party drugs', strategies should not focus on the problem primarily as a drug issue. Where appropriate, interventions need to be culturally sensitive, gender specific and tailored to take into account a range of individual needs and user profiles.

I. The Committee acknowledges that when addressing the issue of amphetamine and 'party drug' use among Indigenous communities, any treatment response must be culturally sensitive and specific to the needs of those communities. The Committee believes that ideally such strategies should be developed and implemented by or in partnership with Indigenous organisations, agencies and community groups.

J. The Committee especially recognises that drug policy and practice can tend to be 'Melbourne centric'. The Committee acknowledges the specific and unique policy, research and service delivery needs of regional and rural Victoria.

K. The Committee acknowledges the reality of 'poly-drug' use among amphetamine and 'party drug' users. Specific drug policies and practice need to be developed to address poly-drug use.

L. The Committee suggests that wherever possible policy and programme development regarding amphetamine and 'party drug' use be informed by the views, opinions and input of the users of those drugs. It is also important that the 'cultures' of amphetamine and 'party drug' use be understood by those responsible for developing drug policy and service delivery.

M. The Committee acknowledges that harm minimisation is a key platform of the National Drug Strategy. For the most part it endorses this approach. The Committee recognises that harm minimisation and harm reduction programmes and strategies form a central part of addressing the problems associated with amphetamines and 'party drugs'. Harm minimisation is a policy in which supply reduction (law enforcement), demand reduction (prevention, education and early intervention) and treatment, rehabilitation and service delivery form equal parts of an overall strategy to address drug misuse.

N. The Committee acknowledges that ongoing and comprehensive qualitative, quantitative and evaluative research should inform policy and practice in the area of amphetamine and 'party drug' use. Such research is fundamental not only to understanding the problem but also in order to develop best practice programmes and responses to address it.

Recommendations

The issue of amphetamine and particularly 'party drug' use has been highlighted in recent weeks due to a series of incidents involving the use of the 'party drug' gamma-hydroxybutyrate (GHB) at the *Two Tribes* dance party held at Melbourne Park.

The recommendations enumerated by the Committee as a result of this Inquiry and the draft of the Final Report were written prior to the *Two Tribes* incident. Nonetheless, as serious as these incidents were, the Committee exhorts policy makers, the media and the general public to be cautious in the way in which it responds to the issue of dance parties and 'raves' and the use of drugs at such events. In terms of numbers, far more incidents involving ambulance call outs or emergency room visits can be attributed to alcohol than to drugs such as GHB. The Committee believes that its recommendations emanating from this Report, particularly those with regard to harm reduction, will assist in preventing or responding to the harms associated with this type of drug use.

The recommendations and the discussion of this Report are guided at all times by the principles of the *National Drug Strategy*. In particular, as stated in the accompanying 'Statement of Principles' the Committee endorses the equal importance of the principles of *supply reduction, demand reduction* and *harm reduction.*

The following recommendations are organised according to broad areas of content and theme as discussed in the Final Report. While there may be overlap between various sections, wherever possible a Part or Chapter number corresponding to where the recommendation is located in the body of the text will be given.

Recommendations with regard to law, policing, law enforcement and supply control

The Committee recommends that the Drugs, Poisons and Controlled Substances Act 1981 be amended to insert a new offence of possession without lawful excuse of an amount to be specified of precursor chemicals and associated apparatus/equipment used for the manufacture of illicit drugs. (Recommendation 20, p.345)

The Committee recommends the amendment of Part 3 of Schedule 11 of the Drugs, Poisons and Controlled Substances Act 1981 to reduce the pure and dilute quantities for amphetamine and methylamphetamine to be in line with methylenedioxymethamphetamine (ecstasy) in order to control trafficking of MDMA. This would reflect the fact that amphetamine is now more commonly sold in tablet form. (Recommendation 21, p.346)

The Committee recommends the amendment of Part 3 of Schedule 11 of the Drugs, Poisons and Controlled Substances Act 1981 to reduce the dilute quantities for pseudoephedrine to be in line with the current amphetamine and methylamphetamine commercial quantities. This would assist in combating pseudoephedrine diversion from pharmacies. (Recommendation 22, p.346)

The Committee recommends that the existing offence for the possession of pseudoephedrine without lawful excuse in Part One of Schedule Eleven of the Drugs, Poisons and Controlled Substances Act 1981 be publicised and enforced. (Recommendation 23, p.346)

The Committee recommends that appropriate legislation be enacted to require photographic identification to be produced to pharmacists or pharmacy staff for the purchase of two or more packets of non prescription pseudoephedrine based medications or products (single ingredient or combination product). In all other cases current Pharmacy Industry guidelines and Codes of Practice should be strictly observed and enforced. (Recommendation 28, p.413)

The Committee recommends that legislation be drafted to protect endangered children, in particular making it a crime of child abuse, as well as a circumstance of aggravation to a drug offence, if a person manufactures, stores or transports chemicals and/or apparatus used to manufacture prohibited drugs in the presence of children. (Recommendation 24, p.363)

The Committee recommends that the current industry Code of Conduct with regard to the sale and diversion of chemical precursors be established in legislation. (Recommendation 26, p.403)

The Committee recommends that the proposed mandatory Code of Conduct incorporate the sale of pill presses, to ensure a consistent approach by all manufacturers. (Recommendation 27, p.403)

The Committee recommends that with regard to 'party drugs' police continue their efforts to reduce supply of these drugs through targeting and prioritising action against trafficking. (Recommendation 30, p.430)

The Committee takes note that state and interstate highways and major roads act as a conduit for the distribution of illicit drugs, including amphetamine. The Committee therefore recommends the increased surveillance of trucks and other motor vehicles. (Recommendation 29, p.420)

The Committee believes that both specialist and general police officers and emergency workers should be aware of the dangers associated with clandestine drug laboratories. To this end the Committee recommends the following provisions with regard to police and community education and training:

a) Police education should ensure that all officers are suitably trained in clandestine drug laboratory awareness and safety procedures.

b) Emergency service personnel should receive appropriate training with regard to clandestine drug laboratories.

c) Existing certification courses for clandestine drug laboratory investigators should be regularly updated to reflect current trends in keeping with the world's best practices. (Recommendation 25, p.389)

The Committee recommends that consideration be given to the creation of a new general offence of 'drink spiking' with a sufficient level of penalty to reflect the gravity of this crime. Such an offence should be in addition to and not in substitution of the provisions of Section 53 of the *Crimes Act 1958* (administration of a drug). (Recommendation 3, p.166)

The Committee recommends that the Sentencing Advisory Council undertakes a wide ranging review of the adequacy of penalties and sentences contained in the Drugs, Poisons and Controlled Substances Act 1981 and other relevant legislation. (Recommendation 31, p.430)

The Committee recommends a wide-ranging and comprehensive review of security issues and security personnel including but not restricted to security personnel and crowd controllers located at nightclubs, dance clubs, venues and 'rave' events. Such a review would concentrate not solely on issues involving security and violence but also those pertaining to health, training and other concerns relating to the industry. (Recommendation 45, p.515)

The Committee recommends that, subject to the findings of such a review, more stringent requirements be placed on the initial issue and ongoing renewal of a Security/Crowd Controller licence to include the following requirements:

a) Training modules developed to give a better understanding of illicit substances, their signs and potential hazards.

b) Training modules developed to give a better understanding of drink spiking, the strategies that can reduce occurrences, and the consequences of non-intervention.

c) Level 2 First Aid qualification must be maintained as current in order to hold licence (renewed every 3 years).

d) CPR Refresher must be maintained as current in order to hold licence (recommended renewal every 1 year).

e) Mandatory reporting of violent incidents involving Crowd Controllers for review of their licence holding.

f) Training in the detection of drug trafficking or distribution at clubs and associated venues. (Recommendation 46, p.515)

The Committee recommends that random drug testing of security personnel should be undertaken by Police on a regular basis. (Recommendation 47, p.515)

Recommendations with regard to education, training and information provision

The Committee recommends that, for the most part, education training and information provision with regard to amphetamines and/or 'party drugs' are most usefully developed for groups, in addition to children and adolescents. These groups should include:

- Teachers and school support staff;
- Parents and parent groups including those from Indigenous and culturally and linguistically diverse communities;
- Police, ambulance officers and other emergency personnel;
- Youth, social and community workers (including culturally appropriate education strategies for those from Indigenous groups);
- Workers from culturally and linguistically diverse communities and agencies;
- Drug and alcohol service workers;
- Residential care workers;
- Doctors, nurses and other health workers;
- Dance club, party venue, outdoor rave staff and promoters;
- Crowd controllers;
- Users and user organisations;
- Local government staff, particularly those working in areas such as recreation, parks and gardens and amenities; and
- Journalists and media representatives.

In particular, these groups and individuals need to be thoroughly informed of the nature and consequences of amphetamines and 'party drugs'. They should also be trained or advised of appropriate ways of assisting a person who appears to be intoxicated through amphetamine and 'party drug' use. (Recommendation 35, p.475)

The Committee recommends that relevant professional bodies should examine the adequacy of current training regarding amphetamine and 'party drug' use and should determine the basic level of knowledge on amphetamine and 'party drug' use appropriate to their professions. (Recommendation 36, p.475)

The Committee recommends that in-service and multi-disciplinary training on drug issues include amphetamine and 'party drug' use. Within training and education programmes for personnel working in the field, instruction should be provided giving accurate and comprehensive knowledge of harm minimisation policy and practice. (Recommendation 37, p.475)

The Committee recommends that sufficient and appropriate ongoing training be given to medical, nursing and ancillary staff with regard to amphetamines and 'party drugs'. (Recommendation 38, p.475)

The Committee recommends that the curricular for medical, nursing and health workers incorporate sufficient information, education and training on alcohol and drug-related issues, in particular amphetamine and 'party drug' issues. (Recommendation 39, p.476)

The Committee recommends that users, including occasional users and poly-drug users, should be provided with accurate and relevant information in relation to the effects of amphetamine and 'party drug' use and how to obtain help when needed. Such an approach provides pathways and access points to treatment services. (Recommendation 40, p.486)

The Committee recommends that strategic and targeted information about amphetamines and 'party drugs' which is tailored to a range of users in different settings and contexts (eg. clubs, raves, schools, universities, workplaces, sports and community clubs) be made readily available, particularly to young people. (Recommendation 41, p.486)

The Committee recommends the provision of a diverse range of relevant and available information and harm reduction messages to individuals. These should be facilitated through a variety of avenues including written guidelines, websites, email alerts and mobile telephone messages, and be accessible through peer networks. (Recommendation 42, p.486)

Recommendations with regard to harm minimisation and harm reduction

The Committee strongly recommends that the Government initiates the introduction of retractable single dose syringes. (Recommendation 60, p.557)

The Committee believes that increasing access to blood-borne virus prevention equipment is of priority and recommends a number of strategies to be implemented including:

a) Establishment of new Needle and Syringe Program outlets including pharmacy-based outlets;

b) Further and ongoing funding for after-hours Needle and Syringe Program services;

c) Attaching Needle and Syringe Program services to other after-hours services. (Recommendation 61, p.557)

The Committee recommends that as a hepatitis C prevention measure, Human Services Victoria supplies Needle and Syringe Program outlets with a range of sterile injecting equipment including sterile water and filters for distribution to clients. (Recommendation 62, p.557)

The Committee recommends that a regulatory framework for dance and club venues and indoor and outdoor 'raves' be established that mandates the appropriate management of these facilities and locations. This should include but not be restricted to:

Mandatory licensing conditions to be developed to govern patron health and safety at venues and events, including:

a) Adequate ventilation and sensible climate controls (generous airflow, and ambient temperature around dance areas to be of a comfortable level for high exertion).

b) Well ventilated seated areas ('chill-out' space) sufficient for the expected patronage.

c) The ready availability of free potable cold tap water, and where appropriate isotonic drinks.

d) For venues or events that cater for less than 500 patrons, a Level 2 First Aid qualified staff person should be in attendance. The requisite standard of first aid equipment should be provided.

e) For venues or events of more than 500 patrons, a Level 2 First Aid (or higher) trained staff member should be assigned the specific duty of patron care (monitoring for concerning signs of drug influences, intoxication or overdose and providing appropriate care).

f) Venue managers and promoters should take responsibility for the care of drug affected patrons where health risk is imminent until such patrons are delivered into the care of ambulance officers, emergency services workers or other suitably qualified staff. In particular, venue or event staff should not evict patrons who appear to be drug affected or at risk until the first aid staff person has been consulted.

g) It is recommended that a comprehensive manual of patron care be developed to govern the detailed management and treatment of patrons who may be affected by amphetamine, 'party drug' and/or poly-drug use. (Recommendation 48, p.515)

The Committee recommends that appropriate licensing agents regularly inspect clubs and associated venues for compliance with the regulations as established in Recommendation 48. (Recommendation 49, p.516)

The Committee acknowledges the valuable contribution of peer network organisations such as RaveSafe in providing information, training and practical assistance at events, clubs and other venues. The Committee recommends that these services be expanded and adequately funded to meet the current needs. (Recommendation 50, p.525)

The Committee recommends that the provision of accurate information in relation to the contents of pills submitted for testing be available to medical support staff, through a system of 'alerts' provided by Victoria Police Forensic Science Laboratories. (Recommendation 58, p.554)

The Committee recommends that pill testing kits should not be available to the public as they are potentially a dangerous and inaccurate tool to measure the content of particular pills. (Recommendation 59, p.554)

The Committee recommends that appropriate educational material in a variety of forms, including signage, leaflets and posters, be clearly displayed and available at clubs and associated venues, including 'raves'. Such material and signage should include warnings and alerts as to the risks associated with amphetamine and 'party drug' use. (Recommendation 51, p.528)

The Committee recommends that commensurate with their powers and responsibilities, local councils should ensure raves, dance parties and clubs and other venues fulfil the appropriate regulatory requirements applicable to the conduct of such activities. These include but are not restricted to issues such as the availability of medical advice and support, ventilation and appropriate use of space, availability of free drinking water, food, toilets, chill-out spaces, transport and general amenity considerations (such as parking and noise). (Recommendation 55, p.540)

The Committee recommends that those local government authorities, licensees and club owners who have not produced or are not currently a member of a Licensee and Safety Accord or equivalent should endeavour to formulate or become part of such an accord. (Recommendation 56, p.540)

The Committee recommends that all accords should also include reference to and strategies for managing illicit drugs, particularly amphetamines and 'party drugs'. To date, most Licensee Accords concentrate solely on alcohol. (Recommendation 57, p.540)

The Committee recommends that a Review of the current provision of public and private transport services, including taxi services, be undertaken with the aim of ensuring that adequate provision is made so people, especially young people, can return to their homes directly after attending nightclubs, dance venues and outdoor 'raves', particularly in high activity precincts. (Recommendation 43, p.510)

The Committee recommends that consideration should be given to the extension of public transport hours that service such high activity precincts. (Recommendation 44, p.510)

The Committee recommends that a manual be developed for events managers and promoters which details all appropriate legal, regulatory and harm reduction strategies required in organising events such as raves and dance parties. (Recommendation 52, p.528)

The Committee recommends that consideration be given to the Transport Accident Commission providing voluntary testing of people for both alcohol and amphetamine at 'raves' and outdoor dance parties. (Recommendation 53, p.528)

The above recommendations recognise that the use of 'party drugs' does occur. They do not, however, condone such use. Instead, in accordance with harm minimisation principles, they seek to prevent adverse or dangerous reactions and consequences for the user or other affected party.

Recommendations with regard to the media

The Committee recognises the valuable role the media play in disseminating information on important issues and its contribution to social policy debates.

However, the Committee exhorts the media to report amphetamine and 'party drug' use sensitively and responsibly. In particular the Committee urges that the media:

- avoid publishing or presenting 'how to' primers on amphetamine and 'party drug' use;
- avoid targeting particular ethnic groups in its coverage of amphetamine and 'party drug' use;
- avoid stigmatising and marginalising young people who engage in drug use; and
- do not identify particular young people or their families without their express and informed consent. (Recommendation 32, p.458)

The Committee acknowledges that there are divisions of opinion as to the appropriate nomenclature to refer to 'party drugs' and their use. Indeed, the Committee recognises the problematic use of the term 'party drugs' in itself. Nonetheless, the Committee recommends that the media should not in any way use terms or refer to these drugs in such a way that glamorises, appears to condone or encourages their use. (Recommendation 33, p.458)

The Committee recommends that the peak agencies in alcohol and drug service delivery and information provision develop more sophisticated and informed responses and advocacy to the media on the issue of amphetamines and 'party drugs'. (Recommendation 34, p.458)

Recommendations with regard to partnerships, networking and collaborative strategies

The Committee recognises drug-related issues will not be resolved without community awareness and participation, cross-agency partnerships and collaboration between all tiers of government, research bodies, service providers, user groups and peer networks, clubs, event organisers and promoters, and local communities. A well-informed community can respond to the complex issues in a more flexible and resourceful manner. The Committee recommends that this can be achieved through the:

a) implementation and better use of formal and informal networks at an international, national, state and local government policy level;

b) public awareness campaigns that are evidence based;

c) targeted information on amphetamine and 'party drug' use tailored to the needs and requirements of individual communities; and

d) meaningful engagement with the media (electronic, print and broadcast) on alcohol and drug issues as outlined in Recommendation 34, p.458. (Recommendation 1, p.16)

The Committee recognises the concerns of many drug service agencies that they do not receive adequate information or data with regard to current trends in amphetamine and 'party drug' related issues or they receive such information far too late to be of practical assistance. The Committee recommends, therefore, the timely and systematic dissemination and sharing of information, data, research findings, evidence of best practice and current trends in the area of amphetamines and 'party drugs'. (Recommendation 2, p.16)

Recommendations with regard to policy, treatment and service delivery

The Committee recommends that the government develop and implement a new strategic integrated framework for the delivery of drug treatment services that should be circulated to all relevant state and local government departments, service agencies and user groups working in alcohol and drug services.

The framework will:

a) be co-ordinated in the Department of Human Services;

b) be supported by sustained and realistic funding;

c) have the capacity to respond to changing circumstances such as the trend of increasing use of amphetamine-type stimulants and 'party drugs';

d) be developed in partnership with service providers and people most affected;

e) incorporate mechanisms to ensure improved co-ordination of services support to individuals;

f) incorporate a research base and evaluation and monitoring processes; as outlined in Recommendation 66, p.629; and

g) incorporate the capacity to map and describe the changing base of services provided in the state.

In developing the framework consideration must be given to current system deficits, particularly:

- crisis response, including quick access to detoxification;
- services appropriate to people with dual diagnoses (see also Recommendation 64, p.611);
- youth-specific services;
- services targeting poly-drug use, especially involving use of amphetamine-type stimulants;
- services appropriate to people from culturally and linguistically diverse communities;
- services relevant to Indigenous people including holistic healing centres (see Recommendation 7, p.224); and

- equitable access to services in rural and regional areas. (Recommendation 63, p.610)

The Committee recognises that there is a high proportion of people who use amphetamine who also have a condition affecting their mental health. Some such people fall too easily 'between the cracks' of government and community agencies dealing specifically with alcohol and drug or specifically with mental health issues. The Committee therefore recommends as part of the Treatment Strategy outlined in Recommendation 63, p.610:

a) That a central body be established within the Department of Human Services to co-ordinate the integration and smooth delivery of services pertaining to people with dual diagnoses of mental health and drug use.

b) That in establishing this body reference should be made to the Western Australian Joint Services Development Unit as outlined in Chapter 20 of this Report.

c) That the proposed body facilitate the training of workers in both the mental health and drug service fields to recognise the issues pertaining to dual diagnoses. (Recommendation 64, p.611)

The Committee acknowledges that there is an ongoing debate as to whether treatment for amphetamine use and addiction requires specialised services. The Committee therefore recommends that a pilot service be established to trial the use of separate facilities and treatment strategies for amphetamine users. (Recommendation 65, p.611)

The Committee recognises that the problems amphetamine and 'party drug' users experience are caused by a range of social and economic variables as well as the use of the drug itself. The Committee therefore recommends that a key focus of Government policy should be the development of programmes which engage vulnerable groups in recreation, leisure, family strengthening and support, and community projects to support health, safety and economic well-being generally. Such programmes should be targeted at a local level.

Such programmes should be supported along the continuum of prevention, early intervention and treatment services for groups and individuals that are vulnerable to substance misuse. (Recommendation 54, p.540)

The Committee recommends that there be a Review of service provision for those young people who, having turned eighteen years of age, can no longer continue to receive assistance or participate in programmes designed to assist them with their amphetamine and 'party drug' use. (Recommendation 4, p.205)

Recommendations with regard to specific groups

The Committee recommends that specific, culturally appropriate training and resources on amphetamine and 'party drug' use be provided to Koori alcohol and drug workers. (Recommendation 6, p.224)

The Committee recommends the need for Koori-specific holistic healing centres to be funded to adequately cater for the specific cultural needs of Indigenous communities with regard to substance abuse issues as described in this Report and this Committee's previous Reports into Public Drunkenness and Volatile Substance Abuse. (Recommendation 7, p.224)

The Committee recommends that the development and funding of Koori-specific leisure facilities, including youth, sport and recreational clubs and programmes, be extended in order to provide structured activities that will engage young people, enhance their self-esteem, promote Indigenous culture and tradition and develop a sense of community. (Recommendation 8, p.224)

The Committee recommends that specific culturally appropriate training and resources on amphetamine and 'party drug' use be provided to parents, families, agencies and personnel working with people from culturally and linguistically diverse communities. (Recommendation 5, p.218)

The Committee recommends that in the development of drug policy and the delivery of drug services, particularly in the area of amphetamines and 'party drugs', the needs and requirements of specific groups, including young people, women, gay men and lesbians be taken into account where appropriate. (Recommendation 9, p.240)

Recommendations with regard to rural and regional issues

The Committee acknowledges that there are significant alcohol and drug problems in rural and regional Victoria. These are seldom acknowledged as matters requiring a specific response that is grounded in an understanding of the local concerns and issues of rural and regional communities. The following recommendations reflect the essential need to incorporate the views and participation of rural and regional based workers, users and local community members in the development of statewide alcohol and drug policies and services. Such an approach empowers rural and regional communities to develop locally specific responses.

The Committee recommends that a specific Rural and Regional Drug Strategy be developed and implemented by Human Services Victoria in collaboration with the Australian Rural Centre for Addictive Behaviours and other relevant rural and regional based agencies and workers. (Recommendation 10, p.327)

The Committee recommends that such a Strategy should provide a 'continuum of response' from prevention, early intervention, treatment and rehabilitation for rural and regional Victorians. (Recommendation 11, p.327)

The Committee recommends that consideration be given to the establishment of specialist drug withdrawal, treatment and residential rehabilitation services in major regional centres, especially for young people. (Recommendation 12, p.327)

The Committee recognises the importance of research into rural and regional alcohol and drug use issues by local researchers. The Committee therefore recommends the establishment of a Rural and Regional Drug Research and Information Institute to be attached to the Australian Rural Centre for Addictive Behaviours based in Warrnambool, Victoria. Such an Institute should collect and disseminate rural and regional data with regard to alcohol and drug use and undertake quantitative, qualitative, social and evaluative research. Such research will inform drug policy and practice to benefit rural and regional communities. (Recommendation 13, p.327)

The Committee recommends that the Rural and Regional Drug Strategy and the Rural and Regional Drug Research Institute be evaluated after the initial three-year period of operation. (Recommendation 14, p.327)

The Committee recommends that the Rural and Regional Drug Strategy, the Australian Rural Centre for Addictive Behaviours (ARCAB) and the Rural and Regional Drug Research Institute be adequately funded. (Recommendation 15, p.327)

The Committee recognises that a considerable amount of rural and regional workers' time is spent in travelling long distances between the home agency and clients or service providers within their region. Additionally, it is acknowledged that workers may need on occasion to travel to Melbourne to attend meetings, training sessions and other work-related commitments. The Committee therefore recommends that any funding of rural alcohol and drug services should provide an adequate amount of specifically allocated funding for travel and training. Staffing levels should also take into consideration the absence of workers and the lost time through travel. (Recommendation 16, p.327)

The Committee recommends that the state Minister for Health propose to the Australian Health Ministers' Council that the federal government give consideration to providing incentives to attract and retain adequately trained and experienced staff in the alcohol and drug area in rural and regional Victoria. (Recommendation 17, p.327)

The Committee recommends that rural and regional representatives be included in all policy and decision making procedures in relation to alcohol and drug issues in Victoria. This should include but not be restricted to membership of relevant policy making committees and decision making bodies. Wherever practicable, such participation should be facilitated via technology that enables the worker or staff person to contribute from their home base. (Recommendation 18, p.328)

The Committee recommends that further investigation and evaluation be undertaken into the desirability and effectiveness of relocating people with drug-related problems from Melbourne to rural and regional Victoria to access services that are already over-stretched. (Recommendation 19, p.328)

Recommendations with regard to ongoing research and/or data collection

The Committee recommends that a research programme and agenda to address amphetamines and 'party drugs' be developed. This should be undertaken by the relevant agency of the Victorian Department of Human Services in association with Turning Point Alcohol and Drug Centre and other suitable research agencies. (Recommendation 66, p.629)

The Committee recognises a substantial level of research has been undertaken in relation to amphetamine and 'party drug' use. Nonetheless, there is a noticeable absence of research that targets specific user groups, treatment issues and the effectiveness of programme delivery. The Committee therefore recommends that the research agenda outlined in Recommendation 66, p.629, should focus its priorities on the research issues which have been identified in the practice and academic literature and also reflected in the expert opinion of those who gave evidence to this Inquiry. Such issues have been highlighted in this Report. (Recommendation 67, p.629)

In addition, there are a number of specific issues that the Committee has identified which form the basis of the following recommendations.

The Committee recommends that there is a need for comprehensive and timely quantitative data that, while centralised and co-ordinated, is also disaggregated at state, rural and regional and local levels. Such data should include that drawn from police, ambulance, hospital and research agencies and community agencies such as Needle and Syringe Programmes. The data will be used to inform evidence based best practice in this area. (Recommendation 68, p.629)

The Committee recommends that such data should be made available and accessible to all tiers of government and appropriate research agencies. This is essential for any ongoing capacity by local governments in particular to address drug and alcohol issues, including those posed by psychostimulant drugs such as MDMA and amphetamines. (Recommendation 69, p.629)

The Committee recommends that emergency hospital presentation and admissions data be disaggregated to more accurately reflect specific drug use, particularly within the rubric of amphetamines and 'party drugs'. Emergency hospital presentation and admissions data currently bundle incidences of drug overdose into the catchall 'other drug' category, unless they are primarily heroin-related or alcohol-related. This aggregation masks rather than illuminates the drug issues associated with amphetamines, 'party drugs', pharmaceuticals and some other substances. (Recommendation 70, p.629)

The Committee recommends that ongoing research continue to be undertaken with regard to the duration and effects of the so-called 'heroin drought' and its aftermath. (Recommendation 71, p.629)

The Committee recommends that research be undertaken into the long-term effects of the ingestion of MDMA/ecstasy including physical, psychiatric, cognitive and behavioural effects. (Recommendation 72, p.630)

The Committee recommends that further research be undertaken into the nature and effects of 'amphetamine psychosis'. (Recommendation 73, p.630)

The Committee recommends that in conducting research on amphetamines and 'party drugs' the complexities associated with poly-drug use need to be taken into consideration in addition to any single focus on specific drugs and/or groups of drugs. (Recommendation 74, p.630)

The Committee recommends that research on the use, impact and diversion of prescription medication such as Ritalin/dexamphetamine for the treatment of Attention Deficit Hyperactivity Disorder among school-age children be undertaken. (Recommendation 75, p.630)

The Committee recommends that research into the possible links between methamphetamine use and violent behaviour be further investigated. (Recommendation 76, p.630)

The Committee recommends that further research be undertaken into effective treatment interventions, including the development of new pharmacotherapies and medications and their appropriate application. Specifically, ongoing research into possible amphetamine substitution treatments be investigated and evaluated if trialed. (Recommendation 77, p.630)

The Committee recommends that more in-depth social research be undertaken into specific populations of users that have been identified as high risk. These may include but are not restricted to groups such as transport and other workers for whom amphetamines serve a 'functional' purpose, party/club drug users, Indigenous people, people of culturally and linguistically diverse backgrounds, homeless and street based drug users, women, gay men and lesbians. (Recommendation 78, p.630)

The Committee acknowledges that there are many uncertainties as to why amphetamine users in particular may or may not access treatment services. The Committee recommends that further research should be undertaken to ascertain the reasons for this reluctance. (Recommendation 79, p.630)

The Committee recommends that further research be undertaken into the difficulties faced by ambulance officers with regard to the transportation to emergency facilities and/or hospitals of people who have overdosed after having ingested amphetamines, 'party drugs' and other drugs. (Recommendation 80, p.630)

The Committee recommends that funding be made available to enable community and local agencies such as Needle and Syringe Program outlets to undertake small-scale research to identify 'hidden' populations of amphetamine injectors and to implement appropriate strategies to reach them. (Recommendation 81, p.630)

The Committee recommends that amphetamine and 'party drug' users should be consulted as part of any research and treatment agenda that is developed, recognising that the demography of the typical 'party drug' users is different from that of those who normally access drug treatment services. (Recommendation 82, p.631)

The Committee recommends that all publicly funded programmes that are established to address amphetamine and 'party drugs' abuse have a requirement for evaluation to determine their effectiveness. (Recommendation 83, p.631)

The Committee recommends the rigorous and ongoing evaluation of all publicly funded school and community based drug education programmes. (Recommendation 84, p.631)

Recommendations with regard to funding

The Committee recommends that to address amphetamine and 'party drug' use it is imperative that adequate funding be provided for:

a) Data collection, research and evaluation initiatives established subject to the proposed research agenda to be co-ordinated by the Department Of Human Services as outlined in Recommendation 66, p.629;

b) Training programmes co-ordinated through the Department of Human Services;

c) An adequate level of ongoing funding for key agencies working in the area of amphetamine and 'party drug' use, including: RaveSafe; Pt'chang Non Violence Group, Youth Substance Abuse Service; DrugInfo Clearing House (Australian Drug Foundation) and the Turning Point Alcohol and Drug Centre; and

d) That budget allocations to drug and alcohol services take into consideration the time needed for workers to undertake professional development and keep abreast of current research developments in the area of amphetamine and 'party drugs'. (Recommendation 85, p.636)

The Committee recommends that funding continue to be provided on a triennial basis wherever possible for appropriate community projects and programmes. (Recommendation 86, p.636)

The Committee recommends that further funding be made available to key Needle and Syringe Program outlets in metropolitan, regional and rural settings to improve their capacity to provide primary health care and other brief interventions to current injectors. (Recommendation 87, p.636)

The Committee recommends that funding for drug and alcohol programmes needs to acknowledge the high probability of 'changing drug use patterns and trends', such as those that occurred as a result of the so-called 'heroin drought'. It is therefore imperative that any funding for drug and alcohol programmes and initiatives, and funding arrangements, are 'flexible' enough to allow agencies to provide services and responses to emerging drug use trends. (Recommendation 88, p.636)

The Committee recommends that the State Government's municipal 'hot spot' drug programmes continue to be funded subject to ongoing evaluation. (Recommendation 89, p.636)

Contents

List of Tables and Figures

Tables

Figures

List of Abbreviations

ABCI	Australian Bureau of Criminal Intelligence
ACC	Australian Crime Commission
ADF	Australian Drug Foundation
ADHD	Attention Deficit Hyperactivity Disorder
ADIS	Alcohol and Drug Information System
AFPLECP	Australian Federal Police Law Enforcement Cooperation Program
AIHW	Australian Institute of Health and Welfare
ANCD	Australian National Council on Drugs
AOD	Alcohol and other drug
ARCAB	Australian Rural Centre for Addictive Behaviours
ATODS	Alcohol, Tobacco and Other Drugs Services
ATS	Amphetamine-type stimulants
ATSIS	Aboriginal and Torres Strait Islander Services
AUSTRAC	Australian Transaction Reports and Analysis Centre
CLD	Cultural and linguistic diversity
DAMP	Drug Availability Monitoring Project (Vic)
DAO	Drug and Alcohol Office (WA)
DASC	Drug and Alcohol Services Council (SA)
DEA	Drug Enforcement Administration (USA)
DPEC	Drug Policy Expert Committee
GAP	Global Assessment Programme
GHB	Gamma-hydroxybutyrate
GLBQ	Gay, lesbian, bisexual and queer
HEBS	Health Education Board of Scotland
IDRS	Illicit Drug Reporting System
IDUs	Injecting drug users
ILIT	Illicit Laboratory Investigation Team
LGA	Local government area
LIV	Law Institute of Victoria
LYHS	Logan Youth Health Service

MA	Methamphetamine
MDMA	Methylenedioxymethamphetamine
NDARC	National Drug and Alcohol Research Centre
NDRI	National Drug Research Institute
NHS	National Household Survey
NIDA	National Institute on Drug Abuse (USA)
OMCGs	Outlawed motor cycle gangs
PAD	Passive Alert Detection
PCP	Phencyclidine
PMA	Paramethoxyamphetamine
RRMA	Rural, Remote and Metropolitan Area
UHCHS	Upper Hume Community Health Service
UNDCP	United Nations Drug Control Programme
UNODC	United Nations Office on Drugs and Crime
VAADA	Victorian Alcohol and Drug Association
VLA	Victoria Legal Aid
VLGA	Victorian Local Government Association
VSO	Victorian State Office
WASUA	Western Australian Substance Users Association
WHO	World Health Organization
YSAS	Youth Substance Abuse Service

PART A: Introduction

1. Scope of Inquiry: History and Background

The misuse of any drugs, licit or illicit, is bound to cause controversy and be subject to misinformation, leading to difficulties and confusion in the policy-making process. Drugs such as amphetamines and other psychostimulants are no exception. Indeed, in recent years there has been much publicity surrounding the use and abuse of 'ecstasy' (methyldioxymethamphetamine or MDMA) in particular. Some of this has been based on misinformation. This is one of the reasons an Inquiry into the use of such drugs is timely.

In the last ten years there have been definite signs of 'a shift in emphasis in the international drug markets away from heroin and cocaine and towards cheaper synthetic drugs, particularly the amphetamines' (Klee 1997d, p.1).[1] Governments, policy-makers and researchers had not kept up with such a shift. There was a:

> [s]ense of frustration in the early 1990s that amphetamine misuse, a chronic and growing problem, was being overlooked... Drug workers and other health professionals were uncertain of how to provide appropriate care – their services were not designed for stimulant users, they were under resourced and there was no research to guide them (Klee 1997e, p.vii).

Changes in the way certain drugs are now perceived are apparent in Australia and overseas. For example, early research in Australia and the United States documented relatively few problems associated with ecstasy use. However, since the mid to late 1990s, many researchers have reassessed such views, particularly in the light of evidence that ecstasy is increasingly used via injection and that the purity of what purports to be ecstasy has been seriously compromised in recent years. In particular, researchers have been concerned about the growing number of deaths overseas and in Australia in which ecstasy has been implicated and the increasing evidence of some psychological morbidity associated with the drug.

1 See also Klee 2001a, 2001b, and 2001c.

This Inquiry

On 15 May 2002 the Legislative Council acting under section 4F(1) of the *Parliamentary Committees Act 1968* passed a resolution requiring the Drugs and Crime Prevention Committee to conduct an Inquiry into Amphetamines and 'Party Drugs' according to the following Terms of Reference.

Terms of Reference

That pursuant to the *Parliamentary Committees Act 1968*, the Drugs and Crime Prevention Committee be required to inquire into and report to Parliament on the use of amphetamines and 'party drugs' in Victoria. In particular, the Committee is required to:

a) examine the nature, extent and culture of amphetamine and 'party drug' use;

b) determine the demographic profile of users;

c) examine the short and long-term consequences of amphetamine and 'party drug' use;

d) examine the relationship of amphetamine and 'party drug' use to other forms of licit and illicit substance use;

e) review the adequacy of existing strategies for dealing with amphetamine and 'party drug' use;

f) consider best practice strategies to address the issue of amphetamine and 'party drug' use, including regulatory, law enforcement, education and treatment responses; and

g) examine national and international legislation, reports and materials relevant to the issue.

On 5 November 2002 the 54th Parliament of Victoria was prorogued, causing the Inquiry to lapse. On 17 April 2003, however, the Governor in Council reissued identical Terms of Reference to the Drugs and Crime Prevention Committee of the 55th Parliament.

Background to the Inquiry

There are several reasons why it was thought that the inclusion of the amphetamine and the 'party drug' components in the Terms of Reference was increasingly important.

First, and most important, it is now recognised that amphetamines are the most widely used of the illicit drugs after cannabis (Commonwealth Department of Health and Family Services 1996; Vincent, Allsop & Shoobridge 1996; Topp & Darke 1997; Vincent et al. 1999; Kamienicki et al. 1998; Makkai & McAllister 1998; Henry-Edwards & Ali 2000; Australian Institute of Health and Welfare 2002). Indicators that substantiate this claim are readily found through the numbers of police and law enforcement seizures of amphetamines and the substantial increase in the number of amphetamine users attending clinical services (Vincent, Allsop & Shoobridge 1996). In South Australia, the problem and prevalence of amphetamine use was considered of such concern that a four-day drug summit, concentrating on amphetamines and 'designer drugs', was hosted by the South Australian government in June 2002 (see South Australian Drugs Summit Communique 2002a).

Second, the use and abuse of a variety of amphetamine, methamphetamine and amphetamine derivatives such as ecstasy is increasing in Victoria, particularly among young people (Department of Human Services Victoria 2001; National Drug and Alcohol Research Centre (NDARC) 2002a).

Third, in Australia the 'proportion of people presenting for treatment with a primary amphetamine problem has doubled in recent years' (Torres et al. 1996 cited in Topp & Darke 1997, p.113). Notwithstanding such concerns, the following comment by researchers Vincent et al. in 1999 is still, it would seem, largely accurate:

> It is recognised that amphetamines are among the most widely used illicit drugs in Australia and there is a growing body of evidence regarding the harms associated with their use. However, effective interventions with this population are yet to be developed and evaluated and, until recently, there has been very little research which has addressed the characteristics of those who seek information, assistance or treatment (Vincent et al. 1999, p.64).

This increase in amphetamine use with the attendant health and social consequences is partly explained by the advent of the 'heroin drought' in Victoria and indeed the country as a whole in recent years.

Fourth, the treatment needs and options for amphetamine users have received very little examination (Burrows, Flaherty & MacAvoy 1993; Wickes 1993a, 1993b; Hall & Hando 1993, 1994; Huber et al. 1997; Kamienicki et al 1998; National Institute on Drug Abuse 1998; Wood 1998a; Richards et al. 1999; Anglin et al. 2000; Baker, Boggs & Lewin 2000; Turning Point Alcohol and Drug Centre 2001; Mundy 2001; NDARC 2001, 2002c; South Australian Drugs Summit Communique 2002a). Treatment for users of amphetamines and 'party drugs' is one of the areas that agencies and other concerned parties in the community have urged the Committee to include as part of its research brief. There is now considerable evidence that a number of physical, psychological and social harms may result from psychostimulant use. In particular, an amphetamine dependence syndrome comparable to alcohol and heroin use is noticeable (NDARC 2002b).

Research into interventions to address amphetamine and 'party drug' use and dependency are extremely limited. The Department of Human Services Victoria states that for some time now drug prevention education, information, treatment and policy has been geared towards the use of opioids.[2]

---

2 Submission of the Department of Human Services Victoria to the Drugs and Crime Prevention Committee, Inquiry into Amphetamine and 'Party Drug' Use in Victoria, August 2002.

This paucity of research applies not only to treatment interventions but also to more general demographic, statistical, epidemiological and social research. As with other areas of substance abuse the Drugs and Crime Prevention Committee has researched, only the provision of accurate, comprehensive and up-to-date data, information and research can inform useful policy development.

Which drugs to include?

In the *Discussion Paper* produced for this Inquiry the problems associated with researching for an Inquiry that includes and indeed couples the wide-ranging terms amphetamines *and* 'party drugs' were canvassed. It was noted that it was not easy to decide which drugs should be included for discussion under the rubric of amphetamines and 'party drugs'. After much deliberation it was decided that the major forms of amphetamine and methamphetamines would be included but not the psychostimulant cocaine.[3] The latter drug is excluded because, unlike Sydney, the use of cocaine is not particularly prevalent in Victoria, despite some recent increases in use. In a submission to the Drugs and Crime Prevention Committee, Turning Point Alcohol and Drug Centre, drawing from work done by Fry and Miller for the NDARC (2002), stated:

> In general, recent evidence suggests that cocaine use remains infrequent amongst IDUs [injecting drug users] in Melbourne due to high prices and the lack of availability in street based markets, as well as the ready availability of good quality methamphetamine.[4]

The Department of Human Services Victoria also stated that cocaine use in Victoria is low due to its prohibitive price compared to ecstasy and amphetamines.[5]

This situation had not changed with the advent of the so-called 'heroin drought' discussed in Chapter 4 of this Report.[6]

As far as 'party drugs' are concerned, the major focus of this Inquiry has been on ecstasy (MDMA). Since approximately the mid 1990s much of what purports to be ecstasy is often not MDMA or is adulterated with other drugs. For this reason other party, dance or designer drugs must also be included. In particular, law enforcement seizures have shown that the derivative paramethoxyamphetamine

3 For a discussion as to what is included under these groupings, see discussion of terminology in Chapter 4.

4 Excerpt from the confidential submission of Turning Point Alcohol and Drug Centre to the Drugs and Crime Prevention Committee, Inquiry into Amphetamine and 'Party Drug' Use in Victoria, August 2002. Quoted with the kind permission and approval of Turning Point.

5 Submission of the Department of Human Services Victoria to the Drugs and Crime Prevention Committee, Inquiry into Amphetamine and 'Party Drug' Use in Victoria, August 2002.

6 Research by the Turning Point Alcohol and Drug Centre in Victoria states that:

'[f]ew participants in Melbourne reported purchasing cocaine, either regularly or as a result of changes in the heroin market. This situation contrasts with New South Wales where an active cocaine market has been reported amongst IDUs [Injecting Drug Users] interviewed for the IDRS...and other jurisdictions where problems with heroin supply have led to the development of the practice of cocaine injecting' (Turning Point Alcohol and Drug Centre 2001, p.16).

(PMA) has been found in drugs passing as ecstasy (Australian Bureau of Criminal Intelligence (ABCI) 2002; Australian Crime Commission 2003). Many of the deaths associated with supposed ecstasy use both here and overseas have in fact been attributed to PMA. In effect, the taking of ecstasy at the present time can be a game of 'Russian roulette'. Given the growing prevalence and serious consequences of these 'substitutes', PMA, other amphetamine/ methamphetamine derivatives, and other 'party drugs' such as gamma-hydroxybutyrate (GHB), ketamine and methylenedioxyamphetamine (MDA), many of which have become popular in their own right, will also be studied as part of this proposed Inquiry.

A table listing the names, properties and intake methods of the most common amphetamines and 'party drugs' used is included in Chapter 4 of this Report.

Structure of the Report

One of the difficulties associated with the writing of this Report has been the bifurcation apparent in the Inquiry title between amphetamines on the one hand and 'party drugs' on the other. Should, for example, different chapters be allocated to the discussion of 'party drugs' as opposed to amphetamines or should chapters and discussion be arranged thematically and according to content. For the most part the Committee has decided to opt for the latter. Thus, for example, a chapter dealing with treatment options will contain discussion as to both treatments available (or not, as the case may be) for both groups of drug, although there may be separation within that chapter where appropriate. Such a schema recognises that there are no clear boundaries between the various drugs in question, but in fact much overlap. Terminology and nomenclature and the problems associated with these are discussed in Chapter 4.

2. The Inquiry Process

The work of the Committee

The Committee has embarked upon an extensive research process in order to canvass the issues and receive input and information from as many individuals, agencies and organisations with an interest in the issues raised in the Terms of Reference as possible.

In conducting the Inquiry the Committee has undertaken an extensive review of the literature on amphetamine and 'party drug' use in Australia and overseas, has called for and received submissions from the community, sought expert opinion, visited various organisations and facilities, prepared a *Discussion Paper*, spoken to key stakeholders in Victoria, held public hearings, undertaken a series of site visits and travelled to Canberra, New South Wales, Queensland, Western Australia and South Australia to meet with the key stakeholders. The Committee has employed a variety of processes and methodologies to produce what it hopes is a comprehensive picture of amphetamine and 'party drug' use in Victoria and beyond. These are detailed below.

Discussion Paper

The Committee prepared a comprehensive and detailed *Discussion Paper*, which contained an analysis of the drugs under investigation and the culture of their use. It also provided a review of current law, policies and programmes in Victoria and other Australian jurisdictions and highlighted the scope and complexity of issues to be addressed. The *Discussion Paper* raised specific questions to be addressed and invited community response. The *Discussion Paper* was circulated widely. A copy was placed on the Committee's web site.[7]

Written submissions

Calls for written submissions were published on 22 June 2002 and 24 May 2003 in the *Herald Sun* and *The Age*. Further calls for submissions were published in both the *Herald Sun* and *The Age* after the *Discussion Paper* was released. Print media and radio interest also alerted the public to the Inquiry. Letters inviting

7 In all, 800 hard copies of the *Discussion Paper* have been distributed and 2165 copies have been down-loaded from the Committee's web site.

submissions to the Inquiry were sent to all local councils and shires in Victoria and key government and non-government agencies in Victoria and interstate. In all, the Committee has received 71 written submissions.[8] These submissions came from a broad range of individuals and government and non-government organisations.

In addition to these submissions, the Committee has taken into account a number of reports, documents, correspondence and formal and informal discussions with a range of key government and non-government organisations, event managers and club owners, experts in the field and young people, including former and current users of amphetamines and 'party drugs', when reaching its conclusions.

Interstate visits and public hearings

The Committee has also travelled interstate to gain information. Meetings were held with key government and non-government agencies in Canberra, Sydney, Brisbane, Perth and Adelaide to discuss approaches to amphetamine and 'party drug' use.[9] Public hearings were also conducted in Melbourne on 6 and 27 October 2003, on 10 November 2003 and also on 11 November 2003 (Knox). They were also held in Benalla on 22 October 2003 and Moe on 23 October 2003. In total, the Committee received oral evidence from 107 witnesses.[10]

Local visits, inspections and seminars

While the Committee's review of the academic literature on clubbing and its relationship to drug use was a valuable exercise it could only give second-hand accounts of the experience of those for whom both clubbing and drug use may be central experiences in their lives. For this reason the Drugs and Crime Prevention Committee endeavoured to gain as much insight as possible from as many participants in the rave and club scene as practicable. To obtain such first-hand information the Committee attended a range of relevant events and interviews. The following brief account outlines these activities.

In Melbourne the Committee met with first aid and harm minimisation officers located at nightclubs, and with police and ambulance officers. A forum was also convened with club, rave and venue operators, promoters and their staff and volunteers.[11] The knowledge gained from this forum, particularly with regard to harm minimisation practices, was invaluable. Committee staff attended a training session held by RaveSafe, which aims to give people who operate or work in club and rave venues best practice knowledge with regard to harm reduction measures and associated information to enable them to make their clubs and raves safe and secure environments. Members of the Committee were

---

8 For a list of the submissions received by the Committee see Appendix 1.

9 For a list of interstate meetings and site visits see Appendix 2.

10 For a list of witnesses appearing at public hearings see Appendix 3.

11 In all, 70 club owners and event managers were invited. For a list of venue operators, owners and promoters who attended see Appendix 4.

also escorted on a night tour of clubs[12] and staff attended 'Earthcore', one of the biggest outdoor 'raves' held in this country, to observe the culture of the event and the harm minimisation practices in place. Most importantly, the Committee has also sought to speak with 'clubbers' and 'ravers' themselves in order to note their observations on the culture of the scene and, in some instances, why drug use may be integral to that culture.

In addition to making these visits and attending these meetings[13] the Committee attended a number of seminars and conferences.[14]

Additional expert witnesses

In order to gain expert opinion and complement the information and testimony received from witnesses at the public hearings, visits to various facilities and information gained from submissions, the Committee periodically invited expert witnesses to address it regarding a range of pertinent matters and issues.[15]

Further research undertaken by the Committee

Rural and regional issues

Throughout the course of the Inquiry the Committee has become aware of the relative paucity of research and lack of attention given to drug and alcohol use and misuse, and specifically use of amphetamine and 'party-drug' type substances, in rural and regional Victoria. In the *Discussion Paper* the Committee called for more information about the prevalence and concomitant cultures of amphetamine and 'party drug' use within discrete sections of the wider community, including rural and regional communities and amongst Indigenous Victorians. The Committee also distributed a set of questions specific to rural and regional contexts with a view to eliciting focussed comment on experiences and issues peculiar to each region, town centre or organisation.[16] In addition, the Committee held Public Hearings in Moe and Benalla and met with Dr Rodger Brough and Suzan Morey from the Australian Rural Centre for Addictive Behaviours. The perspectives, research directives, opinions and evidence that *were* received from individuals, organisations, Shire and City Councils and members of various communities contacted outside the bounds of metropolitan Melbourne have been invaluable in providing the Committee with a greater understanding of the drug-related issues confronting these communities.

The Committee is most appreciative of the time, effort and valuable contribution that all the individuals and organisations have made during the progress of this

12 The Committee is most grateful to Ms Natalie Russell from RaveSafe for arranging the programme of visits and for escorting Members on the tour. For a list of the clubs visited see Appendix 5.

13 For a list of meetings with clubbers, ravegoers and others attended by the Committee and/or staff see Appendix 6.

14 For a list of seminars and conferences attended by the Committee see Appendix 7.

15 For a list of expert witnesses invited to speak to the Committee see Appendix 8.

16 The questions were circulated by the Australian Rural Centre for Addictive Behaviours to all their member organisations in Victoria. For a list of those who responded see Appendix 9.

Inquiry. The submissions, visits, public hearings and research projects have provided insights into the excellent work of various community and government organisations and valuable knowledge into what has turned out to be an extremely complex issue.

3. The Need for a Multi-Faceted 'All of Community' Response

Amphetamine and 'party drug' use, as with many areas of drug misuse, is a complex phenomenon, indeed more complex than this Committee would ever have thought prior to commencing this Inquiry. The Committee agrees with the exhortation of d'Abbs and MacLean (2000) that when something has a complex mix of causes and contextual factors 'the findings themselves should not be considered in isolation from those broader contextual factors' (2000, p.v).[17]

The Committee believes that to successfully address the issues pertaining to amphetamines and 'party drugs', collaborative approaches at national, state, local and community levels must be instigated. Underpinning each of these levels are the harm minimisation principles of the National Drug Strategy which require attention paid equally to *supply reduction, demand reduction* and *harm reduction* strategies.

The national framework

The National Drug Strategic Framework 1998–99 to 2002–03 reaffirms Australia's commitment to harm minimisation as the guiding principle of national drug policy. The draft of the framework for the next National Drug Strategic Framework (2004–2009) is currently at the public consultation stage, but the principles guiding both frameworks are essentially the same.[18] The frameworks aim to improve health, social and economic outcomes for both the individual and the community. The framework includes a variety of integrated approaches. A key aspect of the National Drug Strategy and its subset the Illicit Drug Strategy is the announcement of the funding of a National Psychostimulants Initiative ($2.0 million over two years) in the 2003–2004 budget. This funding will focus upon the challenges faced by the increased availability and use of psychostimulants.

17 d'Abbs and MacLean state this in the context of petrol sniffing among Indigenous Australians but the principles are equally applicable to amphetamine and 'party drugs'.

18 This discussion will therefore be based on the 1998–99 to 2002–2003 Strategy.

One of the primary objectives of the above drug strategy is to develop a partnership approach to drug-related issues. The original National Drug Strategic Framework policy document states:

> The development of a closer working relationship between the three tiers of government and affected communities (including drug users, their families and those affected by drug-related harm), community-based organisations, business and industry, the medical profession, and research institutions has therefore been identified as a priority. In recognition of this, and acknowledging that a partnership approach is still evolving, 'building partnerships' is the theme for this next phase of the National Drug Strategy (Ministerial Council on Drug Strategy (MCDS) 1998, p.21).

Equally important as the National Drug Strategy are national frameworks for Drug Education such as the National Initiatives in Drug Education (NIDE) project. Such national projects have been extremely important in paving the way for support for harm reduction models in school based drug education, particularly among teachers.

The need for state and local policies

While national frameworks provide the 'macro' direction for a national drug policy, the minutiae of programmes and policies pertaining to drug use are usually devised and implemented at state and local level. Policies with regard to amphetamines and 'party drugs' are no exception and many such programmes and initiatives are described and commented upon throughout this Report, particularly in Chapter 19.

Such state-level initiatives that have been developed have specifically incorporated a harm reduction approach to state drug education and associated programmes which recognise that local communities should 'own' local problems, particularly in areas such as rural and regional Victoria, as stressed by the Committee throughout this Report.

The need for local community action has been acknowledged and supported by the Victorian Drug Policy Expert Committee (DPEC). The Committee was established by the State Government in November 1999 to provide advice on the implementation of drug policy. In fact, while recognising the need for broader co-ordination on the part of state and national authorities, the DPEC stated that opportunities to involve local communities had been missed in recent years and called for a systematic response at the local level (DPEC 2000a). The Committee argued that local communities have a distinct role to play because:

- Many actions can only be taken at local level;
- Only local effort can harness local community resources;
- Each community is different and responses will need to be tailored accordingly;

- Communities that act on their own behalf are more healthy (DPEC 2000a, p.4).

The DPEC made a number of recommendations to the State Government with the intention of recognising existing local initiatives and encouraging further local action. The following is an excerpt from the Committee's Stage One Report.

Local drug strategies

That broadly based and multifaceted local drug strategies be implemented as a key element of the Victorian Government's drug policy.

Given the widespread problem being experienced across the State, the Committee believes that it is important that all areas and communities are encouraged and supported to play a role in reducing the impact of drugs on individuals, families and communities.

Recommendation 1.1 The Victorian Government provide support to local governments and communities, to assist them to mobilise community involvement in responding to local drug issues.

Recommendation 1.2 The Victorian Government encourage local governments, which have not done so, to develop formal local drug strategies relevant to the drug use in their communities, including strategies for prevention, treatment and rehabilitation and community safety. Such strategies should be explicitly linked to parallel processes such as municipal corporate plans, municipal public health plans and community safety plans.

Recommendation 1.3 The Victorian Government encourage local government to work with a range of stakeholders in the development of local drug strategies. These stakeholders include:

- drug users;
- Victoria Police;
- residents;
- traders and other local business;
- cultural and language groups;
- local schools;
- community organisations;
- drug and alcohol service providers; and
- other service providers.

Recommendation 1.4 The Victorian Government support communities of interest and the Koori community to similarly mobilise to respond to issues affecting them, wherever possible in association with local government initiatives (Drug Policy Expert Committee 2000a, p.7).

While the above recommendations are relatively broad, the DPEC did propose a number of elements seen to be central to any local drug strategy:

- Improving information provision and linkage between stakeholders;

- Providing youth-focused prevention and early intervention;
- Managing public space;
- Providing advocacy and advice to State Government;
- Intervening to reduce drug-related harms;
- Developing community support strategies (DPEC 2000a, p.4).

In 2001 the State Government accepted the recommendations of the DPEC pertaining to local drug strategies. A team was established within the Department of Human Services to work with local government to develop appropriate strategies for local areas (DPEC 2000b). As part of this strategy the Victorian Department of Human Services (DHS) advertised for submissions for the funding of 'Community Strengthening' projects, 'to enhance the capacity of local communities to prevent drug use and respond to drug issues' (DHS 2001d). Funding was offered for up to three years for projects focussed on drug prevention.

There is clearly financial and political support at all levels of government for local community responses to drug issues. In providing for such responses, the national and state drug strategies acknowledge that those within a local community are often best placed to co-ordinate a response to issues that arise within that community. Indeed, an appreciation of the networks and sensitivities that define a local community's culture is of utmost importance when devising a response to a community drug problem.

The Committee agrees that where there is clearly a demonstrable need for cross-boundary co-operation a co-ordinated and co-operative approach to addressing amphetamines and 'party drugs' is warranted and should be funded and resourced accordingly, wherever possible.

A range of interventions and methods

Such an approach cuts across governmental departments and areas of responsibility. Professor Steve Allsop of Western Australia's Drug and Alcohol Office stressed to the Committee how essential such a collaborative approach is, not only between government departments but also between such departments and community agencies:

> I think it is essential that if we are to respond effectively to drug problems generally that we bring together the various drug specialist services, whether that be the Turning Point, the Drug and Alcohol Office, the Cyrenians,[19] to work collegiately and to manage clients through the system in a more integrated way.
>
> But also [we need to integrate] with the other key players in the general health system, for example, people with drug problems have mental health problems. People with drug problems have legal problems, they have parenting

19 Western Australian based Drug and Alcohol agency.

> problems or children problems. So we actually need to bring those services back together in a much more integrated way. We will get some economy of scale if we are able to do that and in addition to that we will actually have much more effective treatment for people. Then we also need to bring [on board] the other players, the Liquor Licensing staff, the police and so on. I think all of the jurisdictions have done well in that in the last five years but we have still a long way to go.[20]

The Committee also generally agrees that any discussions of amphetamine and 'party drug' use and recommendations emanating from it need to be aware that a *range* of interventions (including primary, secondary and tertiary approaches) will need to be implemented to successfully address the complexity of the issues. There is no 'one size fits all' or shortcut way of tailoring solutions to this area.

Suffice to state at this introductory stage that the Committee would very much embrace interventionist strategies that address the three variables developed by Zinberg (1979, 1984) as 'drug, set and setting'. d'Abbs and MacLean (2000) summarise Zinberg's approach well:

> By these [concepts] Zinberg means: the pharmacological-toxicological properties of the substance (drug); the attributes of persons using the substance, such as personality and physical health (set); and aspects of the social and physical environment in which consumption occurs (setting). No intervention strategy is likely to ameliorate [drug abuse] and the problems associated with it unless it addresses each of these factors, and the interrelated effects engendered by them. This does not mean that a single program must attempt to bring about change in all three domains, even if it could do so. However, it does mean that any intervention strategy, of which particular programs will form a part, must begin by identifying the factors in each of these domains that shape the usage patterns and consequences of petrol sniffing in the community concerned (2000, p.v).

Such theoretical formulations are important and it is essential that they form the basis for well thought out and well funded policy developments. To this end this Committee would also endorse in general terms the principles for government programmes and policies recommended by the recently published report *Structural Determinants of Youth Drug Use* written by the Australian National Council on Drugs.

Although not concentrating specifically on amphetamine and 'party drug' use, the following recommendations with regard to young people and drug use prevention, education and treatment are apposite:

- Invest in core infrastructure. Spending on developmental health should be seen as a social investment, not just a benefit to individuals.
- Improve networks between government departments.

20 Professor Steve Allsop in conversation with the Drugs and Crime Prevention Committee, Perth, 1 October 2003.

- Focus on the critical times in children's development.
- Monitor interventions and their outcomes to assist needs assessments and fine-tuning interventions.
- Adopt better practice in planning, utilising established methods such as those available in the field of health promotion. For example:
  i. Address the multiple risk and protective factors for youth drug use.
  ii. Have specific, measurable, realistic objectives.
  iii. Work at all levels of influence: the individual, the family, and the local and macro environments.
  iv. Take a long-term view – one-shot interventions are not effective (ANCD 2001, pp.x, xi).

The need to 'work at all levels of influence' is particularly important. This has been emphatically reinforced to the Committee by Turning Point Alcohol and Drug Centre:

> Given the nature of drug markets and the patterns of drug use elsewhere in Australia, it is vital for Victoria to develop responses to emerging trends in drug use in the context of other parts of Australia.
>
> There is increasing national focus on policy regarding amphetamine and related drugs by health and law enforcement areas. Victoria has an important role to play in contributing to these discussions and showing some leadership in bringing our information and experience forward. We have a reputation of contributing to the synthesis of research, experience and developmental work in this State. To access future resources being allocated at national level in research, monitoring, evaluation, treatment and workforce development we need to show initiative and be active in these forums.[21]

The Committee concurs with this statement and believes this can be extrapolated more generally to all other forms of illicit drug use. This is reflected in the recommendations at the end of this chapter. The subsequent Parts and Chapters of this Report will also attempt to address why this 'all of community' response is so important.

21 Submission of Turning Point Alcohol and Drug Centre, to the Drugs and Crime Prevention Committee, Inquiry into Amphetamine and 'Party Drug' Use in Victoria, October 2003.

Recommendations

1. The Committee recognises drug-related issues will not be resolved without community awareness and participation, cross-agency partnerships and collaboration between all tiers of government, research bodies, service providers, user groups and peer networks, clubs, event organisers and promoters, and local communities. A well-informed community can respond to the complex issues in a more flexible and resourceful manner. The Committee recommends that this can be achieved through the:

   a) implementation and better use of formal and informal networks at an international, national, state and local government policy level;

   b) public awareness campaigns that are evidence based;

   c) targeted information on amphetamine and 'party drug' use tailored to the needs and requirements of individual communities; and

   d) meaningful engagement with the media (electronic, print and broadcast) on alcohol and drug issues as outlined in Recommendation 34, p.458.

2. Specifically, the Committee recognises the concerns of many drug service agencies that they do not receive adequate information or data with regard to current trends in amphetamine and 'party drug' related issues or they receive such information far too late to be of practical assistance. The Committee recommends, therefore, the timely and systematic dissemination and sharing of information, data, research findings, evidence of best practice and current trends in the area of amphetamines and 'party drugs'.

PART B: The Nature and Extent of Amphetamine and 'Party Drug' Use

As discussed in the beginning of this Report the coupling of a wide-ranging drug category such as amphetamines with an equally broad classification such as 'party drugs' is problematic. It can also be confusing, as in some circumstances a drug such as methamphetamine may be considered a 'party drug' itself. Clearly there may be overlap between and within these drug categories.

Chapter 4 is an overview of the main forms of amphetamine (amphetamine sulphate and methamphetamine) and 'party drugs' (MDMA/ecstasy, GHB and ketamine). It commences by analysing the terminology used and addressing issues pertaining to nomenclature. In particular, this section notes that 'party drugs' is a term that many people in the community feel uncomfortable with. Such critics feel that this term serves to glamorise drug use. This is a concern shared by the Committee.

The chapter continues with a comprehensive review of the individual drugs. Amphetamines are the first group of drugs to come under the spotlight. Their history of use and manufacture, source, form, composition and route of administration are discussed. This section also examines the price, purity and availability of these drugs and briefly discusses whether these factors have been in any way affected by the so-called 'heroin drought'. The chapter concludes with a similar examination of 'party drugs', concentrating on the most popular of these, methylenedioxymethamphetamine (MDMA), more commonly known as 'ecstasy'. Chapter 4 concludes with a brief examination of 'party drugs' which are less familiar to the general public but are growing in popularity. These are gamma hydroxybutyrate or GHB and ketamine.

Chapter 5 examines prevalence rates for the use of amphetamines and 'party drugs'. Chapter 5 is, as its title states, 'A snapshot of international and Australian trend data'. The first part of this chapter examines briefly the extent of use of amphetamine and 'party drugs' from a global perspective, basing its analysis chiefly on United Nations data.

The second section of Chapter 5 is similarly an examination of the quantitative data, however this time from a local perspective. Prevalence data is examined from both national and Victorian sources. Much of this is based on population surveys, although disparate sources such as treatment and ambulance data are also used. The limitation of such surveys, and indeed the problems generally encountered in measuring drug activity, are discussed at length. The chapter and Part conclude with a call for further research that provides more accurate assessments of trends in the use of amphetamines and 'party drugs'.

4. An Introduction to Amphetamine and 'Party Drug' Use

As indicated in Chapter 1, the amorphous area of drug policy and drug studies, and drug practice, results in a difficulty regarding terminology and classification. For example, when we speak of amphetamines or psychostimulants or 'club' or 'party drugs' what are we including? Are we discussing the same thing?[22] The first section of this chapter discusses issues pertaining to nomenclature and sets some boundaries and parameters that will inform the rest of this Report. For example, as discussed in further detail below, the use of the term 'club drugs' or 'dance drugs' in the context of this specific Inquiry is problematic. 'Club drugs' certainly would include ecstasy, GHB, methamphetamine and possibly ketamine in its list, but one could also legitimately include such diverse substances as cocaine, LSD and rohypnol, which are not under review in this Report.

The second part of this chapter will discuss the nature of those drugs or groups of drugs that have been selected as the focus of this Report. This will include an examination *inter alia* of:

- the pharmacological and chemical properties of the drug;
- how such drugs are used;
- the mode of administration;
- a brief account of why some drugs may be seen as 'desirable' by their users; and
- a brief history of use in Australia.

An account of the physiological and toxicological consequences of taking various drugs, in addition to discussion of any psychological and behavioural effects, is analysed in Chapter 6.

22 The Illicit Drug Reporting System (IDRS) considers 'party drugs' to 'include any drugs that are frequently used in entertainment venues such as nightclubs or dance parties, but are not already monitored by the IDRS, including ecstasy, ketamine, LSD, MDA and GHB' (NDARC 2001, p.1).

Terminology and nomenclature

> The planning of appropriate policy responses to the potential for an increase in psychostimulant related harms is currently hindered by the lack of clarity with respect to patterns of the use of these drugs, including terminology, the way in which the various forms are perceived to relate to each other, their appearance, their origin, purchase quantities, their price or the routes by which they are administered.[23]

As the above quote indicates, one of the difficulties pertaining to this Inquiry is that there are various taxonomic or classificatory systems associated with drug policy and particularly psychostimulant use. This can be problematic in deciding what counts as a 'party drug' or a 'dance drug'. Some of these drugs will cross boundaries of pharmacological or chemical groupings. For instance, hallucinogens may or may not be included as a 'party drug'.[24]

The terminology is constantly changing, as is the usage of the terms. For example, it would seem that when analysis is done of the drug being referred to as 'speed', it is for the most part composed of methamphetamine, rather than the amphetamine (sulphate) that it has historically referred to. Similarly, drugs being sold as MDMA or ecstasy have often been found on chemical analysis not to be methylenedioxymethylamphetamine, but may contain additives consisting of other drug types. In fact, an Australian Bureau of Criminal Intelligence (ABCI) report on illicit drug use stated that drugs purported to be ecstasy can contain anything from benzodiazepines and caffeine to agricultural and veterinary drugs or even heroin and LSD (ABCI 2002). Moreover, street drug terminology is, as Miller points out, location specific and not standardised (Miller 1997). That street terms may not accurately reflect or refer to the actual drugs used is another problematic aspect of this type of inquiry.

Such distinctions are not merely semantic; they can have practical consequences. For example, Moore states that it can be difficult to aggregate overall figures for the use of any given drug because of differing data collection categories: 'Some surveys target designer drugs, others examine stimulants, still others look at "psychostimulants"' (Moore 1992a, p.7).

Party or dance drugs

Another way of classifying a range of drugs is that based on the context in which they have been commonly used – in this case a range of drugs thought to be associated with dance clubs and parties, and raves. Such a classification is problematic not only for the wide range of drugs that may be included under this somewhat nebulous category (some of which are not included in the

23 Excerpt from the confidential submission of Turning Point Alcohol and Drug Centre to the Drugs and Crime Prevention Committee, Inquiry into Amphetamine and 'Party Drug' Use in Victoria, August 2002. Quoted with the kind permission and approval of Turning Point Alcohol and Drug Centre.

24 Some drugs such as MDMA (ecstasy), while having chemical properties similar to amphetamines, may also be hallucinogens, thus adding to the confusion surrounding the classification of this drug.

amphetamine 'family'), but also because there are distinct cultural and contextual differences between different settings. For example, a traditional 'rave' may have a different culture of drug use than a more conventional dance club or disco (see the academic work of Lenton, Boys & Norcross 1997; Lenton & Davidson 1999).

Nonetheless, the types of drug often associated with dance and party cultures of one type or another have included:

- Amphetamines
- Methamphetamine
- Ecstasy (MDMA)
- Cocaine
- Ketamine (also known as Special K) – a veterinary anaesthetic
- GHB (gamma-hydoxybutyrate), also referred to as GBH or 'Grievous Bodily Harm'
- Volatile nitrites (particularly in the gay party and club scene).

More problematically, in terms of this Inquiry, using this broader classification of 'party drugs' could include cannabis/marijuana.[25] There is a fairly high use of these drugs at 'rave parties' according to the literature. Synthetic hallucinogens such as LSD and even to a lesser, but increasing, extent alcohol have also been used in conjunction with ecstasy. Certainly the phenomenon of poly-drug use cannot be ignored at these settings.

The use of the term 'party drugs', although commonly referred to as a shorthand associated with clubs, raves and dance parties, is one that some groups feel is less appropriate as the boundary between club drug usage and street drug usage becomes blurred. For example, some commentators note that ecstasy, once a drug predominantly associated with the club, rave and party scene, is now occasionally being seen, distributed and sold on the streets. Moreover, studies such as those done by the Illicit Drug Reporting System (IDRS) report a *slight* increase in the numbers of people who are *injecting* ecstasy in Melbourne (National Drug and Alcohol Research Centre (NDARC) 2002a). Such observations are a salutary reminder that drug use must always be contextualised.[26] However, as will be discussed throughout this Report, these numbers are still very small and not too

25 Measham, Aldridge and Parker 2001 (at p.61) argue that cannabis cannot be viewed per se as a dance drug because it does not have the stimulant qualities needed to sustain the requisite energy levels. It is used, however, as an adjunct to the dance party scene in order to 'come down' after a night of energetic clubbing. See discussion in Chapter 10.

26 The factors of drug, set and setting, formulated by Zinberg (1984) are of utmost importance in this context. This concept is discussed below and in Part D. For example, four settings where amphetamine/methamphetamine use can be discussed and problematised may include:

- Street trade and use
- Party, dance club and rave settings
- Truck drivers and the transport industry and in other occupational health and safety settings
- Amphetamine prescription for children with Attention Deficit Hyperactivity Disorder (ADHD).

much should be made, without further research, of this slight trend towards 'crossover' between party use and street use. Researchers from Turning Point Alcohol and Drug Centre warn that caution must be taken in interpreting these figures:

> Studies like the IDRS in Melbourne suggest that reported lifetime use of ecstasy by injecting drug users is increasing, along with signs that ecstasy injection is becoming more common in this group (as part of polydrug experimentation patterns). While this is indicative of a 'crossing-over' of illicit drug markets (and drug use subcultures) traditionally thought of as separate, further studies will be needed to explore this phenomenon. What is required is contact with different sentinel groups of drug users in addition to the injecting drug user target group (eg. primary ecstasy users).[27]

Some other agencies in their submissions to this Inquiry have criticised the use of the term 'party drugs' in the original terms of reference. For example, the Catholic Education Office submits:

> There is some concern that 'party drugs' may be a confusing description, especially as drugs that may be considered under this heading may not all be stimulants. The term also tends to give the impression that there are drugs that are a positive ingredient in enjoyable 'partying' and are without risk of doing harm.[28]

This is a concern shared by the YWCA in its submission to the Inquiry:

> In preparing this submission, there was much discussion about the term 'party drugs', and trying to determine what this included. In answering the question 'what *are* party drugs?' it seems to YWCA Victoria that the scope of this term is incredibly broad, as it can cover licit drugs including tobacco and alcohol, as well as illicit drugs such as ecstasy, LSD, heroin, amyl nitrate and marijuana.
>
> YWCA Victoria is also concerned by the connection the Inquiry draws between amphetamines and 'party drugs'. The juxtaposition of amphetamines and 'party drugs' in this Inquiry can paint an inaccurate and incomplete picture of amphetamine use, by inferring that amphetamines are only used for 'partying' purposes. In the view of YWCA Victoria, the phrasing of the Inquiry's Terms of Reference unfairly focusses attention onto the actions of young people, and not on the activities of the whole community, by leaving out some significant issues relating to amphetamine usage.[29]

Victoria Police also have their reservations, particularly with the names given to and used for marketing of ecstasy or 'pseudo-ecstasy' tablets:

---

27 Written communication from Turning Point Alcohol and Drug Centre to Committee staff, 18 July 2003.

28 Submission of the Catholic Education Office to the Drugs and Crime Prevention Committee, Inquiry into Amphetamine and 'Party Drug' Use in Victoria, August 2002.

29 Submission of YWCA Victoria to the Drugs and Crime Prevention Committee, Inquiry into Amphetamine and 'Party Drug' Use in Victoria, August 2002.

> A real concern for Victoria Police is the marketing of these products to young people. The manufacturers use designer symbols and labels such as *Calvin Klein* and *DKNY* or have current cultural references such as *Bart Simpson* or *Banana Splits* to appeal to a young affluent market. Additionally, these tablets come in a variety of bright colours and can be easily swallowed. Users do not class themselves as traditional drug users such as intravenous users.[30]

Notwithstanding these reservations, most agencies have stated that 'party drug use' is an appropriate term or descriptor given the context in which much psychostimulant use – predominantly but not only MDMA – takes place. For example, Professor Margaret Hamilton, Director of Turning Point Alcohol and Drug Centre, made the following comments at Public Hearings in October 2003:

> We note that there is some concern about the use of the term 'party drugs'. We are not especially fussed by that, to be honest. It is a phrase that those who use them use and therefore understand. Once you start spending a lot of time on deciding what words we will use and how we will describe this class of drugs, the time can be diverted from some of the other things. It is not something that we want to make a case for, not using that term. We recognise some of the controversy, if you like, about it, but there is some advantage in using the terms that the users use and there are disadvantages in inventing new terminology that then becomes distant from users. [31]

Overarching classifications

One commonly used form of classification is the group of drugs termed 'amphetamine-type stimulants' (ATS).[32] Such drugs, unlike cocaine, may have no botanical raw material but are fully synthetic derived. They include amphetamines, methamphetamines and a loose group of other central nervous system stimulants. Chawla gives a useful account as to the nomenclature of these drugs:

> ATS include two sub groups with slightly different pharmacological properties: the amphetamine group and the ecstasy group. The former includes amphetamine, methamphetamine and methcathinone. Most of them were developed as therapeutic drugs: amphetamine in 1887; methamphetamine in 1919... The substance known commonly as 'ecstasy' (MDMA) has given its name to a whole range of related substances. They are sometimes called the hallucinogenic amphetamines because, in addition to the CNS stimulant effect, they produce effects of empathy, loquacity and serenity (Chawla 1998, pp.1–2).

30 Excerpt from the confidential submission of Victoria Police (Drugs Policy and Services Branch) to the Drugs and Crime Prevention Committee, Inquiry into Amphetamine and 'Party Drug' Use in Victoria, August 2002. Quoted with the kind permission of Victoria Police.

31 Professor Margaret Hamilton, Turning Point Alcohol and Drug Centre, evidence given to the Drugs and Crime Prevention Committee Inquiry into Amphetamines and 'Party Drug' Use in Victoria, Public Hearings (Melbourne), 27 October 2003.

See also the comments of Mr Paul Dillon, National Drug and Alcohol Research Centre, in conversation with the Drugs and Crime Prevention Committee, Sydney, 26 June 2003.

32 For an explanation as to how the term 'amphetamine-type stimulants' is used by the United Nations and the World Health Organisation, see Klee 2000a, p.34.

The latter group of ecstasy drugs may also be described as pure recreational drugs, as opposed to drugs used instrumentally (for example, amphetamines used by truck drivers or students to stay awake) (Chawla 1998). Moore (1992a) states that some Australian scholars have 'argued that to use the term "recreational" to describe illicit drug use may imply that it is "harm-free"'. However, Moore counters this argument by stating that:

> ...at least for some groups the term 'recreational' may accurately describe the orientation of drug use in that [these] drugs are primarily consumed in leisure contexts, eg. at nightclubs or parties (Moore 1992a, p.10).

As Chawla indicates, the difficulty in describing the synthetic designer drugs[33] is complicated by the fact that much of what is sold or passed off as ecstasy is not methyldioxymethamphetamine (MDMA). In discussing ecstasy use in Australia the NDARC stated that 'the term is now so widely used as to be considered virtually generic for any of the ring substituted amphetamine group' (NDARC 1998, p.1). This confusion as to terminology can have serious repercussions for research and data collection, as Gowing et al. explain:

> Identification of exactly which substances are involved when ecstasy use is reported is problematic because of the wide range of substances which are marketed as ecstasy and the fact that tablets may contain mixtures of different substances. In addition, classification of drugs varies from country to country and between studies. Ecstasy may be classified as an amphetamine-type stimulant, synthetic drug, designer drug, dance drug or be listed by name in different data sets... Even when one classification is used comparisons can be misleading. For example, amphetamine-type stimulant use is widespread in most regions of the world but amphetamine and methamphetamine predominate in some regions while ecstasy prevails in others (Gowing et al. 2001, p.4).

Ecstasy or purported ecstasy may contain a number of drugs in substitution to MDMA (aspirin, paracetamol, ketamine, caffeine) or may be an amphetamine derivative that is chemically related or similar to MDMA, such as methylenedioxyamphetamine (MDA), methylenedioxyethylamphetamine (MDEA) or paramethoxyamphetamine (PMA). In referring to ecstasy throughout this Report, at first instance the term will be used to refer to the drug

33 Chesher argues that the term 'designer drug' can be misleading. Traditionally designer drugs (other than those 'designed' for licit purposes by pharmacologists) were those in which 'the psychoactive properties of an illegal drug have been retained, but the molecular structure has been altered in order to avoid prosecution' (Chesher 1990a, p.157). For example, in the United States drugs of abuse have been controlled by classifying, scheduling and proscribing certain compounds as illegal. Until such a process takes place no laws could apply. In recent years many Western countries have changed legislation by making the analogues of scheduled drugs also subject to proscription. To the extent that the analogues are also caught by the legislative proscription they can no longer be called 'designer drugs' (see Shapiro 1989). For an earlier discussion of the inaccuracy and misleading nature of the term 'designer drug', see Buchanan and Brown 1988.

Jenkins argues that 'designer drugs' cause alarm to the general public because of their 'promethean' nature. They are seen as '[r]epresent[ing] the worst hazards of uncontrolled scientific experiment on innocent human victims...' (Jenkins 1999, p.82).

as it is sold on the street unless the context otherwise specifies. If specific reference is required to the pharmacological compound known as 3,4-methyldioxymethamphetamine, the abbreviation MDMA shall be used.

In discussing amphetamines, this Report follows the lead of Burrows, Flaherty and MacAvoy (1993):

> Amphetamine is used throughout this work to denote the sulphate salt of amphetamine [amphetamine sulphate] (the most common form of the drug in illicit use) while 'amphetamines' refers to the range of amphetamine-based psychostimulants (including dexamphetamine and methamphetamine, but excluding MDA and MDMA) (Burrows, Flaherty & MacAvoy 1993, p.1).[34]

In terms of referring to generic drug use for the drugs that are the subject of this Inquiry, the Committee has adopted the term used by the Victorian Turning Point Alcohol and Drug Centre. Its preferred classification as outlined in its submission to this Inquiry is 'psychostimulants'.

The wider classification of psychostimulants is used to reflect 'the diversity of changes to the illicit drug marketplace becoming apparent across Melbourne'.[35] It also avoids some of the problems outlined by Turnbull in the following quote:

> [I]n talking about amphetamines we are clearly faced with a diversity of both substances and users. My main concern here [is] with those stimulants known colloquially as speed – consisting predominantly of either methamphetamine or dexamphetamine. These drugs are used illicitly in Australia by groups ranging from street kids to truck drivers to business executives, and are variously taken as tablets, snorted or injected. It is important to keep in mind, however, that

---

34 The NDARC (2002a) states that until the late 1980s the form of illicit amphetamine most available in Australia was amphetamine sulphate:

'Throughout the 1980s, the form of illicit amphetamine most available in Australia was amphetamine sulphate. During the 1990s, the proportion of amphetamine-type substance seizures that were methamphetamine (rather than amphetamine) steadily increased until methamphetamine clearly dominated the market. In Australia today, the powder traditionally known as 'speed' is almost exclusively methamphetamine rather than amphetamine. The more potent forms of this family of drugs, known by terms such as 'ice', 'shabu', 'base' and 'crystal meth', are also methamphetamine' (NDARC 2002a, p.28, footnote 1).

35 Ryder, Salmon and Walker are leading academics in the field of drug studies. In the book *Drug Use and Drug Related Harm: A Delicate Balance* (2001) they also discuss the difficulties in classifying taxonomies of drugs and drug use. In relation to the more recent drugs that are being used in Victoria, they also prefer the use of the general category 'psychostimulants'. They define this category as those drugs that increase the activity of the central nervous system.

Their category of psychostimulants includes:

- Amphetamines
- Methamphetamine
- MDMA (ecstasy)
- Cocaine
- Nicotine
- Caffeine.

For a discussion of the use of 'alternative' psychostimulants in the German and Dutch club scenes, see Heckmann (1997) and Van Laar and Spruit (1997) respectively. Such 'ecodrugs' taken by a small group known as 'psychonauts' may include guarana, qat, and peyote cactus and are readily available in 'New Age' shops.

> these drugs are closely linked to a range of common stimulants such as ephedrine on the one hand and designer drugs such as MDMA on the other.
>
> *The similarities and the popular confusion between these drugs and amphetamines is a significant factor to be considered in the framing of any strategy.* In some cases it may actually be more effective to address amphetamines as part of a broader psychostimulants strategy (Turnbull 1993, p.98). (Committee emphasis)

Turning Point Alcohol and Drug Centre includes the following in its classification of psychostimulants:

- Amphetamines and amphetamine-type substances
- Methamphetamine (including the powder traditionally known as 'speed' and methamphetamine drugs such as 'ice', 'shabu' (methylamphetamine hydrochloride), 'base' and 'crystal meth')
- Ecstasy (MDMA or its analogues).[36]

Cocaine is also included in this list. Although, as mentioned in Chapter 1, it is argued that:

> In general, recent evidence suggests that cocaine use remains infrequent amongst IDUs [injecting drug users] in Melbourne due to high prices and the lack of availability in street based markets, as well as the ready availability of good quality methamphetamine.[37]

Whatever form of classification is chosen, it is crucial to reiterate that the drugs will need to be studied in their contextual and cultural settings, each of which gives rise to different issues, problems and strategies. For example, the use of amphetamines by truck drivers to stay awake during long transport hauls will raise a different set of issues, risks, strategies and challenges to those facing young people who may use them while 'clubbing'. Moreover, the Committee heeds the advice of Dr David Moore of Curtin University with regard to examining any issues concerning drug use and drug policy:

> If drug policy and practice is to be seriously attentive to specific social contexts, then understanding how drug users themselves categorise these drugs – in and of themselves, and in relation to other drugs – is essential.[38]

---

36 Excerpt from the confidential submission of Turning Point Alcohol and Drug Centre to the Drugs and Crime Prevention Committee, Inquiry into Amphetamine and 'Party Drug' Use in Victoria, August 2002. Quoted with the kind permission and approval of Turning Point Alcohol and Drug Centre.

37 See NDARC 2002a pp.36-37 and Confidential Submission of Turning Point Alcohol and Drug Centre, to the Drugs and Crime Prevention Committee, Inquiry into Amphetamine and 'Party Drug' Use in Victoria, August 2002.

38 Submission of Dr David Moore, National Drug Research Institute, Curtin University, to the Drugs and Crime Prevention Committee, Inquiry into Amphetamine and 'Party Drug' Use in Victoria, November 2003.

The drugs and how they are used

Table 4.1 below lists the names, properties and administration methods of the most common amphetamines and 'party drugs' used. Detailed discussion of the drugs focussed on in this Inquiry follows the Table.

Amphetamines and methamphetamines[39]

Some drug experts, academics, practitioners and policy makers in the late 1980s and early 1990s predicted that there would be a growing trend towards the use of amphetamines in the last decade of the twentieth century. Academic titles such as 'The 1990s: Decade of the stimulants?' (Davies & Ditton 1990) or 'Amphetamine: The new drug problem?' (O'Donovan 1992) were indicative of this phenomenon. And so it came to pass!

Amphetamines are now one of the most widely used drugs in the Western world. In Britain, for example, they have been cited as the second most popular form of illicit drug use, after marijuana (Griffin 1997). According to the United Nations Drug Control Programme (UNDCP), in Japan, Korea and the Philippines ATS account for seven times as much use as heroin and cocaine combined (UNDCP cited in Henry-Edwards & Ali 2003). Amphetamine-type stimulants have been cited as the most commonly used illicit drug in Australia after cannabis. Indeed, the UNDCP is quoted as finding that Australia has the highest prevalence of ATS (primarily amphetamine and methamphetamine) use in the world (UNDCP cited in Henry-Edwards & Ali 2003). Amphetamine use in Australia has also increased markedly since the advent of the so-called 'heroin drought', discussed later in this chapter. Further discussion of the prevalence of amphetamine use in Australia and Victoria is found in Chapter 5.

The term 'amphetamines' in general usage refers to a family of synthetic drugs that are all chemically related to amphetamine and all have similar effects. They are to be distinguished from the classical 'botanical' psychoactive drugs – heroin, cocaine and cannabis.[40] Amphetamines are psychostimulants. Stimulants act upon and increase the activity of the central nervous system and produce effects similar to the body's naturally occurring hormone, adrenalin.[41]

History

Amphetamine (amphetamine sulphate) was originally synthesised in 1887 by German chemists, but only studied and developed to any degree in the 1930s.

It was first used in the 1920s as a decongestant and to treat obesity and depression. Because of its effects in bronchial passage dilation, it was also used

39 For basic factual and descriptive accounts of the various drugs in this section a variety of fact and information sheets produced from several drug and alcohol agencies are available. These include those of the National Drug and Alcohol Research Centre, the Australian Drug Foundation, 'Connexions', the United States Drug Enforcement Administration and Australian State Health Departments.

40 See Chawla 1998 for an account of the emergence and history of synthetic drugs.

41 For an account of the pharmacological properties of (meth)amphetamines, see Derlet and Heischober 1990, pp.625ff.

Table 4.1: Table of drugs
Amphetamines

Common Name	Medical or Chemical Name	Other Street Names	Drug Action	Form	Route of Administration	Comments
SPEED	Amphetamine (Sulphate) Dexamphetamine	Goey or Go-ee Whizz Dexies	Stimulant	Powder, tablet or capsule, liquid	Snorted, swallowed, injected	Speed is often used as a generic name for a 'family' of amphetamine drugs that have been synthesised from approximately the late 19th century. In a general sense, the term amphetamines may also include 'party drugs' such as MDMA. More commonly, however, speed refers to the specific drug amphetamine sulphate and more recently it may also refer to methamphetamines and prescription drugs such as, ephedrine and pseudoephedrine.
METH	Methamphetamine or Methylamphetamine	Speed, Base	Stimulant	Powder, oil or paste (Base)	Snorted, swallowed, injected, smoked	
CRYSTAL METH	Methamphetamine Hydrochloride	Crystal, Ice, Shabu, Crank, Glass	Stimulant	Crystalline powder or crystals	Smoked, swallowed, injected, snorted	Scientists and pharmacists who use the term 'ice' may be referring to the chemical 4-methyl-aminorex. Street ice however is almost exclusively a strong, high purity form of methamphetamine.

cont'd...

Table 4.1: Table of drugs (cont.)

Party drugs

Common Name	Medical or Chemical Name	Other Street Names	Drug Action	Form	Route of Administration	Comments
ECSTASY (MDMA)	3,4-Methylene dioxy methamphetamine	E, Eckies, XTC, Dills, Eggs. Others too numerous to mention	Stimulant (but with hallucinogenic properties) sometimes known as a 'psychedelic amphetamine'.	Pills or tablets Less commonly capsules or powder	Predominantly swallowed. Some trends towards injectable use.	While 'ecstasy' is traditionally associated with the drug MDMA, in recent years analysis has shown what purports to be MDMA may in fact be adulterated or even substituted with other substances – including PMA, methamphetamine, caffeine and/or paracetamol.
GHB	Gamma Hydroxybutyrate Gamma Butyrolactone (GBL) – an analogue of GHB	Liquid E GBH Grievous Bodily Harm Blue Nitro Fantasy Easy Lay	Depressant/ Anaesthetic with sedative properties	Liquid (usually in small vials) Sometimes in bright blue liquid form known as 'blue nitro'	Usually orally, but with some reports of injection	Often used to 'spike' liquids and drinks in order to render victim vulnerable to sexual assault.
KETAMINE	Ketamine Hydrochloride	K, Special K	Hallucinogenic/ Anaesthetic	Tablet or pill, Powder	Swallowed, injected, sniffed	
PMA	Para methoxyamphetamine		Stimulant	Tablets (often purported to be MDMA or 'ecstasy'), Capsules	Swallowed	Not known as a drug of choice, as much as an additive put in tablets purporting to be MDMA.
COCAINE	Cocaine Hydrochloride	Coke, Charlie, Nose Candy, Snow, Charlie, Blow, White Dust	Stimulant	Powder	Snorted, injected,	Cocaine Hydrochloride cannot be smoked as the drug is destroyed at high temperature.
CRACK COCAINE	Cocaine (Freebase)	Crack	Stimulant		smoked	Crack is a freebase cocaine converted to alkaloid form so it can be smoked.

in the 1930s as a nasal spray for treating asthma:

> Subsequent studies showed that the drug was also helpful in providing relief from narcolepsy, reducing activity in hyperactive children, suppressing appetite and enabling individuals (such as students and truck drivers) to stay awake for extended periods of time. In the 1930s and 1940s, amphetamine was used in treating a variety of other conditions and disorders including schizophrenia, morphine addiction, tobacco smoking, low blood pressure, radiation sickness, and even persistent hiccups (Anglin et al. 2000, p.138).

During World War II and the Korean and Vietnam Wars, soldiers on all sides of the conflicts were given amphetamine to keep them awake, to give them more energy and to suppress their appetites.[42] It was also used for the same reasons by the American space programme (Grinspoon & Hedblom 1975).

Amphetamine was readily available without a prescription in the United States until the early 1950s, and amphetamine inhalers were available over the counter until 1960. Prescriptions for amphetamine tablets were one of the major ways of treating obesity and depression during the 1960s. It was only by the 1970s that:

> [t]he dangers associated with the use of amphetamine were better understood, and additional restrictions were placed on the amount that could be legally produced and how it could be distributed. Increased levels of illicit production ensued, originally limited to motorcycle gangs and other independent groups... At the same time, the typical user population changed from white, blue-collar workers to include college students, young professionals, minorities, and women (Anglin et al. 2000, p.138).[43]

---

42 This practice is not apparently restricted to these previous wars if recent newspaper articles are accurate. During January 2003, investigations of American Airforce pilots who had mistakenly dropped bombs on Canadian forces stationed in Afghanistan, revealed that amphetamines allegedly were and continue to be quite commonly prescribed to air force pilots to prevent fatigue. An *Age* article based on a *Los Angeles Times* report states:

'As two pilots face a possible court-martial, the air force says 'go pills' kept tired pilots alive in Afghanistan... As a hearing investigating two American fliers who bombed Canadian forces in Afghanistan entered a third day on Thursday, the air force summoned reporters to hear a pilot-surgeon extol the virtues of the practice of prescribing amphetamines for tired pilots.

"It is the gold standard for anti-fatigue", [said] Colonel Peter Demitry, chief of the US Air Force Surgeon General's science and technology division..."We know that fatigue in aviation kills... This is a life and death insurance policy that saves lives."

Lawyers [for the pilots] have said the pilots' judgment was impaired by amphetamines routinely prescribed by air force doctors...

Colonel Demitry [however] insisted that the drug Dexedrine – called 'go pills' by pilots – "has never been associated with a proven adverse outcome in a military operation. This is a common, legal, ethical, moral and correct application"' (Lianne Hart, 'Air Force rushes to defend amphetamine use in "friendly fire" case', *The Age*, 18 January 2003, p.25).

See also: 'US scientists seek formula to create "super-soldiers"', *The Age*, 6 January 2003, p.10, (no author).

Andrew Masterson, 'More than once were warriors out of their tiny minds', 'The Culture' (Supplement), *The Age*, 21 January 2003, p.1.

43 Jenkins states that before the 1960s, law enforcement agencies such as the FBI were almost totally uninterested in amphetamine pills. Such agencies were much more focussed on heroin, cocaine and marijuana. By 1970, however, the Commissioner of the Food and Drug Administration was to state that half of the legally produced amphetamine pills were being diverted for illicit purposes: 'an amazing four or five billion pills each year' (Jenkins 1999, p.32).

Methamphetamine was first synthesised from ephedrine, itself a form of amphetamine, in Japan in 1893:

> Methamphetamine did not become widely used until World War Two when Japan, Germany and the United States provided the drug to military personnel to increase endurance and performance... [it] was also used in Japan to improve productivity of civilian factory workers in military support industries. Beginning in 1941, methamphetamine was sold over the counter [and] advertised as a product 'to fight sleepiness and enhance vitality'. Widespread abuse occurred only after the war when methamphetamine from surplus army stocks flooded the market leading [in Japan] to the so-called 'First Epidemic' (Anglin et al. 2000, p.138).

It was estimated that at the peak of this 'epidemic' 1.5 million Japanese were injecting methamphetamine (Grinspoon & Hedblom 1975). In a review of the history of amphetamine abuse, Hall and Hando state that similar epidemics of amphetamine and methamphetamine use occurred in Sweden in the 1940s, 1950s and 1960s, the United States in the late 1960s and early 1970s, Japan again in the 1970s to the present day (the 'Second Epidemic'), and the United Kingdom in the late 1950s and the late 1960s (Hall & Hando 1993):

> There are indications that there was a smaller epidemic of amphetamine use in Australia in the middle and late 1960s. During this time there was a large increase in the prescription of amphetamines by general practitioners, increased use of amphetamines among young offenders and young adults attending psychiatric hospitals...and an increase in the prevalence of persons diagnosed with amphetamine psychoses (Hall & Hando 1993, p.59).

By the 1960s the market in amphetamines and methamphetamines had changed from being predominantly licit to illicit. The black market consisted first of the diversion of supplies from pharmaceutical companies, chemists and doctors, then developed into the synthesis, manufacture and distribution of amphetamines and methamphetamines by motor cycle gangs and other criminal gangs and syndicates, particularly on the Pacific Coast of the United States. Clandestine laboratories in California and Mexico are now the primary sources of methamphetamine available in the United States (Anglin et al. 2000).

In Australia, as in Britain, Europe and to a lesser extent the United States:

> [a]mphetamine use was fuelled by a combination of ready availability and perceived safety by users and the medical profession (Hall & Hando 1993, p.60).

It was only when the medical profession began noticing links between heavy amphetamine use and an increase in paranoid psychoses (and to a lesser extent violence)[44] that questions were raised about the advisability of prescribing amphetamines in a relatively unregulated way:

44 For a discussion of the (somewhat tenuous) links between amphetamine use and violent behaviour, see Chapter 7. See also Boles and Miotto 2003.

> Once the abuse potential of amphetamines was recognised...their availability on medical prescription was severely restricted. This had two main consequences. First, the existence of a large market of users provided the incentive for the illicit manufacture and distribution of amphetamines, with a result that many of the later epidemics were supplied by the black market. Second, the development of a black market in turn changed the characteristics of the users. The proportion of amphetamine users who were middle class, middle aged women who used oral amphetamine declined while the proportion of younger male users correspondingly increased. The latter were primarily recruited from the drug subculture, where injection, the most hazardous form of administration, was the preferred route.[45] In this way the changes in the pattern of amphetamine use, and in the characteristics of users, mirrored that which occurred earlier in the century with morphine and heroin use (Hall & Hando 1993, p.60).

Despite such developments, amphetamine abuse in Australia was never as much of a concern, at least in the public realm, as drug issues pertaining to heroin and to a lesser extent cocaine.

However, during the 1990s national Australian drug law enforcement and policy moved away from an emphasis on cocaine to one concentrating on psychostimulants such as amphetamines and MDMA. Burrows, Flaherty and MacAvoy state that by 1990:

> [t]here was general agreement that the use of cocaine remained at a low level in Australia and that the social and economic conditions which have made cocaine such a major problem in the United States do not exist in Australia and are unlikely to develop here in the foreseeable future [and that] ...the use of amphetamines currently represented a larger potential problem for health, welfare and law enforcement authorities in Australia (Burrows, Flaherty & MacAvoy 1993, p.2).

Hall and Hando argue that one of the reasons there was so little known about amphetamines use in Australia was the fears in the mid to late 1980s of a major cocaine epidemic in Australia. These fears turned out to be largely unfounded and 'distracted attention from an emerging home grown amphetamine epidemic' (Hall & Hando 1993 cited in Burrows, Flaherty & MacAvoy 1993, p.61).

> As a consequence, most of what is known about amphetamine use in Australia has been gathered *en passant* in the course of research on the use of cocaine...or on the risks of HIV transmission among injecting drug users (Hall & Hando 1993 cited in Burrows, Flaherty & MacAvoy 1993, p.61).

45 This was not helped by the fact that a liquid form of methamphetamine was being used in the 1960s as a treatment for heroin addiction and 'quickly contributed to a new abuse pattern involving injections of methamphetamine, either alone or with heroin' (Ray & Ksir 1996 cited in Anglin et al. 2000, p.138).

Consequently, in 1991 the national Ministerial Council on Drug Strategy endorsed a National Action Plan on Problems Associated with Amphetamine Use. Under the plan, research into the extent, nature, use and treatment of amphetamines and amphetamine-related problems became a priority.

The IDRS describes the change in traditional amphetamine markets in Australia as follows:

> The amphetamines are a class of drugs that, in chemical terms, are closely related. This family of drugs includes amphetamine sulphate, dexamphetamine, and methamphetamine (also known as methylamphetamine). Throughout the 1980s, the form of illicit amphetamine most available in Australia was amphetamine sulphate. Following the legislative controls introduced in the early 1990s on the distribution of the chemicals used to make amphetamine, illicit manufacturers were forced to rely on different recipes for 'cooking' the drugs. As a result, throughout the 1990s the proportion of amphetamine seizures that were methamphetamine (rather than amphetamine sulphate) steadily increased, until methamphetamine clearly dominated the market. In the financial year 2000/01, 91% of all seizures of amphetamines were of methamphetamines. Most methamphetamine manufactured in Australia is based on the precursor chemical pseudoephedrine[46] (IDRS 2002, p.2).

By the mid 1990s the use of methamphetamines and other ATS was being viewed with growing concern from a global perspective. In 1996 the UNDCP convened two expert meetings to consider ATS use and related problems. As a consequence, a number of regional and global Action Plans dealing with supply and demand reduction of ATS and designer drugs, including ecstasy, were developed (see Henry-Edwards & Ali 2000).

The source of amphetamines in Australia

Other than the clandestine manufacture of amphetamines in underground laboratories, which will be discussed separately in Chapter 14, amphetamines, and particularly methamphetamine, are imported into Australia from East Asia and Southeast Asia and the United States. An account of the sourcing, importation and border control of amphetamines can be found in Part E of this Report and the latest *Illicit Drug Report* produced by the Australian Crime Commission (2003).

Form and composition

Amphetamines were commonly referred to by the street name of 'speed'. Other street names for amphetamines include 'goey' or 'go-ee', 'billy' and 'whizz'. Amphetamines as a generic term (including methamphetamines and 'ice') are also known by names such as uppers, dexies, 'buzz', 'rev', 'crystal', 'meth', 'crystal meth', 'base', 'pure', 'shabu', 'ox blood' and 'ice'. Amphetamine sulphate can

46 See Chapter 14 for a discussion of amphetamine manufacture.

often be adulterated with similar coloured off-white powders such as talc, paracetamol and in some rare cases strychnine (Connolly 2000, p.7).

Today what passes as speed is more likely to be a form of methamphetamine, and to a lesser extent dexamphetamine (a drug sometimes used legitimately to treat Attention Deficit Hyperactivity Disorder (ADHD)). Methamphetamines are similar to amphetamine sulphate in both chemical structure and effects. In addition to the term 'speed', methamphetamines are sometimes referred to as 'meth' and in the United States 'chalk'.[47] Amphetamines and methamphetamines come in many different forms, sizes, colours and shapes.[48] Most amphetamine used for illicit purposes is made in clandestine laboratories by amateur 'chemists'. Unlike cocaine, with its 'centralised foreign production and distribution', methamphetamine in both Australia and the United States tends to be manufactured locally and often in fairly isolated rural pockets (Morgan & Beck 1997, p.135).[49]

A particularly potent form of methamphetamine comes in crystalline form and is colloquially known as 'crystal meth', 'shabu' or 'ice'. This will be discussed further below. Most forms of amphetamine, however, still come in powder form varying from pure white to brown and even orange or purple:

> No matter what form it comes in, almost all the speed available in Australia today is methamphetamine. Methamphetamine is slightly different in chemical terms to amphetamine, but the two have very similar effects. Although the availability and use of crystalline forms of methamphetamine are increasing, most of the speed available in Australia these days still comes in the form of powder. Speed powder can vary in texture from very fine to more coarse and crystalline, and can also vary in colour from white to yellow, pink or brownish. All these variations occur because the purifying process involved in the manufacture of amphetamine is quite tricky and most of the people who make the drug don't have the chemical expertise to do it properly.
>
> This means that, although they're all making speed, they end up with a wide range of products at the end of the manufacturing process which look different and contain different impurities (NDARC 2003, Fact Sheet).

---

47 In Britain, however, although the use of methamphetamines is increasing, amphetamine sulphate remains the most consistently used form of amphetamine.

48 For a good and straightforward summary of the various forms of methamphetamine available on the Australian markets, see Degenhardt and Topp 2003. The authors state there are at least four types of methamphetamine that can be viewed as distinct commodities:

'These are (1) speed, or methamphetamine powder that is locally manufactured, generally of low purity, and is usually administered by snorting or injecting; (2) pills, which are locally manufactured methamphetamine tablets, often mixed with other drugs such as ketamine, that are sold as 'ecstasy'; (3) base or paste, which is a gluggy, pasty or oily kind of methamphetamine powder that is locally manufactured and often has a brown or yellow tinge due to the presence of iodine and other organic impurities and (4) crystal meth or ice which is high purity, imported crystalline methamphetamine that comes in the form of large translucent to white crystals that are usually smoked or injected' (2003, p.18).

49 See Chapter 14 for discussion of methamphetamine production and manufacture.

Methamphetamine abuse has long been viewed as a problem in Hawaii and California but in recent years has also become a substantial problem in other areas of the south, south-west and mid-west of the United States and in big cities such as Denver and San Francisco. By contrast, methamphetamine abuse is seen relatively infrequently in the eastern United States (National Institute on Drug Abuse (USA) (NIDA) 1998).[50]

Route of administration

The NDARC states that most Australians who use speed powder either snort or swallow it, although some people choose to inject it.[51] It can also be added to drinks and swallowed or dabbed from the fingers to the mouth. Some of the people who use the crystalline forms known as ice or shabu smoke it in a special glass pipe.[52] Injecting and smoking of speed are generally viewed as a more harmful route of administration than oral use.[53]

The route of administration and the general rituals and culture of amphetamine use will clearly be dependent on the situation and setting.[54] Those who use amphetamines experimentally or only occasionally are less likely to inject than heavy, dependent or dysfunctional users (see Wickes 1993b, p.2). Such differences may also apply to those who use them for 'functional' purposes such as truck driving, exam performance, weight loss or sports competition.

Hall and Hando completed a survey of 231 Australian amphetamine users in 1994, half of whom injected the drug. They concluded that side effects and adverse symptoms and outcomes were generally greater in the injecting cohort:[55]

> [A]mong heavy chronic users there is a risk of developing a dependence syndrome that is characterised by a prolonged withdrawal syndrome in which

---

50 In the controversial and contentious book *Fast Food Nation*, author Eric Schlosser discusses the increasing 'occupational' use of methamphetamines in various sectors of American industry. This is most graphically described in an examination of the meatpacking and abattoir industries:

'The unrelenting pressure of trying to keep up with the [processing] line has encouraged widespread methamphetamine use among meatpackers. Workers taking "crank" feel charged and self confident, ready for anything. Supervisors have been known to sell crank to their workers or to supply it free in return for certain favours such as working a second shift. Workers who use methamphetamine may feel energised and invincible, but are actually putting themselves at much greater risk of having an accident. For obvious reasons a modern slaughterhouse is not a safe place to be high' (Schlosser 2002, p.174).

51 For a comparison of differences between injecting and non-injecting amphetamine users, see Moore 1992a, particularly at p.49. See also Dornier et al. 2000; Hall & Hando 1994.

52 See Morgan and Beck (1997) for an outline of the relatively prevalent practice of smoking methamphetamine in light bulbs among Latino populations in San Diego, California. In the United States, route of administration follows different regional patterns, for example intravenous use in San Francisco, intra nasal use in other parts of California and smoking in Hawaii (Morgan & Beck 1997, p.136).

53 For a comprehensive and interesting account of the manner of administering amphetamines, methamphetamines and ecstasy, including snorting, smoking, swallowing and 'blatting' (intravenous injection), see Moore 1992a, pp.45ff.

54 For a discussion of Zinberg's (1984) concept of the importance of drug, set and setting, ie. the context of drug use, see Chapter 10.

55 For a general discussion of the physical, psychological and social effects and results of using psychostimulants, see Chapter 6.

> depression, lethargy and irritability contribute to a high rate of relapse to use after abstinence, making it difficult to treat. Secondly, there is a risk, especially among injectors who use large doses, of developing a paranoid psychosis in which loosening of associations; delusions and auditory hallucinations are the most common symptoms. More conjecturally, there is a risk of chronic heavy users committing violent offences, perhaps while in the thrall of delusional thinking... Amphetamine users need to be better informed about the potential adverse effects of amphetamine use, and about ways in which they can reduce their risks of experiencing these harms by avoiding injecting use, and the regular use of high doses of amphetamines (Hall & Hando 1994, p.277).

Howard and Arcuri (2003) found that while ingestion was the most popular method of administration for first use of amphetamine type stimulants among a group of young users of psychostimulants in an adolescent residential treatment agency (25.8% of sample), injection was given as the most preferred *recent* route of administration (55.3%):

> Eighty three per cent of clients who nominated ATS as their primary drug of concern preferred injection as their route of administration. The same pattern may be seen when looking at patterns of cocaine use, where inhalation was the most popular initial route of administration (61%) but injection was the most likely last route (51.4%). Likewise, rates of injection of designer drugs increased substantially from first to last route of administration (from 9.1% to 12.2%) This group of drugs differed to the others in that ingestion was by far the most likely first and last route of administration (from 83.6% to 79.6%) (Howard & Arcuri 2003a in Howard, Stubbs & Arcuri 2004, in prep).

Such views are reiterated in American studies. Dornier et al. also conducted a survey of 427 methamphetamine users in California, 13 per cent of whom were injecting users. Injecting methamphetamine users were found to be more at risk of developing serious health and social problems, including HIV and other blood-borne diseases. Interestingly, methamphetamine users themselves definitely had distinct views about differences between injecting and non-injecting users:

> Overall, this study found several interesting differences based on the route of administration. When the participants were asked if they injected MA many of the non injectors responded adamantly in the negative. There seemed to be a stereotype present within the drug-using population that injectors were 'more dependent' or 'more severe' addicts than other users. This idea that injecting users are more dependent on the drug is growing (Dornier et al. 2000, p.231).[56]

56 Dornier et al. (2000) note that paying attention to the difference between injecting and non-injecting users of amphetamines and methamphetamines may have important implications for strategy development:

'Overall... there are characteristics of injecting users that make them uniquely different from users of other routes. Knowing about these differences can provide useful information for clinicians treating injection users. Possible topics to include or emphasise in an injector's treatment plan are HIV concerns, legal issues, and a greater focus on depression, suicide and hallucinations' (Dornier et al. 2000, p.232).

A 1996 survey study of 100 amphetamine users conducted in South Australia also made some interesting comparisons between injecting and non-injecting drug users. The findings showed that:

- Injection was the most commonly used method for administering amphetamine in the sample, with 77% reporting injecting in the 6 months prior to interview. Forty-three percent of the sample had not used any other method during that time. Fifty-four percent had snorted amphetamine in the 6 months prior to interview, and 37% had swallowed the drug in that time.
- Amphetamine was the first drug injected for 61% of the sample.
- Greater use of injecting as a form of amphetamine administration in the 6 months prior to interview was significantly associated with a lower level of education, a greater number of days on which tobacco and benzodiazepines were used, a more frequent use of amphetamines, greater quantity of the drug used in a day, a younger age at first use of the drug, a younger age at first injection of amphetamine, and a younger age at first injection of any drug. This variable was also associated with a decreased tendency to use condoms for anal sex, and a higher self-rating of concern about the risks of contracting HIV, hepatitis B, and hepatitis C.
- Significantly, over half of all of those who had injected amphetamines in the 6 months prior to interview (n=38) had experienced difficulty in obtaining sterile injecting equipment. The majority of these people (n=20) said that the lack of a needle exchange within easy access had been a problem for them, and 15 people said that the opening hours of these services were often an issue (Vincent, Allsop & Shoobridge, 1996, p.376).

Thus the effects and dangers of psychostimulant use and misuse are very closely connected with how they are used:

> The importance of the route of administration of the psychostimulants rests not only with the bioavailability of the drug (a term used to describe the proportion of the administered dose which reaches the bloodstream), but also with the rate of its delivery to the site of action in the brain (Chesher 1993, p.14).

Mundy states that as well as the physical act of administration the context is all-important in terms of the consumption of methamphetamines, as with all drug use. Discussing methamphetamine use in Sydney she states:

> Methods of administration appear to be dependent on 'community norms'. For instance residents in the Sydney beach suburb of Manly who use this drug seem to prefer smoking it, whereas Kings Cross users are more likely to inject (Mundy 2001, p.2).

For further discussion comparing injecting and non-injecting use of amphetamine, see Chapter 9.

'Base'

Base is a form of methamphetamine that resembles an oily, sticky or waxy powder or paste, often of a yellow or brownish shade. It can also be colloquially referred to as 'wax', 'point', 'pure' or 'paste'. Unlike the sophisticated chemistry knowledge needed to produce 'ice' (see next section), base can be and is produced in Australia by amateur 'chemists':

> It is oily because the pseudoephedrine to methamphetamine conversion produces the base form of methamphetamine, which is oil. An oil is not highly marketable in illicit drug markets, because it cannot be easily injected or snorted. Therefore, manufacturers attempt to purify methamphetamine base (oil) into methamphetamine hydrochloride (crystal). To successfully complete this process requires considerable chemistry expertise, and few illicit manufacturers in Australia have such expertise. The result is an oily powder ...[with organic impurities]. These organic impurities, which would not be present if the conversion and purification were performed accurately, also prevent the substance from forming into the large translucent crystals typical of 'ice', so the appearance of these two forms of methamphetamine is quite different (IDRS 2002, p.3).

Base can be administered by swallowing, smoking snorting and injecting, although its oily consistency makes dissolving for injection difficult without the application of heat.

'Crystal meth' or 'ice'

'Ice' is a particularly strong methamphetamine, which in the past five years has become more widely available and used on the streets of Melbourne and other Australian cities. Generally the drug that is referred to as 'ice' is a high purity form of methamphetamine that comes in crystalline form and may also be called other names such as 'shabu', 'crystal', 'crystal meth, and 'crank' or 'glass' in the United States.[57]

History

Methamphetamine, including 'ice', was developed in the early twentieth century from the parent amphetamine drugs. It was used in licit form in nasal decongestants and bronchial inhalers (see Derlet & Heischober 1990; Safe & Sager 1990).

The history of ice production, the changes in the way it is used and misused and its impact culturally on a population is interestingly expressed in the following quote that outlines the history of the drug in Thailand:

---

57 'Shabu' is a Japanese word that is used to refer to ice in the Phillipines, where the use of ice has a long history. See NDARC 2003, Fact Sheet. For an account of the 'crank' trade and 'crank' use in the United States, see Kirn 1998.

> In Thailand methamphetamine was available first as a pharmaceutical product (methedrine), known colloquially as *ya khayan* (which translates as 'diligence pill'). Use was popular among long distance lorry drivers and other occupational groups but abuse led to strict government controls. Illicit manufacture and distribution followed the restrictions and an illegal trade grew; the drug was renamed *ya-ma* (horse pill) in view of a horse's head being stamped on each tablet. By the mid 1990s methamphetamine became re-branded as *ya ba* (mad/crazy pill) referring to its adverse psychological effects, and it was estimated there were over 250,000 people with methamphetamine dependence across Thailand. Initially the major proportion of drug production was based domestically but the focus of production is now thought to be on the Thai/Myanamar border and in the Yunan province of China (Farrell & Marsden 2002, p.771).

Ice was once very popular in the United States gay communities, particularly in the dance scene, due to its ability to keep users awake for long periods and its sexual disinhibition effect.[58] It spread quickly into mainstream cultures. Truck drivers and bikers have also been known to use meth and ice to keep awake on long journeys.[59]

Most of the 'ice' in Australia is clandestinely manufactured in China and transported to Australia via other Asian countries such as the Philippines or Indonesia. The illicit importation of ice has grown in recent years. According to NDARC, in the 2000/01 financial year the Australian Customs Service seized more than 80 kilograms of ice at the Australian border:

> When there is more good quality ice being imported, it puts pressure on the people who manufacture methamphetamine in Australia to produce a higher quality product, so the purity of methamphetamine powder ('speed') made here has been increasing over the last few years (NDARC 2003, Fact Sheet).

As indicated in the previous section, pure crystalline ice is rarely made in Australia, as clandestine manufacturers do not have the necessary expertise. What is produced is more likely to be 'base', as referred to in the previous section:

> Sometimes people who make or sell speed in Australia will call their product ice or shabu to make it more attractive to buyers so they can charge a higher price. This only leads to confusion among users as to what they've actually bought. Real ice is a big colourless crystal, but often people buy white powder that they've been told is ice (NDARC 2003, Fact Sheet).

---

58 In Australia as well, 'ice' is also associated with the male gay community and 'overwhelmingly within the context of the dance party/club environment' (Degenhardt & Topp 2003, p.19). In a recent study by Degenhardt and Topp that examines the use of crystal meth in Sydney, 58% of the sample identified as homosexual and 16% as bisexual. This is despite the fact that the study was not specifically targeted at the gay community (Degenhardt & Topp 2003). See also Lewis and Ross 1995; Reback and Grella 1999; Klitzmann et al 2000; Murnane et al 2000; Semple et al 2002; Shoptaw, Reback and Freese 2002 and the detailed discussion in Chapter 9 of this Report.

59 For a discussion of amphetamine use among truck drivers, see Chapter 9.

Form and composition

Ice is described as having large, translucent to white crystals or being a crystal coarse powder. It can sometimes have a blue, green or pinkish tinge as a result of the manufacturing processes. Ice is usually sold in 'points' (0.1 gram) because it is so strong that only a tiny bit is used at a time.

Route of administration

Ice has traditionally been smoked in a glass pipe similar to the kinds of pipes that crack cocaine is smoked in. This has particularly been the case in countries where ice has had a long history of use, especially Japan, the Philippines and Hawaii[60] (see NDARC 2003, Fact Sheet; Derlet & Heischober 1990).

Some people who use ice in Australia smoke it through this kind of pipe, whereas others mix it with cannabis and smoke it through a bong ('sno cones'), or 'chase' (heat) it on aluminium foil and inhale the vapours. But many people who use ice in Australia inject it or swallow it, and some people also snort it. Snorting ice leads to nasal damage because the crystals are sharp and can cause nosebleeds (NDARC 2003, Fact Sheet).

Price, purity and availability of amphetamines and methamphetamines

The IDRS annually monitors emerging trends in illicit drug use in Australia. In particular it gauges trends in the use, price, purity and availability of major drugs such as heroin, methamphetamine and cannabis. To a lesser extent it also concentrates on ecstasy and other 'party drugs'.[61]

> A key advantage of the IDRS study is that it replicates core methods across each state and territory. At the national level, this permits the identification of emerging jurisdictional differences with respect to the operation of illicit drug markets, and enhances the capacity of health and law enforcement sectors in all jurisdictions to develop proactive responses to illicit drug problems (NDARC 2002a, p.viii).

Nationally, with regard to methamphetamines, powder and base were considered easy to obtain and availability was stable. Crystal methamphetamine was more difficult to obtain in some jurisdictions. All forms of methamphetamine were cheapest in South Australia. Indeed evidence given to

---

60 It is interesting to note that in Hawaii:

'Ice was developed and distributed completely independently from the U.S mainland methamphetamine networks, so for several years, users and some law enforcement officials assumed ice was an entirely different drug from methamphetamine' (Joe-Laidler & Morgan 1997, p.164).

61 The methodology of the IDRS and its data collection methods are based on a threefold process. First, a survey of injecting drug users is undertaken. This is supported by a survey of key informants, expert professionals in the illicit drug field. Finally, existing indicator data on drug issues is analysed. These may include household and school surveys, law enforcement, hospital and ambulance databases, needle exchange programme data and other relevant secondary indicators. A triangulation of this data avoids the problems associated with relying on secondary indicators of themselves, most notably the fact that they are by their very nature *lag indicators.*

the Committee by Mr Mal Hyde, Chief Commissioner of South Australia Police, highlights the prevalence of amphetamine in that state. Discussing national research[62] being conducted on drug use within police watch-houses and gaols he comments:

> [t]he researchers operate within police watch-houses, and when people are charged and lodged in custody, they, with their consent, get a urine sample, which is analysed. The research has been running for about 18 months now. We have two sites here in South Australia: one is in the city at the Adelaide watch-house; the other is at Elizabeth. Amphetamines use features very highly in both areas. In one area it is close to 40 per cent; in the other area close to 30 per cent. There is no doubt that amphetamines and the other synthetic designer type drugs are readily available. They certainly are in South Australia. That is borne out by at least two things. Firstly, the price is quite low in South Australia. Secondly, we are locating an increasing number of clandestine laboratories; the number is going up quite rapidly.[63]

The use of methamphetamines among injecting drug users (IDUs) has decreased or stabilised in most jurisdictions, possibly as a result of an increase in the availability of heroin in most jurisdictions compared to 2001 and the 'worst' days of the 'heroin drought' (discussed later in this chapter). Cocaine use has decreased in prevalence and frequency in its traditional stronghold of New South Wales. In all other jurisdictions 'it remained relatively uncommon and infrequent' (NDARC 2003b, p.12 and see also the discussion on pp.90ff.).

The median price for a gram of methamphetamine powder ranged in 2002 from $A50.00 (SA) to $A250.00 (WA). The median price for a point (0.1 gram) of 'base' ranged from $25.00 (SA) to $50.00 in most other states.[64] According to the IDRS (NDARC 2003b), the availability of base has increased in Australia in recent years but prices have remained relatively stable. A point of crystal methamphetamine ('ice') varied from $25.00 in South Australia to $80.00 in the Northern Territory and $50.00 in most other states (NDARC 2003b, pp. 15-16).[65]

---

62 The Drug Use Monitoring in Australia (DUMA) surveys conducted by the Australian Institute of Criminology; refer also to discussion in Chapter 7.

63 Mr Mal Hyde, Commissioner of South Australia Police in conversation with the Drugs and Crime Prevention Committee, Adelaide, 3 October 2003.

64 Interestingly, the price has been costed at only $30.00 per gram in South Australia. See IDRS 2002, p.3; NDARC 2001, 2002c; NDARC 2003b, p.15.

65 A submission from Anglicare Victoria, an organisation working with young, often homeless, people states that in their experience the cost of amphetamines and indeed 'party drugs' such as MDMA is beyond most of the young people in their care:

'Young people do not like using amphetamines as these are prohibitively expensive and cannot afford them. Those few who use amphetamines...fund their habit by engaging in criminal behaviour such as theft and trafficking. In general, young people would, however, use whatever drugs they can access. Some people are accessing amphetamine related substances, which they can get from Ritalin...prescribed for children with Attention Deficit Hyperactive Disorder (ADH)' (Submission of Anglicare Victoria, to the Drugs and Crime Prevention Committee, Inquiry into Amphetamine and 'Party Drug' Use in Victoria, October 2003).

The IDRS states that there is no clear trend to gauge the purity of various forms of methamphetamine.[66] However, the majority of IDRS respondents in all jurisdictions reported that it was easy or very easy to obtain and that, unlike heroin, availability was generally stable, with some variations in availability of crystal meth (more difficult to obtain in NSW, ACT, Vic and Tas).

This recent summary of trends (2003 – reporting figures for 2002) contains very little specific information pertaining to Victoria. A separate paper prepared by Turning Point Alcohol and Drug Centre, which conducts the research for the Melbourne arm of the IDRS project, outlined its summary of 2002 trends.[67] It found:

> In 2002, the different forms of methamphetamine – speed, base, and ice – were separated out for the purposes of analyses, making comparison with previous years somewhat difficult. However, more comprehensive analyses will be possible in future years of the IDRS.
>
> The 2002 IDRS study found that 73% of IDU [Injecting drug users] had used some form of methamphetamine (either speed, base or ice) in the preceding six months, a proportion comparable to that of the 2001 IDRS (76%). Separating out the forms of methamphetamine, 70% reported using speed, 19% reported using base and 26% reported using ice in the preceding six months. The median number of days on which speed had been used in the preceding six months was 24, while for base it was 10, and ice 6 days.
>
> The most common quantity of speed purchased was a 'point', and the majority of respondents paid $50 for this amount. The most frequently reported price per gram of speed was $200, and these prices have remained the same since 2001. Over half of the respondents (59%) also reported that the price of speed had been stable over the last six months. Although it is difficult to draw any conclusions about the price of base and ice from the small sample sizes who were able to respond to these questions (base n=4, ice n=13), the most commonly purchased amount of both forms of methamphetamine was a 'point', and the median prices reported by IDU were; base $35 and ice $50.
>
> Eighty-five percent of IDU commenting on speed thought that it was easy or very easy to obtain and 65% thought availability had remained stable in the preceding six months. Only six people were able to comment confidently on the availability of base, however of these, three respondents thought it easy to obtain, and four people thought availability remained stable. Nine of the 13 IDU commenting on ice reported that it was difficult to very difficult to obtain. Five of the 13 people who could comment on ice reported that availability had remained stable, and another five that availability of ice had become more difficult in the last six months.

---

66 In past years, purity has been noted as markedly increasing, particularly in Victoria (McKey 2001, p.17).

67 At the time of finalising this Report IDRS/NDARC trend data for 2002-2003 was still some weeks away from publication. Therefore figures for 2001/2002 are the most recent available.

> It is apparent from recent IDRS surveys that there has been a cross over between the traditionally separate heroin and methamphetamine drug markets and that the recent reduced heroin supply created favourable conditions for this. While current IDU in this study have been able to provide some information about methamphetamine trends in Melbourne, a clearer picture would be gained through contact with other sentinel groups (NDARC 2003c pp.ix–x).

Purity of the drugs for the period 2001/2002 was said to have decreased since previous years. Seizures by Police and Customs officials in Victoria indicate that average purity had increased from five per cent in 1996/1997 to 21 per cent in 2000/2001 (NDARC 2002a, pp.31–32). However, in 2001-2002 the Victorian component of the IDRS survey states that:

> Participants used a variety of methamphetamine forms during the last six months, including speed powder 70% (74% in 2001), liquid 8% (7% in 2001), base 20% (32% in 2001) and ice 28% (52% in 2001). Although similar numbers of IDU used powder and liquid in both 2001 and 2002, it is evident from IDRS data that there has been a decrease in respondents using ice and base.
>
> In terms of purity, generally respondents reported it as medium, however the majority believed that it had decreased in the past six months. This is in comparison with 2001 data where respondents felt purity had either increased or remained stable (Fry & Miller, 2002 cited in NDARC 2002c pp.22-23).

NDARC breaks down the purity figures for the various types of amphetamine as follows:

> **Speed**
>
> The majority of respondents reported that the purity of speed was low (35%), to medium (32%), while 16% reported that it was high and 12% fluctuating. In 2002 most thought that purity had either decreased (31%) or remained stable (26%), while 22% thought that it had fluctuated and 16% increased.
>
> **Base**
>
> Of the six people who answered this section, three felt that the purity of base was medium, two reported that they didn't know about the purity, and one respondent claimed that the purity was low. Three people reported that the purity had decreased over the last six months and one person reported that it had remained stable (two did not know).
>
> **Ice**
>
> Nearly half (46%, n=6) of the respondents felt that the purity of ice was high, three people reported medium quality, and one respondent claimed the purity was low (three respondents did not know). Perceptions about the changes in purity of ice over the last six months were evenly spread amongst the ten respondents who had some knowledge of purity, with equal numbers (n=3) reporting that purity had been stable, decreasing or fluctuating, with only one respondent reporting an increase in purity. (NDARC 2003c, p.23).

> Nonetheless, despite the views of the survey respondents that purity of methamphetamine was decreasing, NDARC also states that Australian Bureau of Criminal Intelligence records of the purity of methamphetamine seizures made by the Australian Federal Police in Victoria show that the average purity of the small number of seizures tested (n=16 of ≤ 2 gms) during July 2001-June 2002 was 79.9% (NDARC 2003c, p.23). Admittedly, the numbers in this sample were relatively low.

The above trends provide valuable information but some caveats must be noted. First, as acknowledged by IDRS itself, '[t]he distinction between amphetamines and methamphetamines in Melbourne has become problematic and many of the respondents appeared unsure of the distinction' (2002, p.x). This confusion between amphetamine (sulphate) and various forms of methamphetamine has the potential to skew the data. Second, the above figures for Victoria have to be read subject to detailed new figures for 2003 yet to be released. In particular, the apparent 'relief' of the heroin drought will need to be factored. It may be that an increasing availability of heroin will impact upon the amount of amphetamine used.

It is timely here to discuss briefly the effect of the 'heroin drought' on the use of amphetamines and 'party drugs'.

A note on the 'heroin drought'

From approximately December 2000 a reduction in the availability of heroin in Australia, partly due to an edict forbidding opium cultivation in Afghanistan, has meant an increase nation-wide in the use of other illicit drugs, especially amphetamines and to some extent benzodiazepines, such as temazepam.

It may be that this phenomenon will be merely a 'historical curio', as anecdotal evidence suggests that increased amounts of heroin are being seen back on the streets of Australian cities. Nonetheless, this section will discuss the linkages between increased usage of ATS as a result of the 'heroin drought', as it appeared until approximately the end of 2002.[68] In the most recent survey of illicit drug trends compiled by the ABCI, it was stated that:

> Increased amphetamine-type stimulant use as a direct result of the lack of heroin has been particularly noted in the Australian Capital Territory, Queensland, South Australia, Western Australia and some areas of New South Wales. In particular, police in the Lake Illawarra, Shoalhaven and Monaro Local Area Commands of New South Wales noted increased usage of crystalline methylamphetamine amongst traditional long-term heroin users. This raises concerns because of the increased propensity towards violent behaviour

68 The most recent Victorian Drug Trends Component of the IDRS (NDARC 2002a) indicates that at the time of the interviews of participating IDUs (June 2001) there may have been a slight shift in perceptions of availability:

'77% of respondents indicated that the availability of heroin had not yet returned to normal, while 20% reported that it had. Reports varied as to the timing of the return of heroin availability with 8%...suggesting that it had returned in June 2001' (NDARC 2002a, p.59).

> associated with crystalline methylamphetamine use. There has also been a significant increase in property offences in those areas, which is correlated with increased consumption of crystalline methylamphetamine.
>
> Researchers from the National Drug and Alcohol Research Centre (NDARC) noted the increased prevalence of crystalline methylamphetamine being smoked by users in Sydney (NDARC 2001). This was also a trend noted in the Footscray area of Melbourne where traditional heroin smokers have turned to smoking crystalline methylamphetamine due to the reduced availability of heroin (Tregear 2001). NDARC also reported instances of methylamphetamine base being swallowed due to the difficulty of injection or intranasal use of the drug in that form (2001) (ABCI 2002, pp.46–47).

Commissioner Keelty of the Australian Federal Police has also posited some reasons why international drug syndicates may have decided to move from heroin production to amphetamine manufacture.[69] These include:

- higher potential market for amphetamines in comparison to heroin
- the vulnerability of opium crops to location by satellite or other aerial surveillance
- opium growing is subject to the vagaries of weather
- ready availability of precursor chemicals in Asia
- there is a shorter, less intensive production and distribution chain for synthetics
- higher profit margins – methamphetamine enjoys a considerably higher mark than opiates
- impending world shortage of opium due initially to Taliban; and more recently a drought in Burma.[70]

A study of the 'heroin drought' conducted through Turning Point Alcohol and Drug Centre by Miller, Fry and Dietze (2001) stated that the 'impact of the reduced Australian heroin supply has been the most pronounced in the state of Victoria'. Turning Point Alcohol and Drug Centre states further that the consequences of the drought have been both positive and negative. A survey of drug-using participants reported:

- A decrease in the availability of heroin
- Increases in the price of heroin and amphetamine
- Decreases in the purity of heroin and amphetamine
- Few changes in the availability of amphetamine...
- Increases in the reported use and injection of pharmaceuticals (especially benzodiazepines) and amphetamines

---

69 See also discussion in Chapter 14.

70 Quoted in the submission of Youth Substance Abuse Service to the Drugs and Crime Prevention Committee, Inquiry into Amphetamine and 'Party Drug' Use in Victoria, October 2003.

- Increases in number of people reporting involvement in criminal activity (including both property and violent crime)
- Reports of a generalised increase in 'danger' for drug users (Turning Point Alcohol and Drug Centre 2001, pp.vi–vii).

The survey sample showed that for 55 per cent of the drug users interviewed, heroin was the drug most often injected. This was in stark contrast to the IDRS (2000) findings:

> These findings suggest that the 'drought' is best understood as an interruption to the steady supply of heroin evident in Melbourne over the late 1990s (Fry and Miller 2001), rather than the absence of the drug from Melbourne drug markets. The change from the 2000 IDRS findings, where 92% reported heroin as the last drug injected prior to interview, was however dramatic (Turning Point Alcohol and Drug Centre 2001, p.11).

The most recent evaluation of Victorian Drug Trends by the NDARC supports the findings of increasing use of amphetamine in Melbourne and other major Victorian centres:

> Amphetamines and methamphetamines have...become the identified drug of choice for a group of people who were primary heroin users and there [has been] an increase in the number of people reporting injecting amphetamines from 50% from the previous year to 75% for the current study [2001]... It was noted that both amphetamines and methamphetamines were readily available... Both were reported as becoming easier to obtain. These trends demonstrate a *major shift in illicit drug use* and require further research to understand the nature of this change (NDARC 2002a, p.xi). (Committee emphasis)

It is not only amphetamines that have been affected by the 'heroin drought'. Fry and Miller, reporting for the NDARC on the most recent Victorian illicit drug trends, state that:

> Victoria Police key informants reported that ecstasy has become of greater interest since the previous IDRS and that greater resources are being allocated to its detection and seizure, particularly due to the heroin drought (NDARC 2002a, p.51).

Treatment agencies have also noted that the 'drought' has had some discernible effect on the reasons clients may be presenting for medical treatment:

> Graph 1...shows the changing patterns of primary drug of use of those seeking treatment between July 2000 and June 2003 [due to in part the 'heroin drought']. It can be seen that the number of clients seeking treatment for amphetamine use more than doubled from 244 in the first quarter of 2000/2001 to 497 in the final quarter of 2002/2003. The number of clients seeking treatment for heroin use fell from 2,170 in the second quarter of

2000/2001 to 1,506 in the third quarter of 2001/2002, before rising to 1,897 in the third quarter of 2002/2003.[71]

Figure 4.1: Primary drug use

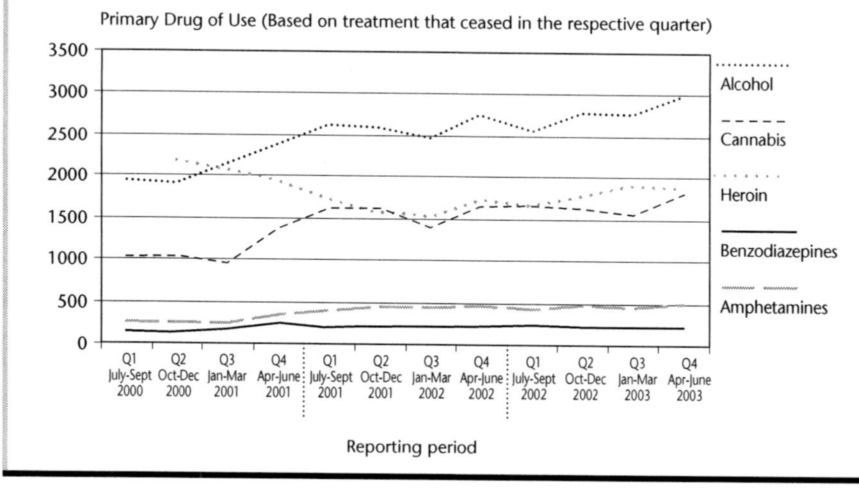

Source: Alcohol and Drug Information System 2003.[72]

Rowe's study of injecting drug use in the Melbourne suburb of St Kilda paints a picture of heroin users reluctantly turning to amphetamine as a second-class substitute for heroin. The testimonies of a variety of research participants suggest that for this group at least, amphetamine was by no means their first drug of choice:

> In the most recent *Australian Illicit Drug Report 2001-2002* (Australian Crime Commission 2003) it was noted that, as a result of continued reduced availability, the street-level purity of heroin had remained relatively low and the price high. This was linked to increasing numbers of intravenous drug users injecting amphetamines (as well as illegally obtained pharmaceuticals and other drugs) (Australian Crime Commission 2003). This was reported by a number of research participants who also drew attention to the negative consequences associated with the increased use of amphetamines.
>
> 'A lot of users, in the drought, there was no heroin but they started using speed and stuff like that. They never used to like speed and speed is a totally different drug to heroin – which meant a lot of people went crazy as well because people were thinking they can use speed like they could use heroin, in big amounts which ended up sending them all crazy. That 'ice' at the moment, it's a very evil drug. It really gets into your head' (21-year-old male, squatter).

---

71 Included in the submission of Department of Human Services Victoria to the Drugs and Crime Prevention Committee, Inquiry into Amphetamine and 'Party Drug' Use in Victoria, November 2003.

72 Submission of Department of Human Services Victoria to the Drugs and Crime Prevention Committee, Inquiry into Amphetamine and 'Party Drug' Use in Victoria, November 2003.

> 'There was no more gear in Cabramatta. You were seeing, 20, 30 users all following each other just trying to find a dealer that was on and the heroin was getting smaller and from there on it was really bad. From Cabramatta we weren't getting nothing proper no more... We had to sometimes travel hours and hours around everywhere just trying to find dealers and stuff... One day we could just not get no heroin so we went and got a shitload of cocaine. Like, the cocaine would usually make you hang out straight away if you're sick but for some reason it just got us up and going and then we started for three of four days using cocaine like the shitload...' (21-year-old homeless male).[73]

Rowe's research tends to bear out the views of Handley that the trend towards increasing usage of amphetamines in the past few years:

> [s]hows that drug users have not gone clean, but are simply turning to other drugs while they wait for the heroin market to improve (Handley 2002, p.14).

However, some respondents to the Inquiry have warned about making too much of the concept of a 'heroin drought' and the idea of amphetamine as a drug substitute:

> [w]hile there has been, to some extent, a displacement effect due to the onset of the 'heroin drought', the use of psychostimulants and other drugs may not fully be the result of drug substitution. That is, for a proportion of current injectors the use of these other drugs was a part of their injecting culture before the 'drought'. This is further corroborated by Thompson's (2003) findings which showed that while all of the Melbourne-based respondents continued to inject heroin during 2002, they were also injecting other drugs.[74]

Rob Kemp, Manager of Queensland Health's Needle Availability Support Program also believes the former abundant supply of heroin masked what was already a pre-existing problem with amphetamine.[75]

Similarly, Professor Jason White of the Drug and Alcohol Services Council in South Australia believes that amphetamine use was independently increasing *prior* to the advent of the 'heroin drought':

> I think the evidence is that it [amphetamine use] was increasing before the heroin drought happened: that you have an upward-rising curve and then the heroin drought came in. Amongst heroin users, a few of them would use a bit of amphetamine, but the vast majority have changed to using morphine. They want an opiate drug; they do not want amphetamine. There may be a little bit of movement between, but I think the increase in amphetamines is reasonably

73 Submission of Dr James Rowe, RMIT University to the Drugs and Crime Prevention Committee, Inquiry into Amphetamine and 'Party Drug' Use in Victoria, October 2003.

74 Submission of Anex to the Drugs and Crime Prevention Committee, Inquiry into Amphetamine and 'Party Drug' Use in Victoria, October 2003.

75 '[W]as in fact the abundant supply of heroin simply masking what was already a pre-existing amphetamine problem? ... I suspect that is probably true. I suspect that it was always there; it was actually the stripping away...the heroin that uncovered this pre-existing issue' (Mr Rob Kemp, Manager, Needle Availability Support Program, Queensland Health, in conversation with the Drugs and Crime Prevention Committee, 27 June 2003).

> independent of the heroin drought and, as I said, I think it precedes it. The increase was only gradual, but I think the curve is exponential, and you saw the beginning part of it prior to the heroin drought. We mainly date the increase to the 1990s, and the heroin drought was later than that; it was after 2000. There may be a little bit of a relationship and trade-off, but not much.[76]

It should be noted that at the time of writing the Final Report, the Committee had heard anecdotal evidence from a variety of individuals and community agencies that the heroin drought 'had broken' and that heroin was now readily available on the streets of Melbourne. If this is the case, it will prove interesting to see what effect, if any, this will have on the trading and consumption of amphetamines in Victoria and the rest of the country. Some speculative comments have been made about increasing amounts of heroin seen on the streets of Sydney and Melbourne:

> Changing levels of heroin availability and their impact upon patterns of injecting drug use are reflected in Australian NSP surveys, particularly when these survey results are viewed alongside Victorian drug trends reported in the findings of the Illicit Drug Reporting System (IDRS)...
>
> Key informants of the IDRS study reported that the increase in methamphetamine use identified in the 2001 IDRS [study] had stabilised to become a regular feature of the Melbourne injecting drug scene. This is reflected in the Victorian NSP figures for 2002. However, NSP survey results in New South Wales and the ACT suggest this may be about to change. As observed in the figures below, the use of heroin by intravenous drug users is returning to pre-'drought' levels in these jurisdictions. Sydney is the primary point of entry for heroin into Australia before it is distributed to other centres (ACC 2003).[77]It would consequently be expected that increasing supplies of heroin would be used to replenish markets close to the distribution centre before spreading throughout other states. Interestingly, figures reported in Queensland also suggest an increase in heroin supplies. The (gradually) falling price and increasing purity of heroin in Victoria may indicate that the dynamics of injecting drug use in this state may be undergoing a similar reversion towards pre-'drought' patterns.[78]

Handley states that if the 'drought' has 'broken' there could be serious health consequences for users who return to using that drug, either in substitute for or alongside amphetamine:

> Most experts seem to agree that the heroin drought is now abating, but the use of other drugs, which came to the forefront during the drought, does not

---

76 Professor Jason White, Director, Treatment and Rehabilitation Services, Drug and Alcohol Services Council, in conversation with the Drugs and Crime Prevention Committee, Adelaide, 3 October 2003.

77 In 2001–02, 31 of the 46 heroin detections at the Australian border occurred in New South Wales.

78 Submission of Dr James Rowe, RMIT University to the Drugs and Crime Prevention Committee, Inquiry into Amphetamine and 'Party Drug' Use in Victoria, October 2003.

> seem to be decreasing. This is a very serious problem, which will no doubt have the government rethinking its current drug-control plans...
>
> Addicts who have been replacing heroin with other drugs during the drought would be at high risk of overdose, as their immunity to heroin would have gone down, but they may not compensate properly for this by injecting smaller amounts. Dr Sandy Gordon [of the Australian Federal Police] said it was highly probable drug users would go back to heroin:
>
> 'These people may have switched to other substances in the interim, but if cheap, pure heroin again comes on to the market, they will likely use it' (Handley 2002, p.15).

The 'heroin drought', then, has clearly resulted in an increase from one injecting form of drug use (heroin) to another (amphetamine). Despite some anecdotal evidence that there has been a slight move toward 'street use' of MDMA/ecstasy, partly as a result of the 'drought', for the most part ecstasy remains a drug associated with oral use in the party and club scene, as the next section outlines.

Ecstasy (methylenedioxymethamphetamine – MDMA)

Ecstasy, often abbreviated to 'e' or 'eckies', is the street term for a number of substances that are 3,4-methylenedioxymethamphetamine (MDMA)[79] or closely related. Pharmacologically it belongs to a family of drugs called the phenethylamines, which also include MDA (3,4-methylenedioxyamphetamine and MDEA (3,4-methylenedioxyethylamphetamine).[80] The latter two drugs are often passed off as MDMA (see Chesher 1990a). Ecstasy/MDMA is also known as an 'empathogen', that is a drug that releases chemicals into the brain that inspire feelings of well being, love, friendship and euphoria.[81] For that reason one of the colloquial names for ecstasy is the 'Love Drug'.

One highly significant fact associated with ecstasy is that, like any illegal drug, there is no 'quality control' during the manufacturing or importation process. Since the 1990s the purity of ecstasy has been highly variable. There is therefore no guarantee that the user is actually consuming MDMA when he or she purchases or otherwise obtains what purports to be methyldioxymethamphetamine:

> Some of the tablets sold as ecstasy in Australia today do not contain MDMA at all, and are more likely to contain methamphetamine, perhaps in combination with an hallucinogenic such as ketamine, an anaesthetic used primarily in veterinary surgery. They might also contain illegal chemicals like MDA, PMA or

---

79 Ecstasy can also be colloquially known as 'eccy', 'XTC', 'doves',' eggs' and many more. For further discussion of the names and nicknames given to ecstasy/MDMA, see Chapter 10.

80 For an interesting account of the history of the pharmacology of designer drugs, see Chesher 1990b; Chawla 1998. Chesher makes the salient point that it is often from articles in scientific and medical journals, which follow years of painstaking research and clinical trials, that many 'street chemists' get their ideas for producing illicit designer drugs and analogues.

81 For an account as to whether ecstasy is considered a 'love' or a 'hug' drug, ie. whether it has aphrodisiacal qualities in addition to being an 'empathogen', see the discussion in Hammersley, Khan and Ditton 2002, pp.59ff and the responses of their interviewees.

> MDEA, or substances like caffeine or paracetamol. Some of the ecstasy tested has contained no active stimulant at all (NDARC 2003, Fact Sheet).

Of particular concern is the fact that in a number of jurisdictions paramethoxyamphetamine or PMA has been known to substitute for MDMA. PMA is generally thought of as a more toxic phenethylamine derivative with more harmful complications than pure MDMA (see for example Byard et al. 1999; Byard et al. 2002; White, Bochner & Irvine 1997; Felgate et al. 1998; Moriarty 2001). Such complications, including death, will be discussed further in Chapter 6, which deals with the medical consequences of the drugs under discussion.

The IDRS reports that few clandestine laboratories or chemists in Australia have the capacity or expertise to make pure MDMA and:

> [a]lmost every tablet that contains true MDMA is imported from manufacturing and distribution points in Europe and Asia. The Australian Bureau of Criminal Intelligence estimates that 80% of the tablets sold as 'ecstasy' in Australia today are actually locally manufactured methamphetamine tablets that are sometimes mixed with other drugs such as ketamine in an attempt to mimic the effects of MDMA. Illicit manufacturers use the reports posted on websites about 'good pills' [to produce] 'fake ecstasy' tablets that are the same weight and colour and have the same logo as real MDMA tablets... Many experienced 'ecstasy' users know that they are unlikely to get real MDMA these days, and sometimes use the term 'pills' in place of 'ecstasy', in a tacit acknowledgment that they don't really know what they are using (IDRS 2002, p.2).

History[82]

Overseas origins

MDMA is generally believed to have first been synthesised by Merck Pharmaceuticals in Germany in 1912 and patented in 1914, originally as an appetite suppressant.[83] Gowing et al. (2001) state that at this time it was never commercially successful or viable and largely was forgotten or ignored until the 1950s:

> [w]hen it was studied by the US Army as a potential agent in psychological warfare. In the late 1960s the drug was synthesised and used experimentally by [Dr] Alexander Shulgin in California, USA. In the 1970s it was increasingly being [legitimately] used in the USA as an adjunct to psychotherapy to help lower inhibitions in patients undergoing psychoanalysis... In 1977 the drug was prohibited in the UK, and in 1985 perceptions of increasing recreational

82 For good general accounts of the evolution, development and history of MDMA, see Solowij, Hall & Lee 1992; Forsyth 1995; Gowing et al. 2001; Grob 2000; Shannon 2002.

83 Gowing states that this account of its origins is disputed by some researchers. Milroy, for example, claims that it was discovered merely as 'an accidental intermediate chemical' (Milroy 1999 in Gowing et al. 2001, p.3).

> use of MDMA and reports that MDA [a structurally similar analogue] had neurotoxic effects in animals, resulted in the USA Food and Drug Administration in 1985 classifying MDMA as Schedule 1 [drug] (no acceptable therapeutic use) (Gowing et al. 2001, p.3).[84]

MDMA's psychotherapeutic benefit was grounded in its reputation as augmenting therapy 'reducing defensive barriers while enhancing communication and intimacy':

> Hailed as a 'penicillin for the soul' MDMA was said to be useful in treating a wide range of conditions, including post-traumatic stress, phobias, psychosomatic disorders, depression, suicidality, drug addiction, relationship difficulties and the psychological distress of terminal illness (Grob 2000, p.551).

Psychotherapists were particularly impressed that MDMA had the ability to facilitate feelings of intimacy, introspection and communication without altering perceptions in body image and sense of self that were typical of LSD:

> MDMA had neither the pharmacological profile nor the provocative reputation of LSD and, so they [psychotherapists] hoped, would not suffer the fate of political reaction and legal censure as the hallucinogens had in the late 1960s (Grob 2000, p.552).

In the early 1980s, 3,4-methyldioxymethamphetamine (MDMA) was reputedly given the name 'ecstasy' by the Los Angeles manufacturer of what was still at that stage a legal drug (Forsyth 1995):

> MDMA was named 'ecstasy' as a marketing ploy... The illicit producer who first used the term said he preferred the name 'empathy', as this word was more fitting with the drug's effects. He believed [however] that the name Ecstasy would sell better than empathy.[85] The name did and the media also 'bought' the story. Had the name of the drug remained MDMA or Adam (its first nickname) it may have been many more years before it came to the attention of the media, followed by the DEA (Drug Enforcement Administration) and made illegal in America (Forsyth 1995, p.194).

By the mid 1980s MDMA was no longer simply the province of a coterie of psychotherapists and psychiatrists. It had been discovered by the counterculture. DEA officials were particularly concerned at its over the bar sales in Texas nightclubs (Forsyth 1995).

---

84 This was despite the objections of many psychiatrists and psychotherapists who championed the drug's therapeutic benefit. For an account of the usefulness of MDMA for psychotherapy, see Riedlinger and Riedlinger 1994; Gowing et al. 2001, 2002. So incensed were some psychiatrists by the listing that they took legal action to rescind it. This action was ultimately unsuccessful and the ban remains. To date Gowing et al. claim: 'There have been no controlled studies of the effectiveness of MDMA as an adjunct to psychotherapy. Claims of effectiveness rely largely on testimonies from therapists and their clients' (Gowing et al. 2001, p.3).

85 Or as Eisner states 'How many people [would] know what it [empathy] means?' (Eisner 1989 in Grob 2000, p.553).

Now popularly known as *Ecstasy,* MDMA had been appropriated by the youth culture for use as a recreational drug. Spurred by media accounts reporting on both its suggested role in treatment and its new reputation as a 'fun drug' among the young, use of MDMA spread. By the mid-1980s the inevitable political response began to take form. With the clear intention of tightening the federal regulatory controls of what was still a legal drug, the U.S. Drug Enforcement Administration (DEA) invoked the Emergency Scheduling Act and convened formal hearings in 1985 to determine the fate of MDMA. These highly publicized hearings, however, achieved the unintended effect of further raising public awareness of the new *Ecstasy* phenomenon, and led to marked increases in manufacturing and marketing of the drug. Media accounts polarized opinion, pitting enthusiastic claims of MDMA by proponents on the one hand, versus dire warnings of unknown dangers to the nation's youth on the other... With growing concerns over the dangers of new 'designer drugs', public discussion took an increasingly discordant tone (Beck & Morgan, 1986).

In the spring of 1985, a series of scheduling hearings on MDMA were conducted by the DEA in several U.S. cites where a collective of physicians, psychologists, researchers and lawyers gave testimony that MDMA's healing potential should not be lost to the therapeutic community. After hearing the duelling sentiments expressed by federal regulators and by those opposed to controls, the DEA administrative law judge presiding over the hearings determined on the weight of the evidence presented that there was in fact sufficient indication for the safe utilization of MDMA under medical supervision and recommended Schedule III status. Not obliged to follow the recommendations of his administrative law judge, however, and expressing grave concerns that MDMA's growing abuse liability posed a serious threat to public health and safety, the DEA director overruled the advisement and ordered that MDMA be placed in the most restrictive category, Schedule I. Since then, with the exception of a three month period in late 1987 and early 1988 when it was briefly unscheduled due to a court challenge, MDMA has remained classified as a Schedule I substance (Young 1986; Lawn 1986).

In the decade following the MDMA scheduling controversy, patterns of use experienced a marked shift. With the failure to establish official sanction for MDMA treatment, most psychotherapists who had used the drug adjunctively in their work ceased to do so, unwilling to violate the law and jeopardize their livelihood through the use of a now illegal drug. In the wake of the highly publicized scheduling hearings, however, use among young people escalated (Grob 2000, pp.553–554).[86]

86 Of great interest, however, is the fact that the wheel seems to have turned full circle recently: 'The [American] Food and Drug Administration and the Spanish Ministry of Health have concluded that the risk/benefit ratio is favourable under certain circumstances for clinical studies investigating MDMA assisted psychotherapy. Both agencies have approved pilot studies in chronic posttraumatic stress disorder patients who have failed to obtain relief from at least one course of conventional treatment... [These] are the world's only on going stud[ies] of the efficacy of MDMA assisted psychotherapy' (Doblin 2002, p.185).

Once proscribed by the DEA, some MDMA manufacturers synthesised another similar substance – 3,4-methydioxyethylamphetamine or MDEA – to circumvent the scheduling:

> MDEA was given the brand name 'Eve' to MDMA's 'Adam'. MDEA was marketed as Ecstasy in an attempt to get round the law against MDMA. This debate was academic in the UK where any substance containing a dimethoxyamphetamine structure was already illegal. Therefore all three of the Ecstasy type drugs – MDMA, MDEA and MDA (methyldioxyamphetamine) – were illegal in the UK before their use [in the UK] had become widespread (Forsyth 1995, p.194).

Because of the scheduling laws, most psychotherapists, however reluctantly, ceased to use the drugs as adjuncts to their practice. Conversely, despite such proscription, or maybe because of it, by the late 1980s ecstasy use was particularly prominent among young people in Britain. As Grob states, the pattern of ecstasy use therefore experienced a marked shift:

> By the late 1980s, the *Ecstasy* scene had attained particular prominence among young people in the United Kingdom. Between 1990 and 1995, British authorities estimated that the use of *Ecstasy* increased by over 4,000 percent. Starting in small London dance clubs, word rapidly spread of the euphoric, mood altering properties induced by *Ecstasy*, leading to larger and larger events throughout the British Isles. Almost overnight an enormous black market for *Ecstasy* was created. Leisure patterns among the young began to change, with *Ecstasy* to an increasing degree replacing alcohol as a generational drug of choice. By the early 1990s, the economic and social certainties of the past in Great Britain had started to change. The free market boom pursued throughout the eighties by the Thatcher government had ended in recession, with increasing unemployment and constricting opportunities, particularly for young people. The freeing of inhibitions, the peer bonding and the sense of community engendered by *Ecstasy's* dance floor pharmacology provided a release from the oppressive social atmosphere and a sense that 'all could be made right in the world'. The *Ecstasy* scene had become, in the eyes of many observers, the largest youth cultural phenomenon that Great Britain had ever seen (Collin 1998 cited in Grob 2000, p.555).

By the mid 1980s ecstasy was being portrayed as a 'horror drug', in the popular press, particularly in the United States:

> Concern about designer drugs reached a new intensity in the spring of 1985. Major stories or investigative reports appeared in all major newspapers and newsmagazines... *Discover* warned of 'The Looming Nature Menace of Designer Drugs' and *Time* examined 'Death by Design' while *U.S News and World Report* featured an alarming report called 'Designer Drugs – Murder by Molecule'. The more extreme reports argues that a new synthetic drug revolution was imminent in which "heroin, cocaine and marijuana are as

> obsolete as the horse and buggy. The drugs of the future have arrived, and they are made in test tubes" Television news programs demonstrated their lamentable tendency to present new drugs in near advertisements... Designer drugs [such as Ecstasy] were a natural theme for the talk shows, which at this point were evolving in a far more sensationalist direction, including material that would once have been condemned as tabloid (Jenkins 1999, p.80).[87]

One of the most profound results of this shift from being a drug used medically and instrumentally to an almost exclusive recreational drug was the diminution of the drug's purity and the adulteration of it with other substances:

> With the rapid expansion of *Ecstasy* culture in the United Kingdom, criminal gangs began to sense the opportunity for amassing large profits and moved in on the developing drug scene, rapidly taking control of the manufacturing and marketing of *Ecstasy*. Motivated solely by financial return and disinterested in the 'purity' of the phenomenon, the quality of distributed *Ecstasy* began to erode (Grob 2000, p.555).

Introduction into Australia

Ecstasy entered the Australian scene in the mid 1980s, although it did not achieve the great popularity it had in Britain and Europe until the late 1980s to the early 1990s. In 1988 a survey conducted by the National Campaign Against Drug Abuse (NCADA) found that of 1,830 Australians surveyed with regard to substance use, three per cent had been offered ecstasy (Commonwealth Department of Community Services and Health 1989).[88] As Solowij, Hall and Lee noted, 'research into the precise nature of Ecstasy use and characteristics of users is greatly lacking' (1992, p.1161). The situation has improved only marginally since that statement was written.

Ecstasy in Australia was and is primarily associated with recreational drug use and the culture of dance parties and to a lesser extent 'raves'.[89] Despite this association with dance culture, the latest survey of the IDRS noted a definite, if small, crossover to ecstasy being used as a street drug, including by injecting drug users (NDARC 2002a).

By the mid 1990s ecstasy and its analogues or substitutes were being viewed with major concern by international drug bodies. In the late 1990s the World Health Organisation's Programme on Substance Abuse developed a project entitled 'Strengthening strategic responses to the health and social consequences of amphetamine type stimulant use (with special reference to MDMA – "ecstasy")':

> This project aimed to give effect to the recommendations of [a] meeting held in Geneva in 1996 and to respond to the priorities of [an] Action Plan relating

87 For further discussion of the way in which ecstasy and other designer drugs have been portrayed in the media, see Chapter 18.

88 In 1987 importing and trafficking in ecstasy was made illegal in Australia under the Customs Act. See Chapter 12 for further discussion.

89 For a discussion of who uses ecstasy and the culture of party drug use, see Chapter 10.

> to raising awareness of the problem of ATS [amphetamine-type stimulant] reducing demand for illicit ATS and providing accurate information on ATS. A further meeting of experts was held in November 1999 in Bangkok to review the nature, extent, context and consequences of ATS use, to further understand the trend of ATS problems worldwide, to create an international network of researchers and relevant partners and to discuss the development of a guide to the use of Rapid Assessment and Response Methods for ATS use (Henry-Edwards & Ali 2000, p.2).

Form and composition

Ecstasy is in the curious position of being classified as a stimulant with hallucinogenic properties. Its stimulant properties speed up the activity of the central nervous system, while its hallucinogenic aspects affect and distort perception and awareness. Marked hallucinogenic effects similar to psychedelic drugs such as LSD are not, however, common unless ecstasy is taken in particularly high quantities.

It is usually sold as a tablet or pill, but is increasingly found in capsule or powder form. The tablets come in a variety of colours and sizes and may carry a branded design.[90] The NDARC states that:

> In recent times well-known brands such as Calvin Klein and Rolls Royce have been found stamped on ecstasy tablets. Despite this identification, there is no reliable method of determining the quality of the drug, since pills with the same stamp can vary widely in the content of MDMA and other substances (NDARC 2003, Fact Sheet).

The active oral dose of the (unadulterated) drug is approximately 75mgs, with most pills containing 80–120mgs (<www.urban75.com/Drugs/e_guide.html>)

A recent IDRS report notes that the availability of ecstasy tablets '[h]as increased markedly over the last few years, and [it] is readily available in most jurisdictions' (IDRS 2002, p.3).

Route of administration[91]

The most common route for the administration of ecstasy is oral,[92] by the swallowing of ecstasy tablets. Taken this way, the pharmacological effects of the drug become evident in 30–45 minutes and usually last 4–6 hours, although this may depend on the context in which the drug is taken.[93] Ecstasy tablets can also

---

90 For a fascinating ethnographic discussion of the shapes, sizes and colours of ecstasy tablets, see Forsyth 1995. Forsyth argues that users of ecstasy have a distinct culture. See also further discussion in Chapter 10 and Appendix 14.

91 For a comprehensive if 'historical' description of the various routes of administration used when taking ecstasy, see Moore 1992, pp.45ff.

92 The 2001 Melbourne IDRS survey noted that the primary route of administration of ecstasy for the group surveyed was oral (34%). However, 31% of the IDUs interviewed reported that they had injected ecstasy before (compared to 15% of the 2000 sample) and 21% had done so within the six months prior to the survey interview (compared to 8% of the 2000 sample) (NDARC 2002a).

93 See discussion on culture of use in Chapter 10.

be crushed and snorted or inserted into the anus to be absorbed as a suppository. Such a practice is referred to as 'shelving' or 'shafting' and avoids causing irritation to the stomach lining. Another practice is that of 'stacking'[94] whereby heavy users of ecstasy may take up to four or five tablets a night as the effects of the previous tablet begin to wear off (see Webb 1998, p.87).[95] Of particular concern in recent years has been a noticeable trend in the use of ecstasy by intravenous injection. This has attendant health consequences that will be discussed in Chapter 6.

Price, purity and availability of ecstasy

Sophisticated quantitative and qualitative data regarding ecstasy use is less readily obtainable than data for other illicit drugs such as heroin and amphetamines.[96] Nonetheless, the Victorian component of the IDRS survey has made some interesting findings.

> A total of 31% of respondents reported ecstasy use within the last six months, and 62% had used it at least once in their lifetime (compared to 65% in 2001, 51% in 2000 and 40% in 1999). Thirty six percent of IDUs interviewed reported that they had injected ecstasy before (31% in 2001, 15% in 2000), and 14% had done so within the six months prior to interview (21% in 2001, 8% in 2000). The primary route of administration of ecstasy for this group during the last six months was oral (28%).
>
> The average purity level of ecstasy seizures analysed by law enforcement agencies in Victoria during the 2001/02 financial year was 31% (range 1% to 82%) which was similar to the previous three financial years: 2000/01 = 31%; 1999/00 = 33.8%; 1998/99 = 28%.
>
> In contrast to the previous IDRS, which found that ecstasy use had increased, most key informants (n=32) reported that ecstasy use had declined in this group and cross overs between traditionally separate drug markets are reported to have declined. Most (n=32) key informants did not perceive ecstasy use to be common among primary heroin users and described most use as opportunistic. All key informants reported that a proportion of their client group had used ecstasy in the past six months. Three key informants reported exclusively on ecstasy use (one outreach worker, one user group representative, and one police officer). Ecstasy

94 For an account of stacking, see Hammersley, Khan and Ditton 2002, p.51 and the discussion in Chapter 6.

95 Average use of ecstasy tablets per session varies depending on the individual, context and setting. A 'neophyte' or novice may only take or need half a tablet to achieve the desired effect, whereas one or two tablets may be average for more 'seasoned' users. See Chapter 10 for further discussion.

96 In recent years, however, the importance of including MDMA and 'party drugs' in data collection and monitoring systems has been recognised. In 2000 the National Drug Law Enforcement Research Fund funded a two year trial in New South Wales and Queensland to 'examine the feasibility of monitoring trends in the market for party drugs using extant IDRS methodology' (NDARC 2002d; 2002e). In South Australia comprehensive monitoring and research into ecstasy use has also been undertaken. (See NDARC 2001, 2002c.) Other states, including Victoria, have now included 'party drugs' such as ecstasy in their IDRS modules.

> use was still perceived to be more prevalent among younger people who were involved in the dance party or 'rave' scenes.
>
> The ecstasy users reported on by key informants were primarily weekend users and other drug users used ecstasy when it was available and affordable, often as a substitute for heroin or methamphetamines. The ecstasy users with whom key informants were in contact were more likely to be male (60%), with one key informant reporting an increase in the number of young women taking ecstasy use (sic). Key informants reported an age range of 12 to 30 years old with an average of 20, similar to previous IDRS studies. Key informants reported an average education level of year 12 or university and that most ecstasy users were in full-time work or study. Whilst the four key informants noted that most ecstasy users experienced few problems associated with their drug use, and did not really consider themselves to be illicit drug users, two key informants reported that more clients were presenting with anxiety and panic attacks after long-term use (5-7 yrs). It was reported that the price and purity of ecstasy had remained stable, that it was easy to obtain and had become easier (sic). Key informants reported that one ecstasy tablet cost $35-50 or $300 for 10 tablets. It was also reported that the purity of ecstasy remained low, however the advent of testing kits (EZ-test) had improved knowledge of what drug was being purchased. Victoria Police key informants reported that ecstasy has become of greater interest than in previous years and that greater resources are being allocated to its detection and seizure, particularly due to the heroin drought.
>
> Ecstasy price reports available from ACC sources for 2001/2002 indicate that one tablet costs around $35, and that price discounts exist for purchases of larger tablet/pill quantities (Australian Crime Commission, in press). (NDARC 2003c, pp.38-39).[97]

Of particular interest is the fact that while the purity of what purports to be ecstasy/MDMA has been seriously compromised by a variety of adulterants[98] since the mid 1990s in most jurisdictions, this does not necessarily seem to have been the case in South Australia. Professor Jason White, Director of Treatment and Rehabilitation Services at the Drugs and Alcohol Services Council of South Australia, when meeting with the Committee advised as follows:

> I know some information has come, particularly from New South Wales, indicating that there is hardly any real MDMA around. That has not been our information in South Australia: there is lots of MDMA around and, when you buy Ecstasy, mainly you get MDMA. The only other component that has been common, although it has declined now, is PMA. The results from the blood samples that were analysed confirm this: they all had MDMA. A lot them had methamphetamine as well, but they probably knowingly took both, although

97 A clearer picture of ecstasy use and trend data will become apparent when a sentinel group of party goers is canvassed. Turning Point Alcohol and Drug Centre is currently conducting research focusing on psycho stimulant use in Melbourne with a different sentinel group of 'party going' drug users. 'It is likely that this expansion of drug trend monitoring will provide a clearer picture of ecstasy trends in Melbourne' (NDARC 2003c, p.39).

98 See Chapter 6 for a discussion of the contamination of ecstasy pills.

> it is possible they had pills with a mixture. But the notion that is put around, particularly from Sydney, that there is very little real MDMA is certainly not true in South Australia. They are absolutely using MDMA.[99]

South Australia, however, would seem to be an aberrant example, at least on the evidence presented to the Committee or found in the literature. In most jurisdictions it appears that the 'data indicate that the amount of MDMA in "ecstasy" tablets is dropping and that dose-effect relationships need to take this into account' (Cole et al. 2002, p.1531). The following table by Cole et al. drawing from a variety of research studies indicates how the purity of ecstasy has diminished over a five-year period (1996–2001). Although the studies are predominantly British there is no reason to believe similar results would not be found in Australia.

Table 4.2 The contents of ecstasy tablets

Study	MDMA	MDA	MDEA	MBDB	Amphetamines	Ketamine	Other	Sample Size
Arimany *et al.* (1998)	48	41	4					*Not specified*
Baggott *et al.* (2000)	54	6	3				29	107
Lenton *et al.* (1997)	30		42					57
Milroy *et al.*(1996)	25		50		25			12
Ramsey *et al.*(2001)	46		3		3	6		156
Rothe *et al.* (1997)	60		32					124
Saunders (1997)	63	3	15		3		9	545
Schifano *et al.*(1998)	90						1	20,000
Sherlock *et al.*	48		16		8	8	16	25

Note One: The data are expressed as the percentage of the total number of tablets tested (as reported by the study authors, therefore the totals do not always equal 100).

Note Two: MDMA = 3,4-methylenedioxymethamphetamine; MDA = 3,4-Methylenedioxyamphetamine; MDEA = 3,4-methylenedioxyethamphetamine; MBDB = N-Methyl-l-(1,3 benzodioxol-5-yl)-2-butylamine

Source (including commentary and notes): Reproduced from Cole et al. 2002, 'The content of ecstasy tablets: Implications for the study of their long term effects', *Addiction*, vol. 97, p.1532.

Other 'party drugs'

Gamma–hydroxybutyrate (GHB)

GHB is naturally produced in the body and is structurally aligned to gamma amino butyric acid (GABA). GHB was first synthesised in 1960 as a hypnotic agent and has been used legitimately as a pre-medication sedative or anaesthetic and as a treatment for sleep disorders such as insomnia and narcolepsy.[100] It has also been trialled as a treatment for alcohol and heroin withdrawal and addiction. Apart from such licit uses, the drug has found favour among discrete

99 Professor Jason White in conversation with the Drugs and Crime Prevention Committee, Adelaide, 3 October 2003.

100 Its role as a sedative was largely discarded 'because of its inability to reliably induce a deep enough sleep for surgery' (Centre for Addiction and Mental Health (CAMH) (Canada) 2002, p.1). This role was superseded by the use of the drug ketamine, later in itself abused for recreational purposes. See discussion later in this Chapter.

groups in the community. During the 1980s, bodybuilders used it for its supposed anabolic qualities.[101] It was (and is) seen as being able to stimulate a growth hormone, release of which aids in fat reduction and muscular development.[102] In some jurisdictions it could be purchased from health food stores and gymnasia.[103] It is also relatively easy to purchase the drug via the Internet (Degenhardt, Darke & Dillon 2002). From the mid to late 1990s it had moved into the club and party scene, because it was esteemed by young people for both its euphoric and sedative effects and its reputation as a sexual enhancer and aphrodisiac. This was particularly true of the gay party scene.[104]

GHB is a colourless, odourless drug that acts as a depressant on the central nervous system, unlike psychostimulant 'party drugs'.[105] It also has anaesthetic and sedative properties. While usually found in liquid form, it has been produced as a powder and in capsule form. It is most usually taken in oral liquid form from small vials or bottles that can be added to water or other drinks. Although it has a salty taste, strong tasting beverages can disguise this.[106] Along with rohypnol, it has become known as the 'date rape drug' due to its disabling effect.[107] It may cause amnesia, impaired movement and speech, and drinks can be spiked without visible trace.[108]

> Some studies have suggested that GHB enhances the CNS depressant effects of both alcohol and other sedative/hypnotic drugs, and may enhance the effects of opioids (Degenhardt, Darke & Dillon 2003, p.199. And see studies cited therein).

Media reports on the drug have largely focussed public attention on this date rape phenomenon (see Nicholson & Balster 2001, p.14).[109]

---

101 For an account of how GHB may be 'home-made' by athletes and bodybuilders, see Sanguineti, Angelo and Frank (1997). The authors quoting from the *Underground Steroid Handbook for Men and Women* refer to a chapter titled 'GHB: A home brew', in which the writer Daniel Duchane gives detailed instructions 'on how to make GHB in your own kitchen' (1997, p.637).

102 Such claims, however, have been refuted by medical scientists. See Centre for Addiction and Mental Health (CAMH) (Canada) 2002.

103 In Britain it is known to be openly sold in sex shops. See www.urban75.com/Drugs/gbh.html

104 Sixty per cent of the sample in Degenhardt, Darke and Dillon's recent research into GHB use among 76 users in Sydney identified as gay or bisexual. Other characteristics of the sample were that they were predominantly well educated, employed and with no history of incarceration (2003, p.98). See also discussion of 'party drug' use among gay and lesbian communities in Chapter 9.

105 For a comprehensive account of the pharmacological, neurochemical and biological activity of GHB, see Galloway et al. 1997; Nicholson and Balster 2001.

106 As a clear and colourless liquid it is also not particularly easy for either medical or police personnel to detect (see Asante 1999).

107 A British Home Office report in June 2000 questioned 123 victims of such drug-assisted assaults and found that 70% of the rapists were known to the victim, 12% were given the drug in their home and 10% on a university campus. One in five victims could not remember the assault while around 70% felt physically unable to resist (see www.urban75.com/Drugs/gbh.html and *The Guardian,* 22 June 2000).

108 A discussion of harm reduction programmes aimed at preventing drink spiking and the harms that can thereby ensue is given in Chapters 7 and 19 (See also Cannon 1999; McKey 2000, pp.21ff.).

109 In March 2000, GHB became a Schedule 1 Controlled Substance in the United States (see Drug Enforcement Administration 2000.) For an account of the somewhat confusing way in which GHB is regulated at both state and federal levels in the United States, see Nicholson and Balster 2001, pp.14ff. The authors note that there is some uncertainty as to its use in legitimate clinical and medical trials as opposed to its abuse potential as a recreational drug.

Other names for GHB include 'Grievous Bodily Harm' (or GBH), 'Georgia Home Boy', 'Fantasy', 'Easy Lay', 'Liquid Ecstasy' or 'Liquid E'. When it comes in bright blue liquid form it is known as 'Blue Nitro' or 'Midnight Blue'. Because it is most often taken in liquid form, it is extremely difficult to gauge how strong, concentrated or toxic any given dose may be. In other words, it is a very fine line between what may be considered a 'safe' dose and one that may cause overdose or even death.[110] Indeed recent research by Degenhardt, Darke and Dillon found that despite their sample of 76 GHB users in Sydney not having had long or extensive experience of GHB use, half (53%) had experienced a GHB overdose (2003).[111] An earlier paper by the same authors somewhat worryingly pointed out that some users did not necessarily view GHB overdose as a negative thing:

> [w]ith many reporting that they had obtained information on this via the Internet and that they felt GHB overdose was not in itself a dangerous thing. These risk perceptions need to be considered in any intervention aimed at minimizing the harms associated with GHB, with efforts aimed at educating users of the risks that may occur after becoming unconscious (eg. falls, injuries, and the risk of choking, particularly if vomiting also occurs) (Degenhardt, Darke & Dillon 2002, p.93).

It is also worrying that some research studies have reported individuals using drugs such as GHB 'specifically in order to temporarily forget safe sex messages they have previously heard' (Bellis, Hughes & Lowey 2002, p.1030; see also Clark et al. 2001).

Of interest is the fact that the education and harm reduction agency RaveSafe (Victoria) reports that GHB is generally not a favoured drug among many of the young people it comes into contact with:

> The intolerance of GHB within the dance scene is of particular interest to RaveSafe in that whilst ketamine appears to be viewed as 'relatively harmless,' the use of GHB is being frowned upon by many users, for fear of overdose, or having seen a user overdose and been taken to hospital.
>
> This variance in acceptance of 'party drugs' demonstrates that there is a hierarchy of 'party drugs.' Ecstasy is well-accepted by partygoer's as a 'safer' party drug and could be rated at the highest end of the scale with GHB as being on the lowest end of the scale and many not tolerant of its use. RaveSafe has observed from discussions with partygoers at events and through responding to questions on web forums, that GHB has a particularly bad reputation amongst 'party drug users' in the dance scene.[112]

110 See Chapter 6 for a discussion of short and long-term effects of GHB.

111 For further discussion of this research, see Chapter 6.

112 Submission of RaveSafe Victoria to the Drugs and Crime Prevention Committee, Inquiry into Amphetamine and 'Party Drug' Use in Victoria, October 2003.

The submission includes as an attachment copies of web site discussion pages which 'demonstrate the arguments the drug creates between party drug users'.

Despite this apparent disdain for GHB among dance club patrons, it is interesting that at the Earthcore outdoor 'rave' held in November 2003, GHB was responsible for multiple side effects and casualties amongst 'ravers'. For further discussion of Earthcore, see Chapter 10.

In sum, there is not a great deal known about GHB (or ketamine) use in Australia. Paul Dillon of the National Drug and Alcohol Research Centre in Sydney suggests that these 'newer' drugs tend to appear in Melbourne some time after they are being used in Sydney. He states, for example, that multiple GHB overdoses were occurring in Sydney in 1997, whereas similar incidents did not occur in Melbourne until 2000.[113] More recently, the survey of South Australian 'party drug' trends found that respondents noted that both GHB and ketamine (discussed below) were reasonably easy to obtain in Adelaide and that availability was stable although price varied enormously depending on the source. Purity of both drugs was reputed to be high (NDARC 2001, 2002c).

In Victoria there has been very little research into GHB use. The need for a greater research profile on emerging 'party drugs' is canvassed further in Chapter 21.[114] This is particularly so since recent events at Melbourne Park put the drug under the spotlight. The issue of GHB at Melbourne Park is discussed further in Chapter 6.

Ketamine

Ketamine Hydrochloride was first synthesised in 1962 by Parke Davis Laboratories[115] as a replacement for the unsatisfactory use of phencyclidine (PCP) as a surgical sedative and anaesthetic.[116] In the United States, in particular, ketamine has most commonly been used as a veterinary tranquilliser (see Jansen 1993; Dotson, Ackerman & West 1995; Cloud 2001; Dillon 2001). It was also used frequently as an anaesthetic in American field hospitals during the Vietnam War (Dillon 2001).[117] Ketamine has also been used legitimately in the treatment of drug addiction, particularly opiate addiction (see Jansen 2001, pp.293ff.).

Jansen, one of the world's leading experts on ketamine, describes it in the following terms:

> Ketamine is not related to heroin, nor is it a form of LSD, amphetamine, MDMA/ecstasy, or cocaine although it sometimes has effects resembling all of these. Ketamine is a complex psychoactive drug with a huge range of possible effects on consciousness, the brain and the rest of the body (Jansen 2001, p.24).

---

113 Mr Paul Dillon, National Drug and Alcohol Research Centre in conversation with the Drugs and Crime Prevention Committee, Sydney, 26 June 2003.

114 The issue of GHB use was, however, thought sufficiently serious for the Victorian Minister for Health, Mr John Thwaites, to issue a press release on the subject in July 2002 warning of the dangerousness of the drug following a spate of admissions to hospitals for GHB overdoses in July 2002 (Thwaites 2002).

115 The actual synthesis was done by American pharmacist Calvin Stevens and the compound was known as CL369 (Jansen 2001, p.23).

116 The use of PCP as a surgical anaesthetic had been known to produce adverse effects such as delirium, hallucinations, confusion, irrationality and even violence (see Dotson, Ackerman & West 1995).

117 Indeed, Jansen argues ketamine had a long and respectable tradition in medical research and still continues to be significant in modern medicine:

'While it does have mysterious aspects, a search of the Mediline database will produce over 6,500 scientific and medical reports containing the known facts about ketamine (including numerous clinical trials in humans), versus a current total of about 800 for MDMA, with almost no sanctioned clinical trials in humans' (Jansen 2001, p.30).

Ketamine is a *dissociative* anaesthetic, that is, it 'induces a lack of responsive awareness not only to pain but to the general environment, without a corresponding depression of autonomic reflexes and vital centres in the diacephelon' (Dotson, Ackerman & West 1995, p.751).[118] It also has few of the emergence problems associated with PCP.[119] In the early 1970s ketamine appeared on the streets in the big cities of the United States in a manner similar to that of its precursor PCP in the 1960s.[120] Despite it being an anaesthetic it 'can be a powerful stimulant at lower doses' (Jansen 2001, p.28).

It comes in a clear liquid and a white or off-white powder form. The liquid can be injected or consumed in beverages.[121] The powder can be injected once dissolved. It goes by the street names of 'Jet', 'Super Acid', 'Special K', 'Green', 'K', and 'Cat Valium'.

Along with the other 'party drugs', ketamine has become popular among young people at dance clubs and 'raves' in recent years.[122] It has been reputed to give the user a powerful 'rush', which may occur very quickly depending on the mode of administration (within a few minutes if sniffed or injected or 20 minutes if taken as an oral pill). It has a relatively short duration of effect:

> Recreational users usually administer ketamine intranasally, and this has an estimated duration of effect of up to one hour... In an evening, ketamine abusers will often self-administer several sequential doses of the drug in order to maintain psychotropic effects over time. The short half life of ketamine would mean it would be eliminated from the body within 24 hours (Curran & Monaghan 2001, p.750).

Recent Australian research has examined patterns of use among 100 Sydney users of ketamine (Dillon, Copeland & Jansen 2003). As with the Sydney GHB study (Degenhardt, Darke & Dillon 2003), a substantial number of the sample identified as homosexual (40%). The authors summarise their research as follows:

> In this sample of ketamine users, ketamine appeared to be a drug that had been added to an already extensive drug use repertoire. They were generally a

118 For a detailed account of the pharmacology of ketamine, see White and Ryan 1996; Curran and Morgan 2000.

119 Patients emerging from anaesthetic use of PCP had on occasion suffered some complications including delirium, hallucinations and catatonic or psychotic reactions. See for example, Smith, Wesson, Buxton, Seymour, Ross, Bishop and Zerkin 1982; White and Ryan 1996, Curran and Morgan 2000.

120 In a curious footnote to the drug's history, Dillon notes that in the 1976 film *Family Plot*, director Alfred Hitchcock 'depicted a kidnap victim sedated with a little-known drug called ketamine. At that time it would have been hard to imagine that more than 20 years later the same drug would be better known as Special K and have little connection with the breakfast cereal' (Dillon 2001, p.11).

121 Thus making it along with rohypnol and GHB a potential 'date rape' drug, particularly given its dissociative effect.

122 This is despite the fact that many educators and drug workers have identified the drug as totally inappropriate to use as a 'dance drug' (see Jansen 1993; Dalgarno & Shewan 1996; Dillon 2001; Dillon & Degenhardt 2001). For an account of ketamine and the early days of dance cultures in Ibiza and Goa, see Jansen 2001, pp.29ff.

> well educated group of people, few of whom were in relationships, and largely had high incomes. They appeared to be an older group of 'party drug' users, in contrast with a sample of regular ecstasy users interviewed in a similar period (Topp et al. 1998)
>
> Workers in the medical field have been identified as a key occupational group of ketamine users in the literature, particularly in terms of ketamine dependence... This sample also reflects the unauthorized use within medical and related professions with 14% potentially having access to a supply of ketamine in the course of their profession (Dillon, Copeland & Jansen 2003, p.27).[123]

The vast majority of the sample (82%) reported that the usual route of administering ketamine was by snorting. The side effects of their ketamine use will be examined in Chapter 6.

Use of ketamine can lead to powerful hallucinations and 'out of body' or near death experiences.[124] This is sometimes known as entering the 'K-hole':

> The diverse subjective experiences of ketamine are collectively termed the K-hole by users and commonly include: the sensation of light through the body; novel experiences concerning 'body consistency' (eg. being made of wood or rubber); grotesque distortion of shape or size of body parts; a sensation of floating or hovering in a weightless condition; absence of sense of time; visions, hallucinations; sudden insight into the riddles of existence and the self; the experience of being at one with the universe; sensations of melting together with people or things in the environment; and 'out of body' experiences (Curran & Monaghan 2001, pp.749–750).

The United States Drug Enforcement Administration (DEA) has commented that the only known source of ketamine for illicit or street use is via diversion of pharmaceutical products from pharmacies in Mexico (DEA 2003). American press reports have also indicated that a significant number of veterinary clinics are being robbed specifically for their ketamine stock (see http://usdoj.gov/dea/concern/ghb.html).

Recognising the dangers of recreational ketamine use, the United States listed the substance as a controlled substance in 1999.

The effects of ketamine and the other 'party drugs' will be discussed further in Chapter 6.

123 See also Jansen 2001, pp.194ff. for a discussion of recreational ketamine use by medical and allied professionals and the ready availability in the course of their work.

124 For a series of case studies on how it feels to be on ketamine, ie. a 'ketamine trip', see Jansen 2001. For an account of ketamine and 'near death experiences', see also Jansen 2001 pp. 100ff.

Conclusion

This brief summary of amphetamines and the club drugs has attempted to give an overview of the major substances other than alcohol, tobacco and heroin being used in both licit and illicit settings and contexts today. Although ecstasy (MDMA) or that which purports to be ecstasy is probably still the major club or party drug to be used by people recreationally, new drugs are being synthesised frequently or 'old' drugs such as ketamine are being discovered or rediscovered by new generations of party goers. As Topp stated in 2001 in the context of 'crystal meth':

> It is important to acknowledge that these [methamphetamine drugs] are not new drugs; some people who have used drugs for decades will say that such drugs have been available, on and off, for years. The change appears not to be the appearance of the drugs themselves, but rather the recent rapid increase in their availability and use across the country (Topp 2001, p.3).

Nonetheless, it is also equally true for Dillon and Degenhardt to claim that for many drug and alcohol workers it is difficult to keep up with new trends and changes in club drug use: 'As new drugs are introduced to the scene, it is important to be aware of these substances and the harms associated with their use' (2001, p.11).

These harms and the medical and social short-term and long-term effects associated with amphetamines and 'party drug' use are examined in Chapter 7.

5. The Extent of Use

There is considerable evidence of an international trend towards the increasing use of amphetamines and ecstasy. Given that drug misuse is a global problem, it is perhaps of little surprise that this trend has also been noted in Australia and Victoria. This Chapter seeks to gain an understanding of these trends and identify the extent of amphetamine and 'party drug' use within Australia and, particularly, Victoria.

At the outset, however, the Committee wishes to caution that any analysis of the prevalence, patterns of use and data relating to the harms associated with amphetamines should be considered alongside other drug use, both licit and illicit. This is not to diminish the harms caused by the use of amphetamines and 'party drugs' and problems created for users and their families but rather to warn against premature responses not premised on evidence-based research.

A snapshot of international data

Sources and limitations of international data on illicit drug consumption

An analysis of international illicit drug trend data is helpful in establishing basic orders of the magnitude of illicit drug use. It can also identify emerging trends of use, facilitate discussion, promote understanding and is also useful for assessing the effectiveness of different drugs policies throughout the world. However, it is important that caution be used in interpreting these trends. As the Australian Institute of Health and Welfare (AIHW) explains:

> ...comparative analyses of drug use in different countries are difficult due to cultural and political differences, and the legal framework of drug laws can differ greatly. In addition, each country has unique surveys and data collection methodologies, which make comparisons difficult (AIHW 2003, p.27).

The following section presents data from the United Nations Office on Drugs and Crime (UNODC).[125] It reports on the use of amphetamines and 'party drugs' internationally and compares this data with Australian figures. The data are drawn from estimates provided by member states of the United Nations via

125 The United Nations Office for Drug Control Policy and Crime Prevention (UNODCCP) became the Office on Drugs and Crime (UNODC) on 1 October 2002. The Office on Drugs and Crime includes the United Nations International Drug Contol Programme (UNDCP).

a range of sources including annual reports questionnaires, government reports, population surveys and research results often collected by the UNODC's field officers.

There are numerous difficulties associated with these statistics, which are outlined in detail in the UNODC's Report *Global Illicit Drug Trends* (2003) (see pp.346–347). As such, assessing the extent of amphetamine and ecstasy use is both extremely difficult and problematic. There were until last year, for example, no questions on ecstasy use in the annual reports questionnaires (UN surveys for member states) and so it is therefore 'not really possible to make comparisons with previous years when reporting ecstasy trends was sporadic' (UNODC 2003, p.155). The UNODC also relies on receiving voluntary information in relation to the prevalence of this drug, which may not be comprehensive (UNODC 2003, p.347). Countries use different methods for collecting data, definitions may vary from country to country and 'in some cases, strongly differing results have been obtained from the same country' (UNODC 2003, p.347). However, despite these difficulties the UNODC believes that the data pooling techniques they use, standardisation of results and the extrapolations they have undertaken are such that, while not guaranteeing an accurate picture, 'should be sufficient to arrive at reasonable orders about the likely extent of drug abuse in the general population' (UNODC 2003, p.347).

Significant findings of the United Nations report on illicit drug consumption

The UNODC estimated that approximately 200 million people consume illicit drugs globally each year: 163 million consume cannabis; 34 million consume amphetamines; 14 million consume cocaine; 15 million consume opiates (of which 10 million consume heroin); and 8 million consume ecstasy. It reported that the strongest increase in use of illicit drugs was cannabis, followed by amphetamine-type stimulants (ATS). The UNODC point out that whilst the drug problem continues to spread geographically 'there are however indications that the rate of increase is slowing down, with the exception of ecstasy' (UNODC 2003, p.13). Other findings included that:

- Abuse of amphetamines is estimated to affect some 34 million people or 0.8% of the global population age 15 and above over the 2000–2001 period. In addition, some 8 million people are estimated to take ecstasy. Abuse of amphetamine type stimulants is thus at a higher level than abuse of opiates (15 million people or 0.3%) or cocaine (14 million people, or 0.3%) though less than consumption of cannabis (163 million people or 3.9%) over the 2000-2001 period (UNODC 2003, p.141).
- About two-thirds of the abusers of amphetamines are found in Asia, mostly in the countries of East and South East Asia. The Americas and Europe account for a quarter of global use of amphetamines (UNODC 2003, p.141).
- While supply of amphetamines in North America, Europe and Asia is largely from clandestine manufacture, supply in South America and

Africa is still supplied from licit channels where the dividing line between licit and illicit consumption is not always clear (UNODC 2003, p.141).

- While in Europe amphetamine is the ATS of choice, in South-East Asia it is methamphetamine which is generally more potent and carries more health risks than amphetamine (UNODC 2003, p.141).
- Ecstasy abuse, after a period of decline, has again shown signs of increase in West Europe. In the USA it declined, for the first time in years, in 2002. In other regions, particularly the Caribbean and parts of South America, Oceania, South-East Asia, and Southern Africa, it seems to be accelerating (UNODC 2003, p.10).
- The main problem drugs in the world, as reflected in demand for treatment, remained opiates, followed by cocaine. In much of East and South – East Asia, ATS are the main problem drugs. In Africa, treatment demand continues to be concentrated on cannabis (UNODC 2003, p.11).

When a comparison is made between the prevalence of amphetamine and ecstasy use in the English-speaking countries of Australia, Canada, New Zealand, the United Kingdom and the United States of America it can be seen that the levels of illicit drug use vary (see Table 5.1). Of particular interest to this Inquiry is that both ecstasy use and amphetamine use is most prevalent in Australia compared to these countries.

Table 5.1: Summary of illicit drug use in 2000-2001: Proportion of the population aged 15 years and over, selected countries[(a)]

Substance	Australia	Canada	New Zealand	United Kingdom[(b)]	United States
			per cent		
Marijuana/cannabis	15.0	8.9	13.4	10.6	9.3
Amphetamines	4.0	Na	3.4	1.6	1.1
Ecstasy	3.4	1.3	2.3	2.2	1.4
Opiates[(c)]	0.6	0.4	0.7	0.6	0.6

(a) Australia, New Zealand and United States 2001; Canada and United Kingdom 2000.
(b) United Kingdom figures for marijuana/cannabis, amphetamines and ecstasy relate to persons aged 16–59 years.
(c) Includes heroin, opium, morphine and synthetic opiates.

Source: Based on tables presented in United Nations Office on Drugs and Crime (UNODC) 2003, *Global Illicit Drug Trends*, United Nations, New York, pp.344–345.

The UNODC noted this disturbing statistic, commenting that:

> ...the ATS phenomenon in Australia is serious and growing. Australia has the highest levels of ecstasy abuse worldwide, and ranks only second after Thailand in prevalence of methamphetamine abuse in 2001 (UNODC 2003).

Prevalence of drug use in Australia and Victoria

To gain the best possible understanding of the extent that amphetamines and party drugs are used in Australia, and particularly in Victoria, three sources of data are accessed: primary data, secondary data and 'other data'.

Primary data refers to use and patterns of use that are reported by population surveys and secondary data provides an indication of the harm that is caused through use. The following chart (Table 5.2) presented to the Committee by Turning Point Alcohol and Drug Centre provides an overview of the data sources available.

Table 5.2: Sources of drug data

Sources of Drug data

Primary data

- Use in general population (eg. Household survey)
- Use in sentinel populations (eg. Students, prisoners, IDUs [injecting drug users])

Secondary data/routine data bases

- Service utilization (eg. Drug/other treatment, NSPs [needle and syringe programmes])
- Drug related mortality (eg. OD deaths, coronial data)
- Drug related morbidity (eg. Accidents, hospital, BBVs [blood-borne viruses])
- Crime (eg. Arrests, convictions, drug seizures)

Other data

- Anecdotal, observation, practice experience, media, participation...[126]

Source: Turning Point Alcohol and Drug Centre, evidence given to the Drugs and Crime Prevention Committee, Inquiry into Amphetamine and 'Party Drug' Use in Victoria, Public Hearings (Melbourne), 27 October 2003.

The primary data which the following discussion draws on includes data from the National Drug Strategy Household Survey, the Australian School Students Alcohol and Drugs (ASSAD) Survey conducted in 1996 and the Victorian School Students and Drug Use Surveys. The secondary data used is from the Alcohol and Drug Information System (ADIS), which monitors clients presenting for treatment across Victoria, the Victorian Admitted Episodes Dataset (VAED), and ambulance attendances collated by the Metropolitan Ambulance Service and Turning Point Alcohol and Drug Centre. Secondary data also includes mortality data collated by the Victorian Institute of Forensic Medicine[127] and anecdotal evidence provided to the Committee.

However, it is important to again emphasise the need for caution when interpreting the figures cited in this Chapter and to give consideration to the weight placed on each level of data. The accurate measurement of drug use from

126 Turning Point Alcohol and Drug Centre, evidence given to the Drugs and Crime Prevention Committee, Inquiry into Amphetamine and 'Party Drug' Use in Victoria, Public Hearings (Melbourne), 27 October 2003.

127 For detailed information relating to these data sources, see Department of Human Services Victoria, *Drug Statistics Handbook 2003*, Department of Human Services Victoria, Melbourne, 2004, pp.97–100.

national surveys, particularly regarding amphetamine and 'party drug' use, is compromised by a number of methodological obstacles that are discussed below. Given the limitations of current measurement techniques, the figures contained within this Chapter are, at best, an approximation of the extent of amphetamine and 'party drug' use. Nonetheless, given the limitations of current research techniques, the data referred to below remain the best available indication of the levels of use within the community.

Measuring prevalence in Australia and in Victoria

Prevalence data is primarily based upon population surveys. Three surveys have been used in order to establish the prevalence of amphetamine and 'party drug' use in Australia and Victoria:[128]

- The National Drug Strategy Household Survey is the largest drug-related survey conducted in Australia. It has been repeated in a similar format every 2–3 years since 1985. In 2001 the survey was conducted by the AIHW and involved the participation of 27,000 people aged 14 years and over (AIHW 2002c). This represented a significant increase on the 10,030 participants who took part in the 1998 Household Survey (AIHW 1999).
- The Australian School Students Alcohol and Drugs (ASSAD) Survey conducted in 1996 was the first national survey of students to obtain data about illicit drugs. It was co-ordinated by the Anti-Cancer Council of Victoria and asked questions of approximately 31,000 school students aged 12–17 years who were selected randomly from government and independent schools. A second survey was conducted with over 25,000 students in 1999. The results of this survey were published in June 2001 (Commonwealth Department of Health and Aged Care 2001).[129]
- The Victorian School Students and Drug Use Surveys record Victorian students' use of over-the-counter and illicit drugs. In 1996 and 1999 surveys were conducted by the Centre for Behavioural Research in Cancer, funded by the Anti-Cancer Council of Victoria and the Victorian Department of Human Services (DHS). Previous surveys in 1992, 1989 and 1985 were conducted by the Department of Human Services. In 1996 this involved 4,700 students who also took part in the 1996 ASSAD survey. In 1999, 4,286 students from Years 7–12 took part. These students were drawn from a representative sample of 67 secondary schools across Victoria (DHS 2001).

128 It should be noted that the survey data reported in this chapter are the most recent currently available.

129 The Victorian component of the triennial Survey of Australian Secondary School Students 2002 is currently being analysed. The Committee awaits with interest its findings.

Limitations of survey data

The measurement of drug activity

The measurement of drug activity will always present significant research difficulties. The use of population surveys as the primary means of measurement inevitably raises questions of validity and reliability. Such problems may arise as a consequence of false reporting or through respondents' misinterpretation of questions asked.

In addition, illicit drug users often go to elaborate lengths to keep their illegal activities hidden. They may, consequently, be unwilling to reveal the extent of these activities to an unknown researcher. Suspicion as to the identity and motives of researchers may further impact upon the accuracy of the research findings. In this respect, the researcher must be prepared to acknowledge that surveys record what respondents *say* about their drug use, and not what they actually *do*. It would be naïve to expect population surveys to generate data that are accurate beyond question (Bourgois, Lettiere & Quesada 1997).

A further concern is the serious doubt as to whether surveys are able to reach a representative sample of the population. Surveys are unlikely to reach those in the community who might be characterised as 'hidden.' The most active drug users and those most likely to suffer from a broad range of health problems would be included within this group (Hopkins & Frank 1991; Jacobs & Miller 1998). There are good reasons for believing that those young people who are more likely to use drugs are the same young people who will be more likely to be absent from school and consequently missed by school-based surveys. Likewise, the homeless, the incarcerated, and those in special accommodation are all populations with disproportionately high reported rates of illicit drug use, and yet they will not be 'captured' by national household surveys, the traditional measure of illicit drug use in Australia.

In addition, the capacity for national surveys to provide regional data is restricted by the sample size of the sample population in any category. The base population used by National Household Surveys, for example, is not of a size that might allow statewide distinctions to be drawn. Similarly, the small number of respondents in categories that address issues of ethnicity or self-identification as an Indigenous person limits the use of resulting data.

Another problem with survey techniques is that they are only able to provide a snapshot of drug use. They provide little information on patterns of use over time, which is an issue of particular importance when considering the increasing nature of amphetamine and 'party drug' use. Similarly they can only provide a representation of past drug use and as such can not be used by themselves as indicative of present use or consumption patterns.

A further problem with both survey data and other forms of secondary data is that:

> ...the majority of indicator data sources by their very nature are *lag indicators*, and therefore insufficient on their own for drug trend monitoring or strategic early warning purposes. Further, these indicators are usually only reported on their own and fail to consider other information sources which can help to provide a more complete picture of illicit drug use (in this case psychostimulant use) in Victoria.[130]

Each of these issues must be taken into consideration when interpreting the survey data reported within this section. It is for the reasons outlined above that the Committee has also drawn on another source of extremely useful information, the Illicit Drug Reporting System (IDRS). The IDRS is a national drug trend monitoring project which is co-ordinated by the National Drug and Alcohol Research Centre (NDARC). The aims of this project are:

1. To provide a reliable method of monitoring emerging jurisdictional trends in price, purity, availability and use of opiates, cannabis, cocaine, amphetamines and other drugs.
2. To inform health and law enforcement sector policy and program responses to illicit drugs, as well as to identify areas/issues requiring further investigation.[131]

Data for this project are obtained from interviews with injecting drug users (IDUs), interviews with experts and professionals who work in the field, other key informants and data routinely collected by other agencies. These data are triangulated and compared against previous years to determine new trends. According to Turning Point Alcohol and Drug Centre the 'key advantage of the IDRS system is that it replicates core methods across each state and territory, and has done so since 1997'.[132] It also enhances the capacity of health and law enforcement sectors to develop informed and proactive responses to illicit drug problems at a number of levels'.[133]

What the national data say

It is important to note at the outset that the 2001 National Drug Household Survey found a very low use of illicit drugs in the community, with approximately only 4 per cent using any illicit drug other than cannabis in the past 12 months, and 13 per cent using cannabis (AIHW 2003).

In relation to amphetamine and 'party drugs', perhaps the most notable finding of the 2001 Survey was the general increase in the use of these drugs by Australians since 1991. Table 5.3 shows that in the category of 'use in the last 12 months', ecstasy/designer drug use increased from 1.1 per cent in 1991 to 2.9 per

130 Submission from Turning Point Alcohol and Drug Centre to the Drugs and Crime Prevention Committee, Inquiry into Amphetamine and 'Party Drug' Use in Victoria, 27 October 2003.

131 Excerpt from the confidential submission of Turning Point Alcohol and Drug Centre to the Drugs and Crime Prevention Committee, Inquiry into Amphetamine and 'Party Drug' Use in Victoria, August 2002. Quoted with the kind permission and approval of Turning Point.

132 Ibid.

133 Ibid.

cent in 2001 and amphetamine use increased from 2.6 per cent in 1991 to 3.4 per cent in 2001. Findings by the Australian Crime Commission (ACC) in the *Australian Illicit Drug Report* supported this trend:

> There is little to no evidence to suggest that amphetamine-type stimulant use in Australia will decrease in the near future. While arrests related to amphetamine-type stimulants remained relatively constant during 2001–2002, other indicators, such as the high availability and increasing quantities seized both at the border and domestically, indicate a continuing if not growing demand for amphetamine-type stimulants in Australia (ACC 2003, p.61).

Table 5.3: Summary of recent[(a)] illicit drug use: Proportion of the population aged 14 years and over, by drug type, Australia, 1991–2001

Substance/behaviour	1991	1993	1995	1998	2001
			(per cent)		
Marijuana/cannabis	13.7	12.7	13.1	17.9	12.9
Pain-killers/analgesics[(b)]	n.a.	1.7	3.5	5.2	3.1
Tranquillisers/sleeping pills[(b)]	n.a.	0.9	0.6	3.0	1.1
Steroids[(b)]	n.a.	0.3	0.2	0.2	0.2
Barbiturates[(b)]	1.5	0.4	0.2	0.3	0.2
Inhalants	0.8	0.6	0.6	0.9	0.4
Heroin	0.4	0.2	0.4	0.8	0.2
Methadone[(c)]	n.a.	n.a.	n.a.	0.2	0.1
Other Opiates[(b)]	n.a.	n.a.	n.a.	n.a.	0.3
Amphetamines[(b)]	2.6	2.0	2.1	3.7	3.4
Cocaine	0.7	0.5	1.0	1.4	1.3
Hallucinogens	1.6	1.3	1.8	3.0	1.1
Ecstasy/designer drugs	1.1	1.2	0.9	2.4	2.9
Injected drugs	0.5	0.5	0.6	0.8	0.6
Any illicit drug	22.8	14.0	17.0	22.0	16.9
None of the above	77.2	86.0	83.0	78.0	83.1

(a) Used in the last 12 months.
(b) For non-medical purposes.
(c) For non-maintenance purposes.

Source: Australian Institute of Health and Welfare (AIHW) 2003, *Statistics on Drug Use in Australia 2002* (Drug Statistics Series No. 12), AIHW, Canberra, p.19.

Australian Customs Service data provides further evidence that the prevalence of ecstasy (MDMA) is increasing in Australia. The data shows that border detections for ecstasy (MDMA) increased from six in 1992–1993 to 308 in 2002–2003. At the same time, the total weight of these detections increased from almost zero kilograms in 1992–1993 to 552 kilograms in 2002–2003 (AIHW 2003, p.62; ACC 2003, p.45).

The following section gives specific data on amphetamine use in Australia and is followed by a corresponding section on 'party drug' use.

Amphetamine use

According to the AIHW study, approximately 1.4 million Australians aged 14 and over had used amphetamines in their lifetime (AIHW 2002c). The study also revealed that amphetamine was the most widely used illicit drug after cannabis. Table 5.3 above shows that 8.9 per cent of the population aged 14 and over reported using amphetamines at some time, and around 3 per cent reported using amphetamines in the previous 12 months. The average age that people first used amphetamines was 20.4 years (see Table 5.4). Between 1995 and 2001 there was little change in the age at which amphetamines were first used (see AIHW 2002a, p.5).

Table 5.4: Summary of illicit drug use in Australia, 2001

Substance/behaviour	Drugs ever used[(a)]	Drugs recently used[(b)]	Mean age of initiation
	(per cent)		(years)
Marijuana/cannabis	33.1	12.9	18.5
Pain-killers/analgesics[(c)]	6.0	3.1	18.9
Tranquillisers/sleeping pills[(c)]	3.2	1.1	22.8
Steroids[(c)]	0.3	0.2	22.5
Barbiturates[(c)]	0.9	0.2	18.7
Inhalants	2.6	0.4	17.6
Heroin	1.6	0.2	20.7
Methadone[(d)]	0.3	0.1	21.8
Other opiates[(c)]	1.2	0.3	n.a.
Amphetamines[(c)]	8.9	3.4	20.4
Cocaine	4.4	1.3	22.6
Hallucinogens	7.6	1.1	19.1
Ecstasy/designer drugs	6.1	2.9	21.9
Injected drugs	1.8	0.6	20.2

(a) Used at least once in lifetime.
(b) Used in the last 12 months.
(c) For non-medical purposes.
(d) For non-maintenance purposes.

Source: Australian Institute of Health and Welfare (AIHW) 2003, *Statistics on Drug Use in Australia 2002* (Drug Statistics Series No. 12), AIHW, Canberra, p.17.

Figure 5.1 shows that males were more likely to have used amphetamines in the past 12 months. However, among the 14–19 year olds, females were more likely than males to have used. Those aged 20–29 years were more likely than those in other age groups to report ever using amphetamines (AIHW 2002c).

Figure 5.1: Percentage who used amphetamines in Australia during 2001

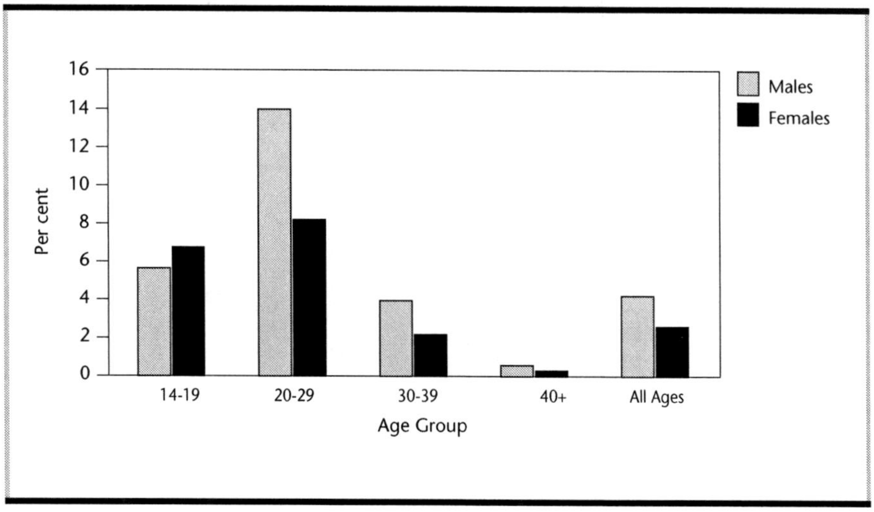

Source: Australian Institute of Health and Welfare (AIHW) 2002c, *2001 National Drug Strategy Household Survey: Detailed Findings* (Drug Statistics Series No. 11), AIHW, Canberra, p.62.

The 1999 Survey of Australian Secondary School Students also reported that young people were less likely to use amphetamines than other illicit drugs. However the results of that study did show that amphetamine use increased with age (see Figure 5.2).

Figure 5.2: Lifetime use of licit and illicit substances by Australian secondary school students, 1999

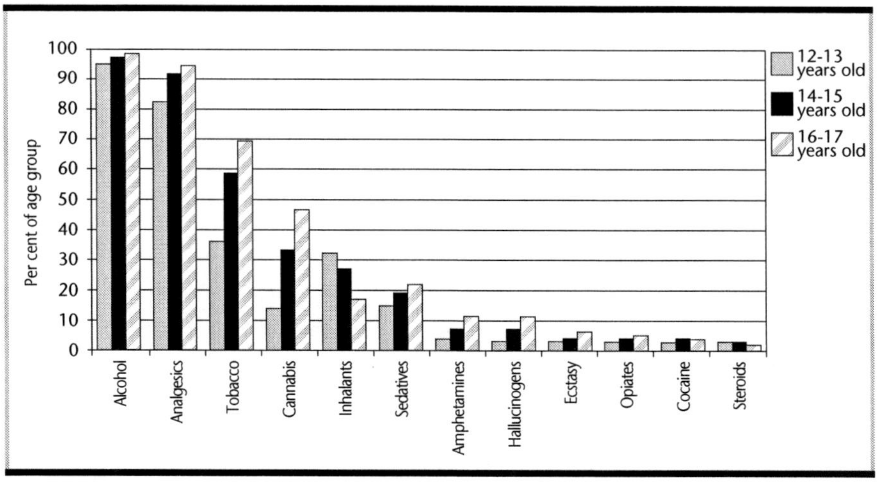

Source: Commonwealth Department of Health and Aged Care (National Drug Strategy Unit) 2001, *Australian Secondary Students' Use of Over-the-Counter and Illicit Substances in 1999*, Commonwealth Department of Health and Aged Care, Canberra, p.28.

Recent users of amphetamines indicated that they also used other drugs at the same time (on at least one occasion). Alcohol was most likely to be consumed at the same time as using amphetamines (87.7%), followed by marijuana/cannabis (71%) (see Table 5.5). This finding certainly supports the academic literature, which suggests that poly-drug use is quite common among amphetamine users. The issue of amphetamines and poly-drug use is discussed in further detail in Chapters 6 and 8.

Table 5.5: Other drugs used with amphetamines, recent users aged 14 years and over, by sex, Australia, 2001

Drug	Males	Females (per cent)	Persons
Alcohol	87.3	88.4	87.7
Marijuana/cannabis	75.0	65.6	71.5
Heroin	3.2	4.1	3.6
Cocaine	15.6	12.1	14.3
Tranquillisers/sleeping pills[(a)]	7.3	6.2	6.9
Anti-depressants[(a)]	2.8	4.1	3.3
Pain-killers/analgesics[(a)]	6.5	5.4	6.1
Barbiturates[(a)]	1.6	1.9	1.7
Ecstasy/designer drugs	43.4	43.2	43.3
Other	3.0	5.2	3.8
None of the above	0.8 *	1.4 *	1.0

(a) Used for non-medical purposes.

Notes

1. Base equals recent users.
2. Respondents could select more than one response.

* Relative standard error greater than 50%.

Source: Australian Institute of Health and Welfare (AIHW) 2002c, *2001 National Drug Strategy Household Survey: Detailed Findings* (Drug Statistics Series No. 11), AIHW, Canberra, p.65.

In relation to amphetamine use through injecting, the AIHW survey found that of those people who injected drugs the first drug injected was amphetamine (60.3%), followed by heroin (30.5%). Similarly, the most common drug recently injected by these users was amphetamine (77.1%), followed by heroin (22.9%).[134]

Ecstasy use

The AIHW survey reported that in 2001 almost '1 million (6.1%) Australians aged 14 years and over had used ecstasy/designer drugs in their lifetime' (AIHW 2002c, p.67). Ecstasy was reported as the fourth most widely used illicit drug ever used, after cannabis, amphetamines and hallucinogens and the fourth most recently used after cannabis, amphetamines and pain-killers/analgesics. On average, Australians first used ecstasy at 21.9 years of age (see Table 5.4 above). The age of initiation has remained relatively stable since 1995 (see AIHW 2002a, p.5).

As illustrated by Figure 5.3 below, the study shows that 10.4 per cent of people aged 20–29 years and 5 per cent of teenagers had used ecstasy in the past 12 months. People in the 20–29 year age bracket were most likely to report ever using ecstasy/designer drugs. Males were more likely than females to have used ecstasy in the past 12 months in every age group; however, the recent use of

134 See Table A in Appendix 11.

ecstasy among females has increased significantly. Between 1998 and 2001, 'the recent use of ecstasy increased both overall and for those aged 20–29 years' but 'among females aged 40 years and over there was a significant decline in the recent use of ecstasy' (AIHW 2002a, p.29). The 1999 Survey of Australian Secondary School Students also reported that young people were less likely to use ecstasy/designer drugs than other licit and illicit drugs. However, the results of that study did show that ecstasy/designer use did increase with age (see Figure 5.2 above).

Figure 5.3: Percentage who used ecstasy in Australia during 2001

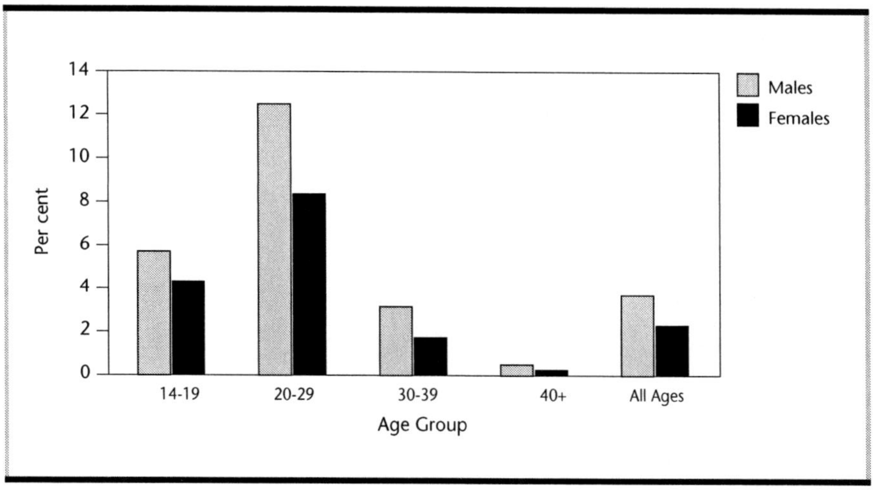

Source: Australian Institute of Health and Welfare (AIHW) 2002c, *2001 National Drug Strategy Household Survey: Detailed Findings* (Drug Statistics Series No. 11), AIHW, Canberra, p.67.

Recent users of ecstasy/designer drugs indicated that they also used other drugs at the same time (at least on one occasion). Alcohol was most likely to be consumed at the same time they used ecstasy/designer drugs (76.5%) followed by marijuana/cannabis (66.2%) (see Table 5.6). This seems to be a significantly different pattern of use from the earlier years of taking ecstasy, when there was little evidence of alcohol being used. At least in the rave and dance cultures, the use of alcohol in conjunction with ecstasy was frowned upon because of the aggression that it could produce in users (see further discussion in Chapter 10). Commentators have noted with concern the increasing use of 'party drugs' and poly-drug use. The issue of poly-drug use will be discussed in Chapter 8.

Table 5.6: Other drugs used with ecstasy/designer drugs, recent users aged 14 years and over, by sex, Australia, 2001

Drug	Males	Females (per cent)	Persons
Alcohol	75.8	77.6	76.5
Marijuana/cannabis	70.6	59.4	66.2
Heroin	0.2 *	2.1	1.0 *
Cocaine/crack	24.1	16.2	21.0
Tranquillisers/sleeping pills[(a)]	8.9	5.9	7.7
Anti-depressants[(a)]	2.1	2.5	2.3
Pain-killers/analgesics[(a)]	4.2	3.5	3.9
Barbiturates[(a)]	1.7 *	0.7 *	1.3
Amphetamines/speed[(a)]	52.6	49.8	51.5
Other	3.4	3.3	3.3
None of the above	5.9	6.2	6.1

(a) Used for non-medical purposes.

Notes

1. Base equals recent users.
2. Respondents could select more than one response.

* Relative standard error greater than 50%.

Source: Australian Institute of Health and Welfare (AIHW) 2002c, *2001 National Drug Strategy Household Survey: Detailed Findings* (Drug Statistics Series No. 11), AIHW, Canberra, p.70.

Victorian drug use

Comparative data

When a comparison is made between all Australian states and territories in the AIHW study, it can be seen that there was low consumption of illicit drugs generally, with 13 per cent using cannabis recently and only four per cent using any other illicit drug (see Table 5.7). The Northern Territory recorded the highest recent use for amphetamines followed by Western Australia, and Victoria recorded the second lowest. The ACT recorded the highest recent use of ecstasy followed by Western Australia. The study reported that nationally there was no significant increase of amphetamine use from 2000 to 2001.

Table 5.7: Recent[a] illicit drug use summary: Proportion of the population aged 14 years and over, Australian states and territories, 2001

Drug	NSW	Vic	Qld	WA (per cent)	SA	Tas	ACT	NT	Aust
Marijuana/cannabis	11.9	11.8	12.7	17.5	14.2	11.9	14.4	24.4	12.9
Amphetamines[b]	3.4	2.4	2.9	5.8	4.3	2.1	4.5	6.3	3.4
Pain-killers/analgesics[b]	2.5	3.2	3.4	3.9	3.1	2.2	3.3	3.8	3.1
Ecstasy/designer drugs	3.4	3.0	1.7	4.0	2.0	0.8	4.8	2.8	2.9
Cocaine	1.8	1.3	0.7	1.5	0.7	*0.2	1.5	*0.5	1.3
Tranquillisers/sleeping pills[b]	0.9	1.1	1.2	1.7	1.4	1.0	1.4	1.1	1.1
Hallucinogens	0.9	0.9	0.8	2.0	1.9	1.0	1.8	1.7	1.1
Injected drugs	0.3	0.4	0.6	1.3	0.8	1.0	*0.3	1.9	0.6
Inhalants	0.5	0.3	0.3	0.6	0.7	*0.2	0.5	*0.5	0.4
Other Opiates[b]	0.2	0.4	0.3	0.6	*0.3	0.7	0.6	0.8	0.3
Heroin	0.2	0.3	*0.2	0.3	*0.1	*0.3	*0.4	*0.1	0.2
Barbiturates[b]	*0.1	0.2	*0.1	0.2	*0.3	*0.1	*0.2	*0.1	0.2
Steroids[b]	*0.1	0.3	*0.1	*0.1	*0.3	*0.1	*0.1	*0.1	0.2
Methadone[c]	*0.1	*0.1	-	*0.1	*0.1	*0.1	-	*0.3	0.1
Any illicit	*15.8*	*16.0*	*16.5*	*22.0*	*17.8*	*14.3*	*18.1*	*29.2*	*16.9*

(a) Used in past 12 months.
(b) For non-medical purposes.
(c) For non-maintenance purposes.
* Relative standard error greater than 50%.

Source: Australian Institute of Health and Welfare (AIHW) 2003, *Statistics on Drug Use in Australia 2002* (Drug Statistics Series No. 12), AIHW, Canberra, p.8.

The findings from the Illicit Drug Reporting System (IDRS) provide further and more recent insights. The report found that 'substantial proportions of IDUs in all jurisdictions continue to use all forms of methamphetamine… [T]he frequency of methamphetamine use decreased from 2001 in all jurisdictions except NSW, VIC, and TAS where it remained stable' (NDARC 2003c, p.81).

As discussed previously, the capacity for national surveys to provide state or regional data is restricted by the size of the sample population in any category. The base population used by National Household Surveys, for example, is not of a size that might allow statewide distinctions to be drawn. The following discussion on amphetamine and 'party drug' use in Victoria is drawn from a range of sources including the IDRS, Victorian Admitted Episode Dataset, the Victorian Institute of Forensic Medicine, Melbourne Metropolitan Ambulance Service and DHS treatment statistics.

Amphetamines – Victorian data

As discussed in Chapter 4, the 2002 IDRS study by NDARC (2003b) has commented about the volatile and changing nature of the amphetamine and methamphetamine markets in Melbourne and particularly the trend, at least in part because of the so-called 'heroin drought', towards increased amphetamine use. The 2002 IDRS study notes that this is a continuing trend with the levels of methamphetamine use among injecting users in Melbourne remaining quite high 'and had consolidated into a regular feature of the Melbourne drug scene'.

> The 2002 IDRS found that 73% had used some form of methamphetamine (either speed, base or ice) in the preceding six months, a proportion comparable to that of the 2001 IDRS (76%). Separating out forms of methamphetamine, 70% reported using speed, 19% reported using base and 26% reported using ice in the preceding six months. The median number of days on which speed has been used in the preceding 6 months was 24, while for base it was 10 and ice 6 days (NDARC 2003b, p.78).

The 2002 IDRS also noted that 'key informants reported that the incidence and prevalence of poly drug use incorporating methamphetamines have increased markedly' and for some 'methamphetamine use was a regular, daily occurrence, whereas in the past methamphetamine use was characterised as sporadic and binge-like in nature' (NDARC 2003c, p.25).

Use of drug treatment services

Human Services Victoria has confirmed this trend towards increasing amphetamine use through its monitoring of clients presenting for treatment across Victoria. Monitoring of clients is via an electronic data collection system – the Alcohol and Drug Information System (ADIS). This System records demographic details as well as some social details of individual clients. Between July 2000 and June 2003 the ADIS recorded the 'primary drug use' statistics which provided the data for Figure 5.4. As can be seen, alcohol was the primary drug of use for clients seeking treatment, followed by heroin and cannabis.

Figure 5.4: Primary drug of use for drug treatment service clients, July 2000 to June 2003

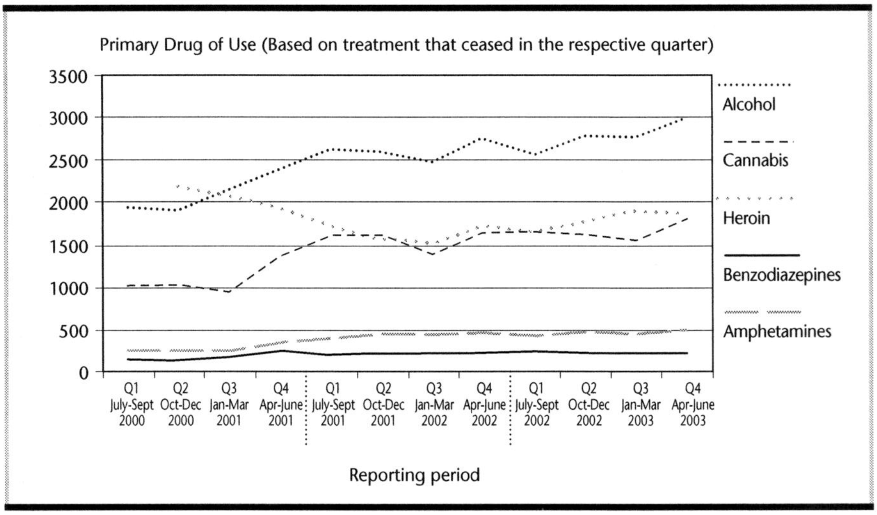

Source: Alcohol and Drug Information System 2003.[135]

135 Submission of Human Services Victoria to the Drugs and Crime Prevention Committee, Inquiry into Amphetamine and 'Party Drug' Use in Victoria, November 2003.

The results of the most recent census of alcohol and drug treatment services conducted in May 2001 reflect a similar trend. Seventy-five agencies took part in the survey that asked them to identify the main drug problem of each of their clients. Sixty-seven per cent of drug-related problems were attributed to alcohol and opioids while only 4 per cent were related to amphetamines.

Figure 5.5: Main drug problem of clients (users) attending specialist drug treatment agencies, Victoria, 2001

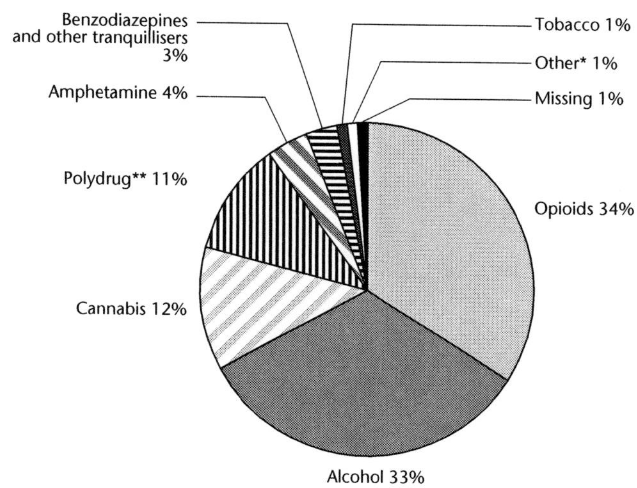

* other drugs = barbituates (1), cocaine (4), Hallucinogens (1), inhalants (5)
** polydrug use = 74 included opiates, 32 excluded opiates

Source: Clients of Treatment Services Agencies (COTSA) 2001, *Census survey*, Department of Human Services, analysis by Turning Point Alcohol and Drug Centre, in Human Services Victoria 2004, *Drug Statistics Handbook 2003*, Human Services Victoria, Melbourne, p.8.

However, it is worth noting that the ADIS data collected by Human Services Victoria indicate that between July 2000 and June 2003 the percentage of clients naming amphetamines as their primary drug of choice has doubled, although the number of clients presenting for treatment remained quite small[136] (see Figure 5.6). The increase during this period is believed to be partly due to the decrease in availability of heroin:

> Amphetamine/methamphetamines have also become the identified drug of choice for a group of people who were primary heroin users and there was an increase in the number of people reporting injecting amphetamines from 50% from the previous year to 75% from the current study (NDARC 2002a).

There has also been anecdotal evidence indicating that amphetamine misuse has become more widespread within the rave party scene. Moreover, it is believed that amphetamines are being used by an increasingly younger age group. This

136 Submission of Human Services Victoria to the Drugs and Crime Prevention Committee, Inquiry into Amphetamine and 'Party Drug' Use in Victoria, September 2002.

evidence is reflected in the 1999 School Students and Drug Use Survey of over-the-counter and illicit substances among Victorian secondary school students.[137]

Figure 5.6: Clients accessing drug treatment services with primary drug amphetamines, July 2000 to June 2003

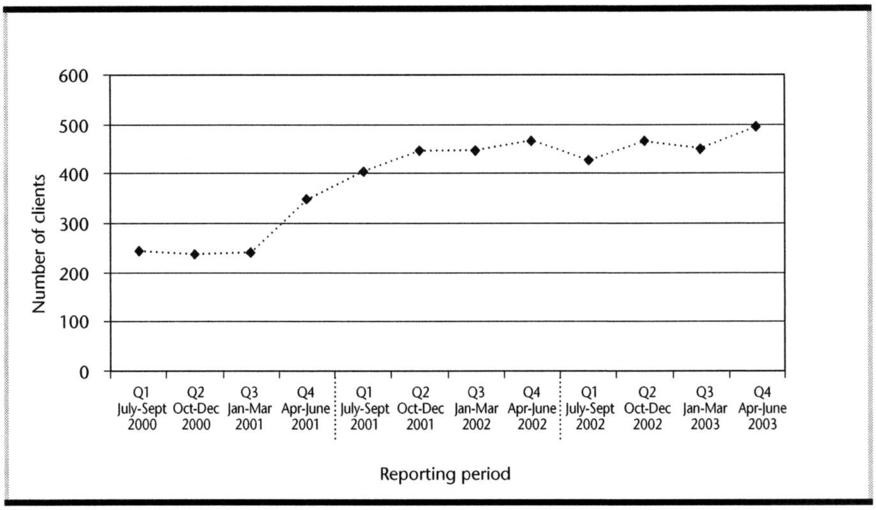

Source: Alcohol and Drug Information System (ADIS) 2002.[138]

Clients whose primary drug of concern is amphetamines access a range of services. According to Human Services Victoria, in 2002–2003:

> ...the most commonly accessed service type was counselling, consultancy and continuing care (901 clients). These services provide a range of services and supports appropriate to the needs of clients, including assessment, treatment and consultancy, referral and ongoing case management. The next most commonly accessed service types were residential withdrawal (233 clients), outreach (166 clients) and outpatient withdrawal (111 clients).[139]

Direct Line

Calls to Direct Line, a 24-hour telephone counselling, information and referral service,[140] show that alcohol, opiates and cannabis are the most frequently mentioned drugs of concern. Nonetheless, calls to Direct Line regarding amphetamines almost doubled between 1999 and 2001 and have remained relatively stable since that time. At the same time calls regarding heroin have more than halved.

137 Ibid.

138 Submission of Human Services Victoria to the Drugs and Crime Prevention Committee, Inquiry into Amphetamine and 'Party Drug' Use in Victoria, September 2002.

139 Submission of Human Services Victoria to the Drugs and Crime Prevention Committee, Inquiry into Amphetamine and 'Party Drug' Use in Victoria, November 2003.

140 This service is for drug users, their families and friends, people requesting drug information and workers from the health and welfare sector.

Table 5.8: Calls to Direct Line by drug type, Victoria, 1999–2003

Drug	1999	2000	2001	2002	2003
Total DL calls	39284	39440	41159	45307	48151
Calls with drug identified	21351	19746	20922	24990	24861
Alcohol	4955	4663	6211	7280	7284
Cannabis	3485	3109	4580	4910	4002
Heroin	7954	6238	3732	3533	3440
Other opioids[a]	3690	4019	3839	6214	6950
Amphetamine	916	1092	1802	1681	1782
BZD & tranquillisers[b]	1216	1087	1461	1341	1372
Ecstasy	438	477	678	699	563

a Other opioids = methadone, narcotic analgesics, LAAM, buprenorphine, slow release oral morphine (unable to determine whether prescribed or diverted)

b BZD & tranquillisers = benzodiazapines and other major tranquillisers

Source: Direct Line, Information supplied by Turning Point Alcohol and Drug Centre Inc, 2004.

Ambulance attendances

During 2001–2002 the Melbourne Metropolitan Ambulance Service attended just under 12,000 drug-related events. There was evidence of stimulant use in 578 of those attendances, 380 of which were for amphetamine use. It should be noted that other substances could have also contributed to these incidents.

Figure 5.7 shows the monthly totals of ambulance attendances between July 2001 and June 2002 for incidents involving evidence of amphetamine use. Fluctuations can be seen during the period which are 'broadly consistent with the patterns observed in previous comparison periods (see Fry and Miller 2002)' and which 'may reflect seasonal patterns of amphetamine usage that peak in the Christmas summer period and decline thereafter' (NDARC 2003c, p.52).

Figure 5.7: Monthly totals of ambulance attendances where amphetamines are mentioned, in Melbourne, July 2001 to June 2002

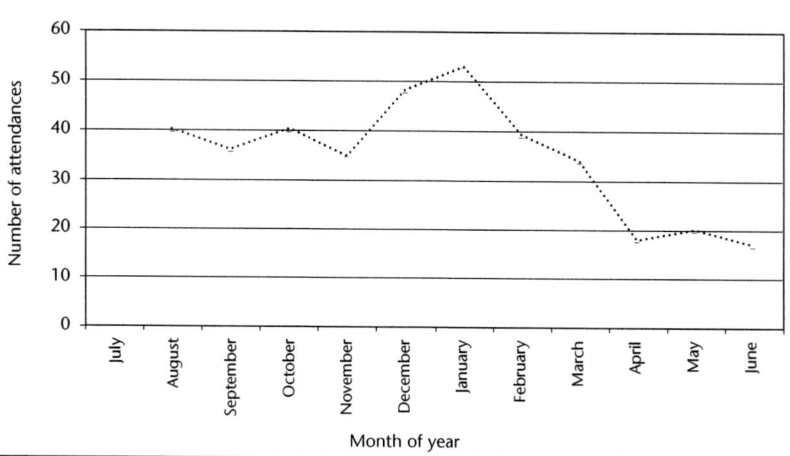

Note: Figures for July 2001 were not collated.

Source: Ambulance attendance data provided by Turning Point Alcohol and Drug Centre

Table 5.9 below provides further information regarding these attendances. Sixty-six per cent of the attendances were for males and 76 per cent of all cases were transported to hospital.

Table 5.9: Stimulant-related ambulance attendances in Melbourne, Victoria, 2001–2002[a]

Main Characteristics	Measure
Type of stimulant	
Illegal amphetamines	380
Licit amphetamines[b]	20
Ecstasy	207
Cocaine	30
Crack cocaine	1
Age of victim	Mean 25.77 years; range 2-55 years
Gender of victim	66% male
Outcome	76% transported to hospital
Total attendances	578

a Data includes August 2001 to June 2002.

b Dexamphetamine sulphate, methylphenidate hydrochloride (Ritalin).

Source: Melbourne Metropolitan Ambulance, analysis by Turning Point Alcohol and Drug Centre, in Human Services Victoria 2004, *Drug Statistics Handbook 2003*, Human Services Victoria, Melbourne, p.34.

Hospital admissions

The Victorian Admitted Episode Dataset that collates information on all hospitalisations in Victoria revealed that between 2001–2002 tobacco and alcohol accounted for 89 per cent of hospital admissions while amphetamines accounted for 0.7 per cent of total admissions.

Table 5.10: Drug-related hospitalisations by drug type and sex, Victoria 2001–2002

Drug	Males	Females	Total
Tobacco	27,181	14,241	41,423
Alcohol	12,626	6,727	19,353
Unspecified	1,036	1,448	2,485
Benzodiazepines [a]	796	1,529	2,393
Opioids	487	447	934
Cannabis	374	220	594
Polydrug [b]	381	150	531
Amphetamines	266	147	430
Hallucinogens	31	16	47
Inhalants	22	3	25
Cocaine	12	5	17

a Includes category 'other sedative/hypnotics (including benzodiazepines).

b Includes multiple drugs or unknown drugs.

Source: Victorian Admitted Episode Dataset, Department of Human Services, analysis by Turning Point Alcohol and Drug Centre, in Human Services Victoria 2004, *Drug Statistics Handbook 2003*, Human Services Victoria, Melbourne, p.9.

According to Human Services Victoria:

> [A]n estimated 430 inpatient hospitalisations were attributed to stimulant consumption during 2001–2002. This represents a 24 percent increase on the previous year's figures. Most of these cases were probably amphetamine – or methamphetamine – related (Human Services Victoria 2004, p.35).

The following chart (Figure 5.8) shows the reason for the stimulant-related hospitalisations.

Figure 5.8: Number of stimulant-related in-patient hospitalisations, Victoria 1998–1999 to 2001–2002[a]

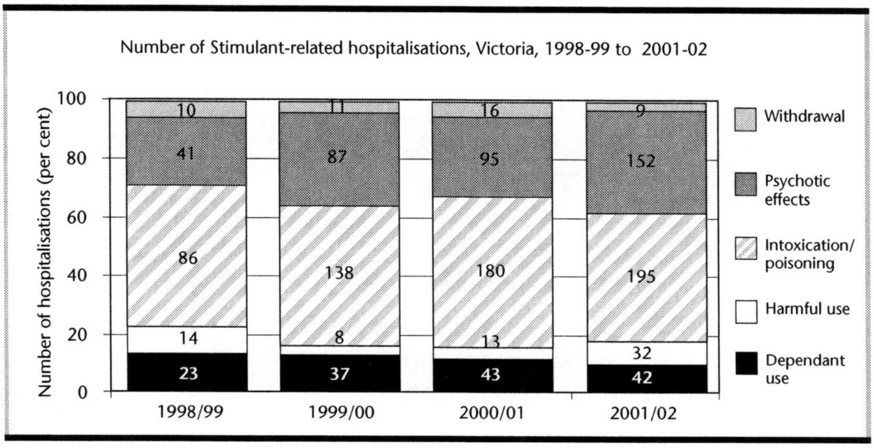

a. Stimulant cases include amphetamines, methamphetamine and caffeine. Cocaine-related cases are also included, although there were only 17 hospital episodes relating to cocaine 2001–2002.

Source: Victorian Admitted Episode Dataset, Department of Human Services, analysis by Turning Point Alcohol and Drug Centre, in Human Services Victoria 2004, *Drug Statistics Handbook 2003*, Human Services Victoria, Melbourne, p.36.

Commenting on these figures, NDARC researchers Jenkinson, Fry and Miller made the following observations:

> These records show that the number of stimulant related inpatient hospitalisations in Victoria have increased from 174 in 1998/99 to 281 in 1999/00 and 347 in 2000/01. Most people hospitalised during 1999/00 were male (67%) and aged between 20–30 years, and around 52% of hospitalisations were for intoxications/poisoning (compared to 50% in 1999/2000) rather than dependence (12% compared to 13% in 1999/2000) or withdrawal (5%). A further 27% (compared to 31% in 1999/2000) of stimulant related hospitalisations during this period were for psychotic, mental and behavioural disorders (2003c, p.50).

Prevalence of amphetamines in deaths

> Tobacco and alcohol were the major cause of drug related death in Victoria 1992–2000, according to figures reported by the Australian Bureau of Statistics. There were very few Amphetamine/stimulant related deaths in Victoria during this period. Only 12 deaths have been attributed to

> amphetamine/stimulant use during the period 1990–2000 (Human Services Victoria 2004, p.36).

Table 5.11: Estimated number of drug-related deaths, Victoria, 1992 to 2000

Drug type a per year	1992	1993	1994	1995	1996	1997	1998	1999	2000
Amphetamines	=<5	=<5	=<5	=<5	=<5	=<5	=<5	=<5	=<5
Inhalants	=<5	=<5	=<5	=<5	=<5	=<5	=<5	=<5	=<5
Opioids	56	48	79	100	107	108	113	28[a]	77
Benzodiazepines/barbiturates	=<5	9	=<5	9	9	7	=<5	=<5	=<5
All illicit drugs	98	84	106	163	160	171	218	257	312
Alcohol	838	735	789	747	776	777	716	748	710
Tobacco	4,762	4,623	4,729	4,709	4,781	4,659	4,599	4,254	4,161
Total	5,698	5,442	5,624	5,619	5,717	5,607	5,533	5,259	5,183

a Changes from ICD 9 to ICD 10 coding systems (in 1999) made it more difficult to specify particular drugs. Aetiological fractions were also applied to illicit drugs for the first time in 1999.

Source: Australian Bureau of Statistics mortality data file, analysis by Turning Point Alcohol and Drug Centre , in Human Services Victoria 2004, *Drug Statistics Handbook 2003*, Human Services Victoria, Melbourne, p.10.

Further evidence that amphetamine use has become more prevalent in recent years can be found in statistics provided by the Victorian Institute of Forensic Medicine and Department of Forensic Medicine at Monash University, which reported an increase in heroin-related deaths involving amphetamine over the period 1997–2001 (see Table 5.12 below).

Table 5.12: Prevalence of amphetamine in heroin-related deaths

	1997	1998	1999	2000	2001	Overall
Morphine plus Amphetamines	7%	10%	6%	10%	22%	11%
Total Heroin Deaths	166	268	359	331	49	

Source: Wallington, Gerostamoulos, & Drummer 2002, Heroin Deaths in Victoria: 2001, Victorian Institute of Forensic Medicine and Department of Forensic Medicine Monash University, Report No. 5, p.4.

While the total number of heroin deaths decreased by 89 per cent from 331 in 2000 to 49 in 2001, the percentage of heroin-related deaths involving amphetamines[141] increased in that year by 12 per cent.

> The use of amphetamines has also increased in 2001 from the previous four years (1997–1999) with 22% of all deaths now involving amphetamine use in addition to heroin (Wallington, Gerostamoulos & Drummer 2002, p.4).

The increase in heroin-related deaths involving amphetamines accords with other research that indicates amphetamine use is on the increase within the drug-using sector.

141 Where toxicological analysis reveals amphetamine in the system in conjunction with heroin.

Ecstasy – Victorian data

Prevalence of use

In the NDARC research paper, *Victorian Drug Trends 2002 – Findings from the National Illicit Drug Reporting System (IDRS) Study*, Fry and Miller conducted interviews with 156 IDUs recruited in Melbourne between June and October 2002. The research identified a total of 31 per cent of respondents reporting ecstasy use within the last six months.

As indicated in Table 5.13 below, 62 per cent of IDUs stated they had used ecstasy at least once in their lifetime compared with 51 per cent in 2000 and 40 per cent in 1999. Fourteen per cent had injected ecstasy within the six months prior to interview compared with, 21 percent in 2001 and eight per cent in 2000 (NDARC 2003c). It is interesting to note, however, that the primary route of administration for those that had used ecstasy in the last six months was oral (NDARC 2003c p.38).

Table 5.13: Trends in ecstasy use

	1999	2000	2001	2002
Ecstasy – lifetime use	40%	51%	65%	62%
Ecstasy injection in last 6 months		8%	21%	14%

Sources: National Drug and Alcohol Research Centre (NDARC) 2002a, *Victorian Drug Trends 2001: Findings from the Illicit Drug Reporting System (IDRS)*, NDARC, p.50; National Drug and Alcohol Research Centre (NDARC) 2003c, *Victorian Drug Trends 2002: Findings from the Illicit Drug Reporting System*, NDARC, p.38.

According to Human Services Victoria:

> It has been apparent in Victoria for some time that there is an entrenched injecting drug culture, which seems to be on the increase with a steep rise in injection of ecstasy between 2000 and 2001. Injecting drugs, particularly those that were not designed to be injected, dramatically increases the risks of blood borne viruses, Hep C and HIV, and can cause vein damage, ulcers and other medical complications.[142]

It should be reiterated, though, that injecting use of ecstasy and ensuing complications mentioned in this quote are comparatively rare. As stated previously most recreational use of ecstasy is administered orally.

Use of treatment services

As Figure 5.9 shows, the ADIS data identified a dramatic increase in the number of clients seeking treatment for problems related primarily to ecstasy use. While the numbers are small, they have nearly doubled during the research period (July 2000–June 2002), as was the case with amphetamines.

142 Submission of Human Services Victoria to the Drugs and Crime Prevention Committee, Inquiry into Amphetamine and 'Party Drug' Use in Victoria, September 2002.

It would seem that the price and availability of ecstasy has been a factor in its increased use. As NDARC researchers Jenkinson, Fry and Millar found:

> It was reported that the price and purity of ecstasy had remained stable, that it was easy to obtain and had become easier. Key informants reported that one ecstasy tablet cost $35–50 or $300 for 10 tablets. It was also reported that purity of ecstasy remained low... (NDARC 2003c, p.51).[143]

Figure 5.9: Clients accessing drug treatment services with primary drug ecstasy, July 2000 to June 2003

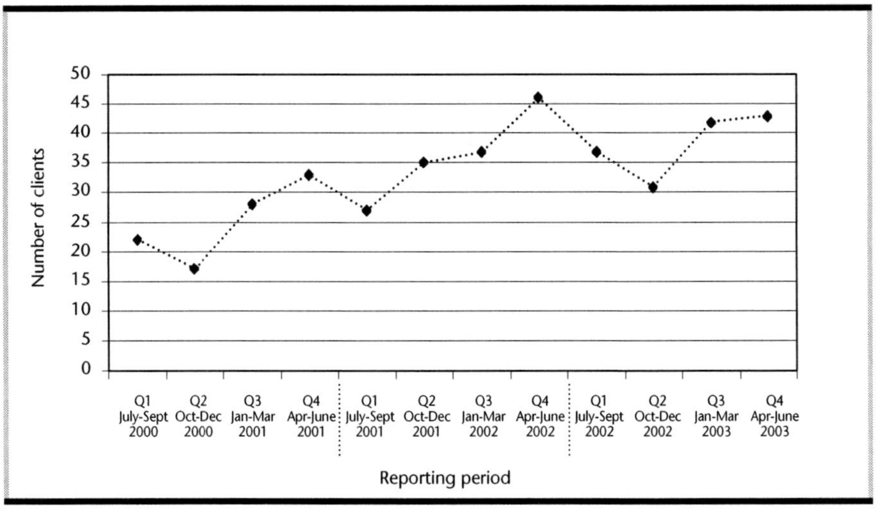

Source: Alcohol and Drug Information System 2002.[144]

Human Services Victoria also notes that as well as an increase in the number of ecstasy users there may be an increase in the amount taken by those who have been using ecstasy for some time, in order to achieve the desired effect. The Department is concerned that:

> A consequence of this will be the increase in the level of contaminants and other drugs that they are ingesting, aggravating what could already be dangerous and certainly unpredictable poly drug use patterns.[145]

Research and anecdotal evidence also indicates that while ecstasy has moved into more traditional drug markets its use is also more widespread among intravenous drug users.

As well, use among young people has increased. In the Victorian Drug Trends 2002 study:

143 In 2003 Turning Point Alcohol and Drug Centre conducted research on psychostimulant use in Melbourne with a different sentinel group of drug users. The results of this study were not available at the time of writing this Report. However, the Committee believes that the results will provide a better understanding of ecstasy trends in Victoria.

144 Submission of Human Services Victoria to the Drugs and Crime Prevention Committee, Inquiry into Amphetamine and 'Party Use' in Victoria, September 2003.

145 Submission of Human Services Victoria to the Drugs and Crime Prevention Committee, Inquiry into Amphetamine and 'Party Drug' Use in Victoria, September 2002.

> Key informants reported an age range of ecstasy users as between 12–30 years with an average age of 20, similar to previous IDRS studies (NDARC 2003c, p.39).

Although the 1999 School Students and Drug Use Report 1999 reported that less than 5 per cent of students had 'ever used' ecstasy, and that use tended to be experimental, the decrease in the age of ecstasy users noted above supports anecdotal evidence within the rave and party scene that ecstasy is attracting younger people, as well as a more mainstream group of users.

Ambulance attendances

During the period July 2001 to June 2002 there were 207 ambulance attendances for ecstasy-related incidents (see Figure 5.10). As was observed with attendances for amphetamines, ambulance attendances for ecstasy also peaked during the period December 2001–January 2002. As NDARC researchers Jenkinson, Fry and Miller explain, 'This summer holiday period is well recognised as the peak time of the year for large dance parties and music festivals' (NDARC 2003c, p.53).

Figure 5.10: Monthly totals of ambulance attendances where ecstasy was mentioned, in Melbourne, July 2001 to June 2002

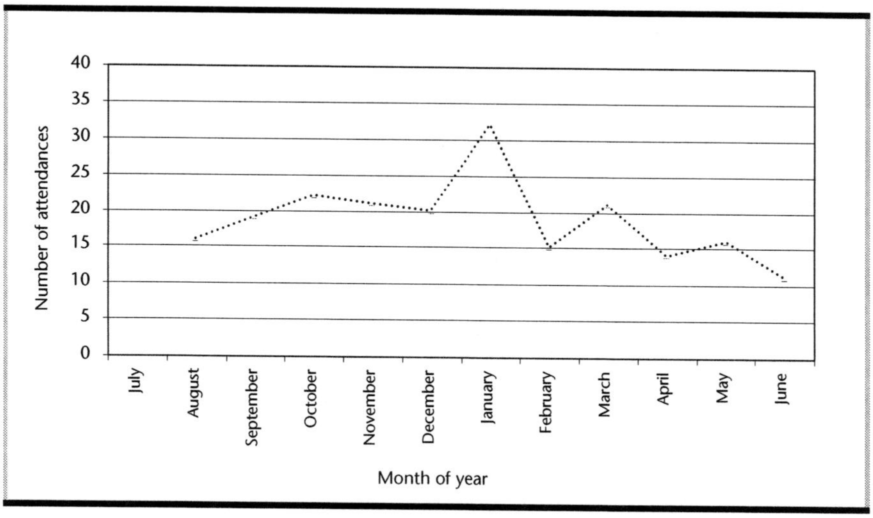

Note: Figures for July 2001 were not collated.

Source: Ambulance attendance data provided by Turning Point Alcohol and Drug Centre

Deaths

There have been very few ecstasy-related deaths in Victoria. Professor Olaf Drummer, Head, Scientific Services, Victorian Institute of Forensic Medicine, provided the Committee with the following report. The table referred to can be found in Appendix 12.

> Since the inception of the Institute in 1989 and to about the end of October 2003 there were 37 cases associated with one or more of the ecstasy style amphetamines. The first case was recorded in 1995. In 1998, 1999, 2000, 2001, 2002 and so far in 2003 there were 2, 4, 2, 10, 5, 4 cases, respectively.

> There were 9 females and 28 males ranging in age from 17 to 44 years old (median 28). The data on these cases is summarised in the attached Table. The inclusion of the data base to the early 1990s provides some historical basis to show the appearance of this drug in coronial cases and the increased incidence over the last few years. Not all cases for 2003 have been completed, hence the incomplete data for last year.
>
> All cases were associated with the use of MDMA and two cases had both MDMA and MDEA. Many of the cases involved the use of other drugs, eg. alcohol, heroin or morphine, Speed (methamphetamine), cannabis etc.
>
> Twenty of the 37 cases were drug deaths in which amphetamines played a contributing role, however most of the drug deaths (n=12) were in association with the intravenous use of heroin. The remaining cases were deaths not caused directly by drug use per se, rather deaths due to car crashes (n=5), victims of homicide (n=5), or successful suicide (n=5).
>
> The place of residence of the cases were located mainly in the more central suburbs of Melbourne, although not exclusively. Two cases had lived in South Australia. The occupations of the 37 deceased cases showed some considerable diversity. Refer to the Table for details.[146]

Anecdotal evidence regarding current trends

The Committee has also received anecdotal evidence that suggests there has been an increase in the incidence of amphetamine and ecstasy use in Victoria during the past two to three years. While this evidence is not statistically based it has provided further insights into the issues and concerns surrounding the use of amphetamine and 'party drugs' in Victoria.

Many drug and alcohol agencies have noted that amphetamine use is not a major reason for their clients seeking treatment, however they note also that there is an increasing trend for amphetamine users to seek treatment.

Uniting Care Moreland Hall is an agency that has provided alcohol and other drug treatment services since 1969 to clients presenting with extensive drug use. In its submission to the Committee it stated that:

> In the two year period from 1st July 2000 to 30th June 2002 there were 4770 treatment episodes across the range of UCMH programs. The primary drug which led people to present for these episodes were amphetamines for 6% of people and ecstasy for 0.5% of people. Amphetamines were also used amongst a range of drugs (ie. not the primary drug) for a further 14% of people, and ecstasy amongst a range of drugs for a further 3.5% of people.[147]

This agency also noted that:

146 Submission from Professor Olaf Drummer, Victorian Institute of Forensic Medicine, to the Drugs and Crime Prevention Committee, Inquiry into Amphetamine and 'Party Drug' Use in Victoria, January 2004.

147 Submission of Uniting Care Moreland Hall to the Drugs and Crime Prevention Committee, Inquiry into Amphetamine and 'Party Drug' Use in Victoria, August 2002.

> As the primary drug amphetamines have roughly doubled in the two-year period (3–4% to 6–8%), however it still remain less than 10% of the presenting primary drug to Moreland Hall. It can be seen that this increase has coincided with a significant reduction in heroin as the primary drug from the July–September 2001 quarter which is most likely due to the 'heroin drought' that has been impacting on the supply of heroin in Victoria since that time. Thus the increase in amphetamine as the primary drug (along with alcohol and cannabis) is likely to be the result of reduced access to heroin.[148]

In relation to heroin users also using amphetamines, the submission added:

> For those people whose primary drug is heroin there has been an increase in them also using amphetamines. In the year 2000/2001, 53% of clients presenting at Moreland Hall had heroin as the primary drug with 14% of these also using amphetamines. In comparison, in the year 2001/2002, 26% of clients presenting had heroin as the primary drug and of these 27% were also using amphetamines. This may indicate increasing numbers of people whose primary drug is heroin using amphetamines when they are unable to access heroin.[149]

Similarly, Open Family Australia, which provides 24-hour street-work services for street children, explained in its submission to the Committee that:

> Illicit drug use has not been exclusive to the city as Open Family Street Outreach Workers in rural Victoria have noticed a considerable rise in the level of amphetamine use in the Hume region over the past couple of years. Staff are seeing an increasing number of young people, especially young women 14–21 years presenting with problematic amphetamine use. Some of the self rationalising perceptions for using amphetamines by young women in rural Victoria are seeing the drug as a social experience and not in any way like taking opiates which they see as 'using drugs'. Amphetamine use is also being used to lose weight and to keep up with social and school life and commitments.[150]

Dr Rodger Brough from the Australian Rural Centre for Addictive Behaviours (ARCAB) also noted that there was 'some evidence that over the past three years in South West Victoria, amphetamine use is becoming an issue for a greater number of people'.[151]

He explained that he had received anecdotal reports from the Western Region Alcohol and Drug Centre (WRAD) counselling staff that:

- Amphetamine use is becoming 'more problematic' (ie. more clients present with 'speed' as the primary problem drug).

148 Ibid.

149 Ibid.

150 Submission of Open Family Australia to the Drugs and Crime Prevention Committee, Inquiry into Amphetamine and 'Party Drug' Use in Victoria, August 2002.

151 Submission of Dr Rodger Brough, ARCAB, to the Drugs and Crime Prevention Committee, Inquiry into Amphetamine and 'Party Drug' Use in Victoria, November 2003.

- Amphetamines are often reported as part of polydrug use but increasingly are the drug of choice.
- Increasing 'local' use of amphetamines being reported (users who report using the same amount or dose in Melbourne also report experiencing a greater effect/more side effects).
- A younger age of first use of amphetamines is an emerging trend (over the last three years the impression is that it used to be 18-20 year olds but is now concentrated in the 16-17 year age group).
- Young women report 'using' as a weight loss measure; shift workers (eg. chefs) and those working long hours are an identifiable sub-population who report amphetamine use.
- 'Ice' starting to be reported being used locally in the past 6 months - possibly coming from Portland.
- Young women tend to snort or drink amphetamines, while men tend to inject.
- Counsellors report noting that the depressed mood associated with ceasing regular amphetamine use tends to last for a protracted period.
- Very few referrals from psychiatric service or clients presenting with acute psychotic symptoms.
- Limited but recent increase in reports of 'local' ecstasy use.
- Ecstasy use is not seen to be problematic by clients. [152]

However, he warned that '[c]onsideration should be given to incorporating data from other rural sites, before drawing conclusions about a "rural perspective" on trends in amphetamine use'.[153]

These findings were not confined to drug and alcohol services. The City of Melbourne was also alerted to the increasing prevalence of amphetamines, as stated in its submission to the Committee:

> However, very recently, Council has become aware of the increasing number of reports from services, police and government departments about the use of amphetamines, in particular, over the last 12 months. Some agencies have noted that this increase in amphetamines use is following a decrease in clients presenting with heroin as their principal drug. Recognising that there are distinctions in the patterns of drug use across and within drug types, amphetamine use is an example where there may be recreational use that differs from the chronic use of this substance… It is anticipated that the use of amphetamines will be identified as an emerging issue when the Drugs Action Plan is reviewed during 2003.[154]

152 Submission of Dr Rodger Brough, ARCAB, to the Drugs and Crime Prevention Committee, Inquiry into Amphetamine and 'Party Drug' Use in Victoria, November 2003.

153 Ibid.

154 Submission of the City of Melbourne to the Drugs and Crime Prevention Committee, Inquiry into Amphetamine and 'Party Drug' Use in Victoria, August 2002.

The experience of the City of Kingston was similar:

> The research undertaken has not identified significant problems with regard to the use of amphetamines and 'party drugs' within the Kingston municipality. However, consultation with relevant service providers and community organisations does indicate an increase in the injecting of amphetamines and benzodiazepines amongst young people who have previously used heroin. Additionally there is evidence of some experimentation and recreational use of inhalants, hallucinogens, stimulants and designer drugs amongst young people.[155]

Human Services Victoria also noted that:

> There has been a recent escalation in Victoria in the misuse of amphetamines and methamphetamines, which has signalled the need for specific policy and program responses... The heroin drought in late 2000 saw an increase in poly-drug use including a perceptible increase in the use of amphetamines.[156]

In addition, the Committee has received evidence that the use of both ketamine and GHB is also increasing. According to the submission from Human Services Victoria:

> Vivaids RaveSafe team advise that GHB 'made a huge appearance' at the New Year's Eve Earthcore party 2000, that 'Ravers often use GHB as a "come down" drug after partying due to its depressant nature, as it purports to relax the mind and body'. It has continued to be prominent in the rave party scene since 2000.
>
> Recently in Victoria 5 'life threatening' cases of 'fantasy' (GHB) overdoses were reported by the Alfred Hospital within 10 days, causing great concern that these might not be isolated incidents.[157]

According to Human Services Victoria there is also anecdotal evidence 'that indicates that currently ketamine is commonly being sold on the streets and in the party scene as ecstasy', and that:

> Ravers have reported sporadically over the past 12 months that ketamine has been sold as ecstasy in pill form (RaveSafe, Safetime, 1999).[158]

Unfortunately the Australian Institute of Health and Welfare study and the IDRS study do not monitor the prevalence of these drugs individually and there is, to the Committee's knowledge, no formal population survey that does. As discussed in Chapter 6, the recent overdoses reported during the Earthcore festival and at Melbourne Park would indicate that GHB is certainly a problem that requires attention.

---

155 Submission of the City of Kingston to the Drugs and Crime Prevention Committee, Inquiry into Amphetamine and 'Party Drug' Use in Victoria, August 2002.

156 Submission of Human Services Victoria to the Drugs and Crime Prevention Committee, Inquiry into Amphetamine and 'Party Drug' Use in Victoria, September 2002.

157 Ibid.

158 Cited in the submission of Human Services Victoria to the Drugs and Crime Prevention Committee, Inquiry into Amphetamine and 'Party Drug' Use in Victoria, September 2002.

Access to accurate and timely data

Throughout the Inquiry the Committee has received evidence from drug and alcohol workers and agencies that they require access to readily available trend data so that they can plan and respond quickly and appropriately to the changing nature of the drug scene. Country witnesses emphasised the need to be informed not only of Victorian trend data generally but of specific local and regional trends.

The City of Monash in its submission to the Inquiry explained:

> Furthermore, a lack of statistical data relating to amphetamine use remains an issue for the development of localised strategies. Information that points to the regularity and impact, both social and health impact, of party drug use remains a challenge for all stakeholders in producing effective programme responses to amphetamine use. Localised data such as ambulance and hospital admissions, Police arrest and offence data, as well as clinical research studies with a particular focus on the local area would assist in the development of evidence based targeted program delivery.[159]

The City of Yarra, based in inner city Melbourne, commented on the problems that exist with current data sets:

> There are several difficulties that local government experience regarding access to relevant data sets and drug trends information which include:
>
> - Restrictions placed upon data collection agencies on their capacity to provide responsive and timely access to research, data and analyses. There needs to be a commitment from state and federal governments to ensure that this information is provided to local government in a timely manner so that local government can plan services and work with local community agencies, services and citizens.
> - Difficulties with negotiating and accessing data from a multitude of government agencies and services. Often the processes in place to access the various relevant data sets are cumbersome, time consuming, fragmented, inconsistently reported (which makes synthesising and integrating the data much more resource intensive and difficult) and not made available unless by request.
> - Other than anecdotal data and ad hoc local research projects in some municipalities – local governments don't tend to be the "keepers" of drug and alcohol data. In the main, secondary data sets are accessed from state government services or government funded agencies such as Turning Point Drug and Alcohol Centre [sic].

159 Submission of the City of Monash to the Drugs and Crime Prevention Committee, Inquiry into Amphetamine and 'Party Drug' Use in Victoria, October 2003.

> The State Government should play a stronger role in coordinating the collection and dissemination of data from its various agencies and funded agencies.[160]

Yarra Council made the following recommendations to redress these problems:

- There is a need for data that is centralised, co-ordinated, and timely and made available and accessible to local government (and also analyses data at local level). This is essential for any ongoing capacity by local governments to address drug and alcohol issues including those posed by psycho-stimulant drugs such as MDMA and amphetamines.
- Quarterly provision and or analyses of these secondary data sets would assist with local governments planning and facilitation role regarding local drug and alcohol issues such as those identified in the Drugs and Crime Prevention Committee Paper.
- Further research into the impacts, behaviours, needs and effects of psycho-stimulants and polydrug use.[161]

Turning Point Alcohol and Drug Centre also has called for more clear data on psychostimulant use in Victoria. In its submission to this Inquiry it stated:

> Given the significant demonstrated potential for health and other harms associated with psychostimulant abuse, there is an imperative for broadening existing drug trend monitoring systems to facilitate a more sensitive mechanism for detecting trends in this area. This may be achieved by extending current monitoring methods to new sentinel groups including gay and lesbian, dance/rave attendees and others (and also through the development of new methodologies). The value of such monitoring is that it may serve as a more sensitive early warning mechanism for emergent psychostimulant trends, and thereby highlight possible areas of focus for future public health response (policy, program and research).[162]

Conclusion

Clearly there are limitations in the accuracy of data on illicit drug use obtained through current research techniques, and therefore caution is needed when considering the available information.

As mentioned earlier, when considering the prevalence, patterns of use and data relating to the harms associated with amphetamine and 'party drug' use it is essential that these be considered alongside the comparative effects of other illicit and licit drug use. When compared to other drug use, particularly the licit drugs alcohol and tobacco, amphetamine and 'party drugs' are less frequently used and cause far less harm to the general community. This is not to diminish

---

160 Submission of the City of Yarra to the Drugs and Crime Prevention Committee, Inquiry into Amphetamine and 'Party Drug' Use in Victoria, October 2003.

161 Ibid.

162 Excerpt from the confidential submission of Turning Point Alcohol and Drug Centre to the Drugs and Crime Prevention Committee, Inquiry into Amphetamine and 'Party Drug' Use in Victoria, August 2002. Quoted with the kind permission and approval of Turning Point.

the harms and problems they do cause to individual users and their families but to put this drug use into context.

However, the research and anecdotal evidence available does point to a trend towards increased use of amphetamines and ecstasy internationally, nationally and within Victoria. It also suggests that both amphetamines and ecstasy are being used by a wider demographic, and while most users are within the 20–29 year age group there appears to be an increase in the number of younger people using, which is concerning. Also of concern is the indication of an increase in these drugs being part of poly-drug use patterns.

It has been suggested that the phenomenon of a so-called 'heroin drought', discussed briefly in Chapter 4, was a significant factor in the increased use of other illicit drugs, and that perhaps this increase will level out as heroin availability increases.

Drug and alcohol workers and agencies have emphasised that in order to plan and respond quickly and appropriately to the changing nature of the drug scene they require access to up-to-date and readily available local trend data, which currently they have problems in obtaining.

Further research is essential for more accurate assessment of current trends in the use of amphetamines and ecstasy, as well as other 'party drugs' such as ketamine and GHB.

PART C: Effects of Amphetamines and 'Party Drugs' – Physical, Psychological and Social Consequences

Discussion on the medical consequences of using amphetamines and 'party drugs' uncovers a paradox regarding research on this topic. On the one hand a search of the medical search engines and databases reveals that there are thousands of articles in medical, health and ancillary journals pertaining to amphetamines and various 'party drugs', of which this Report canvasses many. On the other hand, however, the state of knowledge with regard to the effects of these drugs either on their own or in combination with other drugs is rudimentary or reliant upon anecdotal accounts. Alternatively, academic and clinical findings are subject to debate, disagreement or dissent in the research community.

While a reconciliation of these varying views is beyond both the scope and the expertise of this Report, were such a thing possible, the following Part does at least examine some of the basic and generally agreed upon consequences that may follow from the ingestion of amphetamines and 'party drugs'. The first chapter in the Part discusses the physical and medical sequelae associated with these forms of drug use. It then examines the possible psychological effects of amphetamine and 'party drug' use, an area in which there is much academic debate and in some cases division. For example, can the long-term ingestion of MDMA result in cognitive disabilities? Is there such a discrete phenomenon as 'amphetamine psychosis'?

Chapter 7 raises issues pertaining to the social consequences of using these drugs. In the context of amphetamine use it examines the links between the use of this drug and its association with crime and violence. In particular, it looks at the increasing problem of drink spiking and the use of the so-called 'date rape drugs' such as GHB. Finally, the chapter raises the issue of drug driving, particularly in the context of 'party drugs'.

The last chapter in this Part examines poly-drug use and makes the important point that none of the drugs that are the subject of this Inquiry can be viewed in isolation. It is clearly the case that young people, in particular, take multiple drugs, including alcohol, as part of a wide poly-drug 'repertoire'. The physical and social consequences of this phenomenon require greater acknowledgment and research.

6. Medical Consequences of Amphetamines and 'Party Drug' Use

This chapter contains a detailed but simplified analysis of the medical, physical and psychological consequences or effects of using amphetamines and 'party drugs'. It is an expanded and updated version of the chapter on medical consequences that appeared in the Committee's *Discussion Paper,* taking into account the most recent literature available in the area at the time of writing.

The general (and short-term) effects of the amphetamines, and indeed most of the psychostimulant drugs, can be divided into two basic categories. They provide:

- A sense of euphoria, confidence and well being, and
- Increased energy, often to the point of hyperactivity. This will depend on the amount. Such an outcome is of particular importance to consumers who are using them for instrumental reasons such as long-distance driving or studying.[163]

Physical and psychological consequences – Amphetamines[164]

General and short-term effects of amphetamines

A detailed medical, toxicological and pharmacological account of amphetamines (and 'party drugs') is beyond either the scope or the expertise of this Report. There are also numerous learned journals and texts that the interested and expert reader can consult.[165] What follows is a relatively

163 One reason why amphetamines may be a favoured drug is the belief among some users that they give users: 'a greater tolerance to alcohol. As a result they can drink more cans of beer. For example they [can] drink 12 cans instead of 4. Amphetamines and alcohol are combined regularly' (Submission of Anglicare Victoria to the Drugs and Crime Prevention Committee, Inquiry into Amphetamine and 'Party Drug' Use in Victoria, October 2003).

164 For a list of the toxicological effects of the drugs in question in table form and their interactions with other drugs, see the tables in Appendix 13 (taken from Kong 2000). For an excellent, if technical, account of the medical complications associated with amphetamine, particularly methamphetamine use, see Albertson, Derlet and Van Hoosen (1999). This account covers *inter alia* complications pertaining to the cardiovascular system, the central nervous system, infectious diseases, respiratory system, dermatologic toxicity, renal and hepatic disorders.

165 For example see Kong 2000, and in the context of ecstasy and other 'designer drugs' see Hando, Topp & Dillon 1998 and the references listed therein; Gowing et al. 2001 and the references listed therein.

simplified version of the main medical and physical effects associated with taking amphetamines, methamphetamines and their analogues and derivatives. It should also be noted that there is not always consensus, even among medical experts, as to either the existence of these effects or the severity of the consequences. This is particularly true of ecstasy/MDMA. For example, in a relatively early symposium on psychostimulant use in Australia[166] many of the presenters believed that the effects of psychostimulant abuse had been exaggerated. Chesher, for example:

> ...concludes that most users of amphetamines and cocaine control their use of these drugs and do not progress to dangerous use patterns... In agreement with Chesher, [Dr] Wickes states that, contrary to the impressions gained from the media or medical literature, many psychostimulant users do not suffer any adverse consequences from their use of these drugs. Even when individuals do present to accident and emergency services, few require either pharmacologic treatment or admission (in Burrows, Flaherty & MacAvoy 1993, pp.4, 5).[167]

Clearly the effects of the drug(s) will be dependent on a number of factors, which will vary depending on the individual. These may include the person's size, weight, general and mental health, the amount of the drug taken and whether it is consumed with alcohol or other drugs. Whether the person is a 'neophyte' or experienced user of the drug in question may also have a bearing on its possible effects.

Dangerous modes of administration

The 'dangerousness' or otherwise of using amphetamines may also vary depending on the mode of administration used. As noted in the earlier chapter discussing modes of administration,[168] the general consensus of medical opinion is that those who administer amphetamines through intravenous injection generally run the potential risk of adverse health outcomes associated with that particular form of administration, most notably HIV or hepatitis infection but also abscesses and other serious medical conditions (see Loxley & Macdonald 1990 in Moore 1992; Hall & Hando 1993; Vincent, Allsop & Shoobridge 1996; Vincent et al. 1999; Hando, Topp & Hall 1997). Zule and Desmond, citing European studies, state that:

> [m]ethamphetamine users may be at higher risk of sexually transmitted HIV than heroin users. These findings are consonant with studies that show that methamphetamine and other stimulants enhance sexual interest, while opiates decrease sexual interest (Zule & Desmond 1999, p.1).

166 Despite the various papers presented at the symposium being ten years old, this research collection is still regarded as a key benchmark reference in this area.

167 Chesher had earlier stated: 'If amphetamines are correctly manufactured, if they are adulterated...with safe substances, and if they are taken orally...the potential for harm cannot be described as serious' (Chesher cited in Moore 1992a).

168 See Chapter 4.

This was certainly the outcome of studies by Klee in the early 1990s based on the sexual and social behaviour of amphetamine users in the north-west of England. Her research revealed 'levels of injecting risk behaviour that far exceeded those of respondents who were opiate dependent and also high levels of sexual risk' (Klee 1997a, p.29. See also Anderson & Flynn 1997, p.188).

Although the contraction of the HIV virus is clearly an issue of grave concern, the transmission of hepatitis C through intravenous (amphetamine) injection is equally worrying.

This is of particular concern in Victoria given that there has been a 500 per cent increase in HIV notifications among injecting drug users. Hepatitis C is also the most 'frequently reported notifiable disease in the country'.[169] For this reason Anex, the peak body for needle exchange programmes in Australia, believes 'that as a hepatitis C prevention measure, the supply of other injecting paraphernalia such as filters would be important given the recent increases in methamphetamine injection'. Such a proposal is supported by Leslie Dunbar of the Hepatitis C Intervention Program based at the Streetlink Youth Health Service in Adelaide. She states:

> Amphetamines are usually sold in 'J' bags (small plastic bags with a sealed top), the substance is usually...drawn up directly from the bag. This process is often complicated by not being able to access sterile water, not being able to afford filters, and not having a well lit, safe clean environment in which to self administer.
>
> Filters are usually replaced with scraps of cigarette filters (which contain fibreglass) or hand-rolled pieces of tampons, thus increasing the risk of bacterial and viral contamination...
>
> Needle and Syringe Programmes [should] supply a sterile 1ml syringe pre-loaded with .5ml of sterile water and with a filter needle attached.
>
> Naturally this would significantly increase the cost of equipment supplied... However, minimizing the potential for the transmission of hepatitis C and the resulting health care cost savings in the future would surely justify the initial expense (*Anex Bulletin* 2003, p.8).

Some submissions to this Inquiry have also stated that intra-nasal snorting of amphetamines runs a potential risk of contracting hepatitis C because of the instruments used to share snorting.[170]

Yet even oral use of amphetamines has its risks. The National Drug and Alcohol Research Centre (NDARC) lists some of the most common effects of amphetamine use as follows:

169 See submission of Anex to the Drugs and Crime Prevention Committee, Inquiry into Amphetamine and 'Party Drug' Use in Victoria, November 2003.

170 See, for example, submission of Anglicare Victoria to the Drugs and Crime Prevention Committee, Inquiry into Amphetamine and 'Party Drug' Use in Victoria, October 2003.

Short-term effects

- euphoria and well being
- increased energy and hyperactivity
- talkativeness
- reduction of appetite
- dry mouth
- increased blood pressure and heart rate
- nausea
- headaches.

And in large quantities:

- stomach cramps
- restlessness
- irregular breathing
- sweating
- loss of co-ordination.[171]

Effects of the 'comedown' period

Symptoms such as tension, aggression (even to the point of violence), panic attacks, mood swings, depression and exhaustion may be particularly noticeable during the 'coming down' stage when the (pleasurable) effects of the drug are wearing off. The Australian Drug Foundation (ADF) noted that to combat such effects, users of amphetamines may also use benzodiazepines, cannabis, opiates and/or alcohol.[172] Regular users of amphetamines may also use such drugs to counteract long-term consequences of their use, such as insomnia (ADF 2002, p.2).

Brain function and neurological disorders

A recent paper written by a Victorian hospital radiologist testifies to increasing accounts of immediate adverse effects of amphetamines on the brain and brain functioning. The Committee has met with the author of this paper, Dr Chris O'Donnell of the Frankston Hospital in Melbourne. While it is impossible to extrapolate or generalise from a relatively small sample, Dr O'Donnell stresses the need for emergency room, hospital and other medical personnel to be aware of the possible risks of brain haemorrhage as a result of amphetamine use:

171 This list of short-term effects of amphetamine use was compiled mainly from the ADF 'Fact Sheet on Amphetamines' (2002) and the NDARC 'Fact Sheet – Amphetamines' (2003) as well as other fact sheets and information services.

172 The use of such drugs, particularly cannabis and alcohol is a common way of 'chilling out' during the comedown period of MDMA (ecstasy) use. See discussion below.

> Over the past 12 months or so in my work as a radiologist, I and the neurologist I work with have noticed an increase in patients presenting to the hospital, mainly through the emergency department, with significant side effects from the illicit use of amphetamines. By way of trying to inform my colleagues I prepared a paper, both as an oral presentation and as a poster presentation, for the annual meeting of the college of radiologists in Brisbane earlier this year.
>
> The essence of that paper was that there appeared to be an increasing incidence of these side effects, and the side effects we were seeing were not well documented in the literature. There is lot of medical literature regarding cocaine, for instance, mainly from the United States, but the medical literature really does not provide a lot of information about the side effects of amphetamines in relation to the brain, in particular the radiology of it – the imaging of it. ...
>
> [My] findings are mainly related to the blood vessels in the brain. Amphetamines have a very powerful effect on the blood vessels of the body in general but seem to have a significant effect on the blood vessels in the brain. As a result of that, they can lead to areas of haemorrhage in the brain – that is, the vessels leak blood into the brain and cause areas of bleeding. Alternatively, they can deprive areas of the brain of oxygenation and therefore produce what we call infarction in a medical sense but what is essentially a stroke.
>
> I can observe these findings as a radiologist using pretty sophisticated medical imaging. Perhaps one of the reasons we are seeing this more and more from a radiological perspective is magnetic resonance imaging (MRI), which is increasingly being used to investigate patients who present with these findings.[173]

Dr O'Donnell's work is clearly an important and valuable contribution to research in the area of amphetamine abuse. Nonetheless, as is discussed later in this chapter, much more research is required with regard to the relationship between amphetamine use, brain function and neurological disorders.

Effects of 'bingeing'

One mode of amphetamine use that is documented as being the most potentially dangerous pattern of use is that of 'bingeing' (see Churchill 1991; Chesher 1993; Hall & Hando 1993; Ovenden & Loxley 1996). Bingeing on psychostimulants is usually characterised as 'repeated use over several days involving the administration of high doses by injection' (Ovenden & Loxly 1996, p.33). Bingeing is considered particularly hazardous as it can result in increased dysphoria and toxicity 'potentially producing both behavioural and

173 Dr Chris O'Donnell, Radiologist, Frankston Hospital, evidence given to the Drugs and Crime Prevention Committee, Inquiry into Amphetamine and 'Party Drug' Use in Victoria, Public Hearings (Melbourne), 27 October 2003. Dr O'Donnell adds that amphetamine overdose is the major drug problem being seen in the emergency department and in the Mornington Peninsula area.

cardiovascular [adverse] effects' (Chesher 1993).[174] In the context of MDMA, bingeing has two possible meanings:

> First, "stacking" (ie. taking several tablets at once). Second, "boosting" (ie. taking several tablets but at intervals over a period of time such as evening, or several days). During a binge users may both stack and boost (Hammersley, Khan & Ditton 2002, p.51).

General long-term effects

The long-term effects of amphetamines are well documented in the literature. However, there have been considerable debates over some specific consequences of use. These will be detailed later in this chapter.

According to NDARC these long-term effects of using amphetamine may include:

- sleep problems
- extreme mood swings
- compulsive repetition of actions
- paranoia
- depression and anxiety
- panic attacks
- seizures
- social and financial problems (NDARC 2002a, p.2).

To this list one could add:

- cardiac arrythmias
- headaches
- joint pains
- malnutrition and weight loss (often one reason why amphetamines are used for functional purposes – ie. deliberate weight reduction)
- aggression
- high blood pressure
- reduced resistance to infection, poor immune system functioning (NDARC 2003).

Finally, in terms of general side effects and symptomology, a comprehensive survey of amphetamine and methamphetamine users in South Australia is instructive for the variety of responses it produced. One hundred users of these drugs were surveyed in 1995 and 1996. This wide-ranging survey elicited

174 Research by Anderson and Flynn in the context of methamphetamine use in California suggests that there are 'large numbers of binge or occasional injectors of methamphetamine who may not self identify as injectors and, therefore, not consider themselves at risk for blood borne infections, and ignore infection prevention messages targeted at IDU' (1997, pp.188–189).

responses to a number of questions concerning adverse effects of taking amphetamines. These findings are worth repeating at length. The results showed that:

- Forty percent of the sample reported having experienced health problems which they thought may have been related to their use of amphetamines in the 12 months prior to interview. The most commonly reported problem was an increased susceptibility to infections (such as colds) due to reduced immunity (14%). Others had experienced a variety of problems such as stomach cramps, skin problems, and reduced fitness.
- Thirty percent of participants were taking prescribed medication for health problems at the time of interview. However, younger users were significantly less likely to be on such medication than older users.
- Mental health problems such as anxiety, panic attacks, depression, attempted suicide, mood swings, aggression, hallucinations, and paranoia were extremely prevalent in the sample (ranging from 17% for attempted suicide to 61% for depression). Although participants reported a high rate of these problems before they began using amphetamines, more people had experienced them since starting to use the drug.[175]
- Younger users (aged 24 or less) were more likely than older users to report that they had experienced panic attacks, mood swings, and hallucinations before they started using amphetamines. There was also a greater self-reported prevalence of mood swings since using amphetamines in the younger group.
- Thirty-seven percent of participants had seen a psychiatrist or a psychologist for problems other than drug use in the past. Eight percent of participants said that this was due to behavioural problems while at school, while the remainder had been seen for a variety of problems including depression, eating disorders, agoraphobia, and post traumatic stress.
- Just under half of the women who had been pregnant in the sample had used amphetamines during pregnancy (n=11). Four women said that they had used the drug while breast feeding, and two had actually breast fed their baby while intoxicated with the drug.
- The mean score for the sample on the Severity of Dependence Scale (SDS) was 4.9 (S.D. = 3.7). Using a score of 4 or more as the criterion for dependence, 60% of the sample were classified as dependent on amphetamines.

175 A discussion of 'speed psychosis' and associated mental health problems is given in a later section of this chapter.

- There were no differences between the young amphetamine users (aged 24 or less) and the older users (25+) on the SDS. Both groups had a mean SDS score of 4.9.
- Compared to non-dependent amphetamine users, dependent users had significantly less education, used alcohol, tobacco, and amphetamines on more days in the 6 months prior to interview, used a greater variety of other drugs, used more amphetamine in an average day, had a lower age at first injection of any drug, were more concerned about their risk of catching blood borne diseases, were more likely to inject amphetamines, had experienced more problems from injecting, and had poorer health on all sub-scales of the SF36 (with the exception of 'bodily pain').
- Increasing Severity of Dependence (SDS) scores were associated with a greater likelihood of having shared injecting equipment, having experienced recent health problems related to amphetamine use, being on medication for health problems at the time of interview, and having experienced anxiety, panic attacks, depression, mood swings, hallucinations, paranoia and violent outbursts since starting to use amphetamines. Increasing SDS was also associated with a greater likelihood of having been involved in crime since using amphetamines, as well as a greater likelihood of having experienced other legal problems resulting from amphetamine use. In addition, those with higher levels of dependence were more likely to have been in treatment for their amphetamine use, to have thought about seeking treatment, and to believe that they needed treatment at the time of interview.
- Sixty-one percent of participants had driven a motor vehicle while intoxicated with amphetamines in the month prior to interview, with 45% of these people stating that they had also been drinking alcohol on some or all of these occasions.
- Seventy percent of participants had been involved in some form of criminal activity (not including dealing drugs amongst their friends) since they began using amphetamines. However, 57 of these people had also been involved in crime beforehand. Fifty-one percent of participants had carried out a crime or crimes whilst intoxicated with amphetamines (Vincent, Allsop & Shoobridge 1996, pp.379–380).

Issues pertaining to criminal activity, including driving a motor vehicle while intoxicated, are discussed later in this chapter.

Medical consequences of risk taking

The results of the Vincent survey discussed in the previous section are concerning in as much as they indicate a willingness to engage in risk-taking behaviour, notwithstanding the side effects that many of the respondents had experienced. The particular risk-taking behaviour manifested by the respondents to the Vincent study is shown in the following findings:

- Twenty-two percent of participants had shared a needle with at least one other person in the month preceding the interview. Of these, 3 participants had only received used injecting equipment from someone else, 9 had only given their used injecting equipment to someone else, and 10 had both given and received used injecting equipment.
- There was no significant difference between the number of young injecting amphetamine users (aged 24 or less) who had shared needles in the month prior to interview, and the number of older users (25+) who had shared (44% and 56% of those who had injected in the month prior to interview respectively).
- Ten percent of the sample had shared injecting equipment with their regular sexual partner, 9% had shared with a friend, 3% had shared with a relative, 3% had shared with an acquaintance, and 2% had shared with a casual sexual partner.
- Fifty percent of the sample said that they had shared injecting equipment with another person on at least one occasion in their drug using career, and almost 80% (n=39) of these people had used a needle after someone else had used it. 38% of the sharers (n=19) said that they had done so because they did not have any new injecting equipment.
- Forty-seven percent of the sample said that they were in a steady relationship, although the length of these ranged from 2 weeks to 20 years (median=18 months). Sixty percent of those in a steady relationship (n=28) said that they did not use condoms at all.
- Ninety-one percent of the sample had sex at least once in the 6 months prior to interview, and 82% had sex in the month preceding the interview. Fifty-two percent of participants had done so with only one person, and 19% had two sexual partners. Eleven percent had sex with 3 or more people in the month preceding interview. Only half of those who had sex with two or more people in the month preceding interview had used a condom on every occasion.
- A quarter of participants (n=25) had anal sex at least once in the six months preceding interview. Seven of these people were homosexual males, 13 were heterosexual, and 5 were bisexual. Only half of these participants had used a condom for every occasion of anal sex, and 32% (n=8) said that they never used a condom for anal sex. The remainder said that they used them occasionally. There were no significant differences between younger and older users either in the prevalence or frequency of anal sex, or in the use of condoms for anal sex (Vincent, Allsop & Shoobridge 1996, pp.377–378).

Such findings would seem to indicate the importance of tailoring comprehensive harm reduction strategies to the particular group subject to the intervention. This is a subject that will be discussed further in Chapter 19.

Specific long-term effects

'Speed psychosis'

The National Drug and Alcohol Research Centre suggests that, '[o]ne of the greatest problems experienced by amphetamine users is amphetamine-induced psychosis or "speed psychosis"'.[176]

The symptoms of speed psychosis are similar to those of paranoid schizophrenia,[177] and may include:

- hallucinations
- paranoid delusions
- uncontrolled violent behaviour (NDARC 2002a, p.2).

This state usually disappears after the drug has been eliminated from the body, although the user remains vulnerable to further episodes. If the drug is used again, the psychosis may recur (NDARC 2002a, p.2).

The extent to which 'speed psychosis' is manifested by amphetamine users is a matter of contention, although it is generally agreed to exist (see discussion below in the context of the equally contentious concept of an amphetamine dependence syndrome).

For example, the Youth Substance Abuse Service (YSAS) based in Melbourne has reviewed the literature on the existence of a discrete amphetamine psychosis. In a submission to the Inquiry a representative of the Service states:

> It is unclear whether the mental health problems that many of these young people present with either result from or are associated with their use of amphetamines. The common assumption is that there is a specific, amphetamine-induced psychosis, the most cited study being that of Connell (1958), although he did not describe such a syndrome. Connell actually demonstrated that the psychosis only occurred with intoxication, confirmed by measures of amphetamines in the blood. Brabbins and Poole suggest that psychosis wholly due to amphetamines tends to resolve as the drug is metabolised. Where the psychosis does not resolve, long-term follow-up studies usually find schizophrenia or manic-depression rather than a condition caused by amphetamine. However, Sato (1992) has reported that chronic use of methamphetamine produces a lasting vulnerability to a paranoid delusional

176 Anecdotal evidence suggests that it is 'particularly a problem for young men between the age of approximately 17 to 25' (Richard Bostwick, Director of Clinical Services, Joint Services Development Unit, Western Australian Health Department, in conversation with the Drugs and Crime Prevention Committee, Perth, 1 October 2003).

177 For a discussion of the relationship between schizophrenia and amphetamine psychosis, see Harris and Batki 2000. The authors state:

'Stimulant induced psychosis is common and increasing in frequency... Psychosis can be induced by amphetamine in non psychotic subjects and higher doses of amphetamine may be associated with production of a more complete replication of schizophrenic symptoms. Amphetamine use can also precipitate a schizophrenic episode or exacerbate symptoms in schizophrenic patients. Furthermore, once the psychotic develops with amphetamine use, recurrence can happen in response to psychological stressors without further amphetamine use, making the illness difficult to distinguish from schizophrenia' (2000, p.29).

> psychosis with schizophrenia-like hallucinations, which does extend beyond the excretion of the drug in the urine, and that re-use of methamphetamine and alcohol, and stressors, lead to recurrence of a psychosis with clinical features matching the previous methamphetamine linked episodes. Hall (1998) notes that critics of the hypothesis emphasise the fallibility of clinical judgements about aetiology, the poorly specified criteria used in diagnosing these psychoses, and the dearth of controlled studies. YSAS believes that further research is needed.[178]

This is an exhortation with which the Committee concurs.

Tolerance, withdrawal and dependence

Tolerance

As with many drugs, it is possible for people, particularly regular or dependent users of amphetamines, to develop a tolerance to the drug whereby increasing amounts are needed to get the same effect that a lesser amount achieved originally. As the ADF states: 'The quantity taken can reach a stage at which no further increase in the amount taken will produce the desired effect' (ADF 2002, p.4).

Withdrawal symptoms

Withdrawal symptoms on cessation of use may include fatigue, depression, anxiety or panic and sleep disturbance, including nightmares. Ms Carmen Acosta of the Youth Withdrawal Service based in Perth alludes to the problems clinicians and drug workers face with regard to managing the withdrawal of their clients from amphetamine-type substances as compared to heroin:

> [I]t was almost a very clear cut withdrawal process for heroin users. You know, we could almost time it between that 5 and 7 days and not to say that they weren't suffering after that, you know, cravings are still an issue for months afterwards, sleep patterns are still an issue. Amphetamine use is so unknown still. I mean, we are still talking about a withdrawal process that we still do not understand to the nth degree. It has become particularly challenging for us within the withdrawal service...[179]

Amphetamine dependence syndrome?

Such a contention has been posited for some years now. In an early paper on amphetamine use among heavy and chronic users in Sydney, Hall and Hando state:

> First, among heavy chronic users there is a risk of developing a dependence syndrome that is characterised by a prolonged withdrawal syndrome in which depression, lethargy and irritability contribute to a high relapse to use after

178 Submission of the Youth Substance Abuse Service to the Drugs and Crime Prevention Committee, Inquiry into Amphetamine and 'Party Drug' Use in Victoria, October 2003.

179 Ms Carmen Acosta, Development Manager, Youth Withdrawal and Respite Service, in conversation with the Drugs and Crime Prevention Committee, Perth, 1 October 2003.

> abstinence, making it difficult to treat. Secondly, there is a risk, especially among injectors who use large doses, of developing a paranoid psychosis in which loosening of associations, delusions and auditory hallucinations are the most common symptoms. More conjecturally, there is a risk of chronic heavy users committing violent offences, perhaps while in the thrall of delusional thinking (Hall & Hando 1994, pp.277–278).

Hall and Hando followed up this study with another research project whereby 301 Sydney based amphetamine users were interviewed about their psychological symptoms prior to, and subsequent to, their initiation of amphetamine use:

> The main findings of the study were: that there was a high prevalence of psychological morbidity among a sample of amphetamine users; that the prevalence of most psychological symptoms reportedly increased after the initiation of amphetamine use; and that the severity of these symptoms was related to the frequency of amphetamine use and injection as the usual route of administration. Just under half the sample (44%) showed psychological morbidity suggestive of a psychiatric diagnosis... These results confirm our earlier finding that a transition to injecting is correlated with serious psychological symptoms in amphetamine users (Hall, Hando, Darke & Ross 1996, p.85).

The academic literature has over the years discussed and debated such a phenomenon (see Churchill 1991; Hall & Hando 1994; Topp & Darke 1997; Hall et al. 1996; NDARC 2002b; Turning Point Alcohol and Drug Centre 2002).[180] As with many drugs, such dependence may be physical, psychological or both.[181] Wray argues that:

> People who experiment with methamphetamine tend to use it with increasing frequency and in increasing doses seeking to recover the 'high' much as cocaine users do... (Wray 2000, pp.144).

Burrows, Flaherty and Macavoy, drawing from the work of Wickes, note that the use of a small amount of amphetamine, particularly after a long period of abstinence, may result in a recurrence of psychotic symptoms or behaviour:

> Amphetamines and cocaine can produce a psychosis clinically similar to that which occurs in paranoid schizophrenia. The psychosis may be preceded by pseudo-hallucinations of a persecutory nature, known to be unreal by the user.

---

180 For a relatively early account of an amphetamine dependence syndrome, see Churchill 1991. Churchill based his research on a sample of 101 amphetamine-dependent clients at what was then the Pleasant View Centre in Melbourne and looked at the ways in which the opiate dependence concept could be extended to the amphetamines. Churchill observed that many psychiatric hospital admissions are due to amphetamine-induced psychosis and often mimic the symptoms of schizophrenia (Churchill 1991, p.72).

181 Topp and Darke's review of the dependency literature posits that an amphetamine dependency syndrome similar to that proposed by Edwards and Gross for alcohol and developed into the diagnosis of substance dependence in the *Diagnostic and Statistical Manual of Mental Disorders* (DSM) (DSM 1V, American Psychiatric Association 1994) exists and meets that criteria. In such cases: '[p]hysiological, behavioural and psychological components are all important in defining such problematic patterns of use' (Topp & Darke 1997, p.117).

> True hallucinations – usually auditory or visual, but sometimes olfactory or tactile – may follow. Behaviour may be meaningless and repeated for long periods, and violent outbursts may occur. Once a methamphetamine induced psychosis has occurred, a single small dose after a prolonged period of abstinence may precipitate another psychotic episode. Also psychotic symptoms can last over several years in some methamphetamine users (Burrows, Flaherty & Macavoy 1993, p.5).

Similarly, Wray states that:

> People, places, sounds, smells or moods or things associated with using methamphetamine stimulate a desire for the drug long after abstinence has been achieved (2000, p.145).

Yui et al. have also documented accounts of spontaneous recurrences of amphetamine or methamphetamine induced paranoid hallucinatory states (flashbacks) which may on occasion occur in response to stress (Yui et al. 2000).[182]

More recently, Topp and her colleagues (2002) have also referred to 'the existence and destructive nature of an amphetamine dependence syndrome, comparable to that which exists for alcohol and heroin'.[183]

Notwithstanding such views, in the past there has been some doubt expressed as to whether and to what extent an amphetamine dependence syndrome exists. Dr Nick Lintzeris, formerly Senior Medical Officer at Turning Point Alcohol and Drug Centre, expressed the following cautious view in an interview given in 1997. It is worth reproducing in full:

> 'There's a lot of evidence to suggest that amphetamine users do experience problems. But these are not always necessarily caused by their amphetamine use,' he says.
>
> 'I think that's one of the unfortunate things to come out of some of the research – you go and ask an amphetamine user, "have you ever had problems with...?", and you assume that any problems must be because of their amphetamine use. But that's not necessarily the case at all.'
>
> He asks how often, in the harms described, could amphetamine use actually be a form of self-medication?
>
> 'Are the reported suicidal feelings and depression, for example, caused by amphetamine use, or are they actually using amphetamine because they've been feeling so lousy?'
>
> 'As well, because symptoms are vague and amphetamine users commonly use other drugs, withdrawal symptoms could be due to dependence on any of a number of drugs', he says.

---

182 For an account of the deleterious and costly impact amphetamine use and amphetamine psychotic episodes can have on psychiatric emergency services, see Leamon, Canning and Benjamin 2000. See also Richards et al. 1999.

183 See NDARC 2002b.

> Dr Lintzeris says that linking harm with dependence is wrong, and that the evidence for an amphetamine dependence syndrome is actually 'somewhat shaky'. 'It comes from applying models of dependence that were developed for alcohol and heroin to amphetamine', he says. While such measures may show speed dependence, 'that's not necessarily the best way of describing it'.
>
> Despite the difficulties in determining dependence, Dr Lintzeris is convinced that some people do experience quite specific symptoms related to stopping amphetamine use. However, the level and duration of use required before such symptoms manifest is unknown.
>
> In fact, withdrawal from amphetamine is generally poorly understood...
>
> He described a series of symptoms associated with stopping speed use, the most common of which he called the 'crash' phase. This occurred from day one to three, and symptoms were exhaustion, increased sleep and depression. Following this could come a proper withdrawal period peaking at 7 to 14 days but lasting up to 3 months, during which users may experience decreasing episodic cravings, mood swings, sleep disturbance and increasing appetite.
>
> 'Most people who use a lot of amphetamines will experience that crash phase – but that's not withdrawal. How many people experience full-blown withdrawal syndromes? I think it's a minority of people, but the bottom line is that we don't know' (Dr Nick Lintzeris quoted in Wood 1998a, pp.21–22).

Expert researchers in this area, Hall and Hando, have also been cautious about making too much of an amphetamine dependence syndrome in cases where the user is neither an injector nor a regular user:

> Amphetamines are not the benign drugs many users believe them to be, especially when injected on a regular basis. For those who continue to use amphetamines our advice would be: if you wish to reduce the risks of developing dependence or symptoms of a paranoid psychosis, avoid injection or regular use (say more than once a week), and do not use more than half a 'street' gram by any route. Beware of the increased risks that intoxication with amphetamine and alcohol together poses for motor vehicle and other accidents... If amphetamine use is detected in young adults...practitioners should give factual information about the risks of injecting amphetamine, while being careful to avoid overstating the dangers of intermittent oral use (which may have the unintended consequence of increasing scepticism among illicit drug users about the veracity of all health information about amphetamine). Those users who indicate that they intend to continue to use the drug should be given simple advice on less harmful methods of administration and frequency of use, along the lines indicated above (Hall & Hando 1993, pp.643, 644).[184]

Given that there is still some uncertainty as to the nature and extent of an independent amphetamine dependency syndrome, it is timely and useful that

184 For further discussion of 'harm reduction' techniques, advice and programmes, see Chapter 19.

local authors Morefield et al.,[185] based at the Drug and Alcohol Services Council (DASC) (South Australia), are conducting the Australian component of the World Health Organisation Multi Centre Project on Methamphetamine Induced Psychosis. Similar research is being conducted simultaneously in Japan, Thailand and the Philippines. The authors explain the study in a submission to this Inquiry:

> The major element of this research comprises the interviews that were conducted with 50 inpatients diagnosed with methamphetamine psychosis, recruited from psychiatric facilities within the South Australian Metropolitan area. These interviews investigated patients' past and recent substance use patterns, their experiences relating to methamphetamine use, and their psychiatric symptoms. Secondary data sources were also employed in this research. The treatment provided to the interviewed patients was investigated and the medical records of patients discharged from treating institutions…with a diagnosis of methamphetamine psychosis were also reviewed.[186]

The Committee awaits with interest the final findings of the research project.

Behavioural problems and co-morbidity

Whatever the clinical status of a defined amphetamine dependence syndrome and amphetamine psychosis, at the very least (heavy) users of amphetamine can exhibit behavioural problems. Certainly this is the view of the many drug, alcohol and affiliated workers with whom the Committee has met during the course of the Inquiry. For example, Dr John Howard of the Ted Noffs Centre in Sydney contrasts the presentation with heroin clients to those who have abused amphetamines:

> With the amphetamine [clients] coming in, they are sleep deprived, they are irritable and they are paranoid. So it is not so much physical symptoms other than the symptoms associated with the deprivation of sleep and poor nutrition, and so on. But they are aggressive and much more difficult to manage, and much more difficult to settle in. With [heroin clients] you can do that 'muddley–carey' [sic] stuff around their physical symptoms, but for these ones it is behaviour stuff. So they rub against the rules very quickly; they are much more likely to be thrown out of the program or have to leave because of violence or threats and things like that, so they are a messy population.[187]

Workers at Moreland Hall, Uniting Care Drug and Alcohol Treatment service in Melbourne also testify to the potentially violent nature of some amphetamine clients:

---

185 Attached to a confidential submission from the Turning Point Alcohol and Drug Centre to the Drugs and Crime Prevention Committee, Inquiry into Amphetamine and 'Party Drug' Use in Victoria, August 2002.

186 Submission of the DASC to the Drugs and Crime Prevention Committee, Inquiry into Amphetamine and 'Party Drug' Use in Victoria, August 2002.

187 Dr John Howard, Programme Director, Ted Noffs Foundation, in conversation with the Drugs and Crime Prevention Committee, Sydney, 26 June 2003.

> Moreland Hall staff have observed an increase in clients presenting at Moreland Hall with complex and difficult behaviours, which has been attributed to use of amphetamines. In recent months there have been several incidents involving aggressive behaviour by clients towards other clients and/or staff, some being serious enough to require police intervention.[188]

Carmen Acosta who works with drug affected youth in Perth believes that the combination of adolescence and amphetamine use can be a volatile one:

> [With heroin users] there was no concern about the danger that potentially they could place a staff member in. Whereas [with amphetamine users] that is an equation that is always amongst us and as managers and coordinators we have got to be very, very careful that our staff are very much supported in that process. Policies and procedures, I mean, we have had to really increase those, really tighten them up and it is all around the onset of speed use, you know.[189]

Ms Acosta believes that the problem is exacerbated given that most young people are poly-drug users:

> Whereas adults tend to stick to one drug and use this drug all the time, in my experience, young people, if they can't get what they're wanting will get something else instead. So I think it would be difficult to separate young people in terms of: we'll put the amphetamine users over in this program because they do tend to, like, poly drug use more than what the adult population does. And I think part of it...okay, it is around, it is available, I will use it.[190]

The problem of co-morbidity in relation to drug use and mental health disorders is a serious one in the context of amphetamine use, particularly when they are used in association with alcohol and/or other illicit drugs or indeed licit pharmaceuticals. In the Western Australian context Ms Acosta states:

> I'm not too sure whether these are national statistics but in terms of WA youth and drug and alcohol issues, there is an 80 per cent co-morbidity rate. I don't know how that compares with Victoria but for us it is a good 80 per cent and...I'm including depression and anxiety...so those are things that our young people are obviously needing to deal with on a daily basis and hence our staff are needing to deal with on a daily basis. Suicide ideation, self harm issues, those are just regular part and parcel of what we're doing...very clearly there is this almost enmeshed relationship between the drug use, the mental health issues, the onset of withdrawal and whether that would actually bring on an onset of mental health issues.
>
> Whether the drug use is actually masking the mental health issues and [used as] self-medication, you really don't know what you're dealing with until you start to

188 Submission of Uniting Care Moreland Hall to the Drugs and Crime Prevention Committee, Inquiry into Amphetamine and 'Party Drug' Use in Victoria, October 2003.

189 Ms Carmen Acosta, Development Manager, Youth Withdrawal and Respite Service, in conversation with the Drugs and Crime Prevention Committee, Perth, 1 October 2003.

190 Ibid.

> separate things and people are left without the drug use and starting to deal with what they're dealing with. You don't know what you're going to find.[191]

Richard Bostwick, Director of Clinical Services with the Joint Services Development Unit of the Western Australian Health Department, also gave the Committee some startling estimates as to co-morbidity levels among (young) people when he met with the Committee:

> [P]robably around 60 to 80 per cent of people presenting with a mental health problem have got a co-morbid substance problem and about 50 per cent of people with a drug and alcohol problem have got a co-morbid mental health problem.[192]

Depression

Thus far the chapter has predominantly highlighted the co-morbidity problems associated with psychotic manifestations and behavioural problems. It is apparent, however, that depression also may be a significant consequence of amphetamine use. A submission from Turning Point Alcohol and Drug Centre made two important points with regard to mental health issues and amphetamine abuse.

First, that while there are well documented studies on the links between psychosis and amphetamine use, much more knowledge and research is needed on amphetamine use and non-psychotic co-morbid conditions. And second, that such knowledge and research is particularly important given that a recent Victorian study (Nutting, Lee, Jenner & Davies, forthcoming) has indicated that up to 85% of amphetamine users may suffer depression and/or anxiety compared to 7% who exhibit psychotic conditions. The relationship between psychostimulant use and depression, like that between amphetamine use and psychosis, is unclear and complex. Howard et al. state in this regard:

> A number of researchers have commented on the relationship between excessive psychostimulant use and resultant depression (Weir, 2000; Sussman et al., 1999). The rationale for this being that long term psychostimulant use causes a decrease of certain neurotransmitters in the brain, in particular serotonin and dopamine (Dennis and Ballard, 2002). Other have found that pre-existing depression (self reported) is one of the strongest predictors of young people taking up and continuing use of psycho stimulants (Sussman et al., 1999). Yet, it is also widely acknowledged that depression is experienced during psychostimulant withdrawal (Shearer, Sherman, Wodak & Van Beek, 2002, Mcketin & Mckenna, 2002, Hail, Hando, Darke & Ross, 1997). Obviously, depression is associated with the use of psycho stimulants, but whether use results in depression, or cessation causes depression or simply masks what is already pre-existing is not clear. What is clear, however, is the

191 Ibid.

192 Mr Richard Bostwick, Director of Clinical Services, Joint Services Development Unit, Western Australian Health Department, in conversation with the Drugs and Crime Prevention Committee, Perth, 1 October 2003.

> link with depression and this needs to be taken into account when considering appropriate treatment options (Howard, Stubbs & Arcuri 2004 (in prep)).

This problem of an inadequate and uncoordinated service treatment system for co-morbid disorders is dealt with in more detail in Chapter 20 of this Report.

Cognitive functioning

The ability to which a person's cognitive abilities are affected by the use, particularly long-term use, of amphetamines is also an area of debate. Turning Point Alcohol and Drug Centre refers to recent research by Topp et al. that suggests:

> [h]eavy amphetamine use has been associated with neuropsychological deficits that could not be accounted for by premorbid intelligence, concurrent polydrug use or acute intoxication. This deficit is related specifically to the inability among heavy users to focus attention in relevant stimuli, leading to an increased load on limited attentional resources (NDARC 2002b, p.131).[193]

Simon et al. undertook one of the few studies of cognitive impairment in individuals who are *currently* using methamphetamines. This 1999 study of 65 self-reporting methamphetamine users in San Bernadino, California, noted that methamphetamine users were significantly more impaired than non-users in a variety of cognitive functioning tests, including recall and memory tasks and the manipulation of information. Although the sample was small, the findings were an important 'first step in elucidating the consequences of methamphetamine use' (Simon et al. 2000, p.230). The authors also make the salutary observation that:

> It is important to distinguish between the 'the effects of long term use' and the 'long term effects' of methamphetamines. The former which are the topic of this study are the cognitive effects of using methamphetamines over a long period of time. The 'long term effects' of methamphetamines are the effects of using methamphetamines that persist over a period of time (Simon et al. 2000, p.222, see also Simon et al. 2002).

With regard to the latter phenomenon, clearly more longitudinal research needs to be done with ex-users of amphetamines and methamphetamines.[194]

---

193 And see discussion below for possible links between brain damage, reduced cognitive functioning and the consumption of MDMA (ecstasy).

194 For an interesting study of the links between cognitive deficit, methamphetamine use and people with attention deficit disorders, see Sim et al. 2002. The authors argue that preliminary data suggests that some of the function deficits associated with long-term methamphetamine use 'may be due to the fact that a large proportion of methamphetamine addicts had ADHD symptomatology as children' (p.76). Conversely:

'Some researchers suggest that illicitly used stimulants including methamphetamine may operate in the same pathway as stimulant medications; thus giving similar effects to assist individuals with ADHD to function on executive tasks. It has been suggested that some individuals with ADHD may use illegitimate substances to improve functioning…' (Sim et al. 2002, p.76).

Research by McKetin and Mattick (1997) examined attention, memory and cognitive functioning in a group of illicit amphetamine users (n = 78) in Sydney, Australia.[195] Based on the outcomes of that study and a review of earlier research, the authors state that:

> Dependence on amphetamine has been associated with poor psychological health, especially in younger individuals who frequently use large amounts of amphetamine... Psychological problems reported by amphetamine users included feeling scattered, vague, distracted and problems with concentration that impeded work performance or study. Most previous investigations of neuropsychological functioning in amphetamine users have examined the impact of amphetamine use in the context of poly drug use... The low number of heavy amphetamine users in these studies makes it difficult to infer the neuropsychological impact of amphetamine use per se.... [However] The results of this study show that severely dependent amphetamine users suffer from poor memory and concentration, performing from half to one standard deviation worse on WMS-R indices than less dependent amphetamine users. This study also found preliminary evidence that a history of heavy amphetamine use, particularly injecting more than 3–4 days per week, was associated with impairment of visual memory tasks (McKetin & Mattick 1997, pp.235, 240).

Thus the research into the effect of amphetamines, ecstasy and indeed many illicit drugs on brain functioning and related issues of neurotoxicity is still relatively embryonic. This, as shall be discussed later in the chapter, is particularly problematic in the context of MDMA (ecstasy). At a conference in Chicago in 1998 some of the best academic and scientific thinking on the relationship between psychostimulants and brain functioning and brain behaviour was presented (see the summaries in Battaglia & Napier 1998). In particular, the contributors noted:

> With respect to psychostimulant induced neurotoxicity, the evidence indicates that the amphetamines may produce long term, possibly irreversible, neurotic changes in both dopaminergic and serotonergic neurons, and that the readily observed biochemical changes appear to have a functional counterpart (Emanuele in Battaglia & Napier 1998, p.47).[196]

The Chicago conference also discussed the possibility of amphetamine-related foetal and pre-natal exposure and possible consequent harms, particularly on the foetal brain:[197]

---

195 For an early account of the links between ketamine and memory deficit, see Jansen 1990.

196 For further discussion of the links between methamphetamine use and neurotoxicity, see Cho and Melega 2002.

197 For further discussion of the possible effects of psychostimulant use in pregnancy, see Wickes 1993a, pp.18ff, Wickes 1993b, pp.40ff and the references cited therein.

> [c]onferring on off-spring potential 'neurochemical handicaps' that may render them more vulnerable to developing clinical disorders or patterns of drug abuse during their lifetime (Emanuele in Battaglia & Napier 1998, p.47).

It is salutary, however, to point out, as the Chicago presenters do themselves, that while these possible connections are serious and plausible they need to be addressed by much further research.

The effects of impure drug combinations

The ADF also counsels the need to be aware of the health consequences of using amphetamines that are of impure quality:

> Most amphetamines sold illegally contain a mixture of pure amphetamines and other substances such as sugar, glucose, bicarbonate of soda and ephedrine. These additives can be highly poisonous. They can cause collapsed veins, tetanus, abscesses and damage to the heart, lungs, liver and brain. And because the user doesn't know whether they are using five per cent or 50 per cent pure amphetamines, it is easy to overdose by accident... Due to the unknown strength and mix of street amphetamines, some users have overdosed and experienced strokes, heart failure, seizures and high body temperature. Some have died as a result. Injecting runs a greater risk of overdosing due to large amounts of the drug entering the bloodstream and quickly travelling to the brain (ADF 2002, p.3).

Psychostimulants and medication interactions

One particular problem associated with drug and medical interactions concerns those people who may take medication related to HIV infection, such as antivirals, and simultaneously take recreational drugs. The relatively common use of amphetamines and 'party drugs' at gay dance parties may make gay men with HIV particularly vulnerable. Such a combination is acknowledged to be dangerous and unpredictable, and can have especially damaging results on liver functioning.[198] In general terms, there has been concern expressed, particularly in the United States, about the connection between high risk sexual behaviour and HIV infection among gay and bisexual male methamphetamine users. Research conducted by Frosch et al. (1996) states that:

> Gay and bisexual men represent one group in which the connection between methamphetamine abuse and high risk sexual behaviour appears most pronounced. One study that examined the correspondence between HIV risk behaviours and drug use among gay and bisexual men found increased instances of reported unprotected high risk sex for those men who admitted to drug use, most strikingly those who used amphetamines.
>
> Clinically, urban gay and bisexual males often report that they use methamphetamine to 'intensify' their emotions and sensations, particularly

198 For an account of such interactions and some harm minimisation measures to reduce the risks, see Ryan and Keen 2001, p.4.

> sexual ones...[199] and that methamphetamine is often consumed in highly charged sexual contexts such as bathhouses, sex clubs, and sex work situations. Chronic methamphetamine abuse can result in a specific sexual dysfunction known among users as 'crystal dick', a condition in which men are unable to achieve a full penile erection. Because of this, methamphetamine has been described as a drug that creates 'instant bottoms' [ie.] increased libid.o due to methamphetamine abuse, coupled with an inability to achieve a full erection, can lead to multiple episodes of anal receptive sex with anonymous partners and little or no concern about condom use. Some users further increase their particularly high risk for HIV transmission by administering methamphetamine intravenously, which corresponds to dramatically increased HIV seropositivity rates (Frosch et al. 1996, p.484).

Of particular concern is the fact that numerous studies have shown that use of methamphetamine not only lowers inhibitions among users it can also lead them to engage in high risk sexual behaviours that they would not typically engage in when not using the drug.[200] Some studies have also shown a trend for many homosexual and bisexual methamphetamine users to go on 'meth binges...consuming large quantities of meth for a period of time – "until you run out or just can't physically do it any more"' (Semple et al. 2002, p.151).

Similar cause for concern has been documented with regard to MDMA/ecstasy use among gay and bisexual males. For convenience sake this aspect of ecstasy use is discussed in this section. In a recent study of gay and bisexual men who use MDMA in New York City it was found that:

> MDMA users were found to be younger, less educated, to have had more male partners, more one night stands with men, more visits to bars or clubs and sex clubs or bathhouses, to have unprotected anal sex with a male, to be likely to have been the victim of physical domestic violence... MDMA users thus constitute a group at risk for sexually transmitted diseases, including HIV and other problems. The data suggest that MDMA use is associated with being more 'out', which may be advantageous in helping gay men deal with harmful psychological effects of stigma, but may place individuals in settings that expose them to MDMA...
>
> Media reports suggest that MDMA use is particularly prevalent in the gay community... Indeed in a prior study we found that among the 169 gay and bisexual men recruited from three dance clubs in New York City, 34% had used MDMA in the past month. About half (52%) had used MDMA in the past year,

199 For further discussion of amphetamine and other drug use in gay and bisexual men and its connection to HIV and other health outcomes, see Heischober and Miller 1991; Paul, Stall and Davis 1993; and in the Australian context, Hall and Hando 1994 (Study of amphetamine use and HIV risk taking among young predominantly but not exclusively heterosexual Sydney adults); Murnane et al. 2000; Lewis and Ross 1995; Topp, Hando and Dillon 1999; Degenhardt and Topp 2003.

200 Such behaviours may includes anal sex, multiple partners, casual partners, low rates of condom use and unsafe injecting practices, see Shoptaw, Reback and Freese, 2002; Semple, Patterson and Grant 2002; Reback and Grella 1999.

> and those MDMA users were 2.8 times more likely than non users to have had unprotected anal sex in the past year (Klitzmann et al. 2000). In fact among recreational drugs, only MDMA was found to be associated with unsafe sex in this sample (Klitzmann et al. 2002, pp.115, 116. See also Reback & Grella 1999; Semple et al. 2002; Shoptaw, Reback & Freese 2002).

Of course the experiences of a sample in New York cannot necessarily be extrapolated to the Australian context. However, a comprehensive survey of drug use in the gay, bisexual and lesbian communities of Melbourne suggests that the parallels and circumstances are, at least in part, similar (Murnane et al. 2000, see also recent studies by Degenhardt & Topp 2003). Certainly, both Australian and overseas data suggests, as discussed in Chapter 4, that if the mode of amphetamine administration is via intravenous injection the health-related risks and consequences, including HIV infection, are far greater[201] (Hall & Hando 1994; Vincent, Allsop & Shoobridge, 1996; Vincent et al. 1999; NDARC 2002b). An examination of the patterns of use and the culture of drug-taking among local gay and lesbian communities is found in Chapter 9.[202]

201 Another possible cause for concern arises from some anecdotal evidence that some dance drug users, including gay men, are combining Viagra with stimulants and MDMA to facilitate and prolong sex after dance parties. The side effects of using Viagra in such circumstances may include 'dramatic drops in blood pressure, fainting, blackouts and coma' (see NDARC 'Viagra: the new party drug?' www.med.unsw.edu.au/ndarc/questions/jjjviagra.htm).

202 A comprehensive qualitative survey of gay dance party and club patrons in Sydney highlights the disinhibiting effects of drugs such as crystal methamphetamine and its links with risk-taking behaviour and dangerous sexual practices:

'One of the major and most concerning differences between Ice and Ecstasy, reported by respondents in regards to increased risks of HIV infection, was the degree of hypersexuality they experienced at the same time as impaired judgement. On the one hand they suggested that Ice increased their ability to focus on a task and be in control, and yet on the other they often reported that they were sexually out of control when they used the drug' (Lewis & Ross 1995, p.112).

The very graphic respondents to the Lewis and Ross study nearly without exception recount the complete lack of safe sex precautions taken when sex is practised after having taken drugs such as Ice. The following are representative:

'Most respondents praised the powerful aphrodisiac effects of Ice, including hypersexual stamina, enduring penile erection and multiple orgasms.

Respondent 9 described how this need [for sex] overwhelmed or excluded the concept of safer sex guidelines and survival:

"You don't think to use a condom, because you have feelings of urgency...like you've got to do it NOW!" (p.117).

Respondent 4 [stated]:

"To get a condom would be a hassle, and even if it's only a matter of going outside and asking for [a condom], some people still wouldn't do it...because that's still two minutes out of your life...that you could have got another f***. Are you going to stop and slip a condom on?" (Lewis & Ross 1995, p.118).

The drug or the method? Comparing injecting with non-injecting drug use

In this examination of issues pertaining to amphetamines and 'party drugs', the focus so far has been mostly on the drug or drugs in question. The properties of the drugs and the medical and social effects of the drug have understandably been the focus of the discussion. This section, however, is less concerned with the nature of the drug per se as with the relationship between that drug and the way in which the drug is administered. A bifurcation is noted between the injecting and non-injecting administration of amphetamines and 'party drugs'. A current issue of concern to drug workers and researchers is the extent to which the mode of administration impacts upon the dangers to health of the individual and the harms to the community. Or to put it differently, does the drug itself – be that heroin, amphetamine or cocaine – matter as much as the way in which it is taken.[203] Kaye and Darke have posed the question in recent research:

> It is unclear…to what extent the harm associated with injecting drug use can be solely attributed to injecting per se or to the type of drug that is injected. In other words, does the level of harm associated with injecting drug use vary depending on the drug that is injected? (Kaye & Darke 2000, p.189).

Given the amount of knowledge that has been collected with regard to the spread of blood-borne viruses and other illnesses associated with injection, it seems almost axiomatic that injectors of any type of drugs run greater health risks than those who choose non-injectable forms of drug administration such as oral or intra nasal use. Kaye and Darke recognise that:

> Injecting drug use has consistently been shown to be associated with a greater level of harm than other routes of administration, such as intranasal use, oral use or smoking/inhalation. Injecting drug users are typically more drug dependent, engage in more frequent drug use as well as in more extensive polydrug use, have poorer general health and psychological functioning and exhibit more extensive criminal behaviour than users who employ other modes of administration (Gossop et al 1992; Ross et al 1994; Darke & Hall 1995) (Kaye & Darke 2000, p.189).[204]

Despite such knowledge, Kaye and Darke argue that research has concentrated on:

> [e]ither comparing injectors with non injectors within a particular drug class…or comparing samples of primary heroin and amphetamine users which have included both injectors and non-injectors (Kaye & Darke 2000, p.190).

Their research sought to:

---

203 For some users it may be the 'ritual' of preparing and injecting the drug that is as important or even more important than the drug itself – what Rowe calls 'needle fixation'. See the submission of Dr James Rowe to the Drugs and Crime Prevention Committee, Inquiry into Amphetamine and 'Party Drug' Use in Victoria, October 2003.

204 See also the extensive references listed in Chapters 4 and 6 of this Report.

> [c]larify the extent to which the harmful effects of injecting drug use are confounded by the type of drug injected. [T]he present study examined the drug use history, health, psychosocial functioning, and criminality of primary heroin and amphetamine injectors. Specifically the present study aimed to compare the drug use histories, health, psychosocial functioning, and criminal behaviour of primary regular heroin and amphetamine injectors (Kaye & Darke 2000, p.190).

Other research has concentrated on the 'snobbery' of drug use in which the bifurcation is not between the forms of drug administration but the perceptions of drug users as to what is a clean or cool drug as compared to a dirty or 'loser' drug. This issue will be discussed in more detail in Chapters 8 and 10. Suffice to state at this point that the divide here is generally between opiate and non-opiate users. For example, McElrath and McEvoy's comprehensive research showed that:

> Non-opiate drug users have been known to describe heroin users in stereotypical terms and with scorn. For example, studies of amphetamine users in the North-west of England have shown that those respondents viewed heroin users as 'dirty' (Klee 1998), a finding that was replicated in a London study of recent users of Ecstasy, LSD or amphetamine sulphate (Power et al 1996). Additionally, some amphetamine users have avoided treatment because they did not wish to be associated with heroin users (Wright et al 1999, p.75). In a New York study, researchers found that cocaine users 'felt superior' to heroin users and injectors (Dunlap et al 1990) (McElrath & McEvoy 2001, p.177).

However, some of the respondents to McElrath and McEvoy's survey, most of whom were ecstasy users, distanced themselves from heroin users not only because of the 'dirty' nature of heroin but also because they associated heroin with injection. In other words, the negative perceptions were to do with both the content of the drug and the way in which it was used. One reinforced the other. Injecting use was also perceived as leading to addiction, rather than any properties associated with the drug itself. Some of the responses from the survey are instructive:

> 'I generally think people who inject drugs have a drug problem' (male, age 29, has consumed Ecstasy approximately 100 times during a 2 or 3-year period).
>
> 'Definitely sad, you know that's an abuse of your body...So maybe it's a different type of abuse, but it's obvious what the abuse is...' (male, age 30, has consumed Ecstasy approximately 150 times over a 4-year period) (McElrath & McEvoy 2001, p.181).

For some respondents it was definitely 'the method of consuming the drug rather than the drug itself that contributed to negative perceptions' (McElrath & McEvoy 2001, p.181):

> 'I think they're (injectors) mad. But if they've gone that far down the line (then) they need help, they are addicted to them' (female, age 24).
>
> '...(injecting heroin is like) going down a different path' (male, age 22).
>
> 'Injecting a thing, you're sitting there, tying your arm up, getting a vein out and putting something into your vein which is a lot different than buying a pill...and then dropping in your mouth' (male, age 23) (McElrath & McEvoy 2001, p.181).

The authors point out that in light of their own behaviour and lifestyle, some respondents' perceptions about injectors were hypocritical:

> 'They should be shot – or forced to leave...because they're a drain on the community' (male, age 27, unemployed heterosexual male who had consistently engaged in unsafe sex).
>
> '[Injectors are] totally stupid' (male, age 26, consumed 25 pints of beer and no water during his most recent use of Ecstasy) (McElrath & McEvoy 2001, p.181).

Many researchers that have compared both single populations of drug users (such as methamphetamine or heroin) have found that, despite the mode of administration, methamphetamine users are at greater risk of negative health outcomes because of the properties of the drug. In particular, the disinhibitory effects of methamphetamine can lead to greater risk of HIV and other diseases due to the users being more prepared not to practice safe sex. This issue is discussed in greater detail in Chapter 9. Suffice to state that American research by both Zule (1999) and Anderson and Flynn (1997) suggests that methamphetamine injectors engage 'in more high-risk injection behaviours, with greater frequency than do heroin injectors' (Anderson & Flynn 1997, p.188). Anderson and Flynn also suggest that methamphetamine injectors are more likely to 'binge' inject than heroin users. Particularly worrying to the authors is the fact that 'occasional injectors of methamphetamine may not self-identify as injectors and, therefore, not consider themselves at risk' (1997, p.188). Moreover, Anderson and Flynn found that methamphetamine injectors, whether 'binge' or regular users, were far less likely to access treatment programmes than heroin users, and therefore were 'not accessible in large numbers for harm prevention and risk reduction programmes' (1997, p.187). Zule's studies (1999) concurred with such findings.[205]

Australian research by Hando and Hall (1997) examined, among other research questions, the reasons why non-injecting users of (amphetamine) may change to injecting. This survey, replicating the findings in earlier studies, found that relatively few users of amphetamine inject the drug the first time they use it (23%), snorting being the usual first route of administration. Forty per cent of

205 Zule argues that the major reason methamphetamine injectors were more at risk from HIV infection in particular was due to the fact that methamphetamine and other stimulants increase or enhance sexual libid.o, while the opiates decrease it (Zule 1999, p.1). For further discussion, see Chapter 9.

the sample, mostly males, eventually, however, made a transition to regular amphetamine injection:

> The majority of subjects (69%) reported that they used more amphetamines after beginning to inject, and almost half (44%) reported that they used larger quantities of other drugs, and injected other drugs that they had not previously injected (46%)...
>
> The most common reasons given for changing to amphetamine injecting was liking the 'rush' associated with injecting (88%). The next two most popular responses were that injecting was more economical (23%), and a 'healthier', 'cleaner' way of using amphetamines than snorting (22%) which caused nasal ulcers. The latter reasons are contradicted by the finding that users typically used larger quantities of amphetamines after moving to injection, and so spent more money on the drug, and by the health risks of injecting amphetamine (eg. HIV, vascular problems, psychological problems) which are far greater than for snorting or swallowing amphetamine (Hando & Hall 1997, p.95).

Kaye and Darke's later Australian research study found there was little difference in the harms associated with either form of injecting use:

> While primary amphetamine users had used a wider range of drugs during this period, primary heroin users had used their primary drug much more often and were more likely to have been injecting on a daily basis. The wider range of poly drug use among younger amphetamine users is consistent with an earlier finding by Darke and Hall (1995).
>
> It is of interest to note that while primary heroin injectors were injecting more frequently than primary amphetamine injectors, the two groups were equally likely to have shared used injecting equipment in the month preceding interview. Previous research suggests that amphetamine use is a more social activity than heroin use; with the majority of amphetamine users injecting in the company of their peers (Klee, 1993; Darke et al., 1995) and that, consequently, there may be more needle sharing opportunities for amphetamine injectors. The injection of heroin, therefore, does not necessarily lead to a higher degree of injection-related risk taking behaviour than the injection of amphetamines, even when it is on a more frequent basis (Kaye & Darke 2000, p.193).

However, some workers from the field are not as blasé about the supposedly less dangerous effects of non-injecting use compared to injection as a mode of administration. Paul Dessauer of the Western Australian Substance Abusers Association states:

> I am seeing increasing numbers of people smoking crystal meth and Ice. Virtually every one of them says to me: oh, but I'm not injecting it, and is quite proud of the fact. And obviously the risk of blood borne virus transmission is a lot lower unless you are cutting your lip open on the glass pipe or something, but in terms of the potential, it is just as immediate in effect. If you inject

> something it enters your vein, it goes through your heart and through your lungs, back through your heart and then it is to your brain. You have got 6-and-a-half litres of blood in your body and it does about two or three laps of your body every minute. If you inhale it the same thing is happening, you know. It gets into your lungs, gets straight into your blood stream and away it goes.
>
> The potential for habituation and dependence and the potential for psychosis is just as high with people who are smoking it as with people who are injecting it. A lot of the people that I see who are smoking it take it as often or more often than people who inject it, because they don't have to knock a hole in themself every time they do it. It is a sociable thing to do. We've got a very large population of cannabis smokers in Australia and for a lot of young people the normal social thing to do is pass a pipe or a bong around. Whenever someone new comes over your house you pack it and pass it around again. And I am starting to see this happening with Ice, and that is a real concern because a lot of people who would never have injected methamphetamine will quite happily suck on a pipe all day. This has got the potential to be our crack cocaine, basically.[206]

Professor Jason White of the Drugs and Alcohol Services Council in South Australia also believes there is somewhat a 'myth of the needle' among non-injecting users of illicit drugs:

> Almost all the people that present [with problematic drug use] are injectors, and most people who only use orally think oral is non-problematic. They make a big dividing line between the two: 'If you only use oral, it doesn't matter. It doesn't matter whether you use six or eight Ecstasy tablets a night, four nights a week. It's okay; it's safe.' They make a big differentiation between the two.[207]

Transition from non-injecting to injecting use of amphetamine (and other drugs) is also an issue of great concern for those who work in treatment and programme delivery services. Carmen Acosta from the Youth Withdrawal Service in Perth told the Committee that while there were concerns about putting together one group of drug users (such as amphetamine users) with another group of users (such as alcohol or heroin users), the reality of poly-drug use among young people made such divisions increasingly illusory. The real dangers lie with mixing injectors with non-injectors:

> I think the biggest challenge for our services is the mixture of non IVs with IVs…
>
> Because our biggest issues are around exposure [of young people to drug use] and the management of that… We have got to manage that exposure and then almost ask the questions that are going to potentially give us an

---

206 Mr Paul Dessauer, Co-ordinator, Western Australian Substance Users Association, in conversation with the Drugs and Crime Prevention Committee, Perth, 1 October 2003.

207 Professor Jason White, Drugs and Alcohol Services Council, in conversation with the Drugs and Crime Prevention Committee, Adelaide, 3 October 2003.

> indicator of who is more at risk than another individual of that exposure. I mean, we have got some young people that come to us and are fearful of the needle. There is just no way they're going to go down that road, how could you, you know, how could you stick that in your arm, what are you thinking? Those we know are probably less at risk. Those that are still experimenting and wanting to try it all, those are the ones that we have got to be most concerned about. But the management of that exposure, I think, ...[is] not so much about speed users are separate from others but IV and non IV. And there are not enough resources to go around to warrant [separate treatment/service options] and that is a shame.[208]

There are a lot of mixed messages and indeed confused messages coming out from the various research studies comparing different types of illicit drug use and different routes of administration. On balance, however, the consensus does seem to be that harm prevention and treatment options should concentrate on injecting drug use as the most dangerous form of drug administration, no matter what the drug in question may be. Such concerns are summed up in the work of Hando and Hall:

> From a public health perspective, one of the most worrisome features of the current epidemic has been the relatively high rates of experimentation with injecting as a route of administration. This has obvious relevance to the risks of infectious disease transmission but there is also an increased risk of problems of dependence and psychological disorders arising from daily amphetamine injection. The indications are that these problems are being experienced by regular users, especially injectors, although they are not as yet reflected in a substantial increase in the number of users seeking help (1997, p.104).

Injecting as a route of administration is primarily associated with amphetamines rather than the 'party drugs', which are usually taken orally. This is particularly true of ecstasy. Risks of injecting drug use, such as blood-borne viruses, are for the most part not associated with the use of ecstasy. This does not, however, mean there are no harmful consequences resulting from the use of this drug, as the following section outlines.

---

208 Ms Carmen Acosta, Manager, Youth Withdrawal and Respite Service, in conversation with the Drugs and Crime Prevention Committee, Perth, 1 October, 2003.

Physical and psychological consequences – Ecstasy (MDMA)

General and short-term effects of ecstasy

In Australia and the United States early research documented relatively few problems associated with ecstasy use. For example, comprehensive survey research undertaken by Solowij (Solowij et al. 1992; Solowij 1993) found the most common adverse effects of ecstasy use were relatively minor. These included loss of appetite and a dry mouth. In a recent monograph on ecstasy use produced by the NDARC, Topp et al. summarised some of the academic and medical views towards ecstasy as follows:

> The results of the [Solowij] study confirmed those of early studies conducted in the United States (Beck, 1990; Beck and Rosenbaum 1994; Downing 1996; Petrouka 1990; Petrouka, Newman and Harris 1988). They provided support for suggestions that while the pattern of ecstasy use remained one of intermittent oral use, there was little cause for concern because use was usually self-limited and there were few extreme reactions or severe problems among users (Beck and Rosenbaum 1994; Chesher 1990; Solowij 1993). Such results seemed to confirm the prevailing view that ecstasy was a relatively benign substance with few associated problems (NDARC 1998, p.1).

Since the mid to late 1990s, many such researchers, including Solowij, have reassessed such views, particularly in the light of evidence that ecstasy is increasingly been used via injection and that the purity of what purports to be MDMA (ecstasy) has been seriously compromised in recent years.

It would seem that the 'jury is still out' regarding the extent to which serious medical consequences may follow the ingestion of MDMA (ecstasy). A recent international symposium on MDMA use world-wide summed up the dilemmas for the researcher:

> The capacity for analysis of the health consequences of MDMA is limited by the lack of epidemiological studies. The only current source of information is case reports. Analysis of case reports is problematic as firstly, there is no way to determine whether reported cases are representative of the population of MDMA users and, secondly, there is likely to be significant publication bias, with 'novel' and severe cases being preferred for publication. Furthermore, there tends to be variability in the nature of data collected and reported and outcomes assessed for each case report, often reflecting whatever theme is being debated through scientific and medical literature at the time.
>
> Another limitation is variability in information on drug use preceding the episode. Quantification of drugs in blood and urine samples is not always undertaken, and differing intervals between drug use and presentation for treatment influence the possibility and interpretation of testing. The extent and accuracy of reporting of drug use by the patient or observers, and on medical history prior to the adverse event is also variable (and often limited in cases with fatal outcomes).

A further difficulty in attributing causality of the adverse event to 'ecstasy' is variability in the purity of the ingested substance, together with the tendency for MDMA to be used in conjunction with other drugs (Gowing et al. 2001, p.25 and references cited therein).

Notwithstanding such limitations, some general factors and indications can be given for both the short and long-term health consequences of MDMA ecstasy use.[209]

Short-term effects

According to NDARC the following short-term effects of using ecstasy may include:

- euphoria and a feeling of well-being
- feelings of increased closeness with others
- increased self-confidence
- lack of inhibitions
- tongue and cheek chewing
- teeth grinding (bruxism)[210]
- dry mouth
- increased body temperature
- nausea and anxiety
- sweating
- inability to sleep (NDARC 2002a, p.2).

A number of surveys and research reports have canvassed the short-term effects of ecstasy use, including both during the 'high' and 'come down' stages.[211] Such

209 For an excellent, if technical, account of some of the major short and long-term effects of MDMA use, see Gowing et al. 2001, pp.25ff. This comprehensive examination includes a discussion inter alia of:

Hyperthermia

Hyponatraemia (excessive fluid)

Central nervous system disturbances

Cardiac factors

Cerebrovascular concerns

Respiratory factors

Trauma

Ophthalmic conditions

Liver and kidney damage

Psychiatric sequelae.

210 For a discussion of the links between regular use of MDMA and the excessive wear of the teeth and tooth damage, see Redfearn, Agrawal and Mair 1998. See also Hughes 2000. Hughes gives some practical examples as to how the adverse effects of taking MDMA on dental health can be minimised. For example, the chewing of sugar free gum to 'increase saliva and its associated buffering effects on tooth grinding' (2000, p.209. See also Freese, Miotto & Reback 2002). This Committee has noticed that in many of the clubs and venues it has visited, sweets and lollipops have been on offer as a way of ameliorating the problems associated with bruxism. See discussion in the section 'The World of Clubland' in Chapter 10.

211 See for example, Moore 1992a; Williamson et al. 1997.

surveys are complicated, however, by the fact that many of those surveyed were using other drugs in addition to ecstasy, such as benzodiazepenes, opiates, cocaine and/or methamphetamines. It is sometimes difficult to know whether a side effect or adverse consequence can be isolated to one particular drug or an interaction or combination of a number of drugs (see Williamson et al. 1997). Nonetheless, some adverse effects common to ecstasy use have been frequently noted in such surveys. For example, in a British survey of 158 drug users, subjects were presented with a list of ten adverse effects and asked to rate them in terms of severity when applied to a number of drugs. With regards to ecstasy the authors note:

> Many of the users reported adverse effects after having taken Ecstasy. The frequency with which adverse effects were reported varied from 21% for panic attacks to 79% for loss of appetite. In terms of severity, the majority of effects associated with use of Ecstasy were classed as mild by respondents. Trouble sleeping and loss of appetite scored most highly in severity...along with mood swings and lethargy... (Williamson et al. 1997, p.91).

The severity of the side effects is variable and, as stated by Moore (1992a), is shaped by the quality, quantity and purity of the drug and the individual's reaction to the drug. One might add that the frequency of use, the setting of use and whether or not the drug is used in combination with other substances all have a bearing on the extent or severity of any adverse effects:

> It is also important to note that not all such side-effects will be experienced with each drug episode. For many episodes, few will be experienced; for some episodes several will be experienced; and, on rare occasions, a drug user might experience many of the reported effects. The following then are aggregations of the multiple possibilities.
>
> When taken orally or intranasally, speed and Ecstasy share similar side-effects – excessive sweating, jaw-grinding or clenching, intermittent paranoia, general fatigue (when coming down,) loss of appetite, occasional bouts of nausea and vomiting, skin rashes, anxiety, and blurred or 'glassy' vision (in the case of Ecstasy). Side-effects resulting from trips include 'a bad trip' – an inability to interact coherently with others and to deal with the sometimes disorienting visual and/or mental hallucinations – 'flashbacks' to the tripping state (such as seeing colours or objects moving, although this seems to be a characteristic of people who have used trips with greater frequency), paranoia, painful introspection, and generally unpredictable behaviour.
>
> Injecting speed, Ecstasy or trips may produce bruising at the injection site, the possibility of 'dirty tastes' (from adulterants or unhygienic injecting conditions), 'missing' (when the needle tip slips through or out of a vein leading to injection of the drug into the flesh), and 'trackmarks' (scarred veins), collapsed veins or acute pain (when injecting) from frequent injection in the same site. Such consequences stem from intoxication or manner of administration and are usually considered relatively minor by drug users.

> Unless they become frequent, regular, or painful or detract greatly from the drug experience, they are not generally considered detrimental enough to cease drug use altogether, but may lead to a reduction in frequency or attempts to remain abstinent for a period. For instance, attending a nightclub under the influence of speed may lead to sweating, jaw-grinding and a loss of appetite which, in this setting, will not be considered overly vexatious (Moore 1992a, pp.62–63).

An international symposium on MDMA also pointed to the complex clinical issues pertaining to determining the effect of MDMA on its users:

> MDMA and other similar drugs based on the structure of amphetamine, have been shown to be toxic in animals and humans. It appears, however, that the type and severity of toxicity is influenced by many factors, such as ambient temperature, exercise, concurrent administration of other drugs and hydration... These variables when added to the large number of chemical species sold as 'ecstasy', or found as contaminants of street 'ecstasy', provide a very complex problem for scientists and clinicians alike (Gowing et al. 2001, p.20).

Effects of the 'comedown' period

Some of the worst of the side effects reported by drug users are associated with the 'coming down' period immediately following intoxication. Such a period with regard to ecstasy may last from a few hours to a few days. The ecstasy come down is usually not viewed as anywhere near as severe as that associated with amphetamines or LSD (Moore 1992a). Moore describes the experience as follows:

> Except when used in large quantities for long periods or with other drugs such as speed and/or trips, Ecstasy is distinctive for its gentle 'comedown' (relative at least to speed or trips), particularly after a single dose. Those who have been using it constantly for several days (usually in conjunction with other drugs) may experience unpleasant effects, although it is hard to fathom which drug is responsible for these. After finally going to sleep in the early hours of the morning, those individuals who have used Ecstasy report sleeping well (often with vivid and sometimes pleasant dreams) and waking with a positive outlook on the next day. Ecstasy is held to contribute to a general feeling of well-being which may last several days after the experience. Even those who do experience some 'comedown' from heavy Ecstasy use describe it as being less traumatic than that induced by trips or speed.
>
> The negative effects of 'coming down' are exacerbated by the sometimes massive consumption of alcohol made possible by (in particular) speed, trips and Ecstasy (the number of drinks required to reach a subjective feeling of intoxication is greatly increased), and by the mixing of large quantities of various drugs. For example, one person told me that she consumed Ecstasy twenty-seven times in one week and that this was in addition to the speed and

> trips she has also used. Needless to say, she experienced a severe 'comedown' when consumption ended (Moore 1992a, p.62).

Ecstasy and risk-taking sexual behaviour

Another significant factor that needs to be taken into account, as noted above in the context of amphetamine use, is the possibility that ingestion of MDMA ecstasy may result in a readiness to take risks with regard to sexual behaviour. Klitzmann et al., for example, have noted the potential for greater HIV risk-taking behaviour when gay men in particular have ingested MDMA (Klitzmann et al. 2002, and see also the discussion in Frosch 1996; Moore 1992a). There is also anecdotal evidence that young people – heterosexual and homosexual – who use 'party drugs' '[a]re at higher risk of participating in sexual behaviour which in itself has further issues around sexually transmitted diseases, unwanted pregnancies and regretting their behaviour'.[212]

Research by Topp, Hando and Dillon (1999) that examined the sexual behaviour of ecstasy users in Sydney, both heterosexual and homosexual, showed that a significant number of users would engage in unsafe sex when intoxicated on ecstasy and/or other drugs:

> Among those who had sex with a regular partner during the preceding month [n=123], only one quarter (26%) used condoms on every occasion and the majority (59%) reported that they had never used condoms. Among those who had sex with a casual partner (n=68) over half (59%) always used condoms, although 22% reported that they never used condoms with casual partners...
>
> Half the sample (49%) reported having sex while acutely intoxicated on ecstasy in the preceding six months... Among those who had sex with a regular partner while intoxicated (n=82), 24% used condoms every time, while 50% never used condoms. Among those who had sex with a casual partner while intoxicated (n=41), 49% always used condoms, a lower rate than when not intoxicated. Furthermore, 20% never used condoms with casual partners while intoxicated. Bisexual subjects were significantly more likely than others to have engaged in risky casual sex while intoxicated (Topp, Hando & Dillon 1999, pp.151, 153).

Moreover, this research suggests that ecstasy in particular is associated with such unsafe sexual practices:

> Multivariate analyses also indicated that ecstasy, rather than other stimulants, was specifically associated with the sexual risk taking of this sample, a novel and important finding that...suggests a need for culturally relevant safe sex messages to prevent the spread of sexually transmitted infection among this population as well as among others who may have sexual contact with members of this group...ecstasy users may constitute a special group with

212 Submission of the Shire of Yarra Ranges to the Drugs and Crime Prevention Committee, Inquiry into Amphetamine and 'Party Drug' Use in Victoria, October 2003.

> respect to a greater number of sexual partners as well as an increased likelihood of sexual risk taking (Topp, Hando & Dillon 1999, p.154).

Safe sex messages might be particularly difficult to get across to this population given that 70% of this sample reported that being intoxicated on ecstasy improved sex, lowered their inhibitions (a positive thing) and 'intimacy increased due to improved communication' (p.155). Only 2% of the sample considered one of the 'risks' of ecstasy use was unsafe sex with strangers (p.153).[213]

Two of the most significant of the adverse effects of taking ecstasy are hyperthermia and hyponatraemia. These are discussed in the section below pertaining to ecstasy-related deaths.

Other short-term or general side effects and complications

Finally, in this brief discussion of the short-term side effects of ecstasy use it is worth examining the result of one of the most comprehensive surveys of ecstasy users done in recent times – the South Australian Party Drug Trends study (2001) by Longo et al., auspiced by the Illicit Drug Reporting System (IDRS) for the NDARC (cited as NDARC 2002c). This survey of 70 South Australian ecstasy users questioned the participants as to physical and psychological side effects associated with ecstasy use and the social and legal problems associated with the drug.[214] The results make for interesting reading.

> The mean number of total side-effects reported in the previous six months was 16.5 (SD 4.5; range 9–29). Subjects reported a mean of 10.8 physical side-effects (SD 3.1; range 4–20). The most common were teeth problems (caused by teeth grinding and jaw clenching), loss of appetite, muscular aches, loss of energy, trouble sleeping and numbness/tingling. Many subjects also reported blurred vision, heart palpitations, profuse sweating, hot/cold flushes, tremors/shakes and joint pains/stiffness. A mean of 5.7 psychological side-effects were reported (SD 2.2; range 2–11), most commonly confusion (disorientation, short-term memory loss and vagueness), depression, irritability, visual hallucinations and anxiety. Many subjects also reported paranoia and auditory hallucinations.
>
> There were 22 subjects who reported additional effects they had experienced while taking ecstasy over the previous six months. The most common was a feeling of closeness to others, which included bonding, sharing and connecting, and an increase in tactile and demonstrative behaviour (n=7). Three subjects reported a general feeling of well-being, such as feeling confident, secure and safe, and two reported an increase in energy. Three subjects reported feeling nauseous, and two had experienced distortions in their perception of time.

---

213 The work of Lewis and Ross referred to earlier in this chapter in the context of methamphetamine also refers to unsafe sex practices by gay men after being intoxicated by MDMA, often in conjunction with other drugs (1995).

214 This aspect of the survey is dealt with later in this Chapter.

> Males reported a mean number of 10.9 physical side effects and 5.8 psychological side-effects, and females reported a mean number of 10.8 physical side effects and 5.6 psychological side effects. The number of side effects was thus very similar between males and females. A comparison was also made between the number of side effects in subjects aged under 25 years, and those aged 25 years or more. The younger subjects reported a mean number of 11.1 physical side effects and 6 psychological side effects. In comparison, the older subjects reported a mean number of 9.9 physical side effects and 4.5 psychological side effects. Although there was no statistically significant difference in the number of physical side effects according to age, the younger users reported a significantly higher number of psychological side effects...
>
> The number of side effects reported by subjects were also compared according to whether they had injected ecstasy either recently or in the past, or whether they had ever injected a drug. There were no significant differences found, with one exception. Subjects who had injected ecstasy in the previous six months reported a significantly higher mean number of psychological side effects compared with those who had not...
>
> Many of the physical side effects experienced by subjects were attributed to ecstasy use. The physical side effects that were attributed *solely* to ecstasy use by more than 70% of those who reported them included blurred vision, vomiting, tremors or shakes, numbness or tingling, hot/cold flushes, inability to urinate and loss of appetite. Moreover, side effects such as dizziness, loss of energy, difficulty sleeping, headaches, heart palpitations, stomach pains and teeth problems as a result of grinding and jaw clenching were attributed solely to ecstasy by 50–70% of subjects who reported them... Although muscular aches and pains were experienced by 80% of subjects, only 12.5% attributed this solely to ecstasy use, saying that these effects were predominantly due to the excessive activity and energy that occurs in the environment where ecstasy is often taken, that is dancing at raves and clubs.
>
> In contrast, all of the psychological side effects were attributed solely to ecstasy use by at least 50% of those who reported them, and in most cases by over 70% of subjects. The side effects attributed to ecstasy by at least three-quarters of subjects included depression, confusion, irritability, memory lapses, visual and auditory hallucinations, flashbacks and violent behaviour (NDARC 2002c, pp.37–39). (Authors' emphasis)

Despite these myriad side effects being reported, the authors of the study were most concerned about the concurrent use by the respondents of a wide range of drugs in addition to ecstasy and the unpredictable health risks flowing from this. Such concern accords with that noted by Topp et al. in a 1999 study of 329 ecstasy users in three Australian cities (Sydney, Brisbane and Melbourne) where:

> A broad range of ecstasy users were interviewed, but on the whole, the sample was young, relatively well educated and most were employed or students.

> Patterns of use were varied, although extensive polydrug use was the norm. High rates of intravenous drug use were recorded, which may relate to an over representation of chaotic intravenous polydrug users (Topp et al. 1999, p.105).

Notwithstanding the very real concerns about the use of MDMA, drug experts warn of the need to eschew (media driven) hyperbole in this area. Paul Dillon, expert drug educator with NDARC told the Committee that:

> The reality is that the greatest harm when it comes to most of these drugs is that they are illegal, and if you get caught with them you may have your life ruined. That's not to say they are harmless, but let's be realistic about the harms. Unfortunately what we tend to concentrate on when we actually do anything around harm, is death, and that is so unlikely. What's more likely to happen is a range of problems like dehydration, overheating – and I think where the big area is, is psychological problems. Definitely what I see and hear from young people – and I'm talking very young – [is that they] have severe anxiety problems after taking some of these substances, and sometimes it takes them a long time to recover.[215]

Long-term effects

It was noted in Chapter 4 that when ecstasy first arrived on the scene both in Australia and overseas it gave little cause for concern in terms of its potential for abuse and any deleterious medical or other consequences emanating from its use, particularly in the long term (see Fitzgerald 1991; Solowij, Hall & Lee 1992; Solowij 1993; Hando, Topp & Dillon 1998; Topp et al. 1999, and the references listed therein).

By the late 1990s, however, ecstasy was no longer seen as so benign. There were two main reasons for this, both related to each other. First, a number of deaths had been reported that were attributed to the use of ecstasy or what purported to be ecstasy. Second, according to some commentators, the media was taking a closer and sometimes prurient and irresponsible look at the drug and its associated culture (see Solowij, Hall & Lee 1992; O'Neill 1996; Sweet 1997; Saunders 1998; Lumby 2000; Luckman 2000; Teece & Makkai 2000). The media speculation and hyperbole, always inimical to the development of good public policy, reached its most intense pitch with the death of 15-year-old Sydney schoolgirl, Anna Wood, following on as it did from equally sensationalised accounts of ecstasy deaths in Britain and the United States. The issue of 'party drugs' and the media, including the death of Anna Wood, will be discussed further in Chapter 18. However, it is worth stating here that many media accounts at this time were not helpful in giving an accurate picture of just how dangerous or not the drug MDMA or its analogues was and is. For example, Libby Topp, a researcher with NDARC, found in her interviews with ecstasy users that many young people who take ecstasy were dismissive about legitimate

215 Mr Paul Dillon, Information/Media Liaison Officer, NDARC, in conversation with the Drugs and Crime Prevention Committee, Sydney, 26 June 2003.

health issues pertaining to ecstasy because of the hype surrounding Anna Wood's death:

> She adds that many ravers call a good night out an 'Anna Wood' night, as an expression of their frustration at ecstasy myths. "We really need to get off the idea that everyone who has an ecstasy is going to die" she says, citing a recent European review estimating the risk of dying from taking one ecstasy tablet at one in 3.4 million compared with a risk of one in 84,500 of dying from skydiving... Dr Andrew Byrne, a Redfern GP specialising in drug and alcohol treatment adds: "I get about three calls a year about ecstasy, compared with three calls a day about heroin and cocaine". It is difficult to escape comparisons with alcohol, which contributes to so many traffic and work accidents and to so much ugly violence, apart from not being terribly good for many of our vital organs (Topp quoted in Sweet 1997, p.6).

Certainly medical and research opinion was becoming less sanguine regarding the possible medical side effects of ecstasy by the late 1990s. It should be stressed, however, that much of the concern was and is not so much with regard to pure methyldioxymethamphetamine (MDMA), the ostensible compound that makes up ecstasy. Rather, it was centred on what was being sold or traded as ecstasy but is another drug altogether or is adulterated with more dangerous substances. Samples of ecstasy analysed in earlier years may have been relatively free of contaminants and therefore masked or at least confounded any possible adverse side effects (Fitzgerald 1991). Hando, Topp and Dillon track this change in professional thinking on the subject:

> It was suggested that while the pattern of 'ecstasy' use remained one of intermittent oral use, there was little cause for concern because the use was usually self-limited and there were few extreme reactions or severe problems among users (Solowij 1993).
>
> However, in recent years there has been a growing number of deaths in which 'ecstasy' has been implicated, both in Australia and overseas... Deaths have most often been attributed to heat stroke resulting from the circumstances in which 'ecstasy' is used, such as dance parties. It appears that a combination of sustained physical exertion, high ambient temperatures and inadequate fluid replacement compound a direct pharmacological effect of 'ecstasy' on thermo-regulatory mechanisms, leading to fulminant hyperthermia. This effect is in part a result of 'ecstasy's' neurotoxic effects on serotonergic nerve terminals, but such extreme reactions are idiosyncratic for reasons as yet unknown. On the other hand, some deaths have been attributed to excessive water consumption.
>
> Other risks stem from the consumption of large doses of 'ecstasy' (acute or cumulative), a history of psychiatric disturbance or pre-existing disease... Research has also noted significant psychological morbidity associated with the use of 'ecstasy'.

> Little systematic research on 'ecstasy' related harms has been conducted since the early 1990s. There is also little information about the intervention preferences of 'ecstasy' users necessary for the develop [sic] of public policy (Hando, Topp & Dillon 1998, pp.33–34).

Cognitive functioning

It is still true to state that a paucity of research in this area has resulted in the long-term effects of ecstasy being clouded in uncertainty. It is equally true that there is still a certain amount of disagreement both within and outside the research community as to how dangerous ecstasy is.[216] This is particularly the case with regard to the effect of ecstasy on the brain and brain and cognitive functioning (see for example, Saunders 1998; Concar 2002). Very recent Australian research has explored the impact of regular use of ecstasy on memory function. This study suggests that still no firm results can be posited that links such drug use with memory impairment or deficit (Simon & Mattick 2002).[217]

Another Australian study found a reduction in memory retention and performance in ecstasy users compared to non-users (Dr Jeff Ward and his research team at the Australian National University). This was still the case even for those users who had not taken the drug for two years (quoted in *Youth Studies Australia* 2002, p.15). Such research is, for the most part, still at an embryonic stage.

Despite the doubts of some scientists as to the effect on brain function of ecstasy and other amphetamine analogues, after a comprehensive review of the medical evidence a recent international symposium on ecstasy felt confident enough to state:

> Thus, there is continuing mounting evidence, by a number of independent research groups, supporting the concept of brain damage as a result of recreational use of MDMA. It appears that the most common functional deficit, so far revealed, is in short term memory... Overall, on the basis of animal and human data, it would appear that brain damage is largely irreversible and does not depend on an extensive history of MDMA use. Hence it is likely that the incidence of this irreversible neurotoxicity will be high in all users of MDMA. As this population ages, and normal brain function naturally declines, the effects

216 Saunders argues that both media reporting of and research into drug use generally, and MDMA specifically, is biased:

'Research into drug use is...biased through the grant application process. Funding to study negative effects of illicit drugs is available, while funding to study possible benefits is not. Publication of results is frequently biased, even respected journals reporting negative results of illicit drug use without evidence' (Saunders 1998, p.98).

217 One longitudinal study that does explore the links between MDMA and cognitive disorders is that of Zakzanis and Young (2001). While the authors found that '[c]ontinued use of MDMA is associated with different aspects of memory decline' (p.967), they acknowledged that the results were preliminary and could possibly have been at least in part skewed if the sample group had been taking drugs or substances other than or in addition to MDMA. For research that suggests there is a clear association between MDMA use and impaired memory, see Morgan (1999); Parrott et al. (1998); Parrott, Sisk and Turner (2000); and Freese, Miotto and Reback (2002).

> of previous MDMA brain damage may present itself as a range of neurological and/or cognitive disorders... (Gowing et al. 2001, pp.23, 24).[218]

Long-term effects are also difficult to track and detect because many MDMA users may also be poly-drug users (Beck 1989 in Fitzgerald 1991). Nonetheless, there is a general acceptance, as stated above, that long-term use, frequent use and particularly taking large amounts may have an effect on neurotoxicity,[219] memory and cognition problems, and possibly depression.

MDMA and psychiatric morbidity

Other than problems pertaining to cognition and memory outlined above, depression and low mood 'is reported by users as relatively common in the week following ecstasy use' (Gowing et al. 2001, p.33). Gowing et al. review the published literature on psychiatric sequelae attributed to ecstasy use and find that there are definite connections of varying severity in three groups: altered mental state associated with intoxication; persistent or chronic sequelae; and in a very small number of cases, suicide. They summarise the research as follows:

> Overall, these reports indicate a clear association between ecstasy use and subsequent short-term mood changes. More severe psychiatric sequelae, including depression, panic disorders, psychoses and anxiety, may occur but probably only in those individuals made vulnerable by personal or family history of psychiatric disturbance, by stress or by concurrent use of other drugs (Gowing et al. 2001, p.34; but see also Landabaso et al. 2002; Vaiva et al. 2001 for an argument that MDMA induced psychotic episodes may be more common than otherwise thought).

A British study comparing 12 heavy recreational users of ecstasy, 16 light users and 22 non-ecstasy user controls with group mean ages of 21 was conducted in 2000 (Parrott, Sisk & Turner 2000). The study found that:

> Heavy Ecstasy users reported significantly higher scores than controls on the following SCL-90 factors: paranoid ideation, psychoticism, Somatisation, obsessionality, anxiety, hostility, phobic anxiety, altered appetite and restless sleep, together with greater IVE impulsiveness. Light ecstasy users generally produced intermediate scores, with significantly higher scores than controls on two factors and significantly lower scores than heavy ecstasy users on another two. Previous reports have described various psychiatric and psychobiological disorders in recreational ecstasy users, but it is not known how typical they are, being mainly based on individual case studies. This is the first study to describe

---

218 For specific accounts of MDMA and its links with cognitive functioning, including memory deficits, see Wareing, Fisk and Murphy 2000; Black, Farrell and McGuire 1992. The latter relatively early article questions whether MDMA has the potential to induce psychiatric illness that otherwise may not occur or merely exacerbates it in people already susceptible. For further discussion of the effects of MDMA on the serotonergic system, see Koesters, Rogers and Rajasingham 2002; Tancer and Johanson 2001.

219 Boot, McGregor and Hall state that a review of MDMA studies suggests that 'MDMA can be neurotoxic with those who use two or more doses of MDMA at a time, who inject it, or use it frequently' (2000, p.1818).

> psychological problems in a non clinical sample of young recreational ecstasy users. However, our ecstasy users were polydrug users, with both groups showing significantly greater usage of amphetamine, LSD and cocaine than the controls. These other illicit drugs probably contributed to their adverse psychobiological profiles, while there is also the possibility of pre-existing differences between ecstasy users and non users. However, since repeated MDMA can cause serotonergic neurotoxicity in laboratory animals and man, these problems may reflect reduced serotonin activity inducted by regular ecstasy use (Parrott, Sisk & Turner 2000, p.105).[220]

The concern with regard to poly-drug use among ecstasy users is similar to that found in the South Australian ecstasy use study cited earlier (NDARC 2002c). The psychological and psychiatric side effects experienced by the respondents to that study were profiled for convenience earlier in this chapter (in the section pertaining to physical health consequences of ecstasy use).

In short, it would seem that while there are clearly some minor psychological consequences of using ecstasy observable (predominantly low mood, shifting mood), further research is required into the psychiatric sequelae consequent to frequent, heavy or long-term use of ecstasy, particularly when used in combination with other drugs.

An MDMA dependence syndrome?

There is no reliable, or at least comprehensive, evidence that the use of MDMA is addictive or even with prolonged use can lead to a 'dependence syndrome' similar to that found with opiates, alcohol and some forms of amphetamine (as discussed above). One of the reasons that this may have been the case, at least until recently, is that 'there are simply no reports on individuals who take frequent and large amounts of MDMA for an extended period of time' (Petrouka 1990 in Jansen 1999, p.121). However, Jansen (1999) has noted some case studies where it could be stated that criteria for dependence has now been met:

> MDMA is described as non-addictive, as was amphetamine itself earlier this century... However, there are now reports of individuals who have used large quantities for extended periods... These reports usually focus on adverse effects and rarely consider dependence as a specific issue. [This report describes] ...three cases [that] indicated MDMA can be addictive in certain cases. Identification and treatment is important as there is some evidence to suggest that high intensity MDMA use may cause lasting changes to serotonergic nerve terminals...
>
> A dependence syndrome requires at least three of the following: a strong desire to take the drug; difficulties controlling the behaviour; a withdrawal state;

220 Kish argues that the evidence that ecstasy exposure has toxic effects on human brain serotonion neurons is far from conclusive. He argues that many of the studies that seek to establish this connection are methodologically flawed: 'Until these issues are resolved it cannot be assumed that ecstasy exposure represents a chronic serotonin deficiency condition' (Kish 2002, p.845).

> tolerance, progressive neglect of alternative pleasures; and persisting with use despite evidence of harm (WHO, 1992). These features occurred in all three cases who considered themselves harmed in various ways, made attempts to stop but yielded to a compelling desire to re-use, and listed fatigue, low mood, anxiety and sleep disturbance as withdrawal phenomena. One case was also amphetamine dependent, one was also dependent on benzodiazepines and opioids with a relatively high regular alcohol intake, and one also had a high daily alcohol intake verging on dependence (Jansen 1999, pp.121, 123).

While Jansen's studies are interesting and not without merit, it would seem that far more research needs to be undertaken and similar cases documented for the medical and academic community to be able to pronounce with any certainty that such a syndrome does exist.

Indeed, there seems to be very little authoritative knowledge or understanding of any of the long-term effects of ecstasy. This has flow-on effects to information and education campaigns concerning the drug. As Hammersley, Khan and Ditton state:

> [t]here is considerable ignorance coupled to considerable apprehension about the long-term effects of Ecstasy. It is ironic that the very area that users are most concerned about is also the very area that medical, or other, science is least able to help with information (Hammersley, Khan & Ditton 2002, p.156).

MDMA and mortality[221]

In a recent comprehensive review of the health effects of ecstasy Linda Gowing and her colleagues at the Drug and Alcohol Services Council of South Australia state that although:

> [t]he incidence of serious acute adverse events related to ecstasy is low [i]t is the unpredictability of those adverse effects and the risk of mortality and substantial morbidity that makes the health consequences of ecstasy significant (Gowing et al. 2001, p.53).

Hyperthermia and hyponatraemia

Hyperthermia and hyponatraemia (with consequent cerebral oedema)[222] are the most potentially life threatening of the conditions associated with MDMA

221 For an analysis of Victorian mortality data, see Chapter 5.

222 Concar, drawing from the research of toxicologist and MDMA expert John Henry of St Mary's Hospital, London, explains the relationship between MDMA ingestion and hyponatraemia:

'Henry has discovered that MDMA makes the brain's hypothalamus secrete a substance known as antidiuretic hormone, which stops the kidney producing urine and makes it hard for MDMA users to pass water even if they are drinking pints of it. If they do drink excessively…in rare cases, the blood thins and the brain swells, creating a pressure that in extreme cases pushes the brainstem down the spine where it can no longer support breathing' (Concar 20002, p.31).

For further discussions of the link between MDMA use, hyperthermia and hyponatraemia, see Matthai et al. 1996; Cook 1996; Wilkins 1996; Parr, Low and Botterill 1997; Gowing et al. 2001; Traub, Hoffmann and Nelson 2002.

use. Their manifestation or at least the severity of the outcomes may be in large part dependent on the setting:

> Some MDMA-related complications, such as cardiac arrhythmias and cerebral infarctions, are related to the acute pharmacological properties of MDMA that are shared by a number of amphetamine-type stimulants. Other complications, such as severe hyperthermia with rhabdomyolysis, renal failure and disseminated intravascular coagulation, are more probably related to the use of MDMA in 'raves' and dance parties, where individuals participate in extreme physical activity for prolonged periods in a hot crowded setting (Henry 1992; McCann *et al* 1996).[223] MDMA can produce hyperthermia in quiet surroundings, when taken in sufficient quantity (Green *et al* 1995) but in the setting of 'raves' or dance parties, the toxicity appears to be enhanced; it is probably a combination of direct effects of MDMA and the high ambient temperature, sustained physical activity and inadequate fluid replacement, all reducing heat loss and potentiating the direct effect of MDMA on thermoregulatory mechanisms, that creates the greatest toxicity (Gowing et al. 2001, p.25).[224]

Jones (1998) explains in somewhat distressing detail the ways in which hyperthermia and heatstroke can contribute to MDMA related deaths. While acknowledging that fatalities associated with ecstasy are low in number, they can have severe and dramatic manifestations:

> When MDMA produces problems, they are frequently severe and unpredictable. Generally speaking, the course of events seems to be:
>
> - The victims are out in a nightclub, rave party or concert;
> - They faint or fit;
> - They are taken to hospital where their limbs may be twisted and rigid;
> - Their temperature is recorded at 40–42 degrees Celsius;
> - They bruise easily and drip sites start to bleed;
> - They start to bleed profusely;
> - Death supervenes even where there are multiple infusions of donated blood and clotting factors.
>
> What causes this bleeding to occur? The leading theory is that Ecstasy deaths are the result of the drug and of the setting in which the drug is used. Ecstasy has the tendency, as do many stimulant drugs (Jones & Owens 1996), to alter the body's internal thermostat and incline the body to overheat in hot, ambient atmospheres. In this condition, clubbers dance the night away without the insight of a 'normal' person into their own internal environment.

---

223 For an account of the difficulties in tabulating and defining what is a death attributable to MDMA use, see Gore 1999 and the discussion in Chapter 5.

224 See also Greene et al. for case studies of MDMA toxicity amongst a group of seven nightclub patrons hospitalised in the United States (Greene et al. 2003). For a discussion of the potentially lethal consequences of using MDMA in conjunction with other [pharmaceutical] drugs such as moclobemide, see Vuori et al. 2003. Moclobemide, an antidepressant, is a drug affecting serotonin release. As with other monoamine oxidase A inhibitors there is a strong risk of an adverse reaction if ingested simultaneously with MDMA (see Vouri et al. 2003).

> Nightclubs are often damp, hot places where the high humidity may make sweat evaporation impossible. Add to this the dehydration caused by vigorous dancing, and several conditions coexist:
>
> - Loss of body heat regulation
> - Creation of more and more body heat
> - Loss of ability to dissipate the heat.
>
> This creates a rising core body temperature. Beyond a certain point, the rise in temperature causes problems to develop. The first body system to react is the central nervous system, which is very sensitive to abnormalities in temperature. High temperature caused by Ecstasy-induced heatstroke causes fainting and/or fitting in the victim. Other problems associated with high core temperature (and reported by medical staff caring for Ecstasy victims) include liver and kidney problems, but mainly disorders of the body's clotting system. This involves a condition called DIC (disseminated intravascular coagulation) (Clowes & O'Donnell 1974, Oh 1990), which involves inappropriate formulation of small blood clots across a wide area of the body's blood vessels, causing those components of blood usually reserved for plugging holes to be activated and attracted to areas of clot formation. These clotting promoters are used up faster than they can be produced, causing a depletion of clotting material in the circulating bloodstream. Without clotting material, the patient will bleed spontaneously from nose, mouth and gastrointestinal tract, and in severe cases, will bleed to death. There are blood tests that will reveal that this process is under way.
>
> Certainly the theory that these fatalities are caused by heatstroke could explain the deaths by pointing to variations in the amount of dancing, fluid intake and so on, though it has to be said that, to the writer's knowledge, no empirical study of these variables has been conducted: Did the victim dance a lot? Did the victim drink enough? Was the club hot that night? etc. (Jones 1998, pp.95–96).

The emergence of hyponatraemia as a factor contributing to MDMA-associated mortality suggests that well meaning advice with regard to fluid consumption when ingesting ecstasy needs to be modified or at least tailored to the setting in question. An examination of harm reduction techniques with regard to MDMA is given in Chapter 19 . Suffice to state in this context that the message 'Drink lots of fluids' may not be useful and could be actually bad advice in cases where there is a potential for water overload. As Parr, Low and Botterill state:

> Among the many adverse reactions [to ecstasy] we must now include life threatening hyponatraemia, which may have the same symptoms and signs as MDMA intoxication. To avoid adverse reactions, individuals using MDMA at dance parties are often advised to rest, avoid overheating, wear loose clothing and drink plenty of cool drinks. However, there is no evidence that this prevents adverse reactions. Furthermore, because of the possibility of hyponatraemia, this advice should be modified to suggest ingesting only moderate amounts of liquids (Parr, Low & Botterill 1997, p.137).

Substituting toxic drugs

As indicated earlier, ecstasy use has also been associated with death when what was purported to be MDMA has, on analysis, turned out to be a different more toxic drug. The other drug most usually associated in these circumstances is paramethoxyamphetamine (PMA). Paramethoxyamphetamine is viewed as having 'much more serious adverse effects than other ring derivative amphetamines' (Byard et al. 2002, p.496). Byard et al. state: 'A knowledge of the higher rate of complications occurring with PMA ingestion by users is reflected in…its street name – "death"…' (Byard et al. 1999, p.139). In 1998, six cases of death due to PMA were reported in South Australia (see Felgate et al. 1998; Byard et al. 2002). The pathologists associated with the cases have subsequently commented:

> In 1998, our group warned that although PMA substitution for MDMA appeared at the time to be a local Australian problem, there was a possibility that the manufacture and sale of PMA could occur in other countries. Unfortunately, this prediction has proved accurate, with recent reports of PMA related deaths in the United States, Europe and Canada (Byard et al. 1999, p.139).

Felgate's analysis of the six South Australian deaths in 1998 indicates that PMA is certainly available in localised areas and is of particular concern: 'It is routinely sold as "ecstasy" but would appear to be more toxic than MDMA' (Felgate et al. 1998, p.171). The symptoms of ecstasy poisoning and that of PMA are quite similar, the difference being in the severity of the consequences. One Adelaide study showed:

> [t]hat most people with PMA poisoning present with clinical features that are qualitatively similar to those of people with ecstasy poisoning (ie. hyperthermia, coma and seizures), but that these symptoms occur more frequently and are more severe in those who took PMA (Ling et al. 2001, p.455).

It was thought that in most, if not all, of the PMA deaths reported in Australia the drug users thought they were taking MDMA, when in fact PMA was present as a contaminant (White, Bochner & Irvine 1997).

Such a development gives rise to concern by drug and alcohol workers that taking ecstasy is becoming part of a 'lucky dip' (see for example, Moriarty 2001).[225]

Gowing et al. (2001) reviewed a number of cases of MDMA-related mortality in which PMA was involved:

> It is possible to conclude from these data that, although a number of cases of acute adverse effects involved other drugs instead of or in addition to MDMA, MDMA alone can produce adverse effects. Of the 35 cases in which only MDMA was detected, 21 involved hyperthermia and 10 of these (48%) were fatal. A further eight cases involved disturbances of sodium or fluid balance,

225 For a stark, if at times somewhat sensationalist, account of a young man's death as a result of PMA ingestion, see 'Timeline of a PMA death', *Drugs in Society*, June 2001, p.9.

> with three (38%) fatal. The remaining six cases involved cardiac factors (1 fatal), a cerebral haemorrhage (1 non-fatal), respiratory factors (1 fatal), a sudden collapse (fatal), and trauma whilst intoxicated (2 fatal). Given that hyperthermia and disturbances of sodium or fluid balance generally occur when MDMA is used in nightclub or dance party settings, these data suggest that the acute adverse effects of MDMA arise from the way it is used, rather than solely an inherent toxic effect of the drug.
>
> This may not be the case with PMA (para methoxyamphetamine). There are two major clusters of deaths associated with PMA: nine cases in Ontario, Canada in 1973 (Cimbura 1974) and six cases in South Australia between 1995 and 1998 (Byard *et al* 1998; Byard *et al* 1999). Media reports (New York Times, 30 September 2000, USA Today, 6 October 2000) indicate that a further cluster of PMA-related deaths occurred in Florida, USA and Ontario, Canada in the first half of 2000. Of the 16 published case reports involving PMA, seven involved hyperthermia, five involved seizures, one a cerebral haemorrhage, and three were classed as miscellaneous, largely because of insufficient information. It is notable that in one of the cases reported by Byard *et al*, 'ecstasy' use occurred in a home setting over a 12 hour period and a maximum body temperature of 46.1 was recorded on admission to hospital. This case, together with several others involving ingestion of PMA in home settings, suggest that the adverse effects of PMA may be related more to the action of the drug rather than the way it is used. The higher incidence of seizures associated with PMA is suggestive of a more powerful central nervous system effect.
>
> This makes it impossible to determine whether the apparently high mortality rate associated with PMA reflects the administration of high doses, or whether PMA is inherently more toxic than MDMA (Gowing et al. 2001, pp.30–31).

In a meeting with the Committee Professor Jason White, Director of Treatment and Rehabilitation Services at the Drugs and Alcohol Services Council of South Australia, highlighted the fact that Adelaide may have the less than enviable claim of being the PMA capital of the world:

> We have had a major PMA problem in South Australia, that you may be aware of, over a few years. It has declined in the last 12 months or so, although there was a recent major seizure of PMA, suggesting that it may still be active. The only reasonable explanation is that it is made in South Australia. Why else would Adelaide become almost the PMA capital of the world? We just have more PMA here than anywhere else. At its peak, a little under 50 per cent of the seizures for Ecstasy were actually PMA, and there would be nowhere else that would be like that. The only reasonable explanation is that it is made here; whether because the person found it a little bit easier chemically or because they believed that those effects were desired by people. It was sometimes marketed as Ecstasy; sometimes separately. The attractive trade name of Death was the other name it was marketed under. And some people actively sought

> out PMA, they wanted it, and so the reason for manufacture may have been associated with that.[226]

Whatever the precise linkages between PMA, MDMA and adverse health consequences are, clearly more research is necessary to get a picture of the interaction of these drugs.

Physical and psychological consequences – Other 'party drugs'

GHB and ketamine

Most of the side effects associated with the use of these drugs have been outlined in Chapter 4, however some of the more salient points are repeated in this context.

GHB

A small amount of GHB can produce feelings of exhilaration, euphoria and well being. It may also heighten libid.o or cause sexual disinhibition contributing to its reputation as a 'date rape' drug. Higher doses can lead to disorientation, nausea, blackouts, headaches, seizures, a numbing of the muscles or muscle spasms, loss of consciousness, hypoventilation and vomiting:

> After long term use at high doses, there may be a withdrawal reaction – rapid heartbeat, tremor, insomnia, anxiety and occasionally hallucinations that last a few days to a week. According to the Drug Enforcement Administration [USA], the use of GHB has been associated with 5,700 reported overdoses and 66 deaths over the years, mainly from respiratory depression. The danger seems to come mostly from mixtures with alcohol or opiates (Harvard Mental Health Letter 2001, p.19).

Galloway et al. state that the effects of GHB appear to be 'highly dose dependent':

> The dose response curve for GHB is steep and exceeding the recommended or intoxicating dose can result in severe adverse effects. Effects of GHB in humans include somnolence leading to arousable sleep at 40–50mg/kg and at 60–70 mg/kg, coma for 1–2 hours... The lethal dose has been estimated at 5–15 times that inducing coma (Galloway et al. 1997, p.91)

Particular concern has been expressed regarding the interaction of GHB with other central nervous system depressants, in particular alcohol or MDMA and methamphetamines (Galloway et al. 1997). Again such a mixture makes unsuspecting people, particularly women, vulnerable to assault (Nicholson & Balster 2001).

Sanguineti, Angelo and Frank (1997) also point to the dangers of perceiving GHB as a relatively safe drug when taken in the context of body building or a context outside of recreational drug use. Using a case study of a bodybuilder

226 Professor Jason White, in conversation with the Drugs and Crime Prevention Committee, Adelaide, 3 October 2003.

presenting with visual and auditory hallucinations in addition to depression and anxiety they state:

> The case shows...how misinformation and mislabeling are a main source of the problem with products such as GHB. An athlete or bodybuilder like Mr J who already has a tendency to use illicit safe compounds like anabolic steroids, is lulled into a false sense of security by the way the information is given... The athlete is therefore encouraged to consider these effects as minor irritants from an otherwise natural product and is prone to ingest higher doses than recommended as it appears these doses may otherwise be safe. Symptoms are therefore underreported or unreported (Sanguineti, Angelo & Frank 1997, p.638).[227]

The authors state that this false sense of security is particularly heightened when GHB is marketed in terms of a 'tonic' or 'health stuff':

> Given today's abundance of alternative medical ingredients and the explosion of health stores rich in arcane concoctions, it may be easy for the physician not to recognise the relatively obscure mention of GHB (Sanguineti, Angelo & Frank 1997, p.638).

McDaniel and Miotto have documented five case studies that tend to indicate there is a discrete withdrawal syndrome for GHB use with concomitant dependence on the drug:

> The most common signs and symptoms include anxiety, tremor, insomnia, episodes of tachycardia, affective lability, confusion, paranoia, agitation, delirium, and hallucinations... The observed withdrawal syndrome in these five patients lasted from three to 13 days. In all cases the initial symptoms of anxiety, tremor and insomnia manifested within two to eight hours of last reported dose. Tachycardia was seen within 12 hours of last dosing. In cases of severe withdrawal, psychosis and delirium developed within 48 hours of last use.
>
> The development of addiction in this sample was rapid and unexpected. Patients initially considered GHB or GBL [an analogue] a safe supplement and none expected to transition from short term use to long term dependence (McDaniel & Miotto 2001, pp.146–147).[228]

One of the few recent studies on GHB use in Australia was conducted recently by researchers from NDARC. The study examined the correlates, context and risk perceptions regarding GHB overdose among a survey of 76 users in Sydney and Melbourne recruited in 2001. The survey subjects were divided into those who had overdosed on the drug and those who had not:

---

227 For an account of a (rare) case of psychiatric hospitalisation due to GHB induced delirium, see Hernandez et al. 1998.

228 For case studies of coma induced by the abuse of GHB, in Britain and the United States, see Thomas, Bonner and Gascoigne 1997; Ingels et al. 2000; and Reeves and Duda 2003. The Committee has received much anecdotal evidence from people working within the rave and club scene in Victoria that GHB gives rise to the most problems in terms of medical emergencies. This is the case both in regard to the number of casualties and the severity of the complications or consequences. For example, see Chapters 4 and 6.

> In both groups the majority were male, had a mean age of 27 years, the average education completed was the completion of high school; and around 60% of both groups identified as homosexual or bisexual[229](Degenhardt, Darke & Dillon 2003, p.201).

Of particular importance this study found that:

> Despite only having relatively recent and infrequent use of GHB, *half* had overdosed after using GHB. This suggests that users may be at high risk of overdosing, even after little involvement with the drug (2003, p.202). (Committee emphasis)

Subjects who had never overdosed were far less likely to believe they would ever overdose in any circumstances than those subjects who had already overdosed. However, the authors state that there were very few factors that distinguished an overdose risk situation:

> [o]ther than a tendency for those who had overdosed to be celebrating a special event of some kind. This suggests that harm minimisation messages might be best targeted during periods in which such celebrations are likely to occur (2002, pp.203–204).[230]

Many of the respondents to this Inquiry, particularly those involved with the dance party or rave industry, have expressed serious misgivings about the drug GHB. For example Mr Ben Horan, formerly harm minimisation and first aid officer with ZoS nightclub in Prahran, notes that of all the drug-related first aid incidents seen at dance venues, GHB is the drug most often involved and the one that produces the most serious consequences in terms of injury and/or hospitalisation.[231] Pip Darvall, the chief promoter of the dance 'rave' *Earthcore*, has expressed similar concerns:

> [we] have a lot of medical incidents at the event, more than we have had in the past and basically...over half of the serious incidents were to do with the drug GHB.
>
> It's a serious no-no; it's a stupid drug for people to take. We're going to do a newsletter[232]mail out this afternoon [warning of the consequences of taking the drug]...one girl ended up in a very serious condition as a result of taking a dose...they tell me the dose she took was enough to kill an elephant, well luckily it didn't but one day someone is going to die, guaranteed, it's just the law of averages...
>
> [The newsletter notice]... It will just be a very simple text one 'you guys are being stupid, we can only go so far in our harm minimisation and you guys

---

229 This fact is certainly significant in terms of tailoring education and harm reduction strategies, see also discussion of drug use among gay and lesbian populations in Chapter 9.

230 The Sydney Mardi Gras would be a prime example where this type of overdose might occur.

231 Mr Ben Horan, in conversation with the Drugs and Crime Prevention Committee staff, Melbourne, 25 November 2003.

232 The *Earthcore* event has its own web site with an electronic newsletter and participants forum attached. See www.earthcore.com.au

> need to take care of both yourselves and your mates because we can set the safety net up but we can't stop you falling into the net through your stupidity'. We will give them the basic facts that x number of ambulances came, x number of those were to do with GHB and some day one of you is going to die and if it's not you, its going to be someone you know.[233]

Just prior to completing the writing of this Report, the Committee was concerned to hear of a major incident in which GHB had allegedly featured heavily. On the 7 March during the Labour Day holiday weekend the *Two Tribes* 'Rave' was held at Rod Laver Arena, Melbourne Park. According to press reports, ten unconscious partygoers were rushed to a local hospital in a 'serious condition' as a result of taking the liquid form of the drug.[234] All the victims were later released from hospital.

Predictable responses such as calling for the banning of major dance parties at such venues followed. Yet none of the harm minimisation procedures profiled in Chapter 19 of this Report, including the presence of ambulances on site, appeared to be present. Harm minimisation and reduction strategies and procedures are discussed at length in Chapter 19 of this Report.

Given that GHB is a relatively new drug on the scene, the issues of a GHB dependence and withdrawal syndrome, and the short-term and acute reactions to the drug particularly associated with its use at venues such as raves and dance parties, need to be researched much more comprehensively. Precipitate responses, however, are of little value and serve only to obfuscate serious approaches to the damage caused by such drugs.

Ketamine

There is very little known about the long-term effects of taking ketamine regularly as a recreational drug.[235] Because of its anaesthetic qualities, people have been known to hurt themselves after having taken the drug and not realise until the following day. Ketamine, as with GHB, MDMA and other psychostimulants, should not be taken with respiratory depressants, primarily alcohol, or benzodiazepines because of the potentially lethal consequences of interaction.[236] Large doses could induce unconsciousness, which could lead to cardiovascular failure. Although not physically addictive, some users have developed a strong habit (Drug Enforcement Administration 2003).

---

233 Mr Pip Darvall, in conversation with the Drugs and Crime Prevention Committee staff, 12 December 2003.

234 See for example, Christine Caulfield, Milanda Rout and Paul Anderson, 'Youth put lives on line to party', *Herald-Sun*, 9 March 2004, p.3.

235 Nearly all studies over the past three decades have been with regard to its use in medical science (see Jansen 2001).

236 For a detailed account of the immediate effects on the human body after having taken a dose of ketamine, see Jansen 2001, pp.83ff.

Use of the drug can cause delirium, amnesia, depression, and long-term memory and cognitive difficulties (see Jansen 1993; Dotson, Ackerman & West 1995; Curran & Morgan 2000; Dillon & Degenhardt 2001; Jansen 2001).

Of particular concern is the dissociative symptomology associated with the drug. The out of consciousness or K-hole effect (see Chapter 4) can have dangerous consequences. The physical dangers associated with the drug may, as Dillon and Degenhardt comment, stem not so much from the drug itself as from the context of its use. Jansen explains this further:

> As ketamine has a good physical safety profile and an established place in medicine, within current indications what are the reasons for concern about its non-medical use? The first and most important reason is that ketamine can readily induce a state of virtual helplessness, within the dose range normally taken by users, to a far greater extent than most other substances of abuse. The dissociation can be very dramatic, such that awareness of the environment is completely lost while the user experiences a 'separate reality', a marked reduction in sensory input in all modalities, and difficulty with movement. This is almost never the case with substances such as 3,4-methylenedioxymethamphetamine. The helplessness of the dissociative state may not be a problem for a patient in a protected setting, but at a large social gathering the chances that a disconnected person experiencing incoordination and analgesia may come to harm are substantially increased.
>
> A further cause for concern is that ketamine can sometimes result in a state where the users are unconcerned whether they live or die. This is not a depressive or suicidal phenomenon but is related to the particular effect of the dissociative state upon the mind. "If you have a full-blown experience of K, you can never believe there is death, or that death can possibly influence who you are." Again, this may not be a problem in a protected setting but is cause for concern in a public place.
>
> In some people ketamine has the potential for compulsive, repeated use; cases of self administered injections several times daily over prolonged periods have been reported. Long term use of high doses of ketamine has the potential to interfere with memory, learning, and attentional mechanisms due to blockade of the N-methyl-D-aspartate receptor, although there is no clear evidence of this at present. Ketamine has been associated with recurring phenomena ('flashbacks') although whether these result from drug induced physiological changes or are a functional response to anxiety in predisposed personalities is still unclear. (In these cases flashbacks may involve little more than a 'graininess' of vision under anxiety provoking circumstances) (Jansen 1993, p.601).[237]

237 For example, John C. Lilly, the 'guru' and promoter of ketamine use as a transcendental or mind expanding drug has only contempt for those who use ketamine in a club setting. For a comprehensive account of ketamine as a mind enhancing drug and the role of Lilly in its promotion, see Jansen 2001.

It would seem on the basis of, admittedly meagre, research studies that ketamine use per se is unlikely to have fatal consequences.[238] In New York for example:

> There are very few deaths by pure ketamine overdose recorded (ie. not involving another drug such as alcohol). Of 87 ketamine-linked deaths in New York City, none was solely attributable to the use of ketamine (Dillon, Copeland & Jansen 2003, p.24).

Jansen states that the side effects of ketamine use are very much linked to the setting in which the drug is taken:

> A pleasant set and setting are more likely to have a positive outcome, while an unpleasant set and setting are more likely to have a negative outcome (Jansen 2001, p.72).

A recent research study conducted by the NDARC has identified current recreational patterns of non-medical ketamine use and the potential harms associated with its ingestion. A survey of 100 non-medical users of ketamine in Sydney produced some interesting results. Only one-quarter of the sample reported use of ketamine without any other drug. Conversely, ecstasy had been used in conjunction with ketamine by 71 per cent of the sample. Fourteen of the survey participants reported having accessed the drug at their place of work (doctors, nurses, veterinarians and a pharmacist). The study summed up its conclusions by stating:

> In this sample of ketamine users, ketamine appeared to be a drug that had been added to an already extensive drug use repertoire. They were generally a well educated group of people, few of whom were in relationships, and largely have high incomes. They appeared to be an older group of 'party drug' users in contrast with a sample of regular ecstasy users interviewed in a similar period ...
>
> Many users had experienced significant effects; such that some had either reduced their dose or stopped use altogether. In particular, many users reported regularly experiencing an inability to speak, blurred vision, lack of co-ordination, and increased body temperature. All of these symptoms have potentially serious implications for the safety of the user. However, for many of those who reported experiencing these symptoms, they were seen as the positive effects of the drug (Dillon, Copeland & Jansen 2003, p.27).

Clearly there is a paucity of information associated with ketamine. The Committee would certainly encourage researchers in the field to turn their attention to the recreational use of ketamine used both on its own and in conjunction with other drugs.

---

238 Jansen argues that the number of people who suffer negative effects from ketamine or who 'lose control over their use' is unlikely to exceed 15 per cent (2001, p.166).

Conclusion

Although the medical consequences that follow from the use of drugs such as amphetamines and MDMA are clearly sufficient to give rise to concern, these are not the only adverse considerations that need to be taken into account with regard to their use. The social (or anti-social) costs that may occur through the use of these drugs are also significant. The following chapter will examine the links between the use of the drugs and the possible links with crime, violence and anti-social behaviour.

7. Social Consequences of Amphetamines and 'Party Drug' Use

As with any discussion of drugs and the way they impact upon society, *who* is taking the drug and the use to which it is being put will have a decided bearing on the consequences for the community at large. For example, the truck driver who regularly uses amphetamines to maintain tight delivery schedules may 'cost' the community in terms of road accidents or trauma. For the methamphetamine 'addict' who steals to maintain his or her habit, there is the obvious cost of crime in the community. The examples could be replicated depending on the drug and the reason the person is taking it. This chapter discusses some of the more common and serious social consequences of amphetamine and 'party drug' use. It concentrates on any possible links between the use of these drugs (particularly amphetamines) and the manifestation of crime or violent behaviour. Often such violent behaviour is linked to mental health disturbance, particularly paranoia and the amphetamine psychosis discussed earlier. A discussion of a particular type of criminal behaviour, the unfortunately relatively common practice of 'drink spiking', then follows.

This chapter also examines the links between the use of these drugs and road trauma, including but not exclusive to the use of amphetamines by long-distance drivers. The chapter concludes with a brief discussion of the costs of absenteeism, particularly in the context of 'party drug' use.

Violence, crime and (meth)amphetamine use

It is a truism but nonetheless accurate to state that not all people who abuse drugs turn to crime, just as not all criminals are drug-dependent. There are a range of well documented methodological problems related to drawing links between drug use and crime, not the least of which is that many of the studies that seek to explain the links rely on 'captive samples', usually those in prisons, youth detention centres or drug treatment facilities.[239] Bevan and Loxley warn

239 For an account of drug-related criminal behaviour among detainees in participating watch-houses across Australia, see Weierter and Lynch 2002. The authors analyse data from the Drug Use Monitoring in Australia (DUMA) survey funded by the Commonwealth's Illicit Drug Strategy. For a general review of the literature on the links between substance abuse and violence, see Boles and Miotto 2003.

that '[p]atterns of drug use may differ between incarcerated offenders and those who engage in criminal behaviour but are not incarcerated' (1997, p.65). Having taken heed of these warnings and given the limitations of current research this chapter will in part explore some of the issues that arise with regard to a possible nexus between (amphetamine) use and crime and violent behaviour. Thus the following discussion is very much centred on a particular subset of amphetamine user.

This discussion does not canvass an examination of crime and violence related to MDMA use or its analogues. Nearly all of the profiles done of ecstasy users fail to reveal any links between such use and criminal behaviour (other than the 'scoring' of the drug itself).[240] At most, ecstasy users may generally deal on a small scale to cover the costs of purchase. Often this will be a case of sales to friends and associates and rarely result in any profit (see Moore 1992a, p.630). 'Party drug' users on the whole seem to be law-abiding and non-violent.[241] This is especially the case given that most ecstasy use is primarily experimental and social. 'Most users adopt[ed] patterns and dosages that fail[ed] to produce dependence and significant psychopathology' (Siegel 1986 in Moore 1992a, p.9).[242] This may change of course, as suggested by reports of an increasing trend

---

240 One area where there is cause for concern regarding a link between crime and 'party drugs' is the use of the 'date rape' drugs GHB and rohypnol. Ostensibly these drugs are surreptitiously slipped into unsuspecting people's drinks for the purposes of taking advantage of them sexually (see McKey 2000 and discussion later in this Chapter and in Chapter 19). The Committee has also received some disturbing accounts of violence associated with the nightclub scene in Melbourne, both within and outside the clubs (See also discussion in Chapter 17). It is difficult to know without further investigation whether this violence is drug induced or produced and if so by what type of drugs. Certainly the media publicity surrounding the closure of one particular nightclub in South Yarra, Melbourne, would suggest that there are indeed links between drug use and the nightclub scene, although how much of that is attributable to alcohol as compared to other 'party drugs' is a matter of conjecture.

241 For an account of possible links between ketamine use and violence, see Jansen 2001. Jansen argues that such links (in the United States) are grossly exaggerated. Murders and other forms of interpersonal violence that the American press have associated with ketamine:

'[w]ould not have occurred had the murderer not taken alcohol, crack cocaine or amphetamines. Ketamine is sometimes taken together with these three drugs, and this might increase the risk of violence' (Jansen 2001, p.260).

242 Webb argues that the criminalisation of MDMA and other 'party drugs' creates a frustrating paradox:

'Technically, every MDMA user commits a drug-defined offence. The question then, is whether or not a reason for MDMA's prohibition is that it its use leads to drug-related offences or interactional criminal circumstances. As the Australian Federal Police comments, the "impact of illicit drugs is of particular concern because of the 'flow-on' effect to other categories of crime such as armed robbery, theft and burglary".

Surveys of Australian ecstasy users reveal that around 50% had committed the offence of supplying ecstasy. However, it is paradoxical for the widespread occurrence of drug-defined offences to act as their own justification. These surveys found that apart from dealing drugs, very few ecstasy users were involved in criminal activity. This reflects the growing acceptance that MDMA has minimal harmful effects on the criminal justice system. For instance, a forthcoming report on the link between drugs and crime has found that MDMA use, unlike other illicit drug use, causes low amounts of criminal activity. Further there is no evidence that MDMA causes violent crime by inducing heightened aggression in users' (Webb 2003, pp.108–109).

For further discussion of MDMA 'dealing', see Chapters 10, 12 and 17.

to injecting ecstasy and a perceptible, if slight as yet, shift from ecstasy being used as a 'party drug' to a street drug.[243]

It is thought, not surprisingly, that the heavier the use of amphetamine and methamphetamines the greater the potential for using crime or its proceeds to obtain the drugs. Lintzeris for example, states:

> In general, the more drugs that people use, the more crime they are going to commit and the more severe the types of crime. Thus, an individual is more likely to be committing crimes more frequently when they are using large amounts of illicit psychostimulants compared to periods of more moderate use. Similarly, individuals using large amounts of illicit psychostimulants are more likely to be committing criminal acts than individuals using smaller amounts (Lintzeris 1994, p.152).

But criminal behaviour serves not only such 'functional' purposes (that is, drug acquisition), it can also be a lifestyle by-product of the violent and even psychotic behaviour associated with some, particularly heavy, amphetamine use. The following quote from Wood (1998a) draws on comments by drugs researcher Nick Lintzeris:

> During his work at Victoria's Pleasant View Centre, a treatment service for substance misuse, Dr Lintzeris saw a significant group of heavy users who were involved in crime.
>
> 'These people were using loads of amphetamine – it was definitely their primary drug – and were engaged in quite a lot of serious crime. Their amphetamine use was most certainly a cultural, lifestyle thing. These were heavy dudes, and it wasn't "let's take some speed and go and have fun" [unlike ecstasy] ...speed was not a fun drug for this group' (Lintzeris quoted in Wood 1998a, p.21).

Both the 'functional' and lifestyle links with crime can be seen in the association between amphetamine use, manufacture and trafficking and certain motorcycle gangs in the United States, Australia and Europe, particularly during the 1970s and 1980s. One social cost of amphetamine use, manufacture and trafficking that is often overlooked is the danger and public health consequences to not only those who manufacture the substances but also to police and emergency personnel who are investigating or otherwise responding to emergency events at clandestine laboratories. Such injuries may be caused either by explosions, fires or the caustic, corrosive, toxic or volatile nature of the chemicals associated with the manufacturing process (see, for example, *Journal of the American Medical Association* 2000). A discussion of amphetamine manufacture, including its links to such gangs, is found in Chapter 14 of this Report. One other area of crime that is clearly of relevance is burglary and theft of amphetamines and amphetamine precursors from pharmacies, chemists and pharmaceutical warehouses. This issue will be discussed in full in Chapter 15.

243 See Chapter 9 for a discussion of profiles of drug use.

Research data on links to violence and crime

There has not been a great amount of research investigating any link between (meth)amphetamine use, crime or violent behaviour. Indeed much of the research is equivocal. For example according to Alexander and Tsou:

> Although amphetamines are often said to incite violence, the evidence for this claim is inconsistent. For example, amphetamine treatment reliably *reduces* violence in hyperactive children and sometimes in adult and experimental animals as well. King and Ellinwood (1992) have summarised the evidence as follows:
>
> The overall pattern of research indicates that the effects of amphetamine on aggressive behaviour are complex and that these effects are not solely determined by the pharmacology of amphetamine but seem to be determined by various environmental factors… (Alexander & Tsou 2001, p.109).

Despite such inconclusiveness, the following studies, however, do make some pertinent and useful observations.

University of California Study 1996/1997

A comprehensive survey of methamphetamine abuse and emergency department utilisation was conducted in a California teaching hospital during 1996/1997. This six-month study examined all admissions to the hospital where patients presented positive to a methamphetamine urine toxicology screen (n = 461). This public hospital (University of California/Davis Medical Centre) 'provides health care for a high proportion of uninsured patients and for those patients brought in by police from the street or jail' (Richards et al. 1999, p.198). Thus the findings have to be read subject to this knowledge.[244] The data of the methamphetamine users were compared against a non-using control of all other emergency department admissions for the period. The study concluded that there were significant social and economic costs to the user and the community from methamphetamine use. This included the costs associated with crime and violence, emergency department utilisation, hospital stays, police, ambulance and mental health transportation, costs of care in gaol and mental health facilities and costs associated with road trauma and accidents.[245] The occurrence of such behaviours seems to escalate when individuals have been 'bingeing' over a period of several days. The authors of the study state that:

244 Sixty-nine per cent of the methamphetamine users (MAU) used ambulance transport to attend the emergency room. This was significantly higher than for non-methamphetamine users (NMAU), 22 per cent of whom used ambulances for transport. Twelve per cent of MAU were brought in by police and four per cent by mental health facility transfer. Fifty-eight per cent of the MAU were admitted to the hospital proper from the emergency treatment (compared to 22% of NMAU). Fourteen per cent of MAU were admitted to an in-patient psychiatric facility and 9 per cent to jail. Significantly 386 of the 461 MAU patients had two or more emergency department visits within the previous 12 months (Richards et al. 1999).

245 Very few of the MAU had medical insurance. The economic costs to the hospital and community were therefore great. This of course reflects a major difference in the American and Australian health care systems, universal health cover such as Medicare not being available in the United States.

> Methamphetamine (MAP) is now the most common drug of abuse presenting to emergency departments (ED) in the western United States. Intoxicated MAP patients often present with agitation, violence and loss of self-control and represent a threat to themselves and caregivers. Chronic MAP users often develop paranoia and lasting psychosis as well as deterioration of judgment and fine motor skills, which may predispose them to injury from moving vehicle accidents... Criminal and violent behaviour associated with MAP may lead to blunt and penetrating traumatic injury... Inevitably, increasing MAP abuse translates into more frequent ED visits by this population... Our data suggest MAP users utilise prehospital and hospital resources at levels higher than the average ED population. Based on the current trends, we can expect more ED visits by MAP users in the future... (Richards et al. 1999, p.198).

This survey outlined a variety of serious trauma-related complaints for which emergency treatment was required. Thirty-seven per cent of MAP users as compared to 21 per cent of non-users required such treatment:

> A remarkable association between MAP use and injury from trauma existed in this study. Interpersonal trauma, including gunshot wounds, stabbings and assaults, was responsible for a large number of ED visits... The predisposition for violence and suicide from MAP abuse may account for the large proportion of these cases. This association has been investigated in previous studies. Kratofil and colleagues described self-injury and mutilation by MAP users. Logan reported a correlation between MAP and violent behaviour in drivers arrested for driving under the influence of alcohol. In another series by the same author, 146 deaths involving MAP were reviewed on autopsy, and 27% resulted from homicidal and 15% from suicidal violence. A similar study from Spain also found a high percentage of violent deaths in MAP positive autopsies. Bailey and co-workers reported MAP presence in almost one third of homicides and accidental overdoses in San Diego County. In the subculture of MAP users, in which paranoia, poor judgement, predisposition for violence and access to weapons coexist, any potential misunderstanding or disagreement, however insignificant, may lead to interpersonal violence[246] (Richards et al. 1999, p.201).[247]

South Australia Survey 1995/1996

A South Australian survey of 100 amphetamine users conducted in 1995/1996 across the Adelaide metropolitan region also revealed a relatively strong link between amphetamine use, criminal behaviour and other social problems. Such findings include:

- Sixty-one percent of participants had driven a motor vehicle while intoxicated with amphetamines in the month prior to interview, with 45% of these people stating that they had also been drinking alcohol on some or all of these occasions.

246 This may particularly be the case with 'crystal meth' or 'ice'. See Derlet and Heischober 1990.

247 See also the references cited therein and Leamon, Canning and Benjamin 2000.

- Seventy percent of participants had been involved in some form of criminal activity (not including dealing drugs amongst their friends) since they began using amphetamines. However, 57 of these people had also been involved in crime beforehand. Fifty-one percent of participants had carried out a crime or crimes whilst intoxicated with amphetamines.
- Eighty-two percent of the sample reported having had some form of social problem in the six months prior to interview, which they believed had been caused by their use of amphetamines. Forty-two percent of the sample reported that they had experienced problems with friends, 40% reported problems with their partner, 18% said that they had had problems at work, 9% said that their amphetamine use had caused an accident, and 2% had dropped out of their studies because of their amphetamine use.
- Seventy-five percent of participants said that their use of amphetamines had caused them to have financial problems in the 6 months prior to interview (Vincent, Allsop & Shoobridge 1997, pp.378–379. See also Vincent et al. 1999).

While the authors acknowledge that further and more detailed research into the social problems surrounding amphetamine abuse and the links to crime is required, their findings do suggest a nexus between dependence on amphetamines and poorer social functioning.

South Australian Drugs Summit 2002

A recent summit on amphetamine and psychostimulant use hosted by the government of South Australia discussed *inter alia* the social costs of such drug use. Some of the topics included the community loss due to criminal activity, law enforcement and judicial costs and the loss of quality of life for users and their families. The conference communique summed up the links between amphetamine and other drug use and criminal activity as follows:

> In many circumstances drug use and criminal behaviour are linked, but the relationship is complicated. There are three aspects: users committing crime to obtain money to purchase drugs; crime committed under the influence of drugs; and an overlap between the factors associated with the development of criminal behaviour and factors associated with the initiation of illicit drug use. Whatever the basis of criminal behaviour, it is clear that heroin use results in a significant increase in the frequency of offending. The extent of involvement in property crime among illicit drug users is about 10 times higher than among non-users… Amphetamine use is also associated with higher levels of violent and bizarre behaviour than either opioids or cannabis (South Australian Drugs Summit Communique – *Health Maintenance and Treatment* 2002b, p.3).

Certainly, the 'gut feeling' of police in South Australia is that amphetamine use and production could be responsible for increasing levels of violent crime in that state. When the Committee met with the South Australian Police Commissioner he stated:

> From a police point of view we are also concerned that amphetamine use gets translated into more criminal offending – of a different kind to heroin. A lot of the heroin related crime is about acquiring the money to purchase the drugs and maintain habits.[248] Amphetamine still requires that, but it is not as expensive as heroin, so you do not need as much. But it can produce aggressive and violent type of behaviour. Indeed, we are experiencing more high-speed chases with offenders in stolen cars, and things of that nature. We do not know whether this behaviour is connected with amphetamine use. You can hypothesise that it might be. There are no real studies at this stage to show that there is a link, but it is something we suspect is there. We are looking to see whether this violent or risk-taking behaviour is associated with amphetamine use. Then, of course, it is highly risky in terms of the damage that can be caused to the community, so that is a particular concern. ... it is possible that we are having more violent and aggressive behaviour being displayed because of an increasing amphetamine use in the community.[249]

Turning Point Alcohol and Drug Centre Report 2001

Of interest is the fact that the recent 'heroin drought' has resulted in an apparent increase in drug-related crime in Melbourne. The Victorian Drug Availability Monitoring Project (DAMP), undertaken by Miller, Fry and Dietze from the Turning Point Alcohol and Drug Centre, compared a range of drug use statistics from their own survey work conducted in March/April 2001 with samples from Illicit Drug Reporting System (IDRS) data reported for May/June 2000. While this report has already been discussed in Chapters 4 and 5, in this context the findings are of great interest:

> [P]articipants' reports of involvement in any crime were roughly equivalent to the 2000 IDRS with just over half of the sample reporting involvement in any crime. However, the proportion reporting property and/or violent crime since Christmas 2000...was higher than the proportion reporting such crime in the

248 This distinction between heroin and amphetamine-related crime has been noted in national research conducted by the Australian Institute of Criminology as explained to the Committee by Dr Toni Makkai:

'We have a report before the Commonwealth Attorney-General where we went in and interviewed incarcerated offenders regardless of the offence – in Queensland, Western Australia and Tasmania and the Northern Territory, excluding South Australia. So we had over 2000 offenders that we interviewed. We asked them about their using, their drug use history and we asked them about their criminal history – that is self-report data with all the limitation that go with that. What we found is that those who are primarily violent offenders are more likely to report that they were methamphetamine users and property offenders, and they are more likely when you ask them "Well why did you do the things you did?" to ascribe their offending to the pharmacological aspects of the drug; whereas heroin users are more likely to say, "Well I did it because I needed money for the drugs" (Dr Toni Makkai, Director of Research, Australian Institute of Criminology, in conversation with the Drugs and Crime Prevention Committee, Canberra, 23 June 2003).

249 Mr Mal Hyde, Police Commissioner of South Australia, in conversation with the Drugs and Crime Prevention Committee, Adelaide, 3 October 2003.

> 6 months prior to the 2000 IDRS survey. Given that the timeframe considered in the DAMP study was some 2–3 months less than the timeframe considered in the IDRS, the increase in reported crime involvement is important (Turning Point Alcohol and Drug Centre 2001, p.22).

Fourteen per cent of the DAMP sample reported an increase in the amount of property crime that *they* had committed during the 'drought'. However, 73 per cent of the sample reported that there had been an increase in *other* people committing property crime (Committee emphasis). Fifteen per cent of the sample reported that their dealing of drugs had increased. Moreover, 30 per cent of those sampled who admitted to dealing in drugs reported that they had changed the drugs dealt during the 'drought'. Other relevant data from the survey included the following:

> Respondents were asked a number of questions regarding their perceptions of changes in police activity during the heroin 'drought' and whether these changes had an impact. Most of the respondents (80%) believed that there had been an increase in police activity over the 'drought' period, and over half (53%) reported that more of their friends had been arrested. Over half (58%) of the study participants reported that police activity had contributed to the heroin 'drought'...
>
> The participants in the current study were asked about what other effects they had observed as a result of the heroin 'drought'. Most respondents believed that the 'drought' had led to an increase in the amount of violent crime (68%), property crime (55%), bad deals (68%) and a large minority (38%) believed there had been a significant increase in fraud. Other general impression [sic] reported by the sample included: an increase in sex work (12%), less people using heroin (6%) and an increase in begging (Turning Point Alcohol and Drug Centre 2001, p.22).

What is unclear, or at least can only be the subject of conjecture on the basis of anecdotal evidence, is how much of the increase in crime or violent behaviour reported or perceived to be committed in the sample is due to a switch to amphetamine use in addition to or as a substitution for heroin.

Ted Noffs Foundation 2003

The Ted Noffs Foundation runs the PALM (Program for Adolescent Life Management) residential and rehabilitation units for drug dependent youth in Sydney and other areas of New South Wales. An analysis of admissions data for 2002 found that:

> Residents who nominated either heroin or ATS [Amphetamine Type Substance] as their primary drug of concern were more likely than those who nominated cannabis or alcohol to have committed a property crime in the three months prior to admission...
>
> [c]lients with primary ATS problems were more likely to have committed a crime against the person in the three months prior to admission than

> predominant heroin, cannabis and alcohol users and one hundred percent of these clients [N = 178] felt their use contributed to their offending history...Sexual assaults and risky sexual behaviour were more likely to have been reported amongst clients who nominated ATS as their drug of greatest concern...There is also an increased risk of violence in cases where alcohol and psychostimulants are used (Howard & Arcuri 2003, p.35).

Thus sexual assaults, trauma and other forms of violence were more likely to have been both *committed* and *experienced* by residents who nominated ATS as their drug of greatest concern (Howard, Stubbs & Arcuri 2004, in prep). This accords with recent research conducted in Queensland. A survey of 664 amphetamine users in that state found that the greater the use of or dependence on amphetamine the more interpersonal violence the user experienced (see Buckman, Krenske & Lynch 2003).

NSW Study 1998

Although there is not a strong link established between ecstasy use and crime or violence this does not mean that the use of ecstasy and other 'party drugs' has not resulted in a variety of social problems, particularly when these drugs are used on a regular basis or in large amounts.[250] A number of Australian surveys have examined a range of social problems associated with ecstasy, in addition to the medical and psychological consequences of the drug. A study of 213 ecstasy users in Sydney in 1998 found that a large number of those surveyed reported relationship, financial, legal and employment problems associated with their ecstasy use:

- Almost half (47%) had experienced a relationship/social problem during the past six months with a partner, friend or relative. Most of these (80%) involved relatively minor problems such as arguments, mistrust or anxiety. Minorities reported more serious problems such as ending a relationship (18%) or violence (2%).
- Just under half (46%) of the sample reported a financial problem from their use of 'ecstasy', the most common of which was a lack of money for recreational activities (47%). Minorities reported being in debt (27%) or having no money for essentials such as food and rent (26%).
- Occupational problems were reported by 47% of the sample. Females were significantly more likely than males to report work/study problems... Most of the reported problems (58%) involved trouble concentrating, reduced work performance or feeling unmotivated. Twenty-nine percent reported having to take sick leave or not attending classes. A minority (13%) reported very serious problems such as being sacked, quitting their job or study or not being able to find a job due to their 'ecstasy' use.

250 See also Hando and Hall 1997.

- Seven subjects reported legal problems from their use of 'ecstasy' in the past six months, most having received a caution from police. Two subjects had been arrested (Hando, Topp & Dillon 1998 p.38).[251]

South Australia Study 2002

Similar findings were noted in a recent study of 70 ecstasy users in Adelaide, South Australia (NDARC 2002c):

- In 79% of cases subjects reported at least one problem in the previous six months which they perceived as related, at least in part, to their use of ecstasy. This included relationship and social problems, financial problems, work or study problems, and legal or police problems.
- The most common problems were related to occupation or study, with nearly 63% of the sample experiencing them.... More than half of these problems (52%) involved taking sick leave or not attending classes, and a further 43% involved trouble concentrating (16%), reduced work performance (14%) or feeling unmotivated (14%). A minority (5%) was more serious, such as being dismissed from or quitting a job, or inability to obtain employment.
- The use of ecstasy caused financial problems for 39% of subjects in the previous six months. These subjects specified the most serious financial problem they had dealt with. In 56% of cases the problem was minor, with subjects having no money for recreation or luxuries. In 26% of cases the problem was more serious, with subjects being in debt or owing money to people. In the remaining 19% of cases the problem was extremely serious, with subjects not having enough money to pay for food or rent.
- The use of ecstasy caused relationship or social problems for 36% of subjects in the previous six months. These subjects also specified the most serious relationship problem they had dealt with. In 80% of cases the problem was relatively minor, such as arguments and the development of mistrust or anxiety in the relationship. In the remaining 20% of cases the relationship actually ended as a result of ecstasy use, and in one case this resulted in violence. Three of these subjects also reported conflict within the family as a result of their ecstasy use, including arguments with parents and siblings.
- Only four subjects (6%) reported any legal or police problems related to their use of ecstasy in the previous six months. In one case the person

251 Earlier research conducted by Hando and Hall in the early 1990s among 231 amphetamine users in Sydney showed 'a considerable amount of criminal activity within the sample', although lower than comparative examples of heroin users:

'A quarter of the sample (26%) had been imprisoned previously, 21% had been in a juvenile institution, and 39% had been arrested for a drug related offence. More than half of the sample had engaged in criminal activity such as: dealing in drugs (61%); property offences ...(54% of males and 42% of females); fraud offences (33% of males and 40% of females); and offences involving violence against persons...(31% of males and 22% of females)' (Hall & Hando 1993, quoted in Hando & Hall 1997, p.98).

was arrested by police, another had their car searched by police, and the remaining two reported feeling like they were being followed or were under police surveillance.

- A variety of other problems caused by ecstasy in the previous six months were reported by 19 subjects (27%). Eight experienced problems with their general physical health for several days after taking ecstasy, as well as feeling confused, anxious, paranoid and depressed. Three subjects who had experienced a relationship breakdown due to their ecstasy use also reported conflicts with their family. Two spoke of their increased sexual risk-taking behaviour, saying they have unprotected sex while on ecstasy and "don't care about the consequences". Two reported feeling uncomfortable and alienated in social situations when not on ecstasy, that they have trouble interacting and dealing with people.
- There were no gender differences in the number or type of ecstasy-related problems experienced by subjects. Overall, 82% of females had experienced at least one problem in the previous six months, compared with 76% of males. Similarly, there was no significant difference according to age. Overall, 80% of subjects aged less than 25 years had experienced at least one problem, compared with 67% of subjects aged 25 years or more.
- There were also no statistically significant differences in the number and type of ecstasy-related problems experienced by subjects according to whether they had ever injected a drug. Eighty percent of subjects who had ever injected any drug reported at least one problem, compared with 78% of those who had never injected any drug. Although a higher percentage of subjects who had injected drugs reported financial problems (60% versus 33%), the difference did not quite reach statistical significance ..... Similarly, a higher percentage of subjects who had injected drugs reported relationship or social problems (47% versus 33%) and legal or police problems (13% versus 4%), but again the differences were not statistically significant (NDARC 2002c, pp.41–42).

Summary

While it cannot be said that the social problems related to ecstasy use are as numerous or as severe as those associated with other drugs such as heroin, amphetamines or alcohol, they are not insignificant. They require specific strategies and interventions that are tailored to the particular culture associated with ecstasy use. These interventions will be discussed in Chapter 20.

Drink spiking – A crime of the times?

The issue of the administration of drugs such as GHB or rohypnol into a person's drink as a form of assault has been mentioned briefly in Chapter 4, which outlines the nature and effects of the various drugs. For convenience it is repeated in this context that the common effects of these drugs are intoxication, disinhibition, sedation and memory loss. Such effects clearly make victims particularly vulnerable to rape and sexual assault (see Smith & Temple 2000).

An issue for police, sexual assault and alcohol and drug workers is whether a specifically named crime of 'drink spiking' should be enacted. Drink spiking has been defined as:

> [a] substance placed into a person's drink without their consent or knowledge in order to sedate or incapacitate them. That's pretty consistent throughout all of the literature, and pretty much worldwide that is a consistent message. There are a number of substances used to facilitate drink spiking. They can either be a legal drug or illegal. Your legal drugs consist of prescription drugs and alcohol, and your illegal drugs – that's pretty self-explanatory.[252]

There is no doubt that under current Victorian legislation the act of adding a drug, including alcohol and licit substances, to a person's beverage without their consent in order to commit (sexual) assault or take advantage of the person in other ways is a punishable criminal offence.[253] However, it is argued by some criminologists, lawyers and sexual assault workers that the 'naming' of drink spiking as a discrete crime means that such actions will be taken more seriously as criminal by the police, medical workers and the general community. This is comparable to the issue of family or domestic violence being specifically 'criminalised' rather than being part of the general criminal law of assault (see Thornton 1990, 1995).

As many commentators have discussed, the idea of drugs being used to initiate sexual purposes and rape is hardly new. The scares surrounding women and the white slave trade, whatever the reality of the situation, were premised on such

252 Detective Senior Constable Fiona Hinshelwood, Sexual Crimes Investigation Unit, Queensland Police, in conversation with the Drugs and Crime Prevention Committee, Brisbane, 27 June 2003.

253 For example, see Section 53 of the *Crimes Act 1958* which states:

'A person must not-

(a) administer a drug, matter or thing to a person; or

(b) cause a drug, matter or thing to be taken by a person

with the intention of rendering that person incapable of resistance and

thereby enabling himself or herself or another person to take part in an act

of sexual penetration with that person. (Maximum penalty , 10 years imprisonment)'.

Section 74 of the Drugs, Poisons and Controlled Substances also provides that:

'A person who, without being authorised by or licensed under this Act or the regulations to do so, introduces or attempts to introduce a drug of dependence into the body of another person is guilty of an offence against this Act and liable to a penalty of not more than 30 penalty units or to level 8 imprisonment (1 year maximum) or to both that penalty and imprisonment'.

women being drugged and abducted for the purposes of sexual servitude (see, for example, Jenkins 1999 pp.176ff.).

By far the most frequently used substance in recorded cases of date rape or drink spiking has been alcohol (see Jenkins 1999; Slaughter 2000; Jansen 2001). Certainly, in sufficient quantities the effects of alcohol consumption are comparable to the so-called 'date rape' 'party drugs'. Moreover, contrary to some accounts of 'stranger danger', as the term 'date rape' suggests, the perpetrator of the drug administration and the assault is most likely to be someone the victim knows (see Jenkins 1999; Slaughter 2000; Jansen 2001). Despite the predominance of alcohol as a date rape drug, since the 1990s drugs such as GHB and rohypnol (flunitrazepam) have been most commonly associated with the rape drug concept.[254]

During the course of this Inquiry, the Committee has met with police officers who have been specifically investigating the issue of drink spiking.[255] The work being done by Senior Constable Fiona Hinshelwood of the Sexual Crimes Investigation Unit, Queensland Police was of particular interest. When the Committee met with her in June 2003 she discussed the work of a dedicated programme to combat drink spiking and sexual assault by her unit in conjunction with health, education and community representatives. Ms Hinshelwood commenced her presentation with a discussion of how drink spiking is administered and the purposes for which it is done:

> Methods used: because drugs come in a number of different forms – such as liquid, powder, capsule and tablets – there is no one particular method which people use to spike a drink. Some methods which are used: mixing it up and placing it into an eye dropper, so that when you run your hand over the drink with the eye dropper in your hand, you can just squeeze the liquid into the drink and it's an easy way to put it in; place the tablet straight into the drink or crush it into a powder and put it into the drink, so they are pretty common methods that are used...
>
> There is a theory that offenders are conducting trial runs in nightclubs. So they will go out and spike four different people's drinks in a particular nightclub just to see what amount they need to use, how it will affect people, how the

---

254 Jansen argues that GHB and ketamine have both been proscribed and specifically named as 'date rape drugs' in American legislation, despite extremely tenuous links that the latter drug is in effect used in such a way. On the other hand, pressure from the pharmaceutical industry has resulted in rohypnol not being added to the list of date rape drugs despite evidence that it is much more likely to be used in such culpable ways (Jansen 2001, pp.38ff.).

GHB in particular has been identified as a particularly insidious date rape drug. In the United States, the national 'Hillary Farias and Samantha Reed Date Rape Prohibition Act of 1999' proscribes the possession of GHB with penalties of up to 20 years imprisonment for possession of the drug. See Smith and Temple 2000 and the discussion in Chapter 12 of this Report.

255 Some excellent work in the area of drink spiking is apparently being done by officers of the Victoria Police Sexual Assault Squad in liaison with community agencies. This work is co-ordinated by Detective Sergeant Tony Silver. Unfortunately, for a variety of reasons it was not possible to speak to Detective Silver about this work or meet with other members of the squad.

> bouncers will act, how people's friends will act – so they are giving it a trial run. We are seeing there may be a number of incidents at a particular nightclub, but there won't be any further offence committed, so it will be just a trial run as such.
>
> The purposes of drink spiking: sexual assault, that's probably the most talked about. Robbery, and to facilitate unsafe sex – and we have particularly seen that in the gay and lesbian crowd. As a joke, for a prank – we are seeing that one a lot more. Really the purpose of drink spiking depends on what the MO of the offender is. An example: there was a bloke in Western Australia who went around and spiked women who looked like his ex-wife, so they were all 5 foot 10, blonde. And he didn't want to commit any particular crime, he just wanted to make them look silly in front of their colleagues and he got some kind of sick enjoyment out of it.[256]

The victims of drink spiking and sexual assault are many and varied according to Detective Hinshelwood. One particularly vulnerable group in Queensland are young people taking part in 'Schoolies Week' on the Gold Coast. Backpackers and tourists are also at risk:

> The backpackers: we are seeing that because the backpackers are an easy market; they are quite often in social situations, and they move on quickly. So if they are targeted they may not be aware of what has happened to them; they are still a bit groggy but they have to get up and get on that bus and to the next town before they realise what has happened, and then they are unlikely to report the incident when they are at that next town.[257]

Men, both heterosexual and homosexual, feature as victims of drink spiking in surprisingly large numbers according to Ms Hinshelwood, although they are less likely than women to report the crime or continue with prosecution. Indeed a low reporting rate for this offence is one of the problems associated with drink spiking across Australia. Clinch (2003) states in this regard:

> A lot of drink spiking victims choose not to present or provide samples to a medical practitioner which makes it difficult to collect statistical information on the matter. To be able to confirm drink spiking, victims must report the incident to police or a hospital emergency department as soon as possible, preferably within 12 hours so that blood and urine samples can be taken and drug and alcohol levels can be detected (Clinch 2003, p.10).

Detective Hinshelwood also testifies to the importance of reporting such incidents, particularly in order to collate accurate data on the prevalence of drink spiking:

> One of the reasons we are seeing quite low reporting rates to the police – basically the person may still be suffering the effects of the drug, so they don't realise and put it altogether what has happened to them until a number of

256 Detective Senior Constable Fiona Hinshelwood, Sexual Crimes Investigation Unit, Queensland Police, in conversation with the Drugs and Crime Prevention Committee, Brisbane, 27 June 2003.

257 Ibid.

> hours later – and it may take them 24 hours, 48 hours – and then they may be a little reluctant to come to the police because they think it happened so long ago. Fear of not being believed – "Who is going to believe I've had my drink spiked? I haven't had my blood or urine test, so why would they believe me?" They don't know it is a criminal offence. We have seen that quite a bit. Again with drink spiking, it is very easy in a social situation for anyone to commit the offence, so they really don't have any idea who the offender might be – and embarrassment, that is quite a common one as well.
>
> The Queensland Police stats are not really reflecting the actual offending; we don't really have any statistics because of our low reporting rate. This is pretty consistent throughout Australia in all of the jurisdictions. I would say that there is no jurisdiction in Australia that would have accurate statistics as far as reporting to police. This comes down to some of the factors – meaning that a person might be drink-spiked and then raped, and the offence may go under crime classification of rape...
>
> ... Toxicology base stats are not available. There just aren't enough tests being done and within the right timeframes. [However] There is a project being conducted by Sir Charles Gardiner Hospital in Perth where every person who claims they have had their drink spiked will be tested at Sir Charles Gardiner Hospital. That project started only late last year, so the stats are not really available or measurable yet.[258]

In Victoria there have also been programmes to address the dangers of drink spiking:

> Victoria Police and the Centre Against Sexual Assault (CASA House) is currently conducting a joint 'Drink Spiking' project. The aim of this pilot project is two-fold. Firstly to collect information concerning the offence and those responsible in an anonymous survey and secondly to provide the community with information on how to get help and raise awareness of the issue.[259]

Clearly there is a need for accurate and comprehensive data on drink spiking and associated crimes in most Australian jurisdictions. To this end it is encouraging that the Australian Institute of Criminology has recently commenced a project aimed at ascertaining levels of drink spiking across Australia.[260]

The problem of drink spiking clearly requires interventions that go beyond legal proscription and punishment of offenders, as important as these are. A range of community and harm reduction programmes have been implemented across

---

258 Ibid.

259 Correspondence from Victoria Police to Drugs and Crime Prevention Committee, 29 March 2004. A copy of this Project's Drink Spiking Pamphlet is attached as Appendix 10.

260 The Committee met with Dr Natalie Taylor, the Project's co-coordinator in June 2003. She made the salient point that in examining this issue one needs to go beyond focussing on victims who have reported being sexually assaulted, although clearly they will be an important part of any group affected by drink spiking. However, there will also clearly be a percentage of people who may believe their drinks have been spiked but have not been assaulted (Dr Natalie Taylor, Australian Institute of Criminology, in conversation with the Drugs and Crime Prevention Committee, Canberra, 23 June 2003).

Australia to address both the prevention of drink spiking and ways in which victims can be assisted once an incident has taken place. Some of these programmes and initiatives are discussed briefly in Chapter 19.

In the context of the law, however, this Committee believes that serious consideration should be given to the enactment of a legislative provision that will specifically 'name' drink spiking as a discrete offence with appropriate penalties that reflect the seriousness of this form of violation.[261] Whilst there are certainly legal provisions in existence that make it an offence to administer a drug for the purposes of non consensual sexual penetration[262] the Committee believes that an additional general offence with regard to drink spiking should be enacted. In other words the offence would not be dependent upon the intention of the perpetrator to engage in sexual intercourse with the victim. The mere fact that the perpetrator has intentionally spiked the other person's drink without that person's consent should be of itself sufficient to attract an appropriate penalty.[263] As such the Committee makes the following recommendation:

Recommendation

3. The Committee recommends that consideration be given to the creation of a new general offence of 'drink spiking' with a sufficient level of penalty to reflect the gravity of this crime. Such an offence should be in addition to and not in substitution of the provisions of Section 53 of the *Crimes Act 1958* (administration of a drug).

Road trauma, drugs and driving

One particular problem associated with the use of both amphetamines and 'party drugs' is their use while driving or in control of a motor vehicle. This may be for instrumental reasons, for example the use of amphetamines by truck drivers to stay awake while maintaining punishing delivery schedules, or as a consequence of recreational use, for example getting home from a 'rave' or dance party when there is no public transport available. The user profiles of both amphetamine-using transport workers and 'party drug' use by 'ravers' and 'clubbers' will be discussed in Chapter 9. Nonetheless, it is appropriate at this instance to examine briefly some of the problematic aspects of drug use as it pertains to driving while intoxicated.

Driving under the influence of amphetamines is unfortunately an all too common practice of transport workers (see Mabbott & Hartley 1999). Tight deadlines and turnaround schedules, penalties for late delivery and products

261 See also discussion in Chapter 13.

262 See Section 53 of the Crimes Act 1958 as discussed above.

263 This could cover situations in which the perpetrator spiked the drink as part of a 'practical joke'.

requiring urgent delivery have resulted in the use of 'speed' and both illegal and prescription stimulants by relatively many truck drivers, particularly long-distance or interstate drivers. These are used for staying awake and indeed 'energising' the driver. This can often result in speeding (in both senses of the word) and dangerous driving. Moreover, the abuse of amphetamines, particularly methamphetamines, while driving is not restricted to transport workers. The aforementioned American study of emergency room admissions related to methamphetamine abuse found a clear relationship between methamphetamine use and injury from road trauma. Such injuries may have been sustained by the user, a fellow passenger, bystander or by occupants of other vehicles:

> The deleterious effect of methamphetamines (MAP) on psychomotor and cognitive skills has been well documented. The most notable consequence of this effect is an increased incidence of moving vehicle accidents and falls. In a series of moving vehicle accidents described by Logan et al., poor coordination and judgement was responsible for the majority of crashes, and typical driving behaviours included drifting out of the lane of travel, erratic driving, weaving, speeding, drifting off the road, and high speed collisions. The majority of MAP patients with blunt trauma in our study were involved in car crashes and other moving vehicles, including two MAP users who were riding bicycles and crashed into each other... Crouch and co-workers investigated fatal truck crashes over a one year period and found that an alarmingly high percentage tested positive for MAP postmortem. Although MAP does significantly extend periods of wakefulness, this benefit is quickly negated by poor task functioning. Wiegmann and his colleagues studied the effect of MAP on cognitive processing which deteriorated considerably with extended periods of wakefulness induced by MAP (Richards et al. 1999, p.201).

The practice of driving under the influence of 'party drugs' used for recreational purposes is a problem which is not so well documented.

Of particular concern are the findings of a recent British study (Akram & Forsyth 2000) indicating that, unlike depressant drugs such as alcohol, dance drugs are often perceived (mistakenly) to enhance driving and motor skills.[264] The authors acknowledge that attitudes towards drink driving have changed dramatically in the past few decades but add that 'it is not known to what extent this attitude extends towards drug driving' (p.267). A lack of police roadside testing for drug driving, in addition to the perceptions (partly true) that controlling a car while under the influence of dance drugs is less difficult than when intoxicated by alcohol, has contributed to a false sense of security about 'clubbers' being able to drive safely after having taken ecstasy and/or other 'party drugs':

264 One study (Headen 1994) did show that drug driving was dangerous not only for the driver and any passengers but also to other road users:

'Co-ordination tests on Headen's volunteers showed that driving became considerably more aggressive under the influence of cocaine and ecstasy and judgement of distances between objects (eg. traffic cones) impaired (Headen 1994). Driving skills in general deteriorated especially driving under the influence of ecstasy' (in Akram & Forsyth 2000, p.267).

> The UK dance scene because of its conception in deserted warehouses and outdoor parties may have inadvertently encouraged the practice of dance drug driving. In the early days, party goers would meet at secret rendezvous...in an effort to confuse the authorities as to the whereabouts of the party. This would ultimately result in the return journey, for some, being undertaken whilst under the influence of drugs. Driving therefore became as much a part of the adventure as actually being there. For many, driving under the influence of dance drugs was the only real way of being part of the culture.
>
> Although illegal warehouse and outdoor parties have largely been replaced by town nightclub venues, it is unlikely that this will have stopped the practice of drug driving. One study investigating dance drugs and safety awareness amongst users (Akram 1997) found that 62% of the sample (n = 135) had driven a motor vehicle whilst under the influence of dance drugs. This would suggest that dance drug driving does occur quite frequently (Akram & Forsyth 2000, p.266).

Moreover, Akram and Forsyth state that dance drug driving is not confined to clubs and raves in Britain but is also noticeable in travelling to and from outdoor music festivals:

> The remote rural location of these festivals pose limitations on the availability and accessibility of public transport, resulting in a number of festival goers taking their own transport... It is likely that some festival goers are also under the influence of dance drugs as they drive to and from these sites (Akram & Forsyth 2000, p.267).

Although the culture of 'raving' is arguably not as pronounced in Australia as it is in Britain, there are definite parallels to be noted at a local level. Academic Dr Simon Lenton has done a number of qualitative studies of ecstasy users in Perth, Western Australia, particularly in the context of 'raves'. One study of 83 'ravers' noted that a substantial minority of respondents 'described travelling to or from raves with drivers who were drug affected' (Lenton & Davidson 1999, p.153). Of the 66 respondents in the Lenton study who either drove or were driven to a rave in a motor car, just under half (42%) felt the driver was under the influence of a drug. Twenty-seven per cent of respondents stated they were not concerned whether the driver had taken drugs or not:

> Eight (12%) respondents mentioned taking drugs in the car on the way to their last rave, often in order to reduce the perceived risk of being arrested at, or outside, the rave.
>
> Two respondents expressed the belief that driving under the influence of drugs was less likely to result in being apprehended by police because of the difficulty of roadside detection and four believed that driving under the influence of drugs was safer than driving drunk. *Amphetamines and cannabis in particular were believed to be associated with relatively safe driving.*
>
> Some of the same respondents also mentioned the ease of getting away with driving under the influence of drugs even if pulled over by the police. The view

> was that as long as the driver could maintain a rational conversation and was not weaving all over the road, the police had no way of testing for the presence of non-alcoholic intoxicants at the roadside (Lenton & Davidson 1999, p.159). (Committee emphasis)

The authors view such misconceptions with concern. Of equal concern is the practice of some respondents of driving after consuming drugs on the assumption that they would reach their destination prior to the effects of the drugs taking hold:

> Individual differences, the unknown composition and potency of illicit substances, the possibility of the journey being longer than expected (due to getting lost or police roadblocks near the venue) are just some of the factors which could lead to the driver having to drive while drug affected. Police practices such as road blocks and car searches, which are likely to result in people consuming their drugs to avoid detection and forcing people to drive when events have shut down early, ought to be discouraged (Lenton & Davidson 1999, p.161).

A Scottish study by Neale is equally alarming for the somewhat laissez-faire attitude of the respondents to the issue of driving after drug use where 'Concern about ability to drive following drug use was limited' (Neale 2001, p.315). Of Neale's sample of 61 dance club interviewees almost half (n = 26, 18 men and 8 women) admitted to have driven after having taken MDMA or what was purported to be ecstasy. Fifteen of the interviewees (5 women and 10 men) had driven cars after having taken amphetamines:

> With the exception of one interviewee who had driven home from a friend's house after taking the drug, all [ecstasy users] reported ecstasy driving occurred on weekends following club attendance – that is between 2.a.m. and midday on either Saturdays or Sundays. At these times drivers were invariably accompanied by passengers and making journeys that had the explicit purpose of transporting themselves and their friends home from a night out... Negative experiences of driving on ecstasy [and amphetamine] were very common and included feelings of fear and paranoia; hallucinations; blurred vision, impaired concentration; propensity to speed; and slower reaction times for as long as 12 hours after drug use (Neale 2001, p.319).

Respondents distinguished between driving during different time periods, particularly during the 'coming up' and 'coming down' periods. In the former they were more likely to be stimulated and euphoric behind the wheel, while when coming down tiredness was the overwhelming feeling. One respondent described the experience of driving several hours after ecstasy use as follows:

> Usually by the time you're driving home you're not feeling that well. The road's winding away in front of you and you just want to get home. It's like a doom feeling... You just don't really feel that good... (Neale 2001, pp.319–320).

Neale points to a complex interaction of both personal and environmental factors that contribute in greater or lesser ways to the dangerousness of driving after 'party drug' and/or amphetamine use:

> Drug related factors highlighted include[d] drug type, quantity, strength or purity, and interactions with any other legal or illegal substances consumed (including prescribed medications and alcohol). Individual factors discussed include[d] personal levels of tolerance (due to regularity and extent of drug use, individual metabolism, and/or body size) and the fact that some individuals just seem to be more susceptible to the intoxicating effects of particular drugs or are simply poor drivers. In terms of situational factors, it was argued that the effects of drug use on driving depend on the length of time between substance consumption and driving; the state of mind or mood of the driver whilst behind the wheel; any interference or distractions from passengers; and whether or not the individual is also suffering from a lack of sleep (drug use often being seen as a useful way of countering tiredness) (Neale 2001, p.322).

Conversely, and despite this, 'several individuals (all of whom had driven at least 3 hours after drug use) believed that ecstasy had no major impact on their ability to control a car' (Neale 2001, p.320; see also Aitken, Kerger & Crofts 2000).

Clearly, the results of these types of surveys are worrying. Neale argues one measure that could be used to encourage a change in drug driving behaviour is:

> [m]ore public transportation (including relatively inexpensive coach, bus or minibus services) between venues and residential areas [which] would probably eliminate some of the less frequent and arguably more dangerous forms of drug driving (Neale 2001, p.323).

Certainly access to more public transport and perhaps more importantly more flexible hours in which it is available is one of the key harm minimisation issues identified in the literature and by the respondents with whom the Committee has met. This issue shall therefore be discussed further in the context of harm reduction interventions in Chapter 19.

While most of the British studies that examined driving under the influence of 'dance drugs' concerned MDMA there have been some American studies that have looked at the links between the consumption of GHB and driving impairment. In a recent study by Couper and Logan the authors found that:

> Gamma hydroxybutyrate (GHB) was identified in the blood of 13 subjects arrested for impaired driving... GHB was the only drug detected, and signs of impairment were consistent with those of a central Nervous System depressant, including erratic driving (weaving, swerving, ignoring road signs), confusion, incoherent speech, unresponsiveness, lack of balance, unsteady co-ordination, poor performance on field sobriety tests, and varying states of wakefulness. Given the ability of GHB to induce sleep and unconsciousness, it

> is evident from these cases that recreational use of the drug has the potential to impair a person's driving ability (Couper & Logan 2001, p.919).

The findings and responses of the various surveys and studies outlined have significant implications for policy development, education and in particular harm reduction interventions.[265] These factors are discussed in detail in Chapter 19.

'Speed' kills: New drug driving laws

It is only relatively recently that (Western) legislatures have enacted laws and procedures that penalise drivers who drive with either any or a specified amount of illicit (and licit pharmaceutical) drugs in their system in ways comparable to driving under the influence of alcohol provisions (see Gliddon 2002; Godfrey & Phillips 2003). In a review of driving under the influence of drugs law in New South Wales, Godfrey and Phillips state that the five drug groups which are commonly seen in drug impaired drivers are:

- Alcohol
- Cannabis
- Opiates and opiate derivatives
- Benzodiazepines; and
- Stimulants (Godfrey & Phillips 2003, p.16).

In Victoria the recently enacted *Road Safety (Drug Driving) Act 2003* has amended the parent *Road Safety Act* to include drugs in addition to alcohol for the purposes of random breath testing and the provision of drug driving infringement penalties.

The rationale behind such an enactment is clearly the dangers associated with drug driving and the increasing incidence of drug-related motor accidents in recent years. Peter Bachelor, the Victorian Minister for Transport, highlighted these dangers in the second reading speech of the legislation as follows:

> Drug-driving is now as much a factor in driver fatalities on Victoria's roads as drink-driving.
>
> Research by the Victorian Institute of Forensic Medicine shows that in 2002, drugs other than alcohol were detected in the blood of 27 per cent of fatally injured drivers, almost as many as the 29 per cent who had a blood alcohol concentration above the legal limit of .05 grams per 100 millilitres. The corresponding figures in 2001 were even higher for drugs at 29 per cent, compared to 22 per cent for alcohol.

265 These academic findings are matched by data produced by Victoria Police that also raise concerns with regard to drug driving. The Victoria Institute of Forensic Medicine study of Victorian drivers either fatally injured or otherwise impaired found that in 2001, 2.6% of fatally injured (n = 274) and 23% of impaired when apprehended drivers (n = 57) had methamphetamines detected in their system (cited in excerpt from the confidential Victoria Police submission to the Drugs and Crime Prevention Committee, Inquiry into Amphetamine and 'Party Drug' Use in Victoria, August 2002. Quoted with the kind permission of Victoria Police).

> Over 16 per cent of drivers killed in road crashes in 2001, and over 20 per cent in 2002, tested positive to delta-9-tetrahydrocannabinol (often abbreviated to THC), which is the active component of cannabis, or to amphetamines and other stimulant drugs. In 2002, the use of these drugs was associated with almost 50 driver deaths.
>
> Despite an 11 per cent reduction in the overall road toll in 2002 compared with 2001, there were a similar number of drug-related road deaths in each of those years. In a 10-year study of truck driver fatalities in Australia, the Victorian Institute of Forensic Medicine found that 25.8 per cent of truck drivers killed on the roads tested positive to drugs that could impair driving. Ninety-seven per cent of these drug-positive fatalities tested positive to THC or to stimulants. The majority of these tested positive to either THC or to the illicit stimulant, methylamphetamine (also known as methamphetamine).[266]

Drug is defined in the parent Act as:

> a substance that is a drug for the purposes of this Act by virtue of a declaration under sub-section (3) or any other substance (other than alcohol) which, when consumed or used by a person, deprives that person (temporarily or permanently) of any of his or her normal mental or physical faculties (Section 3, *Road Safety Act 1986*).

Such a definition clearly encompasses both amphetamine and 'party drugs' in addition to licit pharmaceutical substances. Nonetheless, the use of random breath testing will apply solely to *prescribed illicit drugs*, which at this stage will include cannabis and methamphetamine only. According to the Minister:

> These two illicit drugs have been selected for random roadside testing because
>
> - there is clear evidence that drivers using these drugs are at increased risk of causing crashes;
> - they are the impairing substances with the highest incidence, after alcohol, in the blood of fatally injured drivers;
> - neither THC nor methylamphetamine are found in any Australian prescription medicines; and
> - they can be reliably detected in oral fluid samples of drivers at the time that they will adversely affect a driver's ability to drive safely.[267]

There will be no legally permitted amount for these prescribed illicit drugs for the purposes of the Road Safety Act. Even very low levels of these drugs have been shown to have an adverse effect on the abilities necessary to drive safely.[268]

The relevant offence under the legislation is to drive or be in charge of a motor vehicle while prescribed illicit drugs are present in the person's oral fluid or blood (Section 7). New forensic technology will include preliminary roadside

266 The Hon Peter Bachelor, Minister for Transport, *Road Safety (Drug Driving) Bill*, Second Reading Speech, October 30, 2003. Hansard (Legislative Assembly), p.1418.

267 Ibid., p.1419.

268 Ibid.

saliva testing by police or authorised officers and follow up laboratory tests that will be able to prove the presence of such drugs:

> Procedures will closely follow the established random breath-testing model, as do the proposed legislative requirements. The preliminary screening test will be conducted by requiring a person to suck or chew an absorbent pad or other oral fluid receptacle. The oral fluid sample will then be tested using a prescribed oral fluid screening device, which will provide a result within a few minutes.
>
> If the test indicates the presence of THC or methylamphetamine, the driver may be required to provide a further sample of oral fluid. This sample will also be tested on an oral fluid screening device. The device used for this second test and the procedure for its use will be prescribed by regulations.
>
> If this second test also indicates the presence of one or both of the prescribed illicit drugs, this second sample will be divided, with one part given to the driver and the other part sent to a forensic laboratory for evidential analysis by a properly qualified analyst. The result of this laboratory analysis will form the basis of any charge.
>
> As is currently the case under the drink-driving provisions, a driver will have a right to require a blood sample to be taken for analysis. In addition, the police member or authorised officer who required the oral fluid sample will have the power to require a blood sample if the driver is unable to provide an oral fluid sample for the second test on medical grounds or because of some physical disability or condition, or if the testing device is incapable of testing the sample. Blood samples can be taken only by registered medical practitioners or approved health professionals.
>
> Only police members and authorised officers who have been appropriately trained will be able to take a sample of oral fluid for the second confirmatory test and evidential analysis.[269]

Both monetary penalties and cancellation of driver licences may apply in the case of proven infringements.[270]

It remains to be seen how effective such measures will prove. Nonetheless, such laws have been viewed favourably in jurisdictions where they have been enacted. Neale states in the British context:

> For those who use their car on a regular basis, loss of licence is extremely inconvenient and potentially very expensive. Likewise, having a criminal record is likely to be stigmatising and to have social and employment consequences. Certainly, there are many difficulties involved in securing drug-driving convictions. Nonetheless, more overt policing – including routine spot checks

269 Ibid.

270 Fines include up to $600.00 for a first and $1200.00 for a subsequent offence (Sec 7). Offenders may also have their driver licence or permit cancelled for up to three months in the case of a first offence or six months in the case of a subsequent offence (Sec 8).

> at peak drug driving times[271] – would help to improve road safety by countering the dangerous belief that driving after drugs is acceptable simply because the chances of being caught seem very remote (Neale 2001, p.324).

Absenteeism and economic costs[272]

It is exceedingly difficult to quantify the economic cost of illicit drug use to the community. One of the difficulties for economists being: what does one include in the reckoning of what counts as tangible (or even intangible) cost of illicit drug use? Norberry, drawing from the work done by the National Drug Strategy in the mid 1990s, states that in most analyses of drug-related economic data, costs do not include ambulance services, welfare (payments), absenteeism or crime 'as the authors regard such matters as unquantifiable' (Norberry 1997, p.8). She continues:

> About one third of the economic costs [are] law enforcement costs. The balance of quantifiable costs [are] net production costs and health care costs. Production costs are the costs to production that flow from drug related death and illness adjusted for such things as consumption resources made available to the community through premature deaths. Health care costs include the costs of medical services, hospital and nursing home beds adjusted for the savings that result from death and illness due to illicit drug use (Norberry 1997, p.8).

It is beyond the scope of the Inquiry for this Committee to present an expert economic analysis of the cost of amphetamine and 'party drug' production and use to the community. Such an analysis also depends on too many factors that are manifested on a national level and thus beyond the scope of this Inquiry. Nonetheless, there is one related issue that has come to the attention of the Committee that is of concern and does merit some brief discussion.

The Committee is aware of both anecdotal accounts and evidence in the literature that suggests that 'party drug' use and particularly MDMA can be responsible for relatively high levels of absenteeism from the workplace, school or university/college.

As discussed in Chapter 6 the 'comedown' period off MDMA and related drugs can be quite lengthy. Although the amount of time needed to 'recover' from the drug's effects will vary between individuals and will depend upon such extraneous factors as the amount of drug used, the activity performed while using (for example, energetic dancing all night compared to a more mellow 'chill

---

271 Which may include either before or after major raves, rock festivals and outdoor gatherings where long distance driving might be expected. See Chapter 10 for a discussion in the context of festivals such as 'Earthcore'.

272 A relatively recent report produced by the Queensland government estimates the yearly cost of harmful drug use to the nation as being approximately $19 billion. Of this total, tobacco use accounted for $13 billion (67%), alcohol use $4.5 billion (24%) and illicit drug use $1.7 billion (9%) (see Queensland Government 1999). For an analysis of the economic costs of crime to the community and general economic analysis of illicit drug production, see Collins and Lapsley 1996; Norberry 1997 and in the specific context of amphetamines, Pietschmann 1997.

out' experience) and the weight, health and personality of the user, it is fair to state that it is not unusual for a moderately heavy user of the drugs to require at least three days to be operating at optimal performance levels. Apart from paid employment or study, the comedown period may also affect a person's performance of home duties or carer responsibilities for children (Measham, Aldridge & Parker 2001, p.118).

A British qualitative study of clubbers and 'party drugs' found that:

> [a]t least half of our club goers will have recovery periods that overlap with work, study and carer commitments...The comments of some dance drug users to fieldworkers confirmed this overlap:
>
> *It usually took him about four days to recover from taking drugs. He said this affected his work at university as he hardly ever goes in.*
>
> Another dance drug user, when talking about the recovery period, said 'I get up late and lose time sitting around doing nothing'. One interviewer noted the effect of a dance drug user's weekend drug use on the working week:
>
> *It affects his work –'always late and looks and feels like shit' – but he said his bosses are all doing the same sorts of things so it doesn't put his job at risk* (Measham, Aldridge & Parker 2001, p.118).

Measham's results have been echoed in other British studies (McElrath & McEvoy 1999; Shewan et al. 2000; Hammersley, Khan & Ditton 2002). The following response from a participant in the Hammersley et al. study is typical of many with regard to the 'comedown' period:

> So if I took an 'E' on the Saturday, then on the Sunday, I would still have a bit of it in my system, and I feel quite relaxed. But the real come down is on the Monday and the Tuesday, when you're back to reality, and you feel tired because you've been up all night... But then, like, by the time it's Wednesday, I'm fine again. Tuesdays! Tuesday's the worst day. I think maybe on Monday I'm still spaced from the weekend. Then on the Wednesday, I feel a bit better, and on the Thursday, better still, and on Friday I feel really good and then the weekend's there again (Hammersley, Khan & Ditton 2002, pp.81–82).[273]

Measham's study also investigated what the most common after or comedown effects of a period of MDMA use were on the individual. The results are indicated in the table below:

273 For further accounts of 'Blue Tuesday', see Chapter 10. It is of interest that in the 1980s middle-class professions in the United States would 'clear their diaries' two or three times a year so they could enjoy an 'ecstasy weekend'. Such meticulous planning was factored precisely for the reason that their professional lives would not be disrupted. See discussion in Rosenbaum, Morgan and Beck 1999 and Chapter 9.

Table 7.1: The effect of the recovery period on work and study for the dance drug interview sample (n = 317)

	n	%
Affected work/study*	130	41.2
Nature of effect:**		
Tired/fatigue	34	30.6
Performance/quality of work	34	30.6
Absent/time off/late	21	18.9
Mood swings/depression	20	18.0
Lack of concentration/memory loss	19	17.1
Hate day 'X'	15	13.5
Work relationships affected	6	5.4
Sacked/expelled	5	4.5
General health problems	4	3.6
Paranoia/anxiety	3	2.7
Improves work performance	**6**	**5.4**

* 25 respondents had missing responses to this question.

** 9 respondents did not go on to specify the nature of the effect. Base percentage here is respondents who reported at least one effect on work or study (n =111).

Source (including commentary): reproduced from Measham, Aldridge & Parker 2001, *Dancing on Drugs: Risk, Health and Hedonism in the British Club Scene*, Free Association Books, London, p.119.

The authors comment on the results as follows:

> We asked all dance drug users who reported effects due to their come downs on their work or study to tell us the nature of the effect… The most common was fatigue and performance/quality of work (30.6 per cent) followed by absence from work, mood swings and lack of concentration (just under one in five clubbers). More than one in ten (13.5 per cent) clubbers reported that there was a particular day that they experienced the most difficulty with (most often the Monday, Tuesday, Wednesday after the weekend). One fieldworker noted during her interview with a dance drug user: 'Wednesday is usually a wash-out but by Thursday usually getting over weekend drug use'… Smaller numbers (5 per cent or fewer) reported that their relationships at work had been affected, that they had been sacked or expelled, general health problems, or paranoia and anxiety. Interestingly, about 5 per cent volunteered that their weekend drug use when clubbing actually improved their work performance.[274]

In a study of Dutch clubbers, Ter Bogt et al. found that it is exceedingly difficult to combine 'dancestasy' with school and work:

274 Measham argues that harm minimisation strategies and policies should factor in the comedown period in their messages to users:

'The agenda should attempt to appeal to their [users] social responsibilities and encourage them to use flexitime, Friday nights to go clubbing etc' (Measham, Aldridge & Parker 2001, p.189).

> Adolescents who get exhausted during the weekend by drugs and dancing find it hard to function properly at school or work (Ter Bogt et al. 2003, p.173).

There has not to the knowledge of the Committee been any major research in Australia on the effects of 'party drug' use on work, study or other commitments and responsibilities. Certainly some of the young people with whom the Committee has met have confirmed the views expressed by the interviewees in the British studies.[275]

The local agency Anglicare stated in a submission to this Inquiry that for those young people with whom they are in contact:

> [t]aking amphetamines can take up to a week to recover from each 'hit', therefore, they are unable to attend school and cannot concentrate.[276]

It is, however, an issue that policy-makers and researchers have referred to with concern. For example, when the Committee met with Dr Natalie Taylor of the Australian Institute of Criminology, she stated:

> It must be the case that the large companies – most of them have some sort of drug and alcohol service – [would see this type of absenteeism or poor work performance] ...it would be helpful to contact [them] to see if this is an emerging issue for them. They may not have any hard data, but they would be able to say, "Yes, we seem to be having one or two more people coming in".[277]

Although this section of the Report has concentrated on MDMA and 'party drugs' in the context of absenteeism and economic costs, there is no reason to believe that the use of (meth)amphetamines would not result in similar consequences. Unfortunately, there is very little research that specifically examines the links between the use of methamphetamines and work performance or work-related issues.[278] Ironically, as was discussed in Chapter 4, it is common knowledge that amphetamines are used in functional ways to counter fatigue, particularly in workplace environments that demand long hours and concentration (truck driving, assembly line work, students, housework and child care etc). Nonetheless, although psychostimulants may be beneficial in the short term in increasing alertness and staving off a need for sleep, in the long term their prolonged use can have seriously detrimental effects, as discussed in the previous

275 For example, the Committee met with Sean and Emma (not real names), a young couple who were regular attendees of 'raves' and frequently took 'party drugs' such as MDMA. Sean in particular had been continually late for his work as a waiter because of the after-effects of MDMA use and the 'comedown' period. Only one day before his meeting with the Committee he had been given notice from this position. See also discussion in Chapter 10.

276 Submission of Anglicare to the Drugs and Crime Prevention Committee, Inquiry into Amphetamine and 'Party Drug' Use in Victoria, October 2003.

277 Dr Natalie Taylor, Australian Institute of Criminology, in conversation with the Drugs and Crime Prevention Committee, Canberra, 23 June 2003.

278 Most research that the Committee is aware of in this area centres on alcohol. Although alcohol is of a different chemical nature to amphetamine and the effects in part on the user may be different, it is possible to envisage that some of the studies on workplace performance, absenteeism and workplace injury due to alcohol use can be extrapolated to the worker who abuses amphetamines (see for example, WA Chamber of Mines and Energy 1996; Collins and Lapsley 1996; NEACA 2000b; Allsop. Phillips and Calogero 2001). At this stage, however, without specific research such a view must remain conjecture.

chapter. One of these effects is that over a period of time methamphetamine use rather than decreasing tiredness can in fact produce intense fatigue:

> A few hours following use there may be depressed mood, fatigue, and irritability. If use is continued to avoid these effects tolerance can develop, resulting in increased doses of the drug being required to achieve the same effect. Combined use over a period of time is known as a 'run', following which the user will eventually 'come down', sleep for one or more days, and experience *extreme fatigue*, depression, anxiety and lethargy (Ryder, Salmon & Walker 2001, p.235). (Committee emphasis).

One can imagine that at least for the regular or heavy user of amphetamine this cycle of alertness – comedown – more drug – fatigue would eventually result in absenteeism or performance issues related to work, study or family life. It could be posited that this would particularly be the case in heavy amphetamine users who, unlike recreational users of 'party drugs', would not necessarily be in a position to 'plan' their drug use to coincide with a weekend or special event.

Certainly, as more workplaces implement drug and alcohol policies, including *in situ* drug testing, this type of data may become more readily available (see Allsop, Phillips & Calogero 2001). Nonetheless, the Committee believes this is an issue that requires comprehensive research and data collection, both quantitative and qualitative, particularly with regard to methamphetamine use. The costs to both the individual who uses the drugs and the wider community in terms of lost hours and productivity needs to be ascertained and addressed.[279]

Conclusion

This chapter has stressed that the 'costs' of the use of amphetamines and 'party drugs', as with any form of licit or illicit drug, extend beyond purely medical or health considerations. The social costs of drug abuse are many and varied. Moreover, such costs are felt by more than just the individual user of the drug. They impact upon the family unit, friends, co-workers and members of the general community.

One important issue that must be continually borne in mind is that in the current age it is fanciful to speak of the costs, be they physical or social, of any one type of drug. The disturbing reality is that whether drug use is licit or illicit, functional, recreational or a mixture of both, most people who suffer from substance abuse will have been using more than one type of drug. The concept of poly-drug use and its effects on the user and his or her community forms the basis of discussion of the next and last chapter in this Part.

---

279 There are also issues of community safety to take into account if the drug user works in a position where concentration, stamina or alertness is crucial:

'Clubbing hairstylists sometimes advise that Mondays and Saturdays are when they cut their worst styles but more significantly what of those who work in key services who are public transport drivers, doctors, nurses, engineers and mechanics and so on?' (Measham, Aldridge & Parker 2001, p.189).

8. Poly-Drug Use: Compounding the Issues

Throughout this Report it has been noted that users of amphetamines and 'party drugs' rarely use only those substances exclusively (Darke & Hall 1995; Vincent, Allsop & Shoobridge 1996; Boys, Lenton & Norcross 1997; Hando, Topp & Dillon 1998; Kamienicki et al. 1998; Shewan, Dalgarno & Reith 2000; Gowing et al. 2001; Hansen, Maycock & Lower 2001; NDARC 1998, 2001, 2002a, 2002b, 2002c; Henry-Edwards 2002; Von Sydow et al. 2002). In other words, poly-drug use is common among these groups, and indeed most illicit drug users. A submission to this Inquiry from the Department of Human Services Victoria makes the following comment:

> There is much evidence that a range of drugs are used in conjunction with psychostimulants. Nearly all illicit drug users use a variety of drugs at the same time. Most drug users are aware there are risks associated with poly drug use but believe they are far outweighed by the gains. A concern is that many may have no idea of the unintended consequences of this risky behaviour. Drugs used regularly include heroin, LSD, cannabis, alcohol, amyl nitrate and tobacco. Users are known to use GHB, cannabis, alcohol and even heroin when withdrawing from amphetamine.
>
> In Victoria multi or poly drug use is a major problem as highlighted in the Victorian Institute of Forensic Medicine Report No 5...
>
> It is well documented that using many drugs together can cause serious health problems and precipitate drug overdose. The issue is that we do not know the wide-ranging effects of combining a variety of illicit and licit drugs and a range of unknown substances on individuals with very different physical and psychological makeups.[280]

Certainly, the experience of almost all the service providers and agency workers across Australia with whom the Committee has met has been that their clients are poly-drug users. Youth agencies in particular have given evidence about a three-way split in drug use among young people between amphetamines,

280 Submission of the Department of Human Services Victoria (Drugs Policy and Services Branch) to the Drugs and Crime Prevention Committee, Inquiry into Amphetamine and 'Party Drug' Use in Victoria, August 2002.

alcohol and cannabis.[281] One agency warns of the need to avoid 'compartmentalising' responses to drug and alcohol misuse stating:

> It is well known that "poly drug" use (using several different drugs at the same time) is a common practice amongst people who use drugs. For this reason it is important to address the 'complex' and multitude of issues relating to harmful drug use in an integrated and holistic way including:
>
> - Supporting and identifying programs that address the underlying reasons and causes of drug use as well as the harmful behaviours associated with the use of specific drugs.
> - Developing a holistic approach and understanding of harmful behaviours associated with drug use in our community – particularly poly drug use.
> - allowing for greater flexibility for agencies providing services to people who use drugs that incorporates an understanding associated with "complex" drug use patterns and markets.
> - Developing a greater understanding of the changing nature of drug use patterns and drug market trends.[282]

Studies and the findings

A British study on club drug use among young people (Williams & Parker 2001) found that poly-drug use was very much indicative of the 'normalisation thesis' discussed in Chapter 19. That is, young people have internalised drug use, including recreational illicit drug use into a repertoire of accepted (and acceptable) behaviours. Nearly all the research according to Williams and Parker indicates a strong correlation between drinking, smoking and illicit recreational drug use.[283] However, the authors warn that poly-drug use is rarely sufficiently factored into research studies and policy analysis, which tend to favour specific drug types:

> [d]ue to the traditional separation of tobacco, alcohol and illegal drug use in terms of markets, policy and research foci there is little enquiry about combination or consecutive substance taking episodes. So official household surveys and even the national drug treatment data base do not allow poly-drug repertoires to be adequately recorded. Yet when we do enquire about poly drug use, we find high rates and when we profile drug users in treatment its presence is endemic... Given the warnings from the literature on drugs transitions across the adolescent – adult life course and the inter-relationship

281 See, for example, the evidence of Ms Jennifer Lowe, Social Worker, Youth Withdrawal and Respite Service, Perth, in conversation with the Drugs and Crime Prevention Committee, Perth, 1 October 2003.

282 Submission of City of Yarra to the Drugs and Crime Prevention Committee, Inquiry into Amphetamine and 'Party Drug' Use in Victoria, October 2003.

283 Although not heroin which, as discussed in Chapter 6, is seen by recreational and 'party drug' users as a 'dirty' drug.

> between tobacco, alcohol and illicit drug use this is a worrying omission with public health implications (Williams & Parker 2001, p.399).

Prevalence of poly-drug use and the drugs used

When it comes to 'party drugs', the study conducted by the National Drug and Alcohol Research Centre (NDARC) of 213 Sydney based ecstasy users confirmed:

> [w]hat any dance party patron has known for a long time: that ecstasy users are by and large, experienced and concurrent users of many other drugs (Review of the NDARC study by Wood 1998b, p.17).

The NDARC study, conducted by experienced researchers Libby Topp, Julie Hando and Paul Dillon, found that their sample:

> [h]ad experimented with an average of 10.4 drugs, most frequently alcohol, cannabis, LSD, amphetamine, tobacco and amyl nitrate. In the preceding six months, the sample had used a mean of 8.1 drugs.
>
> The study found that almost all the subjects (96.2%) typically used other drugs, both in combination with ecstasy and during the 'come down' period after using ecstasy. While using ecstasy, the average number of other drugs used was 2.4. The most common were tobacco (67.7%), cannabis (43.4%), alcohol (40.4%), amy1 nitrate (11.7%) and LSD (10.3%).
>
> 'Of those that typically drank alcohol while using ecstasy, 45.0% typically consumed more than five standard dinks in an episode. A mean of 1.8 drugs were typically used while coming down from ecstasy, most commonly cannabis (63.4%), tobacco (61.5%), alcohol (19.7%), benzodiazepines (12.7%) and amphetamines', the authors wrote.
>
> The study shows a marked increase in polydrug use among ecstasy users compared with Solowij et al's earlier study. While in the 1992 study 47% of subjects had used ecstasy with marijuana, 41% with amphetamines, 19% with LSD and smaller proportions of the sample with other drugs, the authors found that 24% of users had never taken any other drug together with ecstasy (Discussed and quoted in Wood 1998b, p.17).

Discussing the NDARC survey, Wood comments further:

> It's clear from the studies that many users choose particular drugs to use in certain contexts and for certain effects.
>
> Topp et al report that other drugs were often used deliberately to alleviate the effects of the 'come-down' period after using ecstasy. Most respondents reported doing this (88.7%), using cannabis, alcohol and benzodiazepines for this purpose.
>
> 'The rates of depressant use among a primarily party drug-using sample were surprisingly high, and suggest that ecstasy users are adept at obtaining drugs which help them to self medicate the aversive physical and psychological effects of an ecstasy (and other drug) use episode,' the study states.

> The researchers were surprised at the high level of benzodiazepine use – 60% of the sample had used this drug. Twenty-eight percent had also used heroin (a figure of prevalence that the researchers attributed to its availability, particularly in south-west Sydney where subjects reported smoking it for relaxing or to aid with the side effects of stimulant use), 36% had used other opiates and 20% had used anti-depressants…
>
> Topp et al emphasise the need for better education on the risks of polydrug use.
>
> 'Moreover, half of those who drank alcohol with ecstasy typically did so at binge drinking levels', they wrote.
>
> 'This is a hazardous pattern of alcohol consumption in itself, let alone in combination with a drug known to cause dehydration.'
>
> 'Remarkably high rates of party drug use were also reported, further highlighting the need for a better understanding of the patterns and correlates of such drug use.'
>
> Almost all subjects in this sample had used LSD and amphetamine; over 80% had used amyl nitrate, and more than half had used cocaine, nitrous oxide and MDA, the study states.
>
> 'Given our lack of understanding of these drugs, urgent attention must be given to the possible harms associated with such use' (Discussed and quoted in Wood 1998b, pp.18–19).

Wood also reviews a study of poly-drug use in the Perth dance party scene conducted by Boys, Lenton and Norcross (1997):

> The Perth study found that 80% of its 83 respondents had used a combination of at least two 'dance drugs' – nominated as ecstasy, amphetamines or LSD – during their most recent rave.
>
> 'The most common drug used in addition to ecstasy was cannabis (69.2%), followed by amphetamines (34.6%) and inhalants (34.6%). LSD was used by 26.9% of those who used ecstasy, 19.2% used alcohol and 7.7% reported that they had used tranquillisers of some sort before, during or after the rave', the authors wrote…
>
> Boys et al in Perth found particular patterns of drug use that differed before, during and after a rave.
>
> 'For example, amphetamines were used by many more respondents before or during the rave than after it. Ecstasy and LSD were both used by more people during the rave than either before or afterwards. Cannabis was used by more people before and after the last rave than it was during the event and tranquillisers were mainly used afterwards. As well as choosing combinations of different drugs, the Perth respondents also reported buying tablets reputed to have already been mixed with other drugs, such as opiates, LSD and amphetamines, sold as 'Smack-E', 'Trippy E' and 'Coke-E' respectively (Wood 1998b, pp.18–19).

Both of the studies reviewed by Wood note that 'polydrug use is normal behaviour for ecstasy users' (Wood 1998b, p.19) and comment that very little is known about the possible harmful effects of interacting drugs:

> The authors of the Perth study point to the fact that there is little research on interactions between illicit drugs, and that the many possible specific combinations will continue to make research difficult...
>
> One thing is clear from both studies, far more research is needed before the implications of such polydrug use can be understood or addressed (Wood 1998b, p.19).

A British qualitative study of 76 ecstasy users found that it was impossible to find a single interviewee who could be classified as an 'Ecstasy only user' and that only 37 per cent of the sample could be classified as 'predominant Ecstasy users'. Drug use, both licit and illicit, for dance club patrons was far too intertwined (see Hammersley, Khan & Ditton 2002, pp.3ff.).[284] Another British study of 'dance club enthusiasts' found that many of the sample:

> [w]ere regularly using multiple tablets often consumed in combination with other substances thus exposing themselves to serious health risks, in particular the risk of dose related neurotoxic effects. Seventy per cent [of the sample] were drinking alcohol at hazardous levels... [Alcohol and cannabis] also appear to be the most common drugs used to assist in reducing the comedown associated with ecstasy use (Winstock, Griffiths & Stewart 2001, pp.9, 12).

Comprehensive qualitative and survey research by Measham and her colleagues in Britain also shows that 'clubbers' in particular are willing and able to experiment with drug mixes. Not only do dance club goers have substantially higher rates of tobacco and alcohol[285] use than the general population they are also vastly more experienced in experimenting with and partaking of a wide variety of illicit drugs. This sample of British clubbers at least:

> [h]ave embraced cocaine far more than their predecessors from the early 1990s and have a clear tendency to try 'new' drugs even with problematic reputations. GHB in particular only became easily available at the end of the 1990s, yet we find over one in ten of the [interviewees] having tried it.

284 This survey based on Scottish users of ecstasy in Glasgow crossed social classes and was equally balanced in terms of gender. One of the interesting findings was that cannabis was much more prevalent than tobacco. The survey also usefully asked respondents about the timing of their poly-drug use:

'Irrespective of actual overall frequency of co-use, respondents...indicated whether they took each substance before, during or after taking Ecstasy. The only substance most often consumed *before* Ecstasy use was alcohol, although both cocaine and amphetamine were consumed nearly as often before Ecstasy use as during it. Those drugs used mostly *during* Ecstasy use were tobacco, solvents, mushrooms, LSD, poppers and ketamine. Those used predominantly *after* Ecstasy use were cannabis, heroin...other opiates, temazepam and other benzodiazepines' (Hammersley, Khan & Ditton 2002, p.86) Authors' emphasis.

285 For further discussion of the role of alcohol in the 'party drug' scene, see Measham, Aldridge and Parker 2001, pp.104ff. and the discussion in Chapter 10.

> Similarly, we found that supplies of newly licensed Viagra[286] became quickly available on the club scene during our fieldwork…in autumn 1998…
>
> On the other hand, our clubbers largely continue to eschew crack cocaine and heroin, thereby distinguishing themselves from, as they see it, dependent drug users (Measham, Aldridge & Parker 2001, p.97).

As discussed in Chapter 4, this 'snobbery' of drug use has been well documented. In a study by McElrath and McEvoy (2001) it was quite apparent that non-opiate drug users (including amphetamine users) view heroin and heroin users in negative terms. McElrath and McEvoy found that ecstasy users in particular:

- Distanced themselves from heroin users
- Believed bad experiences with heroin could be attributed to tablets laced with heroin [despite all evidence to the contrary. In particular it would not be cost effective for most dealers to put heroin in ecstasy tablets]
- Describe heroin users in stereotypical terms and with scorn. For example: '*…people living in scum…train spotting type situation, just dirty, just caring about nothing…that's how I imagine drug injecting users*' (female, aged 25)
- '*Injectors are totally stupid*' (male, age 26, consumed 25 pints of beer and no water during his most recent use of ecstasy)
- Avoided treatment because they don't wish to be associated with heroin users (see also discussion in Chapter 20 of this Report)
- Felt 'superior' to heroin users and injectors (McElrath & McEvoy 2001, pp.177ff.).

The authors also found that ecstasy users who in their sample at least were predominantly middle class tended to view heroin as used 'primarily among persons in high unemployment areas' (McElrath & McEvoy 2001, p.178).

In a review of studies of young users of ecstasy by Measham, Aldridge and Parker similar responses were noticed across the board:

> [t]he consensus amongst youth samples studied was that cannabis was benign whilst heroin and crack cocaine were simply never to be tried, being addictive drugs with dreadful reputations (Measham et al. 2001, p.12).[287]

---

286 For further discussion of the use of Viagra in combination with 'party drugs', see Chapter 4. Measham, Aldridge and Parker's research showed that of the survey sample:

'Most reported having taken Viagra simultaneously with illegal drugs...and with alcohol. Amyl nitrite was of particular concern as it is contraindicated for use with Viagra, potentially leading to a dangerous drop in blood pressure. Although this is stated clearly in the product information leaflet, recreational uses of Viagra are highly unlikely to have access to this information or to the advice of their GPs' (Measham, Aldridge & Parker 2001, p.137).

287 The problem with advertising campaigns and policies that buy into fears about drugs such as heroin is, according to Klee, that 'problem users of other drugs are liable to disassociate themselves from the warnings' (Klee 1997a, p.24). Such policies may heighten an already artificial distinction between heroin and drugs such as ecstasy and/or amphetamines (see also Klee 1997b, 1997c).

Problems associated with poly-drug use

The fact that poly-drug use is so prevalent among ecstasy users can often make it difficult to '[d]isentangle the effects of Ecstasy from the effects of alcohol and other drugs consumed during the same episode' (McElrath & McEvoy 2002, p.201). Any negative consequences flowing from drug interactions may in some circumstances be wrongly attributed by the user to a bad 'E'. This may particularly be the case when alcohol is consumed in conjunction with MDMA. For example, Schifano and colleagues in a study of drug treatment patients found that persons who had taken ecstasy in conjunction with alcohol were more likely to suffer negative psychopathological side effects than abstainers of alcohol (Schifano et al. 1998). Cole and his colleagues state that there are a number of 'confounds' or explanatory factors that need to be taken into account when undertaking ecstasy analysis and ascribing any side effects to an ecstasy pill. These include poly-drug use; pre-morbid differences, co-morbid differences, sleep disruption, nutritional status to name a few (Cole et al. 2002, p.1535; see also Sherlock et al. 1999).

Oetting et al. have made similar observations with regard to methamphetamine use among American high school students:

> Methamphetamine users are almost all multi-drug users, with 90% using marijuana and about 90% using a drug other than marijuana and methamphetamine in the past month. The most frequently used drugs by methamphetamine users, outside of marijuana and alcohol, are amphetamines, cocaine and hallucinogens, suggesting a preference for drugs that produce excitement and intense sensations. However, many methamphetamine users also use depressants, downers and heroin.
>
> The finding that methamphetamine users are almost all multi-drug users makes it essentially impossible to determine whether methamphetamine use produce[d] specific drug use consequences (Oetting et al. 2000, p.47).

The findings of Hammersley, Khan and Ditton in a survey of Scottish ecstasy users were similar:

> Such is the spread of illegal drugs, and such is the relatively non-selective take-up of them by consumers, it is well nigh impossible to find respondents who use just one drug. They can tell us – they did tell us – what the effects of ecstasy were (they had all occasionally tried it when they were not using anything else), but given the number of drugs they had used, it was impossible for us to analyse their responses to other questions and thereafter definitively link these general responses (for example, that they felt 'depressed') to their prior use of any one particular drug (Hammersley, Khan & Ditton 2002, p.130).

Degenhardt and Topp's recent study of crystal methamphetamine use among members of Sydney's dance club scene also found that poly-drug use was the norm among the primarily gay sample. The drugs most commonly used were other stimulants and 'party drugs' such as ketamine. Again it was difficult to isolate direct evidence that any negative side effects suffered by the sample were due to the effects of crystal meth alone. Interestingly, however, and in line with other research studies, the participants in the study overwhelmingly attributed their side effects to crystal meth use alone, indicating that many drug users are not sufficiently aware of the dangers of various drug interactions (Degenhardt & Topp 2003, pp.20–21).

Poly-drug use and injecting users

A recent study conducted by RMIT University (highlighted in the submission from Dr Rowe, RMIT University) also testifies to high levels of poly-drug use among injecting drug users, particularly homeless persons in Melbourne. Of interest was the high level of valium (diazepam) being taken by the sample (58.7%: female 68.2%, male 51.2%). Dr Rowe makes the important point that poly-drug use serves an important functional purpose for many users:

> The nature of polydrug use is far more complex than simple drug substitution. A number of street-based users report using amphetamines in order to manage problems of dependency associated with heroin:
>
> *I've been trying to use speed instead of heroin because I'm trying my hardest not to get a heroin habit* (20-year-old female, street sex worker).
>
> *...I have been using 'ice' crystal meth, for a little while now. That's what I used to come down off buprenorphine* (21-year-old male).[288]

The use of amphetamine to 'come off' heroin is not unknown:

> The cost and addictive qualities [of heroin] make it unattractive...and amphetamine replaces it for a variety of reasons, a principal one being to counteract the heroin addiction and perhaps, also, get out of debt. They may then feel strongly attached to amphetamine but occasionally use heroin or a tranquilliser to come down. *Balancing drugs becomes a way of life for some:*
>
> Interviewer: *And when you're actually using speed are you using other things at the same time...?*
>
> Respondent: *Yeah, sometimes I use heroin at the same time, an' all the time I use valium because I really need that, but if I'm on speed I try to cut down on the valium because it seems pointless because valium gives me the same sort of feeling to speed...it gives me a lift... But it's the heroin I need really...even when you're taking speed you miss your other drugs* (Klee 1997b, p.54).[289]

---

288 Submission of Dr James Rowe, RMIT University to the Drugs and Crime Prevention Committee, Inquiry into Amphetamine and 'Party Drug' Use in Victoria, October 2003.

289 The use of amphetamine to come off heroin is also testified to by academic Dr David Moore of the National Drug Research Institute in Perth:

'A common refrain [is] that although using speed did not relieve the symptoms of heroin withdrawal, it did provide the necessary energy with which to deal with withdrawal symptoms' (Submission from Dr David Moore, National Drug Research Institute, Curtin University, to the Drugs and Crime Prevention Committee, Inquiry into Amphetamine and 'Party Drug' Use, November 2003).

'Coming down' drug use

One issue of particular concern in discussing poly-drug use among 'party drugs' users comes to light in a relatively recent Irish study that examines the use of heroin smoking or 'chasing the dragon' by young people when 'coming down' from ecstasy. This Dublin study interviewed 102 young people who were identified as opiate users. Of the sample, 92 had used ecstasy and 68 chased heroin to come down off this drug. The most alarming finding, however, was that:

> Thirty-six reported that their first experience of using opiates was to 'come down' off Ecstasy, 28 citing this as *their main reason for commencement*. Eighty-six of the 102 commenced opiates by 'chasing' heroin, 61 of whom progressed to injecting after a mean of 2.9 years. This was associated with starting illicit drug use earlier, starting heroin earlier, and a history of using Ecstasy (Gervin et al. 2001, p.297). (Committee emphasis)

The authors suggest that chasing heroin to come down would seem to be mostly associated with those who are taking heavier levels of ecstasy. Nonetheless, they acknowledge that further research is needed to investigate the prevalence of heroin smoking in the wider population of young ecstasy users (Gervin et al. 2001, p.299). Certainly, the Committee is not aware of any comparable practices among ecstasy users in Australia. Nonetheless, such practices are disturbing and drug researchers should keep a 'watching brief' on their appearance in Australia.

For ecstasy and 'party drug' users, other drugs such as marijuana and alcohol can be used as a form of 'self-medication' during the comedown stage. As was discussed in Chapter 4, heroin users have been known to use amphetamines and increasingly benzodiazepines in an effort to self-medicate, particularly during the 'heroin drought'. Amphetamine users are also known to use tranquillisers in an effort to self-medicate (see also Vincent, Allsop & Shoobridge 1996; Turning Point Alcohol and Drug Centre 2001; Baker, Boggs & Lewin 2001). This has dangers not only because of the potentially toxic interactions between the drugs, but also because the amounts consumed are far in excess of safe levels.[290] Moore's study of psychostimulant users in Perth found that males in particular consumed enormous amounts of alcohol when under the influence of amphetamines and to a lesser extent ecstasy:

> These drugs seem to suppress feelings of intoxication from alcohol and allow the drug user to drink far in excess of his normal capabilities and tolerance. Consequently, drinking anywhere between ten and twenty standard drinks per

---

290 Williamson et al. conducted a study in Britain of illicit drug users that used stimulants alone and those who used them in conjunction with depressant drugs such as opiates and benzodiazepines. The study found that:

'The stimulant and depressant users were more likely than the stimulants-only users to use stimulants by injection and more likely to report adverse effects associated with stimulant use. The stimulant and depressant users were also more likely to have been treated for a drug problem' (Williamson et al. 1997, p.87).

Henry-Edwards has also noted that the effects of other drugs in conjunction with amphetamine use are marked. In particular, the effects of amphetamine on aggression are accelerated when the user is also affected by opioids and opioid withdrawal (Henry-Edwards 2002, p.3).

> outing…is not uncommon. In an average week, one might attend nightclubs on two or three separate occasions which put the weekly consumption figure somewhere between thirty and sixty standard drinks (Moore 1992a, p.57).

Such studies, however, have been contradicted by others which find that users of ecstasy are inclined not to take it in conjunction with alcohol (at least not during the active phase of the drug) as it counteracts or deadens the effect of ecstasy and may result in unpleasant side-effects (Solowij, Hall & Lee 1992; see also Hansen, Maycock & Lower 2001; Lenton & Davidson 1999). It would seem, however, according to recent and current research, that alcohol use in conjunction with ecstasy is increasingly common, particularly among young people.[291]

There has also been speculation as to ecstasy's potential to act as a 'gateway drug'; that is, initiating ecstasy or other 'party drug' users to so-called harder drugs such as heroin or amphetamines (see Hansen, Maycock & Lower 2001; Von Sydow et al. 2002 and the references listed therein).[292] Research conducted by Pedersen and Skrondal (1999) suggests that such speculation is unfounded.

Hansen, Maycock and Lower suggest rather that:

> Perhaps more significant than ecstasy's potential as a gateway drug [is] the general trend towards polydrug use. Previous studies have suggested that the 'pure' ecstasy user is a rarity, citing significant polydrug consumption patterns… Initiates and inexperienced users tended [in this survey] to use ecstasy in isolation from other drugs, with the exception of alcohol, which was typically consumed in moderation or not at all. It was universal that as users became more experienced, they exhibited a pattern of use that included the consumption of greater amounts of ecstasy and an increasing combination of other drugs. Whether this pattern is a result of physical or psychological tolerance, or simply an experiential expansion along the drug use continuum, is difficult to say without further research (Hansen, Maycock & Lower 2001, p.189).[293]

Drug 'cocktails'

Grob is concerned about the relatively recent trend for ecstasy to be combined with other psychoactive drugs such as ketamine. This has been particularly noticeable in Britain. Commenting on the work of British researcher Valerie Curran, Grob states:

> Curran's work and those of her counterparts in the United Kingdom, have highlighted the degree to which the Ecstasy scene has been pervaded with polydrug abuse. In Curran's study, less than two per cent of her ecstasy

291 As discussed in Chapter 10 of this Report, much of the earlier sociological and ethnographic survey literature on ecstasy use comments that ecstasy users prefer raves precisely because to a large extent they are alcohol free and thereby non-violent and without the 'sleaze factor'.

292 Von Sydow et al. argue that 'it is important to evaluate if ex-ecstasy users who have stopped taking the drug compensate their ecstasy abstinence with an increased consumption of other licit or illicit drugs' (Von Sydow et al. 2002, p.148).

293 For a discussion of the types of drugs commonly used before, during and after 'raves' in conjunction with ecstasy, see the survey of young ecstasy users in Perth done by Lenton, Boys and Norcross 1997; Lenton and Davidson 1999.

> subjects were not polydrug users. An added factor has been the surge in popularity of the dissociative anaesthetic ketamine...ketamine use has increased significantly among Ecstasy using ravers... Excessive use of a variety of powerful psychoactive substances, taken at all night raves under conditions of nutritional and sleep deprivation, were all common histories for the ecstasy users recruited into the British studies...
>
> ...To fully appreciate the degree of public health risk, it is essential for investigators to acknowledge the polydrug context of Ecstasy culture. To mistake the cumulative consequences of multiple drug use for the effects of MDMA alone obfuscates our understanding of this complex phenomenon (Grob 2000, pp.573–574, 578–579).

A drug cocktail (whether because of using other drugs in addition to amphetamines at the same time or proximate in time as the administration of amphetamine or because of the variability in purity or quality of the amphetamines itself) can result in particular health problems. For example, the use of amphetamines or methamphetamines with alcohol can cause increased cardiac and psychological effects.[294] Similarly, 'speedballing' (or the use of amphetamines simultaneously with opiates such as heroin) can increase toxicity (Albertson, Derlet & Van Hoozen 1999, p.215).

Conclusion

This Part has endeavoured to examine, however cursorily, some of the main physical, psychological and social consequences of using amphetamines and 'party drugs'. Given the wide range of drugs and substances that come under the rubric of both these broad classifications, such a task is bound to result in some generalisations.

Nonetheless, the Part has examined a variety of consequences flowing from the use of the main drugs in these categories, particularly methamphetamine and ecstasy. These consequences range from the relatively minor to life threatening.

There are still, however, many 'unknowns' in this particular area of drug knowledge. For example: What effect do amphetamines have on cognitive functioning?

The psychiatric and psychological consequences of amphetamines and ecstasy are still uncertain. For example, is there an ecstasy dependence syndrome? This is one of the many key scientific issues still being debated.

This Part also discussed several social consequences of using these various drugs, including links between amphetamines, crime and violence and the effect of amphetamines and ecstasy on driving and road trauma.

294 A survey by Australian drug researchers Hall and Hando found that:
'An unanticipated health risk among these [Sydney based survey] users was a high rate of concurrent alcohol and amphetamine intoxication. Just over half reported consuming five or more standard drinks when using amphetamines and one fifth reported using amphetamine because it enabled them to drink more alcohol without feeling or appearing to be intoxicated' (Hall & Hando 1993, p.643).

An examination of some of the 'newer' 'party drugs' and their potential for deleterious outcomes was also included. In particular, the alarming trend to use drugs such as GHB as a means for committing sexual assault – that is, as a so-called 'date rape' drug – was noted.

In the final chapter the Part discussed poly-drug use, raising the question: What are the effects of taking other drugs in association with amphetamines or ecstasy?

Clearly one of the main factors to arise from the discussion in this chapter is that more research of both a qualitative and quantitative nature is needed to address some of these unresolved issues and questions. The need to prioritise research in this area will be discussed in detail in Chapter 21 of this Report.

PART D: The Culture and Patterns of Use

The following discussion moves from a quantitative or medical appraisal of amphetamine and 'party drug' use to a more descriptive and qualitative based discussion of the patterns, profiles and cultures of this form of drug taking. It poses the following questions: Who uses amphetamines and why? What is it about the culture of drug use that sustains, and indeed nurtures, that use? What role does music play in the various 'party drug' cultures? What, as one critic has termed it, is the 'folk pharmacology' of 'party drug' use? Such inquiries are properly the province of sociologists and ethnographers. While this Report cannot address all of the possible answers, it does attempt to give a glimpse, however superficial, of the patterns and culture of amphetamine and 'party drug' use. It does this through both a comprehensive review of the literature in addition to incorporating the views of those who can give an insight into this particular world, either through their work in the area or their personal experiences of drug use.

Chapter 9 examines the profiles of varied and discrete groups of drug user. It commences with a discussion of amphetamine use 'on the street', particularly among street workers and the homeless. It then follows with a discussion of amphetamine use as a 'functional' measure, particularly concentrating on those who use it in the transport industry. A section on 'party drug' use in the gay and lesbian community follows. Such a choice is not gratuitous; it is testament to the reality that 'party drug' use is disproportionately high among certain sectors of the gay and lesbian population, which is of great concern to the homosexual community itself. Discussions of amphetamine and 'party drug' use within non-English speaking and Indigenous communities respectively highlight the ways in which addressing drug use in Victoria must be culturally sensitive to the needs of discrete populations. Finally, the chapter examines the somewhat curious case of 'party drug' use among middle-class professionals.

Chapter 10 is primarily a discussion of the culture and profiles of 'party drug' use within the club, dance party and rave scene. Of necessity much of the discussion focusses on ecstasy/MDMA (or what purports to be MDMA) for this is still the predominant drug used within that culture. However, other drugs such as GHB, ketamine and even LSD will also be examined within these 'lifeworlds'.

The Part concludes with Chapter 11, a discussion of amphetamine and 'party drug' use in rural and regional Victoria. Issues pertaining to drug use within country areas of this state, as with so many other areas of health and social policy, have been neglected for far too long. The Committee hopes that its examination of amphetamine and 'party drug' use across the state and the views that were sought from rural and regional stakeholders will, at least in part, ensure that the needs of non-metropolitan areas of Victoria are always addressed and highlighted in proposals, planning or policies pertaining to drug use and misuse.

9. Patterns and Profiles of Use

This chapter recognises that there is no one profile of a drug user or drug abuser. This is true of all drugs, be they licit such as alcohol or illicit such as amphetamines and 'party drugs'. The following sections of this chapter examine a variety of user profiles of discrete groups that predominantly use amphetamines and to a lesser degree 'party drugs' and the reasons for such use. These range from transport drivers who rely on 'speed' and/or prescription drugs to maintain punishing delivery schedules, to women who take amphetamines to 'self medicate' their physical or mental health conditions. Often there may be overlap between those groups. For example, a long-distance transport driver may use amphetamines in order to stay awake to meet deadlines but also may use them or indeed other drugs for recreational purposes. This also reflects the reality that poly-drug use is a prevalent feature of much drug taking in recent years, as discussed in Chapter 8.

The chapter focusses generally on the amphetamines such as methamphetamine. The use of MDMA/ecstasy and other 'party drugs' is profiled for the most part in the next chapter in the context of 'raving and clubbing'. This is because overwhelmingly these are still the contexts in which such drugs are used. As such the culture and profiles of such use merits a chapter of its own. Any discussion of ecstasy use that falls outside this context will be mentioned briefly in this chapter. Such discussion falls into three main groups: These are:

- 'Party Drug' use which forms part of a poly-drug 'repertoire'. For example, those occasions when it may be used as a 'street drug' in substitution for or in addition to a preferred drug such as heroin or methamphetamine;
- 'Party Drugs' that are used *exclusively* by a profiled group outside of the rave or club culture. A section devoted to ecstasy use by middle-class professionals is an example of such use; and
- 'Party Drugs' that are used in addition to amphetamines by a particular group that is defined by some feature and where it is narratively more convenient to include discussion of both types of drugs within the same section. The discussion of both amphetamine and 'party drug' use by women is an example of this type.

Amphetamine users in general

'Street' users of amphetamines, as a separate class of user, are examined briefly in this chapter. There is strong anecdotal evidence of a significant change in the use patterns of and trade in amphetamines, particularly since the advent of the 'heroin drought'. This has resulted in a 'street culture' of use. One should be careful, however, in assuming that a street culture of amphetamine use is necessarily the same as that of heroin or other drug use. The manifestation of a street culture of amphetamine use will clearly display features that are both similar to other forms of drug use but also peculiar to the particular drug in question.

It is erroneous to speak of a 'typical' amphetamine user as it is to speak of a typical drug user per se. However, Kamienicki et al. (1998) note that while it is true that amphetamine users are not a homogenous group:

> [r]esearch has shown that regular psychostimulant users (and particularly amphetamine users) have a number of common characteristics. Namely:
>
> - They tend to exhibit a wider range of polydrug use than opioid users (Darke and Hall 1995);
> - They tend to be younger than opioid users (Darke and Hall 1995; Loxley, Marsh and Lo 1991);
> - They may exhibit a wide range of psychopathology associated with their amphetamine use (Hall et al 1996; Hando 1996; Klee et al 1995; Vincent et al 1996);
> - They are generally highly socially orientated (Hando 1996; Klee and Morris 1994; Vincent et al 1996);
> - They tend to see themselves as different from opioid users, and often won't enter existing treatment services because of the perceived stigma (Klee and Morris 1994; Vincent et al 1997);
> - They are less likely to have experienced treatment for drug use than opioid users (Hall et al 1993), and those who have done so tend to have a more fragile connection with treatment services (Klee et al 1995);
> - Many tend to seek assistance for problems associated with their drug use from a general practitioner in the first instance (Hando 1996; Klee et al 1995; Ross and Miller 1994; Vincent et al 1996) (Kamienicki et al. 1998, pp.7–8).

Despite such factors, it is generally true that one cannot speak of an amphetamine or psychostimulant class of user. One of the reasons why psychostimulant users cannot be readily compared is because amphetamines are a 'family' of drugs rather than one discrete drug and can vary from the prescription medications used to treat Attention Deficit Disorder to weight loss formulae.[295]

295 Indeed research conducted in Western Australia by the National Drug Research Institute has been at pains to warn against constructing a stereotype of amphetamine or other drug use. A survey by Lenton and his colleagues of people who accessed 'Fitpacks' (needle and syringe packs) through pharmacies revealed that over half of the 511 people surveyed injected

The many and varied functions and uses to which methamphetamine is put is well described in ethnographic research conducted by Mayrhauser, Brecht and Anglin (2002). Their research question was primarily: Who are methamphetamine users and what are the circumstances that surround their drug use? Their survey of 260 methamphetamine users admitted to public treatment programmes in Los Angeles revealed a multiplicity of motivations and reasons for using the drug. Twenty-eight per cent of the sample used it because they perceived it as a cheaper, safer, and/or more satisfying drug than other stimulants. Twenty-three per cent used it to stay awake, often by workers in the labouring and construction industries. Invariably if the drug was used for this purpose, increasing amounts of it had to be used over time as tolerance set in. Eleven per cent used it to enhance sexual experience. Ten per cent used it to lose weight. Of most interest and perhaps concern is the fact that twenty-eight per cent of the sample used methamphetamine to help and support people cope with their mental illness, distress or trauma. The use of amphetamines in this way is not restricted to California. Many respondents to this Inquiry have impressed upon the Committee the use of illicit drug use as a form of self-medication.[296]

Professor Jason White of the Drugs and Alcohol Services Council of South Australia stresses the 'heterogeneity' of amphetamine and 'party drug' use:

> We see everybody, from a person who would be a drug user out of central casting, who looks like a street drug user and is a street drug user, through to people who have run into stimulant problems because, for instance, they are businesspeople who have tried to improve their work performance, and they have eventually run into problems with drug use...a lot of the dance party people are very much middle-class kids and they are quite different from your average archetypal drug user. There are also individual little pockets. I have come across people, for example, whose primary drug is alcohol but they use methamphetamine to keep awake. If you take enough alcohol, then you fall asleep and the night ends, essentially. If you use methamphetamine, the night does not end; you keep drinking. They are often much lower socioeconomic people. It is drinking and getting drunk that is the primary activity for them, and methamphetamine is an aid to that. Those people would have absolutely no connection with the middle-class kids going to raves. They would not see themselves in any way as common; similarly, the businesspeople.

---

amphetamine and/or heroin less than once a day and 24% less than once a week (Lenton et al. 2000). Such results suggested recreational use rather than dependent use. As such users did not access treatment programmes it was not necessarily easy to target education programmes at this group:

'"Many IDUs [intravenous drug users) who buy needle packs don't fit the drug-addict stereotype", Dr Lenton said:

The resulting drug user profile countered the common view that users were junkies and were mostly criminals, homeless or jobless' ('Addicts' "middle class"', *The West Australian*, Wednesday 12 March 1997, p.3.

296 See for example the submission of Youth Substance Abuse Service to the Drugs and Crime Prevention Committee, Inquiry into Amphetamine and 'Party Drug' Use in Victoria, October 2003.

> The difficulty for us in the treatment services area – and in the population area – is that you have this very diverse population. We are much more accustomed to dealing with heroin users, where they are not exactly homogeneous but they are a lot more homogeneous.[297]

Because of the variation in the types of amphetamines available and the use to which they are put, it is very difficult to target programmes to meet the particular needs of any particular user, unlike targeting needs in the areas of alcohol and heroin use (Griffin 1997).[298] Exploratory research from southern Queensland conducted by Dennis for the Logan Youth Health Service (LYHS) confirms the difficulties involved in obtaining specific information necessary for targeting programmes:

> Brett Cutting from the LYHS said finding information about amphetamine users was a hard task, which was why the service was forced to conduct its own research.
>
> 'There is little if any discussion about amphetamines at conferences, workshops and seminars.' [Our] study reinforced what we already knew. That amphetamine is on the rise and it is virtually impossible to get it on the agenda at professional level (Dennis 2000, p.12).

However, some distinctions can be made. Although Professor Hilary Klee of the Centre for Social Research on Health and Substance Abuse makes comment on the absolute dearth of research into social profiles of amphetamine users, referring to them as 'this hidden population', she has constructed a typology of what she views as the five main patterns and profiles of use occurring in Britain today. The typology consists of:

- Ravers – young adolescents or people in their early to mid-20s. They used low doses for dancing and partying to capture the ambience of the rave scene and partly because it was cheaper than alcohol
- Drinkers – young men who regularly went out drinking with mates and took speed so they could appear to hold their liquor better
- Young mothers – women who had children at a young age and were working part time. They were rarely injecting users and took speed to give them energy to look after the kids, do the housework and work
- Young experimenters – male adolescents who took a variety of drugs 'in a spirit of adventure' to experience their effects
- Poly drug users – somewhat older than other user groups (Klee cited in Griffin 1997, pp.19–20).

Both research and programme development need to be better attuned to who is using amphetamines and what their specific needs are. In particular:

297 Professor Jason White, DASC in conversation with the Drugs and Crime Prevention Committee, Adelaide, 3 October 2003.

298 See Chapter 20 for an account of the difficulties associated with treating amphetamine-related problems.

> ...Prof Klee nominated certain groups as being particularly hard to reach in campaigns and programmes – 'women with young children, young criminals and any groups that believe that performance is superior if the drug is used' (Griffin 1997, p.19).

There has been insufficient research to state categorically that such a typology can be extrapolated to the Australian context. Nonetheless, anecdotal accounts and some exploratory social research suggest that such comparisons are not without merit.

The LYHS study, although not academically based, did provide some useful information in a poorly researched area. For example, it found that those who used amphetamines were largely uninterested in accessing health and harm reduction information:

> [b]ecause it was viewed as being more relevant to 'junkies' or heroin users. They were classifying speed as a softer drug. They did not see themselves as 'junkies' (Dennis 2000, p.12).

The authors of the report suggested that this 'ignorance' could be combated by an appropriate media campaign:

> An intensive media campaign has been suggested as one solution, as there are often reports about alcohol, tobacco and heroin related health risks. Speed is rarely mentioned and this may be contributing to an almost false sense of security amongst some speed users (Dennis 2000, p.14).

The service found that most of their young amphetamine users commenced their use from curiosity:

> [b]ut other reasons included 'the ability to have the energy to get things done', 'the ability to feel in control', 'the ability to lose weight' and most disturbing was that speed let one user 'escape the reality of my poverty' (Dennis 2000, p.13).

Of particular concern are some suggestions coming from the Logan survey that some young people may be using amphetamines to 'self-medicate' their pain:

> From the information obtained it has been hard to establish whether amphetamines are causing problems or whether they are being used to deal with problems or a combination of the two. The only thing that really helped people to stop using seems to be the high cost of obtaining speed. Fifty-eight per cent of respondents reported that financial cost was the single hardest aspect of continuing to use amphetamines (Dennis 2000, p.14).

To Klee's typology one could also add sportspeople (see Chesher 1990b in the context of 'designer drugs' and amphetamines), and people, particularly children, with attention deficit type disorders[299] and 'bingers' (Ovenden & Loxley

299 The use of the stimulant drug methylphenidate (Ritalin) in the treatment of Attention Deficit Hyperactivity Disorder (ADHD) and similar conditions has come in for much criticism in recent years. Methylphenidate consumption increased by more than 600% between 1989 and 1994 (UNDCP 1996) and prescriptions of the drug are particularly common in the United States and Australia (see Klee 2001a, p.31).

1996).[300] Bingeing on amphetamines, particularly when associated with injectable drug use, has been characterised as one of the most hazardous patterns of psychostimulant abuse (Chesher 1993; Ovenden & Loxley 1996). Studies of binge use of amphetamines show that it is not uncommon for (young) people to use amphetamines repeatedly or continuously over a period of three to four days. In their qualitative survey of binge culture, Ovenden and Loxley argue that an ethnographic understanding of bingeing is important in order to develop appropriate harm reduction strategies (1996, pp.33–34ff.). An interesting finding of their research is that those who inject amphetamines are more likely to binge for longer periods than those who do not inject. Of equal concern is the fact that bingeing has been associated with quite serious poly-drug use (Ovenden & Loxley 1996; Semple, Patterson & Grant 2002).

Unfortunately there is very little research material available of either a qualitative or quantitative nature in the context of sportspeople and bingers. Nor is there comprehensive research that examines the use of these drugs among women, people living in regional and rural Victoria, or people from non-English-speaking backgrounds.[301] In addition, the Committee has received very little information from the community in relation to these groups. The following profiles of amphetamine and 'party drug' use among 'street users', women, people from non-English speaking backgrounds and Indigenous people are therefore limited. More and better research, which draws from the experiences of these people and those who work with them, is therefore essential.

Street users of amphetamines

There have been a number of research studies on 'street use' of heroin. Far fewer have been conducted on the use of amphetamine in a street context. One survey that has recently examined the street use of amphetamines (in the context of other drug use, including heroin) is that of Rowe (2003).[302] Rowe conducted interviews with 150 injecting drug users in the City of Port Phillip (based in St

---

300 A general typology of use could conceivably include licit forms of amphetamine use such as children with attention deficit type disorders and people using the drugs in order to lose weight. Neither of these groups will be discussed in any great detail.

301 A submission from the welfare agency 'Open Family', gives anecdotal evidence that problematic amphetamine use is rising among young women in rural Victoria: It states:

'Illicit drug use has not been exclusive to the city as Open Family Street Outreach Workers in rural Victoria have noticed a considerable rise in the level of amphetamine use in the Hume region over the past couple of years. Staff are seeing an increasing number of young people, especially young women 14–21 years presenting with problematic amphetamine use. Some of the self rationalising perceptions for using amphetamines by young women in rural Victoria are seeing the drug as a social experience *and not in any way like taking opiates which they see as "using drugs"*. Amphetamine use is also being used to lose weight and to keep up with social and school life and commitments' (Submission of Open Family Australia to the Drugs and Crime Prevention Committee, Inquiry into Amphetamine and 'Party Dug' Use in Victoria, August 2002). (Committee emphasis)

302 Dr Rowe's research is described and summarised in a submission by him to this Committee. See Submission of Dr James Rowe to the Drugs and Crime Prevention Committee, Inquiry into Amphetamine and 'Party Drug' Use in Victoria, October 2003.

Kilda, Melbourne). Although not exclusively focussed on amphetamine use, amphetamines were found to be the second most commonly used drug group (107 (71%) of participants reported so using). This was second only to heroin in use.[303] Poly-drug use was the norm for nearly all injecting drug users.

Who are street users?

A number of classifications and typologies have been constructed in characterising who might be considered a 'street user'. Lambert and Wiebel (1990) speak of 'hidden' or disadvantaged and disenfranchised populations including:

> [t]he homeless and transient, chronically mentally ill, high school dropouts, criminal offenders, prostitutes, juvenile delinquents, gang members, runaways and other street people (Lambert & Wiebel 1990 quoted in Klee 1997b).

In their review of amphetamine use in Australia, Hando and Hall include street and sex workers and homeless youth among their disenfranchised populations. They also include people who, while technically not street users (for example, prisoners and juvenile detention inmates), share many of the characteristics of such users or had been using on the streets prior to their incarceration (Hall & Hando 1997).

Rowe in his recent research states:

> [a] 'street-based' drug user is defined as an individual who uses drugs in public (public toilets, alleys and laneways, parkland etc.) through necessity rather than choice. There are three identifiable although certainly not mutually exclusive groups that comprise the majority of street-based users. These are homeless (both those 'sleeping rough' and those living in temporary accommodation), the mentally ill and street-based sex workers, more of who are driven to work such long hours that a significant part of their life is lived on the street (Rowe 2003, p.2).

Rowe reports that some of the research participants did not necessarily like using amphetamine or would not have had it as their first choice, but for the restrictions in their heroin supply:

> [a] number of research participants...[also] drew attention to the negative consequences associated with the increased use of amphetamines.
>
> *'A lot of users, in the drought, there was no heroin but they started using speed and stuff like that. They never used to like speed and speed is a totally different drug to heroin – which meant a lot of people went crazy as well because people were thinking they can use speed like they could use heroin, in big amounts which ended up sending them all crazy. That 'ice' at the moment, it's a very evil drug. It really gets into your head'* (21-year-old male, squatter) (Rowe 2003, p.3).

303 Rowe's fieldwork coincided approximately with the period of the so-called 'heroin drought', which could possibly account for the high levels of amphetamine use. 'Party Drug' use such as ecstasy was relatively low and is not considered further in this section.

Rowe argues that for street users of drugs the patterns of use are very fluid:

> In this respect, it would be inaccurate to refer to an injecting drug user as a 'heroin user' or an 'amphetamine user'. For some injecting drug users, 'needle fixation', the ritual of preparing and injecting a drug, is almost as important as the drug itself (McBride et. al. 2001). This may partially explain the use of amphetamines as a 'substitute' for heroin. It is not so much that they find it difficult to acquire heroin, but rather the use of speed provides the injection 'rush' without the risk of acquiring an opiate dependency (again).[304]
>
> *I tried heroin before I tried speed. Once I'd tried the heroin and I got used to the needle it was like, oh, speed? I'll try it. I went through a stage when my mate came over from Tassie and he knew someone [who could supply] and it was really good stuff and it ended up becoming a weekly thing that we would go and do it. It's not really addictive. The needle is more addictive than what the speed is* (23-year-old male, in transitional accommodation).
>
> The point should, however, be noted, that street-based users would be expected to exhibit greater patterns of fluidity than 'functioning' drug users who have a steady disposable income and established drug 'contacts' whose business transactions are conducted within the relative security and privacy of private accommodation (ensuring a steady supply of one's drug of choice). In comparison, street-based users whose lives may be transient, their income may be limited and their access to certain drugs may be short-lived. Again, the key words are availability and affordability (Rowe 2003, p.8).

Reasons for 'street users' using amphetamines

Dr David Moore of Curtin University argues that in discussing street drug use, the focus shouldn't necessarily be on the particular drug in question. The type of drug (and its effects) are not so important as the reasons why it is used and the antecedents of its use:

> I think what you've got...is a set of people whose primary issues are marginality, homelessness, poverty, low qualifications and so on and so forth so the emphasis shouldn't be so much on particular drugs but on a set of processes that put people in that kind of situation or lead them to that kind of situation and using a whole range of drugs when they get to that situation whereas with the rave kind of scene it's a very different kind of user, a different

304 Relatively recent research by Kaye and Darke compared the demographic profiles of primary heroin and amphetamine users. While there were many similarities in use, there were some interesting differences including:

Primary heroin injectors were older, less educated and more likely to be unemployed, in drug treatment and have a prison record;

Primary amphetamine users were more likely to have a wider poly-drug use repertoire;

The social functioning of heroin users was 'significantly worse' than that of primary amphetamine users;

Amphetamine is more likely to be injected in peer company than heroin, ie. it is a more 'social activity' (See Kaye & Darke 2000).

> social context and so your responses in the way you might think about it need to be quite different.[305]

Nonetheless, there are some reasons why amphetamine may be singled out and therefore needs to be specifically factored in terms of harm reduction approaches. For instance, for many street users of drugs the use of amphetamine has particular instrumental value. The 'functionality' of amphetamine use is discussed in detail in the next section of this chapter. In the context of street use, however, amphetamine serves distinct purposes.

First, it may offer a form of escape or redress from social isolation, mental illness and/or homelessness:

> For some these circumstances may increase the attraction of drug use as a form of self-medication (Mallett et.al. 2003; Neale, 2001). A study of 200 young homeless drug users by Klee and Reid (1998) found 71 per cent had self-medicated with drugs for depression, 23 per cent for aches and pains and 15 per cent for insomnia. Neale (2001) found that drug taking helped to fill the time and diminish the physical and emotional pain of being homeless. Rather than using drugs to transcend ordinary life, as many users of 'party drugs' seek to do, those who use drugs to relieve emotional pain do so to transcend pain and achieve a state that resembles everyday life (Dowsett & Wain 2000 cited in Mallett et.al. 2003) (Quote and references in a submission from Rowe 2003, p.9).

Second, for street users of drugs who are involved in prostitution, amphetamine enables them to work longer hours and serve more clients than they may otherwise be able to. A vicious circle is created whereby sex workers use amphetamine to work longer hours to earn the money to buy more drugs:

> *'It's the girls' boyfriends that's pimping them. They're standing there with their hand out you know and they've got their girl working on the corner you know. I was listening to one guy the other day saying how oh yeah my girl's gotta do this, that's the only way we can survive at the moment, she's got to do this, you know? I'm thinking, she don't have to do nothing I'm thinking to myself, like she's only a young girl she's only 14 or something and he's like 28 and she's only been on the street for about 2 weeks and he's got her out there 24/7 and he's just giving her speed, speed, speed so she can stay awake and she's a mess, absolutely a mess. She wouldn't even know if she got raped you know. Eventually they just lose the plot'* (36-year-old street-based sex worker) (Rowe 2002, p.11).

Many witnesses giving evidence to this Committee have commented that current policy and service delivery does not cater for the needs of street based and injecting users of amphetamine (and other drugs). For example, Moore made the following observations on how the delivery of primary health care services:

305 Dr David Moore, Curtin University in conversation with the Drugs and Crime Prevention Committee, Perth, 2 October 2003.

This was a view also put forward by Dr John Howard of the Ted Noffs Foundation when the Committee met with him in Sydney in 2003.

> [n]eeds to be re-aligned more closely with the often nocturnal temporal rhythms of the target groups. Sterile injecting equipment should be available on a 24 hour basis (via vending machines). Late night 'needle sharing' is shaped by the unavailability of sterile injecting equipment between 11.15pm and 9am (when fixed or mobile NSPs are closed). This is also consistent with epidemiological indicators of street drug market activity indicating St Kilda's higher proportion of overdoses between midnight and 6am when compared with Melbourne's other identified street markets (Dietze, Jolley and Cvetkovski 2003).[306]

The area of service delivery, particularly in the context of harm reduction will be commented upon more fully in Chapter 20. It is, however, worth noting Rowe's views that:

> The experiences of street-based drug users are all too often overlooked in the course of policy and other research. If policy and / or treatment interventions are to be effective in addressing the misuse of illicit drugs by street-based users, they must be sensitive to both the social context in which drugs are used and the related reasons that motivate an individual's use of drugs. It should be obvious to all concerned that those best placed to provide this information are those who live the day-to-day reality of street-based drug use. Until the experiences of 'users' are accorded the priority deserved, then the policy prescriptions of 'experts' and 'specialists', however well-intentioned, will invariably meet with limited success (Rowe 2003, p.3).

Young people in crisis[307]

There is clearly a certain amount of overlap between this profile of drug use and street use of amphetamine. Young people who use drugs are often homeless and/or in state protective care.[308] Sadly they may all too often be street workers. Drug use for many young people at risk may be a coping strategy. The Youth Substance Abuse Service (YSAS) based in Melbourne is very familiar with the reasons why many of the young people in their care may choose to get 'trashed' on drugs or alcohol:

> The 'typical' young person accessing the services provided by YSAS has experienced multiple adverse events in his or her life, apart from and preceding

---

306 Submission of Dr David Moore, Curtin University to the Drugs and Crime Prevention Committee, Inquiry into Amphetamine and 'Party Drug' Use in Victoria, November 2003. See also the submission of Anex to the Drugs and Crime Prevention Committee, Inquiry into Amphetamine and 'Party Drug' Use in Victoria, October 2003, and the discussion in Chapter 19.

307 The 'party drug' use by young people who may not necessarily be 'at risk' or 'in crisis', and are often educated, middle-class clubbers, is not discussed in this section. See instead the discussion in Chapter 10.

Howard and Arcuri stress the need for policy-makers and educators to distinguish between the various patterns of adolescent psychostimulant use. These can be generally referred to as Experimental Use, Rave or Club Scene Use and Problematic Use. The latter group is 'characterised by chaotic use often by injection and often associated with homelessness and criminal behaviour' (2003, p.7). It is this latter group that this section focusses upon.

308 These are not necessarily mutually exclusive categories.

> those associated with their alcohol and/or drug use. The majority of these young people have experienced significant levels of trauma and abuse during their childhood and adolescence. Children who have been exposed to overwhelmingly negative early life experiences suffer from a 're-setting' of their arousal baseline, so that even when no threat is present they remain in a state of physiological alarm. This makes them more 'reactive', increasing the likelihood they will be pushed into a state of terror by quite minor stressors. These changes in arousal levels as a result of abuse and neglect play a major role in the behavioural problems associated with such young people. For these young people drugs provide an escape from unbearable feelings.
>
> Young people accessing the services provided by YSAS also typically present with a multiplicity of mental health concerns such as self-harm, eating disorders, anxiety and depression...
>
> YSAS believes that in seeking to respond to the needs of young people such as these, to simply focus on the drug without understanding the set and the setting is at best irresponsible, and at worst creating more problems than such an approach seeks to solve.[309]

Howard and Arcuri make similar comments:

> It appears then, that young people who develop patterns of regular and problematic or harmful use differ from those who merely experiment or maintain irregular use. Personality characteristics, genetic and biological factors, individual differences in vulnerability, family difficulties, association with substance using peers, differential exposure to substances, shared and non-shared environments, and accumulations of social disadvantage all play a role (Moncher, Holden and Schinke, 1991; Rutter and Smith, 1995; Spooner, Mattick and Howard, 1996). The interplay of these variables in particular cultures and situations, or, more broadly, varying contexts are crucial (Spooner, Hall and Lynsky, 2001). Some sub-groups of young people may be more at risk, for example, indigenous young people, street youth, gay/lesbian/bisexual/transgender young people, those within juvenile justice systems, and young people from war-torn areas and refugees (Howard & Arcuri 2003, p.9).

---

309 Submission of YSAS to the Drugs and Crime Prevention Committee, Inquiry into Amphetamine and 'Party Drug' Use in Victoria, October 2003.

Such a group of clients needs to be distinguished from the other main type of profile of user that YSAS sees. That being young people referred to by the courts or police as a result of being apprehended with an illicit substance:

'[i]ncreasingly young people are coming to us in that capacity, but they do not fit the same profile as the typical young person that we would normally be seeing. In other words, they are reasonably well educated or still in education or in employment, and their use of the substance is not particularly problematic at this point. They are often using it in the context of the party scene' (Mr David Murray, YSAS, evidence given to the Drugs and Crime Prevention Committee, Inquiry into Amphetamine and 'Party Drug' Use in Victoria, Public Hearings (Melbourne), 27 October 2003).

Jurgen Hemmerling, a drug outreach worker in country Victoria, has had vast experience in working with young people who have had a life history of adverse events. When he met with the Committee in Benalla in October 2003 he stressed the need to understand the drug use of young people as meaningful to them:

> The good thing about drug use is: if I drink enough, I will get drunk; if I take enough amphetamines, I will be high; and if I smoke or eat enough cannabis, I will be stoned. That is a 100 per cent given guarantee. There are not many things in this world that can guarantee you that every time, are there? If you have nothing else in the world, your prospects are poor, your education is shot to bits, you are disconnected and alienated from the community, and this works for you.[310]

As with the adult use of amphetamine discussed in the previous section, for some young people, particularly street users of the drug, amphetamine may not necessarily be their first choice of drug. It may simply be a question of what is available at the time:

> When we look at [opiate users with traumatic childhood backgrounds] switching to drugs like methamphetamines we have real concerns, because we are talking about young people who already have anxiety and panic attacks, and who already suffer from the debilitating effects of hyperarousal, and now they are taking a psychostimulant on top of it. That is one of the reasons why…we talk about these changes in drug usage amongst the young people we are looking at as not being to do with their choices. It is market driven rather than choice driven. I think most of them would prefer to use opiates, but the market has changed in such a way that methamphetamines are being pushed onto that old opiate marketplace, so they are starting to take up psychostimulant use. That presents real problems for our residential workers, because we have a very well-established system for dealing with opiate addictions.[311]

This view was reinforced in YSAS's written submission to the Inquiry:

> YSAS staff have observed an increasing number of young people using amphetamines. These young people describe what they are using as either 'speed' (methamphetamine powder) or 'ice' (crystalline methamphetamine). They overwhelmingly tend to inject the drug. While these young people could be described as polydrug users, in the sense that they use a range of drugs (including alcohol, cannabis, and benzodiazepines), few of them ingest more than one substance simultaneously.

---

310 Mr Jurgen Hemmerling, Open Family, Hume Region, evidence given to the Drugs and Crime Prevention Committee, Inquiry into Amphetamine and 'Party Drug', Use in Victoria, Public Hearings (Benalla), 22 October 2003.

311 Mr Tony Palmer, Training Consultant, YSAS, evidence given to the Drugs and Crime Prevention Committee, Inquiry into Amphetamine and 'Party Drug' Use in Victoria, Public Hearings (Melbourne), 27 October 2003.

> YSAS holds the view that drivers of changes in drug markets cannot simply be explained away by recourse to an assumption of individual consumer driven choices. Rather, these choices seem to be driven by global market forces, as demonstrated by the amount of crystalline methamphetamine being detected at the border by the Australian Customs Service increasing from less than 1 kg in 1997/98 to over 150 kg by 2001/02.[312]

Problematic drug use among young people is particularly vexing. As has already been indicated there are a series of risk factors that are associated with the likelihood of young people developing serious drug problems. There are also a number of protective factors that can be developed in young people who are most vulnerable to becoming problem drug users (European Monitoring Centre for Drugs and Drug Addiction (EMCDDA) 2003). These protective factors and associated harm reduction and education strategies designed to prevent the uptake of problematic drug use or lessen the problems associated with drug use that has already commenced is discussed in detail in Part F of this Report. It should be stated at this point that the Committee is concerned that young people who enter drug therapy or rehabilitation or residential programmes not have their involvement with such programmes end abruptly once they reach the age of eighteen as has happened in some instances. As such the Committee makes the following recommendation:

Recommendation

4. The Committee recommends that there be a Review of service provision for those young people who, having turned eighteen years of age, can no longer continue to receive assistance or participate in programmes designed to assist them with their amphetamine and 'party drug' use.

Amphetamine use in the transport industry and by other workers

Amphetamines have long been associated with their functional use of guaranteeing longer and more sustained work performance. Indeed, Klee argues that the amphetamines are the perfect drug for the capitalist economy:

> The amphetamines are ideally suited to the age of economic expansion in a non interventionist capitalist environment as the work load increases and workers need to keep up to stay up in business. Low cost, sustained action and a reputation as harmless, make these drugs acceptable for working people...the value of amphetamine in facilitating performance in certain jobs,

312 Submission of YSAS to the Drugs and Crime Prevention Committee, Inquiry into Amphetamine and 'Party Drug' Use in Victoria, October 2003.

> for example shift work, long distance driving and construction work, had become fairly commonplace (Klee 2001a, p.27).

In a similar way, one American commentator has linked the image of the amphetamine user to the 'most prized American virtues':

> [i]ntense activity, efficiency, persistence and drive, and the desire to excel, to break records, and to move with even greater speed. These are admirable behaviour patterns that are not easily relinquished, even when a drug is required to achieve them (Edison 1978 quoted in Morgan & Beck 1997, p.155).[313]

Despite the focus of this section being on 'truckies' and other drivers, it is not only the transport industry in which the functional use of amphetamines is found. Earlier reference has been made to the use of methamphetamine by abattoir workers in order to maintain strenuous shifts (see Chapter 4, Footnote 29). The World Health Organisation has also recently completed a collaborative study on instrumental methamphetamine use among drivers, factory workers, sex workers and students in China, Nigeria, the Philippines and Thailand. Certainly it would seem countries with the highest poverty rates and lowest per capita incomes have high levels of instrumental/functional drug use among their workers (see Marsden et al. 2000).

Wermuth argues, however, that while workers in developing countries may be particularly dependent on amphetamines to sustain energy levels for long hours of work,[314] such instrumental use is also apparent in developed countries such as the United States:

> Adult pressures are often centered around working long hours while also carrying out family responsibilities. Dual earner marriages are often essential in maintaining middle-class incomes and life styles, and a broad array of individuals feel they need more time and energy to meet life's demands. The economic and time pinches are most intensely felt by single working parents, composed mostly of lower paid women, and by the working poor generally, a growing proportion of the U.S. labor force. Given this social landscape, the appeal of a drug that boosts energy is not surprising. In parallel fashion, perhaps because of Japanese achievement pressures and 'workaholism', a methamphetamine epidemic took hold there earlier than in the United States, resulting in some of the few studies of long term effects (Wermuth 2000, p.431).

Amphetamine use in the transport industry

The occupational use of psychostimulants including amphetamines by one particular group of workers, namely long-distance and other drivers, has been an issue of concern for some time. Early survey research cited by Hall and Hando

---

313 During World War II, Japanese soldiers and industry workers were forced or coerced into using amphetamines in order to increase efficiency and productivity, see Suwaki, Fukui and Konuma 1997.

314 This would particularly be the case in countries where there is no minimal guarantees of working hours or conditions in favour of the worker or worker protection legislation.

(1993) suggested that in both Australia and the United States – countries with huge amounts of territory covered by road transport – between 40 and 60 per cent of long-distance truck drivers had taken stimulants (particularly ephedrine) to remain awake. More recent research reported prevalence figures varying between 20 and 50 per cent, although the higher figures tend to be based on anecdotal evidence (see studies and evidence cited in Mabbott & Hartley 1999, p.117).

A submission to this Inquiry by Victoria Police notes that the number of transport industry drivers charged with amphetamine offences, while relatively low in absolute terms, has been steadily increasing over the last five-year period.[315] Victoria Police state further:

> Traditionally, transport industry truck drivers are not recreational drug users. They may use alcohol and tobacco, but the use of amphetamine away from the work place is not widespread. Fatigue, due to demanding schedules, is a major issue within the transport industry and illegal drugs are often being used to address it.
>
> In 2000 the percentage of truck drivers at fault in fatal collisions was 28%. However, toxicology data shows that 20% of truck drivers' blood tested following a fatal collision was found to contain stimulant drugs. This figure is tenfold higher than for the drivers of motor cars. In 2001 this figure rose to 25%...
>
> While numbers are low, there appears to be an increase in the detection rate for transport industry drivers using amphetamines over the above five-year period. These figures reflect only amphetamine possession and do not include any other stimulants or prescription drugs.[316]

The medical and other consequences of using psychostimulants for these reasons have already been commented on in Chapter 6. However, another major concern of governments and the community alike is the personal and economic costs associated with some fairly horrendous motor vehicle accidents involving heavy transport vehicles in which the drivers were found often to be using excessive amounts of psychostimulants.

An extensive study by Mabbot and Harley aimed to more systematically ascertain the prevalence and nature of psychostimulant use and abuse in the transport industry of Western Australia. One of the more concerning issues outlined by the authors was that since a crackdown on illegal prescription drugs had made such drugs harder to obtain there had been an increase in the amount of illegal street amphetamines being used by drivers. The authors summarised their research as follows:

---

315 From 12 offenders in 1997 to 19 in 2001 and 22 as of May 2002 (Confidential Submission of Victoria Police to the Drugs and Crime Prevention Committee, Inquiry into Amphetamine and 'Party Drug' Use in Victoria, August 2002. Quoted with the kind permission of Victoria Police).

316 Confidential Submission of Victoria Police to the Drugs and Crime Prevention Committee, Inquiry into Amphetamine and 'Party Drug' Use in Victoria, August 2002. Quoted with approval of Victoria Police.

> In July 1997, 236 truck drivers were interviewed at three truck stops in Western Australia. The interviews collected information on driver fatigue and stimulant drug taking as a fatigue countermeasure. Drivers have become more aware of fatigue as a problem within the industry over the last two years, however 27% of drivers reported using stimulant drugs to combat driver fatigue. Interstate drivers use more prescription and illicit stimulant drugs to keep awake while intrastate drivers use more over the counter stimulants. Over the counter stimulants are not perceived as drugs by intrastate drivers because they are easily and legally obtainable and this is reflected in many of their responses.
>
> The most frequent way that drivers obtained stimulant drugs was through a chemist or illegal prescription. Anecdotal evidence from the drivers suggests that increasing pressure from the public and the media to eliminate illegally prescribed stimulant use by drivers has made them harder to obtain. Therefore, without fatigue issues within the industry being addressed, an increase in street purchases of illicit stimulants may occur. Prohibition of stimulant drug use without changing industry practices eliminates a fatigue countermeasure and could lead to a serious increase in fatigue related crashes (Mabbott & Harley 1999, p.115).

Of the illicit substances nominated by the surveyed drivers, amphetamine was the most common substance used. Prescription drugs were often obtained from partners or friends who had obtained them from doctors for weight problems. Illicit amphetamines were acquired from the black market and drug dealers, 'with some responses suggesting bike gangs, hotels and "off the street"' (Mabbott & Harley 1999, p.122).

Many factors contribute to fatigue being a major problem within the road transport industry.[317] These include structural factors within the industry and problems pertinent to individual drivers, including:

- Extended driving periods;
- Tight delivery schedules;
- Penalties for late delivery;
- Lack of rest or sleep prior to commencing long hauls;
- Monotonous scenery;
- Job competition (or taking on more than one job or contract);
- Related to the previous point is undercutting of rates with some operators willing to offer a faster service for the same price or less; and
- Products requiring urgent delivery (such as livestock).

317 American studies have also testified to quite serious cases of amphetamine abuse by pilots and other aviation personnel, particularly in the United States. Drug and Alcohol Testing of personnel by the US Federal Aviation Administration from 1995–2000 demonstrates that people working in safety sensitive workplace occupations such as aviation are being found positive to substance abuse. See for example Canfield et al. 2000.

In addition to such factors, it is disturbing that Mabbot and Harley's study reveals that: 'It is clear from driver responses that little is known about the side effects of stimulant use' (p.127).

Indeed, 81.65 per cent of surveyed drivers knew of fewer than three side effects of listed psychostimulant drugs. As the authors remark, in addition to structural change within the industry (for example, regulated driving schedules etc) there is 'a need for education within the road transport industry on the risk of harmful effects from stimulant drug use' (Mabbot & Harley 1999, p.127).

Psychostimulant use and abuse in the transport industry is by no means a problem restricted to Western Australia. The very nature of interstate road transport and its dependence on long-distance driving make this a nation-wide problem. A submission from the Department of Human Services Victoria is testament to the seriousness with which they view the use of psychostimulants by heavy vehicle drivers and other motorists. They cite recent work done in this area outlining their concerns:

> Heavy Vehicle drivers also continue to be at high risk. Vic Roads safety expert Phillip Swann stated at a recent road safety conference that drugged-out drivers were more dangerous than drunk drivers. Phillip Swann cited a 10 year study by the Victorian Institute of Forensic Medicine, which showed that psychoactive drugs outstripped alcohol among some road-user groups. The Victorian road safety report also cited in the paper 'Psychostimulants in Australia' (Henry-Edwards 2001) indicated that stimulants were found in 21% of dead truck drivers compared with 3.9% of all dead drivers. This would seem to indicate an urgent need for harm reduction strategies to address this continuing problem.[318]

Researchers and writers such as Mabbot and Harley recognise that driver education, particularly with regard to the side effects of psychostimulants, is very important. It is also suggested that prohibition of some psychostimulants may have positive effects (or conversely push drivers into seeking the drugs underground). However, neither of these measures will, according to the authors, prove effective in reducing fatigue-related crashes without a change to industry practices.[319]

Amphetamine use in other industries

The Committee has also received anecdotal evidence that the use of amphetamines is also quite high within the fishing industries of Western Australia and Queensland and among kangaroo hunters in Queensland. Similar factors such as long working hours and tight schedules have been posited as to

318 Submission of Human Services Victoria (Drug Policy and Services Branch) to the Drugs and Crime Prevention Committee, Inquiry into Amphetamine and 'Party Drug' Use in Victoria, August 2002.

319 For a discussion of recent changes to the law in Victorian allowing the testing of motorists for amphetamine, see Chapter 7.

why this may be the case. The following comments of Paul Dessauer of the Western Australian Substance Users Association (WASUA) are pertinent:

> I meet a lot of people in the building industry who take Speed regularly. And I meet a lot of people in the fishing fleets who take Speed regularly as well. And they are using it in a very functional way. They are using it to try and be fit enough to do a hard day's slog every day.[320]

Mr Dessauer also refers to the functional use of amphetamines by workers within the medical profession:

> I have met medical professionals who use amphetamine on occasion. And in fact I have got a little 3 and a half year old daughter and when she was only a few months old, she had febrile convulsions... And so the first time it happened we raced into the children's hospital, terrified that something dreadful was happening to her. And the doctor who treated her, was quite obviously to me, under the influence of amphetamine. Her pupils were enormous and it was quite obvious to me that she had helped herself to some dexamphetamine. This is at 3 in the morning. And I don't know, she had probably been on a 16 hour shift.[321]

Unfortunately, no material quantifying the use of these drugs in such groups has, however, been forthcoming.

The use of amphetamines and 'party drugs' by women

> [I]n drug and alcohol research male experience has often been considered to be normative, and research has traditionally been designed to examine the issues in drug use that are problematic for men (Donath 2004, p.103).

A recently published book on drug use in Australia, from which the quote above is taken, makes a convincing argument that 'women and women's issues remain seriously under-represented in the research literature on alcohol and drugs' (Donath 2004, p.103). This has certainly been the experience of this Committee in researching this Report.[322] This is despite the fact that for both biological and social reasons there are distinct differences in the way men and women use and are affected by drugs.

While it is clear that men are substantially more likely to be users of illicit drugs then women (Dietze, Laslett & Rumbold 2004), this does not mean that the

320 Mr Paul Dessauer, WASUA, in conversation with the Drugs and Crime Prevention Committee, Perth, 1 October 2003.

321 Ibid.

322 Not only has the Committee staff been unable to find sufficient literature on amphetamines and 'party drug' use among women, there has been very little response or input from the community by way of submission or other evidence that details the specificity of female experience with regard to these drugs. This is a regrettable state of affairs as gender focussed research and contributions are an essential element in producing good policy that draws from and addresses women's experience.

effects of such drugs on the women who do so use are any less severe. Indeed for both physiological and social/cultural reasons, it is arguable that the effects may be more profound on women. For example, it has generally been the case that there has been far more disdain shown to women who misuse drugs, both illicit and licit (particularly alcohol), than to males who do so:

> A survey of alcohol and drug treatment personnel in Australia found that most believed that there was more stigma attached to women with alcohol and drug problems than to men (Swift and Copeland 1998). In addition, women with alcohol and drug problems also believed that society looked down on them more than on men with similar problems (Copeland 1996). Women who already occupy a marginalised position in society (for instance Indigenous women, non-English speaking women, lesbians) are even more stigmatised than heterosexual, white, 'Anglo' drug users (Donath 2004, p.107).

In turning to the specific issues of amphetamines and 'party drugs', while it may be true that illicit drug use is generally lower among women than men, international research has shown that over the last 15 years women's recreational or functional use of amphetamine is often as high as that of men (see research studies reviewed in Klee 2001b).[323]

Motivations for using amphetamine

Klee states that the demand of women for amphetamine:

> [w]ill encourage the production of ATS to meet all their needs, which will be different to those of previous generations, namely, for domestic chores, childcare, sexual disinhibition,[324] confidence in social settings, and at work, and for weight loss (2001b, p.86. See also Klee 2001a, p.26).

Similar findings are reflected in American studies. For example, the research of Morgan and Beck highlights the use of amphetamine as an adjunct for what the authors term 'welfare mothers' as a way of coping with mundane tasks such as housework or to relieve the tiredness associated with childcare. One of the women surveyed as part of this study claimed:

> *'I stayed up and did my bills, got my paperwork done, got my coupons organized, started projects I had been procrastinating on, like filling photo albums and doing baby books. Just getting caught up on laundry and housework. I never stopped'* (Morgan & Beck 1997, p.145).

Klee's British research found that for 'young mums' the main aim of using amphetamine:

---

323 Research with regard to methamphetamine use among high school students in the United States indicates that while methamphetamine use is more prevalent among males, use among females is gradually increasing (Oetting et al. 2000). For further prevalence data according to gender with regard to both amphetamine and 'party drug' use, see Chapter 5.

324 In Japan some female misusers of methamphetamine were initiated into use or encouraged to use by husbands and boyfriends wanting to use the drug for a heightened sexual response (see Suwaki, Fukui & Konuma 1997, p.211).

> [i]s to have enough energy to look after the children, do the housework and still have some leisure time. It seems the responsibility of having babies at a young age, with the associated problem of the confinement in the home until the children can be safely left with others, results later in a desire to have a good time while they are still young enough to enjoy it (1997b, p.44).

Despite the use of amphetamines to circumvent tiredness in this way, long-term use of the drugs may result in the opposite effect.[325]

> Unfortunately for most [women] who first tried methamphetamine to improve their work capacity, increased and prolonged use had the opposite effect. Respondents reported becoming increasingly dysfunctional after prolonged use, especially after transitions to a stronger mode of use. For example, one respondent described the difficulties encountered as a hair cutter when she switched from snorting to shooting meth, and bingeing for longer periods of time:
>
> '*You do become dysfunctional. You shake real bad, that's kind of hard when you're cutting hair! ...you think you're going fast but you're going slower. At first you're going real fast and then the more you stay on it, you start slowing up and then your hands start shaking and your vision gets blurry*' (Morgan & Beck 1997, p.145).

In many of the research studies undertaken by Klee a constant factor that arose with regard to women's use of amphetamine was their use of the drug as self-medication for either physical health or more often mental health problems, particularly depression:

> Women confined to the home by children, who have several small children and other responsibilities and are tired, find that not only is their depression lifted, but they [also] have more motivation and energy. It is not surprising that amphetamine is particularly attractive to them, and perhaps gives rise to the reputation of this drug as 'a woman's drug'.
>
> Some women start their drug career early with a prescription from their doctor for dexamphetamine or get the tablets from relatives or friends and then move on to street amphetamine...
>
> Tiredness and depression are the critical features of a self medicating female amphetamine user. The tiredness is often associated with children.
>
> The younger women with partners may be criticised by them for putting on weight, which threatens their fragile self-esteem further. It is difficult to determine how body image interacts with depression – the women get depressed when they put on weight but frequently they have eating habits strongly influenced by depression that cause obesity and the pattern becomes cyclic. Most self medicating women have a history of depression from traumatic life events in childhood or adolescence. However, not all women are introduced to amphetamine by a medical prescription – doctors are extremely

325 As was pointed out in Chapter 7.

> reluctant to prescribe dexamphetamine. The majority start their use, like most amphetamine users, by being offered street drugs (Klee 1997b, pp.61, 62).

The use of amphetamine for self-medication is, however, highly problematic:

> People self-medicating with the drug for depression can find that this worsens when withdrawing, and they easily fall into the trap of continuous dosing in order to avoid it (Klee 1997c, p.311).

Australian research has also found that women with substance abuse disorders have a much higher prevalence of mental health problems, particularly depression:

> Forty four per cent of women with an alcohol dependence or abuse disorder suffer from depression or anxiety or both. For women with a diagnosis of illicit substance abuse or dependence, the rates are even higher, with more than half of these women (55 per cent) suffering from at least one of the mood disorders (Donath 2004, p.109).

Moreover, it would seem now fairly apparent that there are strong links indicating that women who have suffered childhood sexual assault may develop substance abuse problems later in life. The numbers of women with substance abuse disorders who had been sexually assaulted as children has been estimated as at least one-quarter and possibly as many as half (Hodgins et al. 1997. See also Swift & Copeland 1998).

'Party drugs' for pleasure

With regard to 'dance drugs', British studies suggest that while 'gender differences are minimal in adolescent drug using populations' by early adulthood there is a far higher degree of drug experimentation and use among males compared to females (Measham, Aldridge & Parker 2001, p.8). Measham and her colleagues also found that among their sample of clubbers while '[w]omen in clubland tend on average to be younger than men, and to have initiated into drug use at a younger age than men, [our] findings suggest that fewer of them are taking illicit drugs in clubs than men' (2001, p.109). Measham et al. also warns, however, that any 'gendered distinctions of drug use should not overshadow the key finding that both female and male clubbers are remarkably drug experienced' (2001, p.101).

Much of the little research that reviews drug use among women tends to concentrate, somewhat understandably, on the negatives of such use. Very little research reflects on why such drug use, particularly in the area of 'party drugs', may be pleasurable for some women. One qualitative survey that does examine the perceived positives of ecstasy use for women is that of Hinchcliff (2001). Her survey of women clubbers between the ages of 21 and 31 years of age sought to represent women-specific experiences of ecstasy. These women 'used ecstasy for pleasure, believed themselves to be independent in their use, and did not view their actions as deviant – all of which contradict traditional research findings' (2001, p.455).

As has been stressed throughout this Report, evidence based policy and research should ideally start from the position or viewpoint of the user themselves, if strategies are going to be developed that will 'reach' that client group. Hinchcliff's research starts from the basis that the dance scene and its associated drug use was pleasurable for these women. It reflects a change in the 1990s where:

> [a]ttitudes to leisure changed as women openly talked about getting 'off their heads', which may reflect the finding that recreational drug use is normalised for many women (Hinchcliff 2001, p.456).

For these women, according to Hinchcliff, clubbing and the feelings associated with ecstasy use is a 'form of "time out" from the pressures of everyday life' (p.460). Clubbing has dualistic meanings. It enables the women to reach an individual state of altered consciousness yet at the same time experience a communal level of feeling or group celebration and solidarity among fellow women. Another attraction of club dancing for women according to Henderson (1993) was that the energetic forms of dancing on the dance floor are perceived as fun forms of weight control.[326]

Most importantly, although the venues frequented by the women were mixed sex and heterosexual, the women did not feel either intimidated by men or pressured into attracting a partner. This lack of objectification was heightened both by the feeling of collectivity among the women and the relative lack of alcohol at these clubs. These feelings are represented in the quotes of some of the survey participants:

> *'I'm sure that it is a big attraction for a lot of women on the dance scene, that they can go out, have a f****g good time and just not be hassled by men...you feel more relaxed as a woman going out and that means you can get off your head without worrying, you know if you get too drunk at a normal club then you're a victim aren't you, they home in on you'* (Kate).
>
> *'...[i]t's really to good to get off your head because you forget everything...this club culture thing they've sussed it – if you can have a night where you're not worrying about things and shitting yourself over bills, and you just forget everything for one night and feel absolutely fantastic'* (Ann) (Hinchcliff 2001, pp.459, 460).

For the women in this group the drugs could not be separated from the setting in which they were taken. Many:

> [h]ad used other drugs but none had the same influence, implying it was more the social context of ecstasy use rather than the drug alone which had this effect. Whether regular participation in dance events means that the experiences and emotions felt in that context permeate into life when ecstasy

326 This was viewed as an increasingly important consideration also for gay and heterosexual men alike (see Measham, Aldridge & Parker 2001, pp.35ff.).

> is not being used is an aspect that requires further investigation (Hinchcliff 2001, p.462).

While some of the women in the study did consider the potential negatives of ecstasy use, the benefits were considered to far outweigh the costs, particularly as no one in the group had experienced a harmful encounter with the drug. Earlier research into women clubbers by Henderson (1993) resulted in very similar findings. The young women in her study eschewed the alcohol driven nightclubs or pubs with the 'beer monsters' with their tell-tale 'beer bellies' who appeared in stark contrast to the lean and toned male clubbers of the 1990s (quoted in Measham, Aldridge & Parker 2001, p.38). Dance clubs were (and are) perceived as safe and fun:

> [t]he young women occupied this social space with confidence, circulating and meeting new people independently...[clubs] provided an exciting, exhilarating, but also 'safe' social space for them (Henderson 1993, p.125).[327]

Amphetamine and 'party drug' use in communities of cultural and linguistic diversity[328]

If it is thought that there is little information or research about drug use patterns among women in Australia, this is even more the case for people from non-English speaking or ethnically diverse backgrounds. Certainly, specific material with regard to amphetamines and 'party drug' use is very difficult to ascertain. Most academic or research work is generalist. Unfortunately the Committee has also not received any input from the public about experiences of amphetamine use in non-'Anglo' communities.

Prevalence of use

Generally speaking, epidemiological research and systematic data collection indicates that people from non-English speaking or culturally and linguistically diverse (CLD) communities have lower rates of alcohol and drug use than those from Anglo Australian backgrounds. The 1998 National Drug Strategy Household Survey (Australian Institute of Health and Welfare (AIHW) 1999; see also AIHW 2001) showed:

> Reports of having used drugs in the previous year were substantially lower for:
>
> - Alcohol (50 per cent versus 81 per cent for the general population)
> - Tobacco/cigarettes (12 per cent versus around 23 per cent)
> - Any illicit drug use including cannabis (16 per cent versus 46 per cent) (AIHW 1999, p.5).

---

327 Malbon's study of club culture found that for some women clubbing could almost be seen as a form of 'safe sex'. Flirting and sexual display were for these women as much about 'flirting for [themselves] as about being with others' (1999, p.44).

328 The term cultural and linguistic diversity, usually abbreviated to CLD, is seen as a useful shorthand reference to '[d]ifferences in identity, social affiliation, cultural practices and language as a result of immigration' (Rowland, Toumbourou & Stevens 2003, p.3).

Nonetheless, despite this data and other research which suggests 'misuse of alcohol and other drugs is not a major issue in CLD communities', Rowland, Toumbourou and Stevens 2003 warn that '[t]his general conclusion masks some "pockets" in which there do appear to be more serious issues'. Such examples may include analgesic and tobacco use among Arabic Australians and heroin use among some young Vietnamese men (Rowland, Toumbourou & Stevens 2003, p.5).[329]

Given the above qualifications as to the quantum of drug use among CLD communities, and the fact that there may be many commonalities between CLD and non-CLD users, particularly young people, as to why they use drugs, it is also true that 'there may be specific factors such as migration and integration that increase the risk of initiation into drug use by [young] people from CLD backgrounds' (DrugInfo Clearinghouse 2003, p.20).

A recent study conducted by Rowland, Toumbourou and Stevens interviewed 11 practitioners working in the field of drug prevention within CLD communities in Victoria. Given the dearth of rich material available in this area, the findings and responses were particularly instructive:

> Practitioners recognised that harmful levels of alcohol and other drug consumption did take place within Australian CLD communities. While practitioners believed that specific factors were associated with harmful levels of drug and alcohol consumption within CLD communities...practitioners considered immigration and integration issues to be the principal issues associated with general alcohol and drug use in CLD communities.
>
> In relation to integration and immigration, it was suggested that immigrants who were refugees and/or victims of torture, war or other trauma used alcohol and other drug to relax or forget about the past. It was also suggested that immigrants often had difficulty integrating into Australian society if they lacked proficiency in English and/or their overseas qualifications were not recognised in Australia. These hurdles made it difficult to get a job and thus placed these immigrants, especially young people, at risk of taking up alcohol and other drugs (Rowland, Toumbourou & Stevens 2003, pp.7–8).

The interviewed practitioners were somewhat sceptical about research findings that suggest low rates of substance abuse among CLD communities:

> [p]ractitioners believed that illicit drug use was probably higher among Australians from non-English speaking backgrounds because of the higher number of risk factors they are exposed to. Scepticism focused on the validity of research findings. It was mentioned that research into CLD communities hinged on how CLD status was defined and recorded, with practitioners suggesting that researchers often defined CLD status poorly.

329 There is a reasonable amount of research collected on (injecting) drug use among Vietnamese youth. Most of it, however, focusses on heroin. See for example, Kelsall et al. 1999; Louie et al. 1998; Reid et al. 2002.

> It was also suggested that for many immigrants drug use was perceived as a stigma, thus many individuals with CLD background did not report drug use by self or family members. As a result, drug prevalence and use within CLD communities has been under-reported.
>
> Practitioners suggested that this theory could be supported with the anecdotal evidence indicating a greater proportion of second generation CLD individuals taking up drugs, when compared with first generation immigrants (Rowland, Toumbourou & Stevens 2003, p.6).

Reasons for use

Drug use among young people from CLD communities reflected a mixture of issues that were specific to youth or generational issues on the one hand and ethnic or culturally specific issues on the other. In the first case:

> Many young people from CLD backgrounds participated in licit and illicit drug use because, like other Australian young people, they too wanted to take risks and push boundaries imposed by their parents and society in general (Rowland, Toumbourou & Stevens 2003, p.7).

Intergenerational conflict and the pressures on the family unit (particularly if both parents worked) also were viewed as risk factors:

> A recent Victorian government report (Department of Human Services 2000) suggested that risk factors in some families included poor parenting skills, specifically ineffective discipline practices, and parent-child conflict, perhaps related to differential acculturation. In other cases, poor family communication and associated low family supervision were key issues. In some cases, children may have been placed under unrealistic pressures to succeed...
>
> Other research also supports the view that higher rates of drug use within some CLD communities may stem from family factors including family isolation (Louie *et al.* 1998), family disruption associated with traumatic refugee experience (Groves 1993) and/or loss of parental control over adolescents due to differential acculturation and role reversal (Kumpfer *et al.*1998). On the other hand, having rules and good parental supervision has been found to be protective against substance use among adolescents from some ethnic communities (Maher *et al.* 1998)...
>
> ...Consistent also with research findings were practitioners' views that lack of parental control often led to drug use by young people from CLD backgrounds. It was suggested that the Western-oriented culture of Australia, often characterised by notions of freedom and independence in youth, was difficult for many recently migrated individuals from CLD backgrounds.
>
> In particular, it was suggested that parents from CLD backgrounds needed education in how to communicate effectively, and how to manage issues around drug use by young people (Rowland, Toumbourou & Stevens 2003, p.7).

Given the importance of the factors mentioned by Rowland, Toumborou and Stevens in the above quote the Committee makes the following recommendation:

Recommendation

5. The Committee recommends that specific culturally appropriate training and resources on amphetamine and 'party drug' use be provided to parents, families, agencies and personnel working with people from culturally and linguistically diverse communities.

One issue that is not mentioned in Rowland et al.'s review of the Department of Human Services Report is the issue of young refugees who have arrived in Australia without parents or other family members. Anecdotal evidence would suggest that this is also a major risk factor that could contribute to drug use among young people from refugee backgrounds.

Culturally specific factors that compounded drug use by young people included frustration and boredom at school:

> [d]ue to difficulties with language and literacy. As a result, they are unable to sustain their interest in school or in other daily activities. In order to alleviate the frustration and boredom the young person may take up use of drugs... (Rowland, Tomourou & Stevens, p.7).

Practitioners also perceived drug use by young people from CLD backgrounds as being compounded by ethnic cultural factors in their use of drugs to gain membership or acceptance by desirable social groups. Specifically, drug use by many young people from CLD backgrounds appeared to provide a 'gateway' into peer groups and broader social networks.

Another major project conducted by researchers at the Burnet Institute in Melbourne (Reid 2003, 'Drugs in a Multicultural Community') examined the use of illicit drugs by members of CLD communities from 1998 to 2001. Similar to other studies conducted both here (see DrugInfo Clearinghouse 2003) and in the United States, the authors found that vulnerability to being involved with illicit drug use was related not so much to ethnicity *per se,* but rather as a result of economic and social disadvantage:

> [t]hat *stemmed* from language difficulties, high unemployment, inadequate education and cultural pressures. These factors render ethnic minority groups less able and, in many cases, less willing to utilise services which exist to reduce drug-related harm.[330]
>
> It appear[ed] that people of *any* background were made vulnerable to illicit drug use and more likely to participate in street-level selling of drugs, by the

330 For a discussion of some Victorian community projects which do seem successful in addressing harm prevention and other drug-related issues among CLD communities, see Part F of this Report.

> fact of their *youth*, strong influence on their behaviour by peers, high unemployment and poor literacy. The socio-economic handicaps of ethnic minority served to exacerbate those tendencies (Reid 2003, p.3). (Committee emphasis)

The determinants according to this school of thought are not so much ethnicity as economic position and social class. According to some commentators, this is also the case among members of the Indigenous communities who use licit and illicit drugs.

Amphetamine and 'party drug' use in Indigenous Victorian communities

While there is a plethora of literature and information about drugs such as alcohol and volatile substances among Indigenous people, there is very little material pertaining to amphetamine use and virtually none with regard to 'party drugs' in this population. One must therefore somewhat unsatisfactorily extrapolate from general principles and hypothesise that the underlying reasons why Indigenous people may misuse alcohol or sniff petrol are, at least to some extent, the reasons why they may use other drugs.

A submission received from the Victorian State Office (VSO) of Aboriginal and Torres Strait Islander Services (ATSIS) highlights this knowledge deficit:

> The VSO notes the relative absence of accurate data on the levels of illicit drug use amongst Indigenous Victorians.
>
> Despite this absence, the VSO is of the opinion that amphetamine and 'party drug' use within Victorian Indigenous communities is an issue that needs to be addressed. However, the VSO believes that the numbers of people involved in amphetamine and/or 'party drug' use, and the frequency of this use, are significantly lower than in the wider community (as a proportion of the respective populations), and are significantly lower than those associated with other drugs/substances, namely alcohol, marijuana and volatile substances. This has implications for the prioritising of resources for responses to different sectors and programs.[331]

The submission from the Victorian State Office of ATSIS also includes some recent data presented at the Victorian Aboriginal Justice Forum which makes for disturbing reading:

- illicit drug use is more widespread among the Indigenous urban community than in the general community
- 50% of members of the Indigenous urban community have tried an illicit drug compared with 38% in the general community

331 Submission of State Office (Victoria) of ATSIS to the Drugs and Crime Prevention Committee, Inquiry into Amphetamine and 'Party Drug' Use in Victoria, November 2003.

- 24% of members of the Indigenous urban community are current users [of illicit drugs] compared with 15% in the general population, with marijuana being the most popular drug
- in a recent study, 63% of Indigenous participants under 20 reported sharing needles
- heroin accounts for 12% of drug use by Aboriginal drug users, compared to 22% for non-Aboriginal drug users.[332]

A recent Report discussing injecting drug use among Indigenous South Australian found the following:

> A Report on injecting drug use among Aboriginal people in the Lower Murray region of South Australia revealed that injecting drug use contributed to poor health, and negative social and legal outcomes for those members of the community who injected, and their families. Additional consequences associated with injecting drug use included the transmission of blood borne viruses, assault, violence and potential for suicidal behaviour. The report also revealed higher rates of unsafe practices such as sharing needles and other equipment, despite knowing the associated risks, as they had the belief that the Aboriginal cultural concept of sharing belongings included sharing injecting equipment. [333]

The indigenous Health Web Site 'healthinfonet' notes the following with regard to Indigenous injecting drug use:

> A number of studies have found that injecting drug use is more prevalent within urban Indigenous communities, rather than in rural Indigenous communities and consequently the majority of studies on injecting drug use within Indigenous communities have been conducted in urban areas. In 2001, the Aboriginal Drug and Alcohol Council (ADAC) conducted the largest single study of Indigenous people who inject drugs in Australia. Through this study it was established that heroin or speed (or both) was most frequently stated as the drug most often injected by Aboriginal injectors. There was widespread belief amongst consultants of the project that injecting drug use impacted the whole of the Aboriginal community. It was reported that injecting drug use was increasing the social disadvantage of the Indigenous community, and was contributing to Aboriginal people's low self worth, generalised poverty, and poor health. Injecting drug use was said to be affecting families who were already struggling – interfering with parenting, causing disruptions within families, stress and shame. Another issue raised throughout the study was the devastating effect on the community, and the grief and trauma associated with overdose deaths. Consultants of the project believed that poor relations between Aboriginal people and the police contributed to reluctance to call for an ambulance to attend an overdose. Lack of knowledge of resuscitation

332 Ibid.

333 Quoted in *Summary of Injecting drug use and its health consequences among Indigenous people* www.healthinfonet.edu.au

techniques amongst Aboriginal injectors was believed to be a contributing factor in overdose deaths. In addition to the lack of knowledge about responding to overdose, it was also identified that there was a lack of knowledge among Indigenous injectors regarding overdose prevention. Prison release (lowered tolerance) and poly-drug use were the most common factors relating to Indigenous overdose. [334]

Reasons for use

Some of the factors put forward by ATSIS can help to explain their figures quoted in the previous section:

> The VSO submits the following matters as key factors contributing to drug use amongst Indigenous Victorians, and therefore considers these key matters to be addressed in any attempts to reduce drug use within this community:
>
> - Low school retention rates
>
> Retention rates for Indigenous youth are abysmally poor. This is a result of a culturally insensitive education system alienating and failing to nurture Aboriginal young people while at school, a lack of support for young people when outside school and inadequate support and encouragement form family and their own community. These issues, combined with racism and the distraction of family problems (including poverty), cause many young Aboriginal people to miss significant periods of schooling. The result is high numbers of Aboriginal youth with considerable time on their hands, few constructive alternatives, and no sense of building a future for themselves.
>
> - Family dysfunction – arising from substance abuse, violence, poverty
> - Lack of options for dealing with problems
>
> Given the range and seriousness of problems faced by many Indigenous people, there is a need for culturally-sensitive support services to assist people to cope with and overcome these problems and the pressures they cause. Most Aboriginal communities lack the capacity to provide the complex and resource-intensive assistance required. Mainstream services are often inaccessible for cultural reasons and most Aboriginal-specific services (like many mainstream services) are already stretched.
>
> - Racism
> - Family disconnection
> - Lack of positive role models
> - Unemployment
> - Lack of opportunities to develop and utilise skills
> - Lack of social activities (ie. as constructive alternatives to risk-taking activities such as drug use)
>
> These factors contribute to boredom, loss of identity, lack of aspiration/sense of purpose, feelings of worthlessness and incompetence, depression, which many

334 Ibid.

> Indigenous Victorians experience. In turn, these states of mind can, and often do, lead people to search for an 'escape' which is commonly achieved through drug use.[335]

As with youth from CLD communities, it can be posited that it is not so much the fact of Aboriginality per se that contributes to relatively high levels of illicit drug use but more the high degree of economic and social disadvantage that results from being a member of the Indigenous community. A fine distinction but a real one nonetheless.

In the deliberations for this Inquiry, the Committee sought to meet with representatives of the Victorian Indigenous community to discuss amphetamine use in those communities. It was generally agreed that 'party drug' use was not a major problem if for no other reason than Aboriginal youth would be unlikely to regularly patronise the types of clubs and venues where such drugs are accessed or taken. Attitudes as to whether 'speed' was a significant problem in Indigenous communities differed. When the Committee met with staff members of Indigenous health agencies in the Latrobe Valley, some workers believed it was a problem, others had not seen it. Mr Rick Henderson, Acting Executive Officer of the Central Gippsland Aboriginal Co-operative, Latrobe Valley, was most emphatic that amphetamines *are* a huge problem for Indigenous Victorian communities: He told the Committee:

> In the Koori community this [amphetamines] is a big thing. It is not only here [in Gippsland] but also in Shepparton, Robinvale, wherever, in a Koori community, amphetamines are a big thing. Morwell and probably Robinvale and Moe are the worst-off communities in the state.[336]

Mr Henderson was at pains to stress, however, that in addressing any issues pertaining to drug use in Aboriginal communities attention must be paid to the heterogeneity of those communities. Just because Indigenous amphetamine use may not be prevalent in one corner of the state does not mean it is not problematic in another area:

> Drugs, substance abuse, employment, education, family violence, all those sorts of things. It was put to me that the things that happen in this community [Latrobe Valley] do not happen in Shepparton and would never happen in Shepparton. It was put to me by my mother-in-law that that is because there has been a group of leaders over the last 20 years in Shepparton who have taken control of what has gone on and have led the process. But here, what I hear is that there are people who will do things but will not go that extra step.
>
> ...What happens in Shepparton does not even happen in Echuca, which is only 40 minutes away. As I say, it is two different communities. Even though across all communities issues are similar, there are differences.[337]

335 Ibid.

336 Mr Rick Henderson, Acting Executive Officer, Central Gippsland Aboriginal Co-operative, evidence given to the Drugs and Crime Prevention Committee, Inquiry into Amphetamine and 'Party Drug' Use in Victoria, Public Hearings (Moe), 23 October 2003.

337 Ibid.

Whatever their differing views on amphetamine use in Indigenous communities, all workers were agreed, however, that alcohol, marijuana (*yandi*) and chroming (paint inhalation) were the predominant issues of concern among Indigenous youth.

Interventions

Given the paucity of information with regard to Indigenous injecting drug use, and particularly the use of amphetamines and 'party drugs', there has also been a corresponding lack of initiatives developed to target this particular form of drug abuse. Most drug related programmes relating to Indigenous people throughout Australia concern alcohol use. The Indigenous health web site healthinfonet notes in this regard:

> Interventions aimed at reducing injecting drug use and associated harms have focussed on two areas: health education programs (usually delivered in schools or prisons), and the provision of safe injecting equipment through Indigenous community-controlled needle and syringe programs. The first needle and syringe program targeted at the indigenous community was established in 1992 by Nunkuwarrin Yunti in South Australia. Since this time, another six indigenous focussed needle and syringe programs have been established. Nunkuwarrin Yunti also established the first methadone maintenance program specifically for Indigenous injecting drug users. Since the establishment of this program, several intervention projects have been established, in both residential and non-residential locations. Despite the presence of these services, recent research has identified a lack of appropriate detoxification and rehabilitation facilities for Aboriginal injecting drug users. THis is particularly true for young injecting drug users, and for those living in rural and remote areas, who are hesitant to seek treatment if it means they will have to be away from family and country.
>
> Access to services, and a lack of culturally appropriate services is a common theme in Indigenous health. This is no different when assessing the prevalence and influence of services for injecting drug use in the Indigenous community. While Aboriginal people are able to access mainstream services, these are not always appropriate or accessible. Through one particular study a criticism of provided services was that few workers were knowledgeable about injecting drug use, and that services were generally male focussed and staffed. In another recent study, consultants stated that Aboriginal clients viewed the atmosphere of mainstream drug and alcohol services as uninviting and impersonal, adding that there were not enough Aboriginal workers for clients to identify with. Other issues identified as barriers to accessing were believed to be: lack of confidentiality, reassurance, lack of awareness of services, and location (services not being where clients live). Isolation from family and community recommendations for services included the introduction of a clinic that would ideally be managed by Aboriginal people, and would be relatively informal. It was also suggested that the service should provide methadone

> maintenance therapy, counselling, medical and health assessments, food parcels and overnight accommodation. Workshops on drug use, the presence of an outreach worker, qualified and dedicated alcohol and drug workers and activities to alleviate boredom, were also perceived as important components of a service targeting injecting drug use.[338]

The committee believes that more research with regard to injecting use by Indigenous people in both urban and rural communities needs to be undertaken. Such research should specifically focus upon the use of amphetamines, and where appropriate or relevant, 'party drug' use in these communities. Any strategies or initiatives developed alongside or consequent to such research needs to be culturally specific to the communities it is targeted at. The Committee believes the following recommendations are 'first steps' to addressing and hopefully eventually resolving some of the problems faced by Indigenous communities with regard to licit and illicit drugs generally and amphetamines and 'party drugs' in particular:

Recommendations

6. The Committee recommends that specific, culturally appropriate training and resources on amphetamine and 'party drug' use be provided to Koori alcohol and drug workers.

7. The Committee recommends the need for Koori-specific holistic healing centres to be funded to adequately cater for the specific cultural needs of Indigenous communities with regard to substance abuse issues as described in this Report and this Committee's previous Reports into Public Drunkenness and Volatile Substance Abuse.

8. The Committee recommends that the development and funding of Koori-specific leisure facilities, including youth, sport and recreational clubs and programmes, be extended in order to provide structured activities that will engage young people, enhance their self-esteem, promote Indigenous culture and tradition and develop a sense of community.

Amphetamines and 'party drugs' in the gay and lesbian community[339]

Drug use at dance clubs and parties is not of course an issue restricted to gay culture, but it is definitely *part* of that culture. Indeed much of the mixed or 'straight' dance, music and club scene that grew up in the 1980s 'rippled out from a predominantly gay base…the embryonic features of the gay dance club

338 Quoted in *Summary of Injecting drug use and its health consequences among Indigenous people* www.healthinfonet.edu.au

339 This section predominantly is a profile of the use of 'party drugs' within the gay community; for an account of the harms associated with the use of such drugs, particularly methamphetamine, see Chapters 6 and 8.

scene were evident in gay and lesbian clubs many years earlier' (Measham, Aldridge & Parker 2001, pp.56–57).

'Liberating' effects of 'party drugs'

Gay raves and dance parties are seen as safe venues where gay men and lesbians can be themselves, free of homophobic threats.

Ryan and Keen explain the attractions of the gay party scene:

> The [gay] dance party scene has developed along with post-Stonewall gay culture. Many of the bigger parties in Australian cities have grown out of gay and lesbian community events. Some gay and lesbian dance parties are part of a lineage of mass celebrations where people come together to participate in a life-affirming expression of communal identity and beliefs...
>
> Such celebrations are often characterised by ecstatic, orgiastic release; extreme and unusual behaviour is allowed and things are generally turned on their heads. They are a time out of time. They simultaneously provide space for self expression, and participation in a collective articulation and affirmation of a shared identity...
>
> Many modern gay and lesbian dance parties contain elements which are similar to ancient events: spaces are constructed to exclude the (real) outside world and create a new, artificial world – partygoers step into different identities and roles through costume; normal states of consciousness and perception are disturbed through drug use; and people dance all night instead of going to bed (Ryan & Keen 2001 (1999), p.4).

Drug use, particularly 'speed', serves several purposes for gay men and lesbians in similar ways that it does for heterosexuals. It gives dancers the energy to stay on the dance floor all night. It has an aphrodisiacal effect. It lowers inhibitions allowing a person to 'succumb' to the aphrodisiac. It also, has been suggested that it provides them 'with an escape or sanctuary from unrelenting homonegative [sic] attitudes and discrimination in their everyday lives' (Lewis & Ross 1995, p.73).

In a survey of recreational drug use, with a focus on ecstasy use in Perth, Moore (1993) comments on the experience of young gay men with whom he conducted several interviews. To a certain extent their 'party drug' use was very much a product of their feelings about being gay and their experience of 'straight' society:

> [these men] ...describe and understand drug use in terms of 'altered states', of experimentation, and of rejecting 'straight' society in favour of a coherent, well organised alternative value system in which their sexuality is not a mark of derision or exclusion. In their shared understandings about drugs, themes such as sharing the experience with friends, of grasping new perspectives on their lives while under the influence of drugs, and of thumbing their noses at the conservative, homophobic majority appear frequently (Moore 1992a, p.32).

The sense of 'other worldliness' testified to by Ryan and Keen, while one of the attractions of the gay dance scene and the taking of 'party drugs', also:

> [c]reates an interesting dilemma for partygoers, promoters, and health educators: when everyone is trying as hard as they can to go beyond and outside their normal selves, how can everyday concerns – such as safe sex, safe using and adherence to HIV therapies – be properly incorporated in people's party planning and experience? (Ryan & Keen 2001 (1999), p.4).

A recent survey of drug and alcohol use in the Victorian gay and lesbian community (see Murnane et al. 2000) attests to the central role of drug use in some parts of the gay community and culture:

> Historically in both Australia and other developed countries, drug use has been at the centre of the establishment and the 'coming out' of the gay and lesbian community as a whole. Initially, sympathetic bars and clubs were the sole places where gay men and lesbians could socialise. Later Mardi Gras and a variety of dance parties became a way of celebrating the community and developing a sense of unity and strength. MacEwan and Kinder (1991) described a 'tripartite family system' made up of family of origin, an intimate partner and a close network of gay and lesbian friends, the latter being 'the major support for identity formation and maintenance'. Whilst not all gays and lesbians frequent pubs and nightclubs, it appears that such venues play a different role than in the general community. A qualitative investigation of the gay dance party phenomenon in Sydney identified a number of themes: that drug use is prominent at such events, there are established etiquettes and rituals around drug taking at these events, people in the age range 14–46 years attend the parties, attending the events and taking drugs has strong meanings for both individuals and the communities around belonging, defining and celebrating community (Lewis & Ross 1995 in Murnane et al. 2000, p.11).

Risks for users

Despite the 'liberating' aspects of much gay dance and party culture, concerns have been raised as to the extent, type and level of drugs being used at dance parties and nightclubs within the gay, particularly male homosexual, community.[340] More importantly, such concerns have been expressed by members of that community. Drug and Alcohol Researcher, Paul Dillon, writes:

> Recent studies have found that particular drugs are used by a sizeable percentage of homosexually active men, with men who identify with the

340 See for example, Hando and Hall 1994; Lewis and Ross 1995; Frosch et al. 1996; Morgan and Beck 1997; Reback and Grella 1999; Topp, Hando and Dillon 1999; Degenhardt and Topp 2003; Degenhardt, Darke and Dillon 2003; Semple et al. 2002; Shoptaw, Reback and Freese 2002; Murnane et al. 2000; Klitzmann et al. 2000.

Many of these concerns have been raised in Chapters 4, 6 and Chapter 8 (Poly-Drug Use).

> lifestyle of the gay community far more likely to report recreational drug use than those who are not involved in that community.
>
> However, experts believe that it is difficult to quantify how rates of drug use among gay men compare with those among the heterosexual population.
>
> Research examining gay men has identified that their potential alcohol and drug abuse may be due to a number of factors including drinking styles, stress or the cultural importance of bars.
>
> Gay men's involvement with the nightclub and dance party scene and the influence this has on increasing levels of drug use has also been examined. Dance parties have become increasingly popular in gay communities around the world, while nightclubs and bars have been long associated with gay culture (Dillon 2000, p.10).

Dillon (2000) comments that ecstasy would appear to be far the most popular dance club drug associated with gay men, but amphetamines, LSD and ketamine have all appeared on the scene. In more recent years GHB has proven particularly popular in gay circles, at least in part due to its reputation as a sexual enhancer. Of particular concern is that GHB has a reputation for being a drug that is taken to 'forget' any safe sex messages that a user may have previously internalised or abdicate any responsibility for them (Bellis, Hughes & Lowey 2002; Clark et al. 2001; Jenkins 1999). Equally worrying is the fact that high risk behaviour was not attributable to ignorance about safe sex guidelines, as many men in various samples were well informed (see Lewis & Ross 1995 and the studies reviewed therein).

Just as research on drug use among the heterosexual population reflects concerns about the relationship between drug use and unsafe practices, international studies have expressed dismay also at the relatively high correlation between drug use and high risk behaviours within the homosexual population. Much of this research has concerned injectable drug use, unsafe sex and HIV risk but more recent studies have examined links between the use of 'party drugs' and high risk behaviours. For example, Klitzmann et al. (2002) examined the patterns of use of 733 gay men using MDMA/ecstasy in New York City. MDMA use, particularly at night and dance clubs, was found to be directly associated with unsafe and unprotected sex. The authors state:

> ...MDMA users are a group at risk that are young, are engaging in high risk sexual behaviours that may expose them to HIV or other STDs...and are using MDMA which may cause neurotoxicity. MDMA users as a group thus may face several important threats to their health. Part of the public health problem may lie in the fact that MDMA may be perceived as being safe because it is non addicting. Clearly, there is a need to research perceptions of the drug as safe or unsafe and in what ways it is or is not seen as posing risks.
>
> MDMA use presents particular challenges in terms of possible interventions. MSM [Men who have sex with men] users [of MDMA] are more out and involved in the gay community than MSM non-users. Being 'out' can thus be

> psychologically advantageous in terms of dealing with stigma, but may also place individuals in settings where MDMA is used. Indeed, for many men, MDMA use may be a part of a process of entry and socialisation into gay culture itself (Klitzmann et al. 2002, p.124).

An American ethnographic study by Reback and Grella found that methamphetamine use was extremely high among gay and bisexual users in Los Angeles or in gay operated and owned institutions such as sex clubs, bars and saunas.[341]

> The men in this study reported that they had incorporated methamphetamine use within their sexual activities and described methamphetamine as the vehicle for greater sexual risk taking. The ability to have continuous sexual encounters and multiple sex partners was viewed as a beneficial function of the drug, particularly for those men who exchanged sex for drugs or money.[342] Further, HIV positive men in the study were less likely to use condoms than HIV negative men. Methamphetamine was central to the self identity of the men in the study, for whom sexuality has been fraught with the threat of HIV. Using methamphetamine enabled them to be sexually active within the context of this risk and to reclaim a sense of pre-AIDS sexuality (Reback & Grella 1999, p.156).[343]

Similar findings were found in a study of gay methamphetamine users in San Francisco. For such males 'methamphetamine use was inextricably entwined with their sexual behaviour' and had a functional purpose if they worked as 'hustlers' or 'escorts' (Morgan & Beck 1997, p.141). Also in the United States, the drug's aphrodisiac effects:

> [W]ere blamed for undermining safe-sex campaigns which had been successfully reducing the number of new AIDS infections. A British journalist observed in Los Angeles that "crystal has in recent years become a gay men's drug. It has a liberating as well as a stimulatory effect. Its disinhibitory effect means users temporarily forget about safe sex".
>
> By the mid 1990s, crystal was being cited as a factor in roughly half of all new AIDS cases in Los Angeles County (Jenkins 1999, p.103).

---

341 In Australia a high and early profile of HIV/AIDS prevention that worked in tandem with the gay community has for the most part meant that gay operated venues are more likely to co-operate in disseminating harm reduction messages and providing harm reduction information or materials such as condoms, lubricant etc than may be the case in the United States.

342 Part of the functional or instrumental use of amphetamines as discussed above. A later study also based in Los Angeles found that the long-acting stimulant qualities of amphetamines enabled users, particularly street workers, to:

'[e]ngage in sexual activities with one, two or many partners while using methamphetamine. Homeless street users report that the drug has functional aspects; its use enables them to increase their number of paid sexual customers' (Shoptaw, Reback & Freese 2002, p.93).

343 Reback and Grella used outreach workers to gather the data for this study. They believe outreach interventions are a crucial strategy for disseminating harm reduction messages to these populations. For further discussion of such interventions, see Chapters 19 and 20.

Australian researchers have also worried about the link between methamphetamine use and new HIV infections:

> [The] data indicate that whilst previous intervention programmes were successful in imparting safer-sexual and drug related information to a large proportion of gay men, they have been less efficacious in changing these risky behaviours among a minority of younger gay men (Lewis & Ross 1995, p.3. See also Murnane et al. 2000).

The concern is particularly felt with regard to young gay men, as indicated in the above quote. Some young men who use drugs and have sex with other men, particularly if they have not 'come out', put themselves at greater risk of HIV or other diseases. One 'experienced' participator of gay dance parties comments on:

> The lack of safe sex in the toilets, at the dance parties. Particularly if they are young and aren't actually in the gay scene. They don't have the same understanding of the dangers of risky sex (Lewis & Ross 1995, p.87).

Other young men may naively view themselves as 'invincible' or their 'discriminative capacity [is] over-ridden by their need for experimentation and sexual gratification' (Lewis & Ross 1995, p.87).

Risk taking is encouraged by what Lewis and Ross term the 'eroticizing effects of set and setting'.[344] They believe the risk taking at dance parties is compounded by four impairing conditions:

> [a]n erotic environment, the over-use of consciousness changing substances, the loud background party music and the lack of conveniently placed condom machines or facilities within this context... (Lewis & Ross 1995, p.89).

Lewis and Ross' research is now almost ten years old and it would seem that in the interim there have been great improvements in addressing the dangers flowing from drug use and its relationship to unsafe sex in the male gay community. Of particular importance is that this issue has been addressed by the gay and lesbian communities themselves.

Extent of use

Community forums have been held by various AIDS Councils and also by the Sydney Gay and Lesbian Mardi Gras to discuss drug use among the community (Haire 1999; Dillon 2000). Although there has not been a great deal of research into the drug patterns, and particularly 'party drug' use, in the Australian gay community, research by Erica Southgate at the University of New South Wales indicates there is a high rate of recreational drug use in the gay community:

> ...[t]he Sydney Men and Sexual Health Report showed that 78% of men surveyed had used illicit drugs in the last six months, and 12% had injected drugs... "From [Drug Use in Gay Men, a qualitative study], we've identified patterns of drug use within the gay community. The most prominent pattern

344 Lewis and Ross are drawing from the work of Zinberg (1984) in this context, see Chapter 10.

> is around partying – dance parties or clubbing", said Southgate... (quoted in Haire 1999, p.19. See also Knox et al. 1999).[345]

Despite this fairly high figure, Southgate believes that most members of the gay and lesbian community adhere to harm reduction practices (including the use of needles to inject drugs) and have 'a commitment to controlled drug use'[346] (Haire 1999, p.19).

Although most of the Australian research focusses on gay men, the University of New South Wales is broadening its research profile to study the drug use of lesbians and women attached to the gay community.

Victorian research on 'party drug' use within gay and lesbian communities

A major research project on drug and alcohol use among gay and lesbian communities in Victoria was conducted recently.[347] This study developed a project to identify patterns of drug use and associated harms within the gay community and the consequent development of appropriate harm minimisation strategies.[348] A detailed analysis of the findings is beyond the scope of this Report, however some general findings give an important insight into the role drugs and alcohol, and in particular ecstasy, plays in certain gay, lesbian and queer communities. In 1998 a questionnaire survey of 518 members of the Victorian gay and lesbian community established that:

- Overall the alcohol and other drug use within the GLBQ [Gay, Lesbian, Bisexual, and Queer] communities is two to four fold higher than in the general community [compared to figures in the National Household Survey 1998];
- Many respondents referred to past drug and alcohol problems. These were often associated with low self-esteem, depression, anxiety, paranoia, confusion around sexuality, and the stress of 'coming out' to family, friends and work colleagues;
- Alcohol and other drug use was associated with particular subcultures or contexts, for example ecstasy, amphetamines and LSD were strongly

345 Certainly recent work conducted by Degenhardt and Topp indicates that drugs such as 'crystal meth' are used 'overwhelmingly within the context of the dance party/club environment' and that substantial amounts of users 'identif[ied] its effects on sexual arousal and feelings of sociability as positives of the drug' (Degenhardt & Topp 2003, p.19).

346 In this regard Lewis and Ross (1995, pp 29ff.) stress how important the role of the dance party organiser or promoter is in the context of safe sex and drug use information. This is particularly so with regard to the huge warehouse parties often organised by the gay and lesbian communities. Promoters and organisers should be utilised as conduits for harm reduction measures, information and materials. This is equally true for heterosexual dance parties. Of interest is the fact that while homosexual saunas have been criticised for promoting unsafe and 'promiscuous' sexual practices, it is arguable that in some at least there is better provision of safe sex information, condoms and lubricant than at the dance parties in which drug use may be prevalent and sex happening in unsafe places in unsafe ways (see Lewis & Ross 1995). For further discussion of the role of dance parties and dance party organisers in the context of harm reduction strategies, see Chapter 19.

347 See *Beyond Perceptions: A Report on alcohol and other drug use among gay, lesbian, bisexual and queer communities in Victoria* (Murnane et al. 2000).

348 Conducted jointly in partnership with the Australian Drug Foundation (Centre for Youth Drug Studies), the ALSO Foundation and VicHealth.

associated with the 'dance party scene'. Poly drug use was common with different drugs used to achieve different effects;

- Illegal drugs are normalised to such a degree for some members of the GLBQ communities that their illicit nature is barely recognised;
- For some respondents drugs were seen as integral to creating and celebrating a sense of community and belonging. Some described it as a 'rite of passage'... (Murnane et al. 2000, p.7).

When examining ecstasy use in particular, the survey found that 65 per cent of men in the age group 20–29 had ever used the drug (23.9% in the last month prior to completing the survey) compared to 13 per cent of men aged over 50 (1.8% in the last month) (see Tables 9.1 and 9.2). This compared to 36 per cent of women having ever used ecstasy in the age group 20–29 and 7.1 per cent in the over 50 age group. Generally men were twice as likely as women to have used drugs of any type (except ketamine, where gay men were six times more likely to have used this drug compared to women).

Table 9.1: Percentage of respondents ever having used ecstasy

		National Household Survey 1998		GLBQ	
	Age	Women % by age	Men % by age	Women % by age	Men % by age
Ecstasy/	20-29	11.9	19.1	36.0	65.2
Designer	30-39	3.7	9.5	24.6	59.1
Drugs	40-49	0.0	0.0	2.3	36.7
	50+	1.6	1.9	7.1	12.7

Note: Men in the 20–29yr age group were four times more likely to have ever used ecstasy or designer drugs at 65% compared to men 50+, 13%. This percentage was considerably higher than the proportion of young men in the National Household Survey (NHS) sample (19% for 20–29) and 2% for 50+.
The percentages decreased from 36% of women (20–29) to 25% (30–39) then dropped substantially to 2.3% (40–49) and rose again to 7% (50+) with respect to ever having used ecstasy. It is difficult to explain this rise in the older age group. It did not occur in the male data. The difference in proportions between women in the Gay, Lesbian, Bisexual and Queer (GLBQ) sample and the NHS is considerable with 36% compared to 12% for women (20–29). The difference for men is also substantial, particularly within the 20–29yr old group, with 65% in the GLBQ sample compared to 19% in NHS. The difference continues in the 30–39yr, 40–49yr and 50+ groups.

Source: (including Note commentary): Adapted from Murnane et al. 2000, *Beyond Perceptions: A report on alcohol and other drug use among gay, lesbian, bisexual and queer communities in Victoria*, The ALSO Foundation, Centre for Youth Drug Studies, Vic Health, Melbourne, p.36.

Table 9.2: Percentage of respondents using ecstasy in the last month

		National Household Survey 1998		GLBQ	
	Age	Women % by age	Men % by age	Women % by age	Men % by age
Ecstasy	20-29	1.6	1.6	4.0	23.9
	30-39	0.0	0.5	0.0	13.6
	40-49	0.0	0.0	0.0	3.8
	50+	0.7	0.0	0.0	1.8

Note: For men in this GLBQ sample, ecstasy use ranged from 24% (20–29), 14% (30–39), 4% (40–49) and 2% (50+). Ecstasy use was only reported by 4% of women in the 20–29 age group and not by any women in other age groups. This is supported by the qualitative data, which indicated that ecstasy use is associated with the commercial and dance party scene, in which the greatest participants are gay men (although young women seem to be starting to become more involved in this in recent years). In comparison to the NHS the highest percentage was 1.6%, found for young women and men (20–29), which again could be associated with their involvement in the rave culture.

Source (including Note commentary): Adapted from Murnane et al. 2000, *Beyond Perceptions: A report on alcohol and other drug use among gay, lesbian, bisexual and queer communities in Victoria*, The ALSO Foundation, Centre for Youth Drug Studies, Vic Health, Melbourne, p.44.

The percentage of gay men using ecstasy, particularly in the age group 20–29, was far higher than that for the heterosexual cohort based on the National Household Survey (NHS) (19% for the 20–29 age group and 2% for the over 50 age group).

With regard to ketamine, 24 per cent of the 20–29 year age group of young men had ever taken ketamine compared to 1.9 per cent of the over 50 group. Only four per cent of lesbians in the 20–29 year age group took ketamine and no women over that age took ketamine (see Table 9.3). In the last month, 2.2 per cent of gay men aged 20–29 and 1.1 per cent of women aged 30–39 had taken the drug. No men in the higher age bracket and no women at all had used ketamine in the last month (see Table 9.4). There were no figures available for NHS data (Murnane et al. 2000, pp.36–37).

Table 9.3: Percentage of respondents ever having used ketamine

		National Household Survey 1998		GLBQ	
	Age	Women % by age	Men % by age	Women % by age	Men % by age
Ketamine	20-29			4.0	23.9
	30-39			0.0	20.5
	40-49			0.0	11.4
	50+			0.0	1.9

Note: In this GLBQ sample approximately a quarter of the (20–29) males reported having used ketamine and this then decreases to 21% (30–39), 11% (40–49) and 2% (50+). This exhibits a very different pattern to women's where the only use of ketamine reported is in the 20–29yr group at 4%. In the qualitative data references are made to the effects of ketamine as, 'get so blotto' and 'you loose [sic] your perception of time'. Although not mentioned in the qualitative data, ketamine is now being identified in some of the tablets sold as ecstasy. There are no data available for NHS comparison.

Source (including Note commentary): Adapted from Murnane et al. 2000, *Beyond Perceptions: A report on alcohol and other drug use among gay, lesbian, bisexual and queer communities in Victoria*, The ALSO Foundation, Centre for Youth Drug Studies, Vic Health, Melbourne, p.37.

Table 9.4: Percentage of respondents using ketamine in the last month

		National Household Survey 1998		GLBQ	
	Age	Women % by age	Men % by age	Women % by age	Men % by age
Ketamine	20-29			0.0	2.2
	30-39			0.0	1.1
	40-49			0.0	0.0
	50-59			0.0	0.0

Note: Use of ketamine was only reported by 2.2% by men (20–29) and 1.1% (30–39). This indicates that although the drug is used rarely its use is specific to the gay male community. No comparison with NHS is available.

Source (including Note commentary): Adapted from Murnane et al. 2000, *Beyond Perceptions: A report on alcohol and other drug use among gay, lesbian, bisexual and queer communities in Victoria*, The ALSO Foundation, Centre for Youth Drug Studies, Vic Health, Melbourne, p.45.

Finally, with regard to amphetamines (methamphetamine) gay men in the sample were much more likely to have used amphetamines than those in the National Household Survey (76% of the GLBQ survey compared to 20% of the NHS cohort for the 20–29 year old age group). The percentage of lesbians having ever used amphetamines (48% in the 20–29 year old age group) was also substantially higher than the NHS sample (18% of women aged 20–29). It was noted that for both men and women in the GLBQ sample, amphetamine use was likely to decrease with age (see Table 9.5).

Table 9.5: Percentage of respondents ever having used amphetamines

		National Household Survey 1998		GLBQ	
	Age	Women % by age	Men % by age	Women % by age	Men % by age
Amphetamines	20-29	18.4	20.7	48.0	76.1
	30-39	10.3	21.9	44.9	64.8
	40-49	4.3	7.0	17.4	50.6
	50+	1.6	1.9	7.1	14.5

Note: The number of respondents reporting ever having used amphetamines decreased with age. Thus young men at 76% in the 20–29yr age group were five times more likely to report using amphetamines compared to 15% for (50+). Further, the proportion of 76% (20–29yrs) for this GLBQ sample of males is much higher than the 20% reported in the NHS. At 15% for (50+) this percentage can still be considered notable for men in this age group when compared to the NHS sample of 2%.

In comparison, women's reports of ever having used amphetamines were generally lower than men's, with 48% of women 20–29yrs compared to 76% of men (20–29). This percentage is still considerable however, with almost half of the women respondents having used. This percentage is also substantially higher than the NHS figure of 18% for women (20–29yrs).

These data are supported by numerous references in the qualitative data to widespread use of amphetamines, along with other drugs, typically at nightclubs and dance parties. Mention was made by a number of respondents of the difficulty individuals experience when trying to withdraw from amphetamines.

Source (including Note commentary): Adapted from Murnane et al. 2000, *Beyond Perceptions: A report on alcohol and other drug use among gay, lesbian, bisexual and queer communities in Victoria*, The ALSO Foundation, Centre for Youth Drug Studies, Vic Health, Melbourne, p.35.

In the last month, 17 per cent of gay men compared to two per cent of the National Household Survey sample in the 20–29 year old group had taken amphetamines. While lesbians took amphetamines far less frequently than gay men, their use was still high compared to the women in the National Household Survey. Eight per cent of women in the 20–29 year old GLBQ group compared to one per cent of women in the National Household Survey took amphetamines in the last month (see Table 9.6).

Table 9.6: Percentage of respondents using amphetamines in the last month

		National Household Survey 1998		GLBQ	
	Age	Women % by age	Men % by age	Women % by age	Men % by age
Amphetamines	20-29	1.2	1.6	8.0	17.4
	30-39	0.0	0.5	2.9	14.8
	40-49	0.0	0.0	0.0	2.5
	50+	0.0	0.0	0.0	1.8

Note: 17% of men in the 20–29 yr in this GLBQ sample compared to 2% of the NHS survey used amphetamines in the last month. The percentages for women were lower than men, at 8%, but still substantially higher than women of the same age in the NHS, at 1%. Interestingly, 2% of men in the 50+ age group had used within the last month compared to nil in all the other groups of that age.

Source (including Note commentary): Adapted from Murnane et al. 2000, *Beyond Perceptions: A report on alcohol and other drug use among gay, lesbian, bisexual and queer communities in Victoria*, The ALSO Foundation, Centre for Youth Drug Studies, Vic Health, Melbourne, p.43.

The survey makes some interesting comparisons with the data collected and what is known from an ethnographic and social perspective about the gay community and dance culture, particularly as it applies to age:

> The reports of ever having used most drugs declined very rapidly with age. Thus among men, those aged 50 or more were five times less likely to report ever having used amphetamines, four times less likely to report ever having used ecstasy or designer drugs, and three times less likely to report ever having used cocaine. Similar patterns were apparent among women. This suggests that the use of such drugs has become much more common within the communities within the last 30 years, the period of major development of the commercial lesbian and gay worlds (Murnane et al. 2000, p.32).

The Murnane survey is a useful document that shows how a mix of qualitative and quantitative data and methodologies can point the way to informed policy development with regard to drugs and particular harm reduction programmes, be they used in the gay and lesbian or wider communities. Harm reduction, education projects and associated policies will be discussed in greater detail in Chapter 18. One of the challenges for the gay and lesbian communities and indeed the wider policy field is to address what Lewis and Ross termed almost ten years ago the 'incongruency between knowledge and risky behaviour' (1995, p.205). In other words, what education and harm reduction strategies can be implemented to minimise the dangers occurring to gay men who continue to engage in unsafe sex and drug behaviours, notwithstanding their relatively high levels of knowledge and awareness of the dangers flowing from their sexual practices?

Some of the techniques being currently implemented by gay communities are having positive results in addressing harmful drug use. Such strategies also have implications for 'mainstream' Victoria. As Dillon states, 'many of the drug trends identified within the gay dance scene eventually emerge in the general community' (2000, p.11). They are therefore worth paying close attention to.

Middle-class professionals and ecstasy use

Early studies by Rosenbaum, Morgan and Beck (1989) examine a different cultural profile of ecstasy use, namely the middle-class professional who does not fit into the stereotype of 'junkie' or 'raver'. During the course of their research the authors noted that several middle and upper middle-class professionals used ecstasy on a regular basis:

> This group, we discovered, has been able to integrate drug use into their busy lives, scheduling it in much like any other appointment or activity. It is, in the words of one respondent, 'controlled hedonism' for the ability to choose selectively where, when and how one experiences a...moment of 'time out' behaviour with drug induced altered states of consciousness (Rosenbaum, Morgan & Beck 1989, p.17).

Ecstasy use as 'time out' and 'therapy'

Like the ravers in Lenton and Davidson's study (1999) and that of Shewan, Dalgarno and Reith (2000) these respondents testified to the importance of planning the drug experience. The acquisition, use of and aftermath of these professionals' ecstasy use were meticulously planned to the last detail.

The motivation in using ecstasy for these professionals was the reward it gave for a punishing and hectic work schedule. It was also contrasted with other drugs such as heroin, which were not seen as conducive to a busy professional lifestyle:

> *'To me this is time out behaviour. My life is very full and I have lots of responsibility. I've got a lot of work that I need to do, I have a lot of deadlines. So to me it's like time out...it's like taking a vacation to Mexico for a week, only I'm going to do it in a day, because that's all I've got'* (Female aged 38, quoted in Rosenbaum, Morgan & Beck 1989, p.17).

Ecstasy was also viewed as part of the 'good life' in much the same way as good movie, a fancy dinner party or a ballgame. It also was seen as a way of 'depress[ing] time and accelerating interpersonal processes'. This point was particularly important for those whose workloads did not allow for frequent socialisation:

> *'In addition to making you open, it seems to depress time and the ability to cover a lot of ground in this flurry of experience that you might take quite a long time to or may not get to without it. I think the world we live in right now seems too busy with our lives'* (Male aged 30, quoted in Rosenbaum, Morgan & Beck 1989, p.17).

For other members of the sample, ecstasy had a therapeutic benefit which allowed them to do 'two years of therapy in one afternoon' (Rosenbaum, Morgan & Beck 1989, p.17).

Planning and preparation

The demographic of these users is clearly different to those in the rave or club samples. For instance, they are on average much older, usually in their 30s and 40s, having already completed tertiary education and built up professional careers. The importance of their careers is highlighted in the meticulous preparation put into arranging an 'ecstasy weekend':

> When a professional is planning his or her [first] trip, much research on the drug and its effects is done. These individuals have a healthy respect for the power of drugs, and want to know exactly what to expect. They tend not to like surprises and do not want to lose control. Consequently, they attempt to learn as much as possible about the drug before taking it (Rosenbaum, Morgan & Beck 1989, p.17).

Moreover, a combination of hectic schedules and the need for recovery time militates against having more than a handful of 'trips' in a given year:

> [b]usy professionals do not have the time necessary to do more than three or four trips per year. They are too busy, too discriminating and a bit too old. Professionals cannot afford to lose sleep. Thus although it is understood that a 'trip' technically lasts four hours, with boosters of more MDMA or marijuana, it can be extended to eight or ten hours. Thus people very often take ecstasy early in the day, often between noon and 4.00pm and rarely later than 6 or 7pm.[349] This requires scheduling a whole day and night, rather than just an evening. Given that many of these people, aside from having demanding jobs, also have children, finding a mutually acceptable day and night can be quite a task. They report that usually five or six appointment books have to be consulted in order to find a date that works. And then numerous arrangements have to be made, clearing of calendars, procurement of babysitters, hotel accommodations if the group is going away for the trip...
>
> ...Often trips are planned in three day increments, so that the first day can be spent 'resting', the second for the actual trip, and the third for recovery and gearing up for the following week's work... (Rosenbaum, Morgan & Beck 1989, p.17).

Some of the respondents to the Rosenbaum, Morgan and Beck survey note that the planning can even extend to goals and objectives pertaining to relationship issues that can be 'worked through' while under the influence of ecstasy. In this respect ecstasy has an instrumental purpose that goes beyond merely getting 'high'.

> If the professional is planning an Ecstasy trip for specific goals such as personal growth, awareness or building or patching up a relationship/friendship/ marriage, often lists are made of items to address. Many professional couples,

349 Which is a major difference from the patterns of use of the young person who uses ecstasy as a club or rave drug.

> for example, use this opportunity to explore issues and/or problems in their relationship (Rosenbaum, Morgan & Beck 1989, p.18).

Thus the profile of user and the reasons for taking ecstasy are somewhat different when comparing the professional and the raver or clubber. The professional user is much more likely to use ecstasy as an adjunct to inward reflection than the clubber. As such it may be used in conjunction with ambient music, a beautiful setting such as a beach and/or talking with friends or loved ones (Rosenbaum, Morgan & Beck 1989, p.18).

It should be noted that Rosenbaum's research is over ten years old and the debates surrounding ecstasy have changed in the intervening period. For example, as has been noted in a previous chapter, ecstasy, particularly if it is not pure MDMA, is not viewed as the benign drug that it was hitherto. Nor can the American experience be simplistically extrapolated to the scene in Australia.[350]

Nonetheless, it still remains true that the sample of users profiled by Rosenbaum is testament to the importance of drug, set and setting (Zinberg 1984). The dangers associated with using ecstasy in a calm and peaceful environment may be of a different order than that used in an overheated nightclub while dancing in an energetic manner. Moreover, a United Nations report on ecstasy in the mid 1990s found that a high proportion of recreational use of ecstasy was by people in the middle and upper classes (UNDCP 1996). Professor Klee, one of the world's most authoritative experts on amphetamine-type substance use has also commented that:

> The use of MDMA and new drugs will continue to extend beyond the dance scene particularly to the intimacy of home environments partly because the earlier generations are getting older (Klee 2001, p.85).

Often price may be seen as the main determinant of who uses the drug. For example:

---

350 Solowij et al. in their earlier survey of ecstasy use in Sydney compared their own survey findings to that of an American survey (Beck et al. 1989). While many of the respective findings were comparable, an account of user profiles and 'culture' of use was in some ways quite different:

'While the study of Beck et al and the present study approached the subject matter from differing theoretical perspectives, a number of factors regarding the recreational use of Ecstasy have emerged consistently in both studies, and thus in both cultures. These include the motivations for use, patterns of use, mode and context of use, the nature of the experience itself (including effects, side effects and residual effects), abuse potential and issues of tolerance. Perhaps the only area on which the Australia and American samples differ is the hierarchies of user typologies. This may in part be due to this Australian sample being primarily an inner city one, while the American one was somewhat broader. In this Sydney sample at least, the most predominant users of Ecstasy were the dance party crowd and recreational drug users in general whose main reason for using ecstasy is to have "fun". It appears that Ecstasy has not penetrated the social world of the "New Age" spiritualists to the same extent in Australia as it has in the United States. While Australian users do seek the therapeutic effects of Ecstasy, it is in a way more akin to a "fortuitous therapy" user group with therapeutic effects being the secondary bonus rather than the primary reason for taking the drug' (Solowij et al. 1992, p.1169).

There is nothing substantial in the literature to suggest that this difference in user profiles has changed to any extent in the ten years since Solowij et al. conducted their study. In other words, ecstasy is still not used to any great extent as a primary therapeutic or 'New Age' drug.

Whereas Ecstasy sells on the street for less than 20 pounds per tab in the United Kingdom and approximately A$50.00 per tab in Australia, the average street price for a single tab of Ecstasy in New Zealand is around NZ $90.00. This is outside the discretionary buying power of many people, particularly young people (Webb 1998, p.88).

Conclusion

The patterns and profiles of ecstasy and amphetamine use are constantly changing. Recent qualitative evidence, for example, suggests that at least in Australia the social demographic of ecstasy users is getting younger:

> [The evidence] indicates that the age of Ecstasy users may be dropping, and the proportion of female users may be increasing. On the whole, the sample [of Sydney ecstasy users] was young and well educated. Ecstasy was reported to be used in a variety of social contexts. It was often linked to dance events such as nightclubs or dance parties, but was also used at pubs, friends' houses and at home. Most of the Sydney sample emphasised that Ecstasy users were just ordinary people who were not necessarily part of any particular 'scene' (Webb 1998, p.88).

Similarly some of the most recent research surveys of ecstasy use in Australia (NDARC 1998; Hansen, Maycock & Lower 2001) have also found that the patterns of ecstasy use are changing.[351] While ecstasy is still highly, even primarily, associated with dance parties and to a lesser extent 'raves', at least in the public eye, the authors note that it has also moved in recent years into the mainstream, being used by a much more diverse range of people.[352]

---

351 Data from recent Australian research suggested that ecstasy was increasingly being consumed by a more demographically diverse group of people than has been previously recorded (NDARC 1998). This trend was also evident in data taken from Western Australia (Australian Institute of Health and Welfare 2001; National Drug Strategy Household Survey 2000). The majority of self-reported ecstasy users were aged between 20–29 years of age; however, a significant number of users were aged 30 years and above, with approximately 11% of users belonging to the 40+ age group (National Drug Strategy Household Survey, 2000). All age groups, except the 30–39 years group, revealed little to no variation in the number who reported having ever used and having used in the past year. This suggests that there is a small but dedicated number of "older" (40+) ecstasy users within the Perth community. Despite this evidence, much of the research and many of the intervention programs have focussed on the rave/dance music scene and youth, thus ignoring a significant "hidden" population of ecstasy users. This study purposively selected a sample of ecstasy users to represent the pattern of age use in Western Australia, with the intention of broadening the current understanding of popular recreational ecstasy use in community settings' (Hansen, Maycock & Lower 2001, p.182).

352 A comprehensive survey of international ecstasy use also attested to this change in patterns of use and demographics of use:

'There is evidence from a number of countries that ecstasy has spread beyond the rave culture and is also used in a variety of other situations (European Monitoring Centre for Drugs and Drug Addiction 1999; Forsyth 1996; Gamella 1999; Handy et al. 1998; Klee 1999; Liu 1999; Luna 1999; Moskawiecz et al. 1999; Smart 1999; Topp et al. 1997, all citations quoted in Gowing et al. 2001, p.10).

Recommendation

9. The Committee recommends that in the development of drug policy and the delivery of drug services, particularly in the area of amphetamines and 'party drugs', the needs and requirements of specific groups, including young people, women, gay men and lesbians be taken into account where appropriate.

As noted in Chapter 4, there has also been a slight but apparent shift from oral recreational use of ecstasy to injectable street use:

> [Survey] Participants were asked to nominate a 'type' of ecstasy user with which they most identified. This proved a somewhat ambitious undertaking as some participants were reluctant to categorise or 'pigeon-hole' themselves, and some were unable to name a single scene or type with which they identified. While many participants identified with various dance scenes, the item provided a flavour of the wide range of ecstasy users in Australia and refuted the common view that ecstasy is *exclusively* a dance drug. Participants identified with a broad range of 'types' or 'scenes' of ecstasy use, although the validity of such a 'typology' cannot be evaluated using survey methodology. Ethnographic research would be preferable to develop a typology of ecstasy users, similar to that described for amphetamine users [developed by] Klee 1997 (NDARC 1998, p.33). (Authors' emphasis)

As discussed earlier in this chapter, Klee's typology on amphetamine use is supported by little grounded research that gives much useful information about profiles of those who use amphetamines. As this chapter has discussed, there is a noticeable lack of information on amphetamine and 'party drug' use as it applies to women, Indigenous Victorians and people from culturally and linguistically diverse backgrounds. The paucity of research, both qualitative and quantitative, for both amphetamines and 'party drugs' is the subject of detailed comment in Chapter 21.

Throughout this chapter there has been reference to the amphetamine use by young people. Most of the discussion, however, has been with regard to problematic use, particularly of methamphetamine and in contexts such as street use. The chapter has not focussed to any degree on the recreational use of psychostimulants such as MDMA or other 'party drugs'. It is the profile of this type of user and an examination of these types of drug that is the subject of the following chapter in this Part.

10. The Culture of Use – Clubbing and Raves

> *DJs are the high priests and priestesses of the rave ceremony, responding to the mood of the crowd, with their mixing desks symbolising the altar, the only direction towards which ravers consistently face is the DJ box* (Newcombe 1992, p.5).

The previous chapter examined a diverse variety of profiles of amphetamine and 'party drug' use in Victoria. This chapter concentrates on one profile or pattern of use only. It is a discussion of those who may use amphetamine or more commonly 'party drugs' such as MDMA ('ecstasy') in the culture of raving or clubbing.

It should be observed from the outset that there is a notable dearth of good qualitative and ethnographic research detailing the cultural and sub-cultural aspects of drug use, particularly amphetamine use. While there has been some excellent ethnographic work conducted in the United Kingdom (Forsyth 1995; Malbon 1999; Shewan, Dalgarno & Reith 2000; McElrath & McEvoy 2001; Measham, Aldridge & Parker 2001; Hammersley, Khan & Ditton 2002; Deehan & Saville 2003),[353] there has been not a great deal of this type of research undertaken in Australia.[354] One of the comprehensive qualitative studies that was undertaken is Moore's ethnographic observation of networks of young recreational drug users in Perth. Although ten years old, the following observation is both salient and salutary:

> There appear to be two worlds of illicit drug use – the world of the clinic and the world of the general community with the latter category receiving

353 In Britain much of the (academic) writing pertaining to clubbing and drug use is in the area of cultural studies. Much of this literature is by younger academics with direct access to or participation in clubbing (Measham, Aldridge & Parker 2001 and the references therein, particularly Chapter 2 of that text). In Britain there is also a noticeable 'rave fiction' that explores the worlds of clubbing, raves and drug use. The most well known exponent of this sub-genre being Scottish writer Irvine Welsh. The rave and clubbing scene in Australia has also been explored from a fictional and artistic viewpoint in the recent film *One Perfect Day*, directed by the Melbourne film maker Paul Currie.

354 Some work currently in progress is that of Dr Cameron Duff of the Australian Drug Foundation who is examining the place of 'party drugs' in Australian youth culture. Mr Shaun Baxter, a Monash University medical student, is also looking at the context of 'party drug' use, examining a group of university law students as a cohort. Papers on both these research projects were given recently at the Victorian Alcohol and Drug Association's Party Drugs Symposium – *Beyond 'e': Exploring the impact of party drugs on everyday youth and culture'*, held in Melbourne on 23 June 2003.

increased attention in recent years. One of the many terms used to describe drug use within the community is 'recreational'. Anecdotal evidence suggests that recreational drug use, particularly of psychostimulants such as amphetamines and Ecstasy, is on the increase. Yet information on the nature, meaning, expressive styles, extent, cost, routes of administration, and overall circumstances of recreational drug use is sparse. The paucity of research data on drug use in natural social settings precludes both the conceptualisation of a clear framework for understanding its nature and the development of appropriate harm reduction strategies (Moore 1992, p.1).

Defining a culture

When one speaks of a culture or sub-culture of drug use, in a sense one is referring to membership of a group that is mainly distinguished by the narrow focus of drug use. As will be discussed in greater depth later in this chapter, this may be less true of a drug such as ecstasy which, at least in some contexts, may be seen as one aspect of a cultural phenomenon or as a means to an end. For example, in terms of 'rave use' it may be seen as an adjunct or contributor to a total transcendental experience which usually includes music, dance, visual images, lighting etc (see Melechi 1993; Moore 1995; Nolan 1998). Siokou states that: 'Although ravers may be viewed as a subculture, they are not a homogenous group and come from diversified backgrounds' (2002, p.12).

Conversely, at least in a 'traditional' rave context (for example large, often open-air, dance parties), other drugs such as alcohol may not be tolerated as it is associated with aggressive behaviour not conducive to the feelings of 'communality' expected of the 'love drug' (see Nolan 1998). Rather than speak of a culture or sub-culture of drug use, Moore's valuable study of amphetamine and ecstasy use in Western Australia prefers to refer to 'situationally specific shared understandings' or 'a sort of sub sub-culture':

> These are the specific understandings shared by a small set of people about a particular activity in which they engage regularly with one another in particular social situations and which has relative little impact on their membership of other social scenes (Moore 1992, p.31).

Moore and his colleagues observed a close network of young drug users in Perth over a 12-month period. The social contexts of their drug use showed that many of their 'subjects' had very diverse backgrounds and 'share few common understandings other than those pertaining to the particular focus of network activity'. Moore continues:

> On subjects such as politics, the importance of money, the intrinsic value of material objects such as cars or fashion clothing labels, sexuality and a number of other social issues, there was little or no consensus amongst the recreational users I studied. Some did not appear particularly impressed with material things while others were; some held conservative political views, others were more radical and others still virtually apolitical; and so on. To some extent this

> variety was reflected in their membership of other sets of people outside the narrow focus of drug use (Moore 1992, p.31).

When it came to their drug use, however, the network shared a very marked set of specific understandings about such use:

> [For example] Most were familiar with the idea of 'taxing' drugs (removing a small amount for one's personal consumption before passing it on to the buyer) either as a buyer or a seller, whatever they thought of such a practice. What was meant by the term 'junkie' was another oft-discussed theme. Some felt themselves to be junkies, others viewed it as a term of abuse, others felt it did not apply to them. Definitions of the term also changed over time. The point is that within a particular set of shared understandings, themes such as taxing and junkie-ness were commonly discussed and accepted as part of 'the way we use drugs' (Moore 1992, p.31).

In a different paper presented at an Australian symposium on psychostimulant use, Moore again outlines the importance of understanding the 'social world' of the drug user, particularly for policy development:

> Drug use occurs within specific social contexts and social networks which are constantly evolving, competing, collapsing, interacting and expanding. Drug users are embedded in ever changing social networks which do not consist solely of other, like drug users. The social world of a drug user is also likely to include employers or employees, workmates, partners, relatives, clients and sporting associates, some of whom use the same illicit drugs, others who use different illicit drugs and some who do not use illicit drugs at all. It is within these fluid social settings that individuals, as members of social groups, interact with one another and interpret, construct and negotiate the *shared* cultural means underlying their drug use.
>
> If one accepts the principle that to reduce drug-related harm we must first understand the 'insider' view of drug use, then ethnographers must locate themselves within the specific social contexts in which drug use occurs. They are then ideally positioned to describe and interpret the social processes which underlie drug use, the social meanings of drug use fashioned during social interaction and the harm minimisation practices currently employed by drug users to reduce drug related harm.
>
> Many aspects of psychostimulant use are...understandable with reference to broader themes in social life. The importance of social relationships and their management, the ways in which some individuals seek to assert their superiority within social groups, the processes by which individuals maintain their membership of these groups and the importance of the social context are all hallmarks of much human activity, drug related or otherwise. We should always pause to consider these complexities before resorting to simplistic explanations for drug use and before implementing simplistic policies (Moore 1993, p.88). (Author's emphasis)

Therefore the reasons for using different drugs will be as varied as and as inextricably related to the cultures or sub-cultures of which they are part. These reasons are discussed at appropriate points throughout this chapter. However, an initial comment is that the reasons why people take amphetamines or 'party drugs' are of course as diverse and varied as the reasons people take any form of drug, substance or stimulant.

The reason why a drug is taken may be instrumental or functional as much as recreational, as was discussed in the previous chapter. It may even be a mixture of both motivations. Similarly, some drugs such as ketamine or nitrous oxide may have functional purposes (anaesthesia) or be used to get 'high', often by those very persons responsible for administering the drug in a legitimate setting, for example doctors and nurses.

One of the most formative and influential theorists to discuss drug use from a social context perspective was Zinberg (1979, 1984). Zinberg noted that policy development in the field of drugs had to take into account the variables 'drug, set and setting'. The concept of 'drug', 'set' and 'setting' is of primary importance in determining why different 'classes' of user may administer a particular substance.

d'Abbs and MacLean (2000) summarise Zinberg's approach well:

> By these [concepts] Zinberg means: the pharmacological-toxicological properties of the substance (drug); the attributes of persons using the substance, such as personality and physical health (set); and aspects of the social and physical environment in which consumption occurs (setting). No intervention strategy is likely to ameliorate [substance abuse] and the problems associated with it unless it addresses each of these factors, and the interrelated effects engendered by them.[355] This does not mean that a single program must attempt to bring about change in all three domains, even if it could do so. However, it does mean that any intervention strategy, of which particular programs will form a part, must begin by identifying the factors in each of these domains that shape the usage patterns and consequences [of substance abuse and drug taking] (d'Abbs & MacLean 2000, p.v).

Rave and club culture and its relationship to ecstasy use

As discussed in Chapter 4, ecstasy has been described as an 'atypical' drug that does not fit within traditional pharmacological groupings, as it possesses both hallucinogenic and stimulant properties. Nor are ecstasy users necessarily 'typical' or at least stereotypical of 'drug users'. The recent survey of ecstasy users in Adelaide, South Australia, conducted by the National Drug and Alcohol Research Centre (NDARC) found that they:

---

355 Although d'Abbs and MacLean are discussing Zinberg's theories in the context of volatile substance abuse, their views are equally applicable to other forms of licit and illicit drug taking.

> [t]end on the whole to be young, well educated, heterosexual, from English speaking backgrounds and likely to be employed or engaged in studies. Most subjects had not had contact with police or other social authorities and did not come from socially deprived backgrounds, and few engaged in crime other than drug dealing. None were currently in treatment for a drug-related problem, and only one had a criminal conviction (NDARC 2001, p.vii).

British research indicates that there is a particular relationship between the 'clubber' and 'party drug' use that distinguishes them from other types of drug user:

> The [clubber] population is made up of devotees from a wide variety of socio-economic backgrounds but with students and employed people being strongly represented. What distinguishes this overall population from their peers is the emphasis on the consumption of music, dancing, tobacco, alcohol and drugs. The dance drug users thus stand out from an already conspicuous lifestyle group by being extremely drug experienced. They are poly drug users, who routinely combine tobacco, alcohol and illicit drugs. Yet in turn they are distinguished and distinguishable from most problem drug users by social class, employment and education, criminality, frequency and quantity of use and drugs imbibed, although the rise in cocaine use may fray this bifurcation between addictive and less addictive drugs (Measham, Aldridge & Parker 2001, p.11).

The 'double' effects of ecstasy – that is, as both stimulant and euphoric producing but 'controlled' hallucinogen – seem to be one of the reasons that ecstasy is such an attractive drug for its users. Solowij et al.'s early research on ecstasy use in Sydney found that:

> Ecstasy is an appealing drug to recreational drug users in that it provides an 'added bonus'. That is, for those seeking primarily stimulant effects it also induces the positive mood, euphoric and intimacy effects; for those seeking an enlightened experience or perhaps emotional therapy and insight it provides feelings of intimacy and closeness to others plus the stimulant-like alertness, talkativeness and energy.
>
> Further, it is a drug experience in which one feels that one can remain in control of one's thoughts and actions rather than the drug being in control... Shulgin and Nichols described [the controlled altered state of consciousness] as an 'easily controlled altered state of consciousness, with emotional and sensual overtones' and this was apparent in the responses of a large proportion of this sample, often being given as a reason for preferring Ecstasy over more 'mind bending drugs' (Solowij et al. 1992, pp.1169–1170).

A relatively recent study of ecstasy use in Australia (NDARC 1998) produced similar findings to the earlier survey work done of Sydney ecstasy users (Solowij et al. 1992) as to the reasons young people in particular use ecstasy:

> A range of motivations for ecstasy use were reported, many consistent with those reported in the Solowij et al. (1992) study. In both studies, participants reported that a combination of curiosity, availability and having friends who used encouraged them to experiment with ecstasy. Ecstasy-induced euphoria was the overwhelming reason for continued use. Other reported reasons for continuing to use reinforced the nature of ecstasy as both a stimulant and an hallucinogen, as well as an 'entactogen' or 'touchy drug' (Hermle, Spitzer, Borchardt & Kovar, 1993; Solowij et al., 1992). Thus, energy, confidence, heightened sensations, the group experience of warmth and friendship, improved communication and empathy, and insight and clarity of thought, were all important reasons for continued use in the present sample. Further, these effects of ecstasy were most often described as the best things about the drug.
>
> These effects also relate to the activities undertaken while intoxicated, which were more extensive and varied than just dancing at clubs or raves (Henry, 1992; Forsyth, 1996). They included socialising and meeting new people, feeling emphatic and close to friends, touching, relaxing, 'hanging out' at home, having sex and thinking. Its enhancement of social events makes ecstasy conducive to use in many situations, ranging from using at home with a partner for empathy and intimacy, using during the day with friends to go shopping or to the beach, to taking small doses before the cinema or dinner parties. Although the social effects of ecstasy, in combination with the hallucinogenic and stimulant effects, made dancing in an aurally and visually stimulating environment a favourite activity for many participants there were many participants who had never used the drug in a dance environment.
>
> Ecstasy is a drug used within a particular context. Few participants in either sample reported that they used it alone, with their dealer or acquaintances. Most used with small groups of friends, larger groups of friends or partners. Participants described extensive networks of friends who used the drug, with a majority of both samples indicating that most of the people they spent time with currently used ecstasy. The majority of those in the present study with regular partners reported that their partners also used. The social nature of ecstasy use also relates to the sources from which the drug is obtained; almost all participants (91%) usually obtained ecstasy from their friends (NDARC 1998, pp.35–36).

The Department of Human Services Victoria is concerned about the reasons young people use ecstasy and their lack of understanding of potential harms, as stated in its submission to this Inquiry:

> Ecstasy has always been associated with the rave and dance party scene, which seems to attract young people from all cultures and socio-economic backgrounds, apparently with plenty of money to spend on drugs. In the main however, people who attend rave parties are well educated, employed or involved in studies, extremely sociable young people most likely from the middle and upper classes. They have not usually had involvement with the criminal justice or the drug treatment system. The drugs are considered as much a part of the rave party culture as the music and the clothes.

> "Many young people in the rave subculture are coming into contact with drugs for the first time. This becomes more apparent as the rave subculture grows in numbers and many more people under the age of 18 join the scene. People younger and younger are having to make decisions about whether or not they are going to take drugs" (RaveSafe Safetime 1999).
>
> "Ecstasy is very much a social drug that decreases inhibitions, enhances social experience and allows people to share emotions together" (RaveSafe Safetime 1999).
>
> It is evident that impressionable young people with little experience or knowledge of drugs are becoming involved in a culture of which they have little understanding and are introduced to drugs purporting to be ecstasy, which may contain a harmful cocktail of other drugs and substances.[356]

The NDARC Topp survey found that contrary to popular opinion:

> [e]cstasy was used in a wide variety of situations, rather than being exclusively a dance drug. Ecstasy appears to have become a 'mainstream' drug in Australia, used by a demographically diverse range of people in a variety of contexts, not all dance oriented (NDARC 1998, p.viii).

Nonetheless, ecstasy is still very much a drug to be found and used at raves and dance parties and these are the contexts with which it is most associated. It is to this context that this section now turns.

The rave and club scene

In Australia, the emergence in the late 1980s of 'raves', often open-air or 'secret' dance parties associated with acid house music,[357] often brought with it, at least in the public and media mind, a concomitant use of 'party drugs', particularly MDMA (ecstasy) (Ryder, Salmon & Walker 2001, pp.242–243).

The early rave scene was:

> [l]inked to the mobility of clubbers, who could live anywhere in the country, drive to dance venues and consume illegal drugs with (relatively) little fear of prosecution. This mobility was the result of both the location of dance venues and the consumption of illegal drugs. Firstly, from the early days of raves in disused warehouses, fields and caves, access to transport was important...[358] Party venues were revealed on telephone answering machines or pirate radio stations on the very night of the dance event in order to evade police

356 Submission of Department of Human Services Victoria (Drug Policy and Services Branch) to the Drugs and Crime Prevention Committee, Inquiry into Amphetamine and 'Party Drug' Use in Victoria, August 2002.

357 Acid House is an eclectic music style originating in the United Kingdom. It draws from and incorporates modern and cool jazz, 1970s funk, house or dance music, soul, hip-hop, fusion and reggae. It became popular in the underground, rave and dance scenes in London, soon spreading to most other (Western) music and dance scenes in the 1980s.

358 This issue of transport to and between venues is still an important issue, see discussion in Chapters 7 and 19.

> detection, necessitating driving many miles to remote locations (Measham, Aldridge & Parker 2001, p.49).[359]

By the 1990s a shift was observed whereby ecstasy use was more associated with a music and dance scene located in mainstream night clubs, discos and licensed premises (Fitzgerald 1992; Lenton & Davidson 1999; Boys, Lenton & Norcross 1997).[360] Such a shift was not restricted to Australia but was also noticeable, somewhat earlier, in the United Kingdom and to a lesser extent the United States.[361] Measham, Aldridge and Parker have termed the period 1988–1998 the 'decade of dance' It was the era of 'enormous changes within club culture [with] diversification and fragmentation from a single underground rave scene into a myriad of sub-genres'(2001, p.19). Garratt states in this regard:

---

359 Ravers and to a lesser extent clubbers still rely on fairly unpublicised ways of accessing events, particularly the more 'hardcore' ones. It is not unusual to see posters 'advertising' raves that invite patrons to access venue or location details by Internet or phone on the day, although this is not necessarily the case with large-scale and arguably 'commercial' raves such as Earthcore, which are well advertised in a number of fora (record shops, Internet, trade magazines) months before the event. For a discussion of Earthcore, see later in this chapter.

In the American context this eschewal of traditional media is described as follows:

'[t]he advertising is designed to appear semi-spontaneous and underground. Events are usually announced no more than a month in advance and might use word of mouth, handbills, recorded phone messages, the Internet and/or the worldwide web to target the desired clientele.

Police intervention can represent a serious threat to a rave. One avoidance technique involves notifying potential participants of the date and the time of the event over the Internet and providing a phone number for further information. Only those recognised as properly referred when they call are told where the event is held. This modern day technology based procedure serves a similar function as the classic visual check and verbal interrogation through the slot in the door of a speakeasy' (Golub et al. 2001, p.1702).

360 Lenton, Boys and Norcross (1997) note the suggestion that since the rave/dance culture has become located in more mainstream settings there is a danger that particularly younger users may not heed the 'safe' drug use messages adhered to by some members of a more 'traditional' rave culture:

'[t]he risk of harm has increased due to ill-informed, inexperienced users who do not have the knowledge informally held within a more entrenched drug culture. Many new ravers were found to have romantic, positive beliefs about effects of ecstasy, LSD and speed and were effectively blind to the more negative effects including needle sharing and risky sex. There is also a risk that novice ecstasy users, unaware that the drug can take an hour or so to take effect, may think that they had bought a 'dud' and go in search of alcohol or some other drug with serious interactive effects' (1997, pp.1328–1329).

A discussion of harm reduction campaigns as they apply to rave and party goers is given in Chapter 19.

361 The American experience of clubbing and 'raves' seems to be at least in some respects different from countries such as Australia and Britain. The patrons tend to be wealthier than their British/Australian counterparts and a wider range of hallucinogens, particularly LSD, is on offer (see Golub et al. 2001; Jenkins 1999). Raves per se have not had nearly the same popularity in America as in Europe. They have largely been introduced by European expatriates and mostly restricted to cities such as New York and San Francisco (see Jenkins 1999 pp.163ff.).

For general accounts of raving, clubbing and their relationship to 'party drugs' from an international perspective, (the 'internationalisation' of clubbing) see Gowing et al. 2001 and the numerous references therein. For accounts from a specifically European perspective, see Tossmann, Boldt and Tensil 2001; and particularly Ter Bogt et al. 2002 for an account of 'dancestasy' in Holland. For an American account, see Jenkins 1999; Golub et al. 2001 and the references in both these texts. For an interesting cross-cultural account of 'clubbing' and ecstasy use in Hong Kong, see Chan Wai Leung 2003; Gosling 2003. Some good British sources on clubbing and raving are Malbon 1999; Measham, Aldridge and Parker 2001; Hammersley, Khan and Ditton 2002; Deehan and Saville 2003. These latter references have been drawn upon extensively in this Chapter.

> By 1990, it was no longer possible to talk of one single 'scene', but far from weakening the growing club culture, this fragmentation only served to make it stronger. As everyone took the basic ingredients and adapted them to their own needs, backgrounds, tastes and drugs of choice, the music began to mutate endlessly, splitting off into interlinked scenes and sub-cultures that continue to influence and feed back into each other in the most unexpected ways (Garratt 1998, pp.258–259).[362]

Much of the trends later found in the mainstream club scene could, as has been pointed out in a previous chapter, be seen much earlier in the gay dance clubs and discos.

> The 'counter-culture' of the club scene is viewed not so much as political as hedonistic. As celebration and escapism rather than about protest or rebellion (Measham, Aldridge & Parker 2001, p.27).

Alternatively, some commentators have viewed the dance party counter-culture as being simply a different form of 'politics', another type of 'revolution'. A tolerant form of politics where inter-racial, inter-sexual and inter-sexuality differences are subservient to the unity of the vibe:

> [A]ll youth cultures, inasmuch as they stake out a space, an 'investment in society', are inherently political... Yet, this does not necessarily mean that all youth cultures are political in a *mega*-political, 'anti-authority' sense, although some do appear to be so. The practices of youth cultures can be as much about *expression* as about resistance; as much about *belonging* as excluding; as much about temporarily *forgetting* who you are as about consolidating an identity; as much about gaining *strength* to go on as about showing defiance in the face of subordination; and as much about *blurring* boundaries between people and cultures as affirming or reinforcing those boundaries (Malbon, 1999, p.19). (Author's emphasis)

Tossmann, Boldt and Tensil, commenting in the context of the European 'techno' scene, view this shift from a traditional rave-type culture to a more commercial scene as part of a general shift whereby young people are consumers of a 'specific consumption/leisure industry' in which choice of clubs is as important an aspect of conspicuous consumption as the purchase of clothes,

362 For an account of the different types of music and dance genres noticeable in club and rave scenes, including mellow house, acid, hardcore, jungle, trance, bass and goa, see in particular Malbon 1999; Measham, Aldridge and Parker 2001. Golub et al. comment that these forms of music have evolved to enhance the drug/club experience:

'Fans and musicians alike describe these forms of electronic music as simultaneously futuristic (computerised, innovative, disorientating) and primitive (percussive, overwhelming and communal). This "future-primitive" music effectively releases participants from their restrictions to the here and now and enhances psychedelic drug experiences that are often saturated with memories, associations, and hallucinations that seem like revelations. In this manner the club drug scene draws symbolic ties between music and drugs that catalyse drug-like trance states' (Golub et al. 2001, pp.1702–1703).

music, magazines and travel (2001, p.2).[363] Clubbing is now part of a global cultural industry and overwhelmingly an urban form of leisure (Malbon 1999).[364] With an increase in disposable income for many young people, 'dance music tourism' to rave and club hotspots such as Ibiza are not uncommon, particularly for the British or European clubber (see Bellis, Hughes & Lowey 2002). Given this fact, it has been argued that any harm reduction policies aimed at clubbers and ravers must draw from the experience of, and consult with, travel and tourism organisations at international level. This is particularly the case given that there are added dangers for clubbers and ravers with regard to their drug use when they are on holidays, particularly in foreign countries (see Winstock, Griffiths & Stewart 2001).[365]

Ecstasy use and club dance culture appears to be part of an international (youth) trend and 'while there are some exceptions, descriptions of ecstasy users in the literature are remarkably similar between countries and regions' (Gowing et al. 2001, p.11).

A recent global survey of ecstasy use auspiced by the United Nations makes the following comments:

> Ecstasy users tend to be middle class, socially well integrated, well educated, are more likely to be employed than other drug users and less likely to have a criminal record. In Australia, the Netherlands, the USA, and Canada, ecstasy users are predominantly white, although use is increasing among other ethnic groups in the USA (Anonymous 1998; Anonymous 1999d; Forsyth 1996; Gamella 1999; Luna 1999; Smart 1999; Topp *et al* 1997b). In the Philippines, users predominantly come from wealthy families or are professional entertainers (Sunga 1999). Associations between ecstasy use and sex workers are reported in a number of countries including China (UNDCP Regional Centre for East Asia and the Pacific 2000), Spain (Gamella 1999) and the USA (Luna 1999). In spite of these trends, ecstasy use is found across the whole range of socioeconomic backgrounds and unemployed youth are considered to be at high risk (Henry-Edwards & Ali 1999; Liu 1999; Luna 1999)...
>
> Ecstasy originally became popular as a party drug in association with so-called 'raves' at which large groups of young people gathered to listen to specific types of music and dance all night (Milroy 1999). This association has continued and rave attenders have the highest reported prevalence of ecstasy

363 Indeed these commodities are essentially intertwined. The purchase of CDs and music magazines are clearly related, as is fashion. For example many 'ravers' at the outdoor rave Earthcore wore a particular 'uniform': baggy, colourful and often expensively custom-made trousers and jackets appliquéd with 'smiley' symbols and motifs. The carrying of little teddy bears and 'glowsticks' was also popular. For an account of 'XTC' fashion see Ter Bogt et al. 2002. See also discussion later in this chapter.

364 In an age of 'designer' everything, clubbing too has its own particular cachet. Designer clothes, designer music, designer clubs and designer drugs – so pervasive on an international level that even young people in the former Soviet bloc are 'intent on following the newest trend of youth culture in the western democracies' – including their illicit drug sub-cultures (Heckmann 1995, p.240).

365 See also Bellis, Hughes and Lowey 2002 and the discussion in Chapter 19.

> use. Ecstasy has also spread into regular nightclubs, discos and parties although prevalence of use in these settings tends to be lower (Anonymous 1999f; Anonymous 1999d; European Monitoring Centre for Drugs and Drug Addiction 1999; Forsyth 1996; Gamella 1999; Handy *et al* 1998; Klee 1999; Liu 1999; Luna 1999; Moskalewicz *et al* 1999; Smart 1999; Sunga 1999; Topp *et al* 1997b). Some users also use at home and in other venues but use seldom occurs alone (Handy *et al* 1998; Topp *et al* 1997b). (Quote and all references therein cited in Gowing et al. 2001, p.11).

While it certainly seems that much of the club culture surrounding ecstasy use has to a certain extent become commercial and mainstream, Lenton's research suggests that, at least in the west, there is a move back to the 'rave experience' by ravers who are disillusioned with the commercialisation of the nightclub scene:

> In Western Australia, as disenchantment grew with what many in the scene experienced as commercialisation and exploitation, a movement back to underground and unregulated events occurred with those in the scene reclaiming the scene by running their own events. These became known as 'Doofs', onomatopoeic for the heavy bass of music heard while approaching a rave held in a, usually clandestine, outdoor setting (Lenton & Davidson 1999, p.154).

Motivations for attending raves

The motivations for attending raves and the attraction of the rave (and club) scene centre on a combination of music, dancing, lighting and the pleasurable and euphoric feelings produced by the drugs taken, particularly 'ecstasy', although similar descriptions have been attributed to ketamine at raves (see for example, Dotson, Ackerman & West 1995).

Stimulating atmosphere

Champness (2000) describes the compelling nature of a (Victorian) rave in the following terms:

> The thumping tribal beats at rave dance parties, which attract the dedicated music fans, provide more than a good excuse to dance. There's an inherent sense of community, of being taken away from reality to another dimension, an altered state of being where the surreal becomes truth.
>
> At a rave, the DJ is shaman, controlling psychic musical voyages by manipulating music and working beats and samples into a mind bending tapestry of sensory overload.
>
> Together with visual stimuli, and more often than not, drugs, the experience elevates one to an altered state of physical or psychological existence (Champness 2000, p.50).

Gowing's international survey of ecstasy use reflects similar observations:

> Sociability is a major characteristic of ecstasy use. It is almost exclusively taken in a social setting with partners or groups of friends. Users particularly seek the

> feelings of empathy and closeness with others, which result from ecstasy use, to foster a group identity and sense of belonging (Anonymous 1998; Gamella 1999; Klee 1999). Friends have a major influence on ecstasy use with the majority of users reporting that they were introduced to ecstasy by friends, and decided to try it because friends were using. A significant proportion report that they continue to use because their friends are using (Gamella 1999; Sherlock & Conner 1999; Topp *et al* 1997b).
>
> There is a strong influence of youth culture, lifestyle and fashion trends on these social networks and groups of friends. Ecstasy is associated with a variety of specific cultural trends in particular networks where the importance of the group is emphasised. These groups have been likened to tribes which go out together, share the same taste in music or dance and develop the same norms (Anonymous 1998; Luna 1999). There is fairly universal acceptance of drugs as a component of the music and dance scene among these groups (Gamella 1999; Klee 1999). The gay club and party scene and the 'techno' music scene are two examples of particular subcultures in which ecstasy use is popular (Gamella 1999; Luna 1999; Anonymous 1998). In the UK, there are large differences in drug use at nightclubs and parties depending on the type of music played, with 'rave' and 'techno' music most associated with ecstasy use (Anonymous 1999f; Forsyth *et al* 1997; Klee 1999). In spite of the significance of drug use within the club and party scene, users in the UK rate drug use as only the fifth most pleasant experience after music, socialising, atmosphere and dancing (Klee 1999) (Quote from Gowing et al. 2001, pp.11–12).

Reduced 'sleaze' factor – feeling safe and free

One of the perceived attractions of the rave for those who attend, particularly women, is the lack of a 'sleaze factor' and a generally non-violent ambience. This is partially attributed to far fewer people being intoxicated by alcohol than at other types of venues such as bars, nightclubs and pubs:

> People who go are all going to have a good time, and very rarely are they drinking, and I think that helps to keep away people [who are] being really sleazy, really aggressive. So people are generally really friendly to everyone, really social, no one gets aggro, everyone is very accepting of different people, colour, sex, size, age, whatever they're like, because its such a broad angle of people going to raves (Male aged 19, quoted in Lenton & Davidson 1999, p.154).[366]

Although it would certainly seem, as discussed later, that the consumption of alcohol in conjunction with 'party drugs' such as ecstasy has markedly increased in recent years.

366 Further discussion on the difference between 'drug clubbing' and 'alcohol clubbing' is given later in this Chapter.

Siokou (2002) researched ecstasy use in the Melbourne rave scene and also found among her respondents that one of the main attractions of the rave culture was a 'sense of feeling free and safe':

> Over 90% of interviewees stated that they felt safe at raves and had never been harassed by anyone. One female interviewee, Anna (aged 26), stated: "I feel safe at raves even if I come alone and I have never been hassled by anyone. I would be too scared to go to a nightclub alone"... There is a low level of consumption of alcohol at raves and combined with a focus on the music and dancing rather than 'picking up' this clearly creates a feeling of safety for participants that they do not experience in other forms of night time entertainment (Siokou 2002, p.14).

Non-homophobic atmosphere

Raves were also seen as not creating a homophobic atmosphere. Even at dance parties that were not exclusively gay or lesbian, same sex couples were not frowned upon.[367] Conversely, at dance parties and raves catering for homosexual people in particular, there tended to be a relatively high percentage of heterosexual people in attendance.[368] This phenomenon testified to the fluidity of a youth culture predominantly based on music, fashion, books and dance rather than sexuality per se.[369] The move to rave parties enhanced by the use of 'party drugs' indicates a cultural swing that reflects a change from pub-based hard rock to acid house and techno dance parties. Dr John Fitzgerald of Melbourne University's Politics Department has stated that all things being equal, ecstasy can be seen as a relatively constructive social development for young people at least compared to alcohol and the 'suburban beer barns and meat market clubs' (quoted in Sweet 1997):

> 'What we've got is a generation of young people who've experienced social relations where a lot of the gender based distinctions are overturned', he says. At dance parties, men don't stand around awkwardly, waiting until they're plastered to hit the dance floor (Sweet 1997, p.11).

Webb states that ecstasy use explains why:

> [S]ocial drugs have become appropriated into mainstream youth culture, where they operate as both coping devices and ready-made identity badges... As one reviewer [United Nations Drug Control Programme] has commented:

367 Measham's British research found among the clubbers sampled in the study there was a 'strong commitment to tolerance of other people's lifestyles, particularly in respect of sexuality and drug use' (Measham, Aldridge & Parker 2001, p.7).

368 In the context of gay specific clubbing, the dance party was seen as an affirmation of group identity and cohesiveness. A respondent to Lewis and Ross' survey of gay dance party culture states:

'The parties are a celebration of life... It's a community and the dance parti[es] originated out of the gay scene...a group of people who are constantly oppressed through no fault of their own...and [are] rejected constantly. The dance party brings all these people together...and not have any restrictions upon them' (1995, p.129).

369 For a discussion of amphetamine and ecstasy use in the gay community, see below.

"On the one hand they offer possibilities for coping with today's performance-oriented society and social pressure on adolescents. On the other hand, they are used as representations of integration and socialisation, of a fashionable lifestyle and collective identification" (Webb 1998, p.92).

Communality and unity

Lenton and Davidson's survey research of 83 people who attended raves in Perth found that over a quarter of the sample (27%) described a 'sense of community' as being one of the chief attractions of the rave scene:

> 'Everyone's, it's like a big family sort of thing...you get to know everyone from the raves, when you get to see them every single rave and that. You feel like you're somebody, you feel like you belong somewhere' (Female aged 17, quoted in Lenton & Davidson 1999, p.155).
>
> Ecstasy in particular is seen as promoting group solidarity and togetherness:
>
> 'Ecstasy is the classic, because it enhances that group atmosphere, lots of people I know talk about the "mass breathe" where everybody's almost breathing as one, it's one of the things with Ecstasy, it makes your respiratory system go mad. You can be in a crowd of 1000 people, feel like you're all taking in the same breath sort of thing' (Male aged 22, quoted in Lenton & Davidson 1999, p.157).[370]

Research studies in both Australia and Britain, particularly, have established that a person is more likely to have taken their first ecstasy tablet at a club than anywhere else and usually through friendship networks (Solowij et al. 1992; Hammersley, Khan & Ditton 2002; Measham, Aldridge & Parker 2001). For most (young) people initiation into ecstasy use was not a solitary experience. It was usually taken in a group of friends and, as has been mentioned in this chapter, often it is introduced to the novice by a more experienced user who can 'mentor' the initiate.

For some people ecstasy use in a club context may also be an 'antidote to adolescent anxiety about peer rejection and coping with social relationships' (Klee 1997b, p.40). According to Klee it may give some young people the 'confidence to get up and dance uninhibitedly in front of others and be able to talk easily to others' (1997b, p.40). Unity and a sense of 'belonging' is particularly important for women (Hinchcliff 2001, p.459).[371]

---

370 While drugs such as ecstasy may indeed promote group cohesiveness and unity, research into the gay dance club scene also suggests that the clubbers 'need to belong to a group [and their consequent use of drugs such as ecstasy] often overwhelmed their personal autonomy and discriminative capacity' (Lewis & Ross 1995, p.46). One of Lewis and Ross' clubbing respondents testifies to the powerful group dynamics of the club scene:

'I took Ecstasy because my friends took it, and I knew it would be fun to do. On one occasion I didn't really want to take [LSD] [but] we were all going out and my friends were taking it too' (1995, p.46).

371 See also the discussion in Chapter 9.

Ecstasy is perceived as the 'great leveller' (Hammersley, Khan & Ditton 2002, p.37). This sense of belonging, unity, community and ritual[372] is what Nolan in her study of rave culture in Townsville, Queensland, calls 'communality': 'Communality can be defined as a sense of unity or oneness with other rave participants' (Nolan 1998, p.7).[373]

Paul Dillon from NDARC testified to this sense of connectedness among young people in particular when the Committee met with him in June 2003:

> I think we have to go way back about connectedness, and actually instilling connectedness into young people is really difficult. But I think that is what is really interesting about these drugs – particularly ecstasy – I would urge you as a group to sometime or another try to go to an event to actually see the connectedness that exists in an event where these drugs are used. Particularly ecstasy, if you understand how it works and the empathy it creates between people – you can walk in a room of young people who are so connected. Now it is artificial, it doesn't last very long, but for that brief time they feel more connected than they do at any other time in their life. And I think that is why this drug has just taken hold of a generation.[374]

Moore also observes this sense of collective consciousness among his sample of psychostimulant users in Perth (Moore 1992):

> An individual basking in the euphoric glow of Ecstasy, experiencing the kaleidoscopic sensory whirl of a trip, or internally racing under the influence of half a gram of speed, may positively vibrate to the pumping sound of contemporary dance music, the pulsating lighting displays and the mass of thrusting, sweating bodies in such close physical proximity. Any minor physical side effects such as sweating, jaw grinding or mild nausea will be largely ignored in such contexts.
>
> One pharmacological property of stimulants well suited to nightclubbing is the ability to remain awake and 'up' for several hours. After injecting half a gram of speed, or dropping a trip or an 'Eckie' mid evening (say 10pm), one is likely to be still awake at dawn or even later the next morning. The afternoon is then used to rest or alternatively, phone calls are made, prices and quantities are agreed and arrangements made for procuring further drug supplies for the coming evening. If there are few demands from the 'straight' (non drug using) world, such as an employment incompatible with little sleep or a social appointment with non using friends or relatives, sleep may be dispensed with

372 For a cross-cultural and trans-historical discussion of ritual in the context of group dancing and clubbing, see Lewis and Ross 1995.

373 Although as many commentators have pointed out, once the effects of ecstasy wear off some users of the drug may quickly discover they have nothing else in common with their fellow clubbers or ravers (see for example, Malbon 1999, p.41; Hammersley, Khan & Ditton 2002, pp 37ff.).

374 Mr Paul Dillon, NDARC, conversation with the Drugs and Crime Prevention Committee, Sydney, 26 June 2003.

> altogether for several days, until one's money, source of drugs, desire to consume further or stamina run out (Moore 1992, p.52).

Commentators of the rave scene have observed that a sense of oneness or collective consciousness is an exclusionary as well as an inclusive concept. Sarah Thornton's academic study of clubbers suggests that the majority of clubbers (or ravers) define themselves *against* the mainstream (Thornton 1994).[375] Malbon also discusses how the 'hard core' ravers or clubbers would never use mainstream entertainment guides such as *Time Out*[376] to find out which clubs to attend. Instead such clubbers/ravers would rely upon the Internet, flyers, friends or word of mouth (Malbon 1999, p.62).[377]

Some of the most interesting qualitative research on ecstasy use in Australia comes out of Western Australia (Moore 1992; Lenton & Davidson 1997). A relatively recent survey of users of ecstasy in Perth (Hansen, Maycock & Lower 2001) stresses the importance of friendship networks to the casual user of ecstasy:

> A range of factors was important when making the decision to use, however the friendship groups and social support network were revealed to be of particular importance. All participants initiated their use in the company of close friends, partners or a relative. These friends were either fellow initiates or they were previously experienced and thus were accorded the role of guide and mentor. In this role they were responsible for reducing feelings of anxiety, monitoring the effects (physical and psychological) and enhancing the experience of the new user. Feeling comfortable, relaxed and secure were universally reported as essential to ensuring a positive introductory experience. The presence of friends in itself did not, however, serve to meet those needs. Typically, the initiate sought out information concerning the effects, risk of adverse events and strategies to minimise those risks from experienced acquaintances prior to making the decision to use. This was either done directly, by asking experienced individuals, or through observation of users in situ.

---

375 A cautionary note should be sounded, however. While this sense of unity, oneness or 'communality' appears to be very real among 'ravers' and to a lesser extent 'clubbers', a phenomenon that has been often noted in the literature and observed by the Committee itself (see discussion later in this chapter), it is also true to state that it is not going to affect all people who attend clubs or raves to the same degree or in the same ways. As Tossmann comments in the context of the European 'techno' scene, 'for one person techno may represent a lifestyle, while for another person, techno is simply a type of music he or she occasionally enjoys dancing to' (Tossmann, Boldt & Tensil 2001, p.21).

Paul Dillon from NDARC in Sydney also testified to the need to bear in the mind the heterogeneity of the dance party scene as well as its unifying features:

'[i]n my experience within the club-drug setting there are so many different sorts of cultural groups. You have your ravers, you have your people who go to nightclubs, you have your gay dance party users, you will have your gay club users, and you have your Asian clubbing users, who are very different from the others. So you've got all of these different groups who all have different rituals, who all use drugs in different ways' (Paul Dillon, NDARC, in conversation with the Drugs and Crime Prevention Committee, Sydney, 26 June 2003).

376 The British equivalent of journals such as the *The Age's* EG (Entertainment Guide).

377 Malbon adds, however, that even within the 'scene' there will be variations and degrees of taste and style: 'what is "cool" for one clubber' may be the epitome of 'un-cool' to another (1999, p.38).

> The appeal for ecstasy users appears to be controlled freedom, a loss of inhibitions, affirmation of friendships and...a range of sensory sensations linked to enjoyment and pleasure. Ecstasy is the drug of choice because it provides the fun, confidence and companionship that the users seek without the negative consequences associated with other recreational drugs. In fact, a significant proportion viewed ecstasy as an alternative to alcohol and preferred its effects. The preferred effects included the lack of aggression (physical and sexual), the sense of retaining control, the absence of a hangover, the positive feelings experienced during the ecstasy high, the loss of inhibitions (in particular dance-related inhibitions for men), the sense of intimacy and the desire to dance. Essential to the popularity of ecstasy is the sense of control that the users maintain, as the following quote highlights:
>
> 'I don't like being not in control. I've always whenever I've had stuff before I've always been able to control what I'm doing. With 'e's you always know what you're doing. You can always remember what you did' (A.J., aged 23) (Hansen, Maycock & Lower 2001, p.187).

Overcoming boundaries – cultural, sexual, sectarian

An even more fascinating study of the communality found among ecstasy users is that of McElrath and McEvoy (2001). The authors conducted in-depth interviews with 50 users of ecstasy in Northern Ireland. Their paper explores the folklore of ecstasy use 'as it relates to the social relationships of drug user lifestyles' (p.1). Of particular interest is the fact that the communality produced by 'ecstasy', 'the loved-up drug', at least for the duration of the time it is being used, crosses sectarian boundaries of religion, culture and class in 'socially estranged' (and highly demarcated) communities such as Belfast. In other words, according to some of the study's respondents, the use of 'E' and the dance/rave scene has a positive impact on intercommunity relations between Protestant and Catholic. Take some of the following responses for instance:

> 'I think Ecstasy has had a very positive effect. I have to say living where I do which would be perceived as a Protestant loyalist area, I hadn't had much dealings with Catholics you know. I have to say I have made a couple of good friendships through it [Ecstasy] and it doesn't matter to me now whereas before I would have put my flag out on the twelfth and this sort of craic. Now I don't bother putting my flag out.'
>
> 'I'm a Catholic myself, I used to fight with the Protestants out in the park like but since we've took drugs like we don't give a fuck and people we used to scrap with, we go out and party with.'
>
> '[Ecstasy] greatly changed my socializing. Before, I wasn't much into religious mixing ... you would have known and talked to people but you wouldn't have gone out with somebody from the other religion and [Ecstasy] changed your perspective, you meet people you realize it's not all everybody's been saying, you know, talk to them. I know some guys I knew turned from being in bands

> and being staunch loyalists into mellow people who started having Catholic girlfriends and all.'
>
> 'Ecstasy has bridged that gap socially... You would have had Catholics and Protestants but you would [also] have had loyalists and some republicans and to have them housed in one place was amazing like, you know? And they couldn't have done that unless they were off their faces, you know?' (All respondents quoted in McElrath & McEvoy 2001, pp.13–14).

Siokou (2002) has examined the rave culture in Melbourne, Victoria. Drawing from earlier work by Hopkins (1996), she explores the concept of collective and multiple identities and a sense of unity as it applies to rave culture:

> Rave parties are events at which participants enter a fantasy world, which is dominated by loud techno music and utterly different to their everyday lives. There is a paucity of academic studies of raves...this paper focusses on theoretical issues to do with the construction of identity by the participants in raves... These questions about unity and identity are significant in the context of raves. Many ravers I have met during the past six years have asked me, "Has the party got the vibe?" as a way of asking whether the crowd is feeling unified and emotionally part of something larger than themselves (Siokou 2002, p.11).

The music factor

Siokou, as with many of the commentators on ecstasy and the rave scene, stresses the importance of music to the overall collective experience:

> Music played at raves is generally provided by a DJ. It is very loud, electronic and has minimal vocals. The ravers all dance facing the DJ...rather than each other, which is more often the case at clubs. Malbon's (1999) comment that music "provides us with an intensely subjective sense of being sociable...it both articulates and offers the immediate experience of collective identity" may be applied to the Melbourne rave scene. Many of my interview respondents stated that through the experience of dancing to electronic music at a rave, 'the vibe' or collective identity is created among the crowd. This is exemplified when a classic or anthem song is played (Siokou 2002, p.13).[378]

In Siokou's study of the Melbourne rave scene, 75 per cent of her respondents had taken ecstasy and 60 per cent had taken some form of amphetamines and

---

378 Siokou states that the Melbourne rave scene is bound to change once warehouse or 'dock' parties cease at the Melbourne Docklands due to redevelopment:

'The location shift will alter the Melbourne rave scene because many of the raves will be subsequently held at licensed nightclubs, which have a different atmosphere compared to dock parties which are held at huge warehouses colourfully decorated, with a DJ pumping extremely loud music through the speaker systems. "Chill out rooms" with quieter music and comfortable seats and cushions provide space for a break from dancing and offer people a chance to recuperate and talk.

The atmosphere at dock parties may be considered more underground compared to nightclubs which are generally smaller and more restrained. Furthermore, alcohol is not generally sold at the Docklands, whereas it is the main commodity at nightclubs' (Siokou 2002, p.13).

marijuana. Alcohol use was rare and there was little or no use of heroin or cocaine. Siokou writes:

> Many ravers described drugs such as ecstasy and amphetamines as enhancing their appreciation of the music and their ability to dance, so that they literally 'feel' the music through their bodies. Ecstasy enhances empathy and lowers social inhibitions. Sheila Henderson (1997) notes that "it is curious that a drug which can increase emotional closeness, enhances receptivity to being sexual and would be chosen as a sexual enhancer, does not increase the desire to initiate sex" (Siokou 2002, p.15).[379]

While drugs such as ecstasy are undeniably used at raves and dance clubs, according to Lenton and Davidson (1999) and contrary to much popular and media belief raves are not 'drug supermarkets'.

Perhaps surprisingly only 17 per cent of the Lenton and Davidson sample mentioned drugs as one of the attractive aspects of the rave scene, despite the fact that it was believed the majority of attendees used drugs at the rave. Many of the respondents commented on the synergy produced between the drug and its effects, the music, dancing and lighting:

> Techno [is the] sort of music to listen to on drugs because it just sort of goes with it. The whole thing, little things just add up, like the lights and the atmosphere, a hypey atmosphere hypes you up and gets you going, and that sort of like relates to the drugs, what the drugs do to you anyway, they sort of hype you up, but that sort of adds to it (Male aged 20, quoted in Lenton & Davidson 1999, p.157).

As the authors state, however, it is not that drug use is seen as a necessary part of the rave experience as much as the rave experience is viewed as being enhanced by the use of drugs, particularly ecstasy.[380]

> 'I've been to raves straight and I've been to raves off my face as well. The connection is well, you can have a good time if you're there and you're not under the influence of any drugs, but if you are, you have a better time because the lights are three times more brilliant, and the music is more impressive, you get disorientated and you've got a challenge to try and get your orientation back. I suppose it's...an environment conducive to taking drugs. You don't have to, but it is definitely a better time if you do' (Female aged 21, quoted in Lenton & Davidson 1999, p.157).

379 A study of British club and rave culture finds there has been a change in attitudes towards sex to some degree within those cultures over the last ten years:

'[c]ommentators have noted that with the popularisation, commercialisation and fragmentation of the dance scene there was also an increasing sexualisation. The late 1990s have been characterised by the re-emergence of the traditional heterosexual narrative, with the atmosphere in clubland shifting from 'luv'd up' to 'sex'd up' (Measham, Aldridge & Parker 2001, p.46).

380 A different paper produced by the authors based on the same sample noted that 'poly-drug use' was prevalent among the sample, including amphetamines, ketamine, cocaine and nitrites. Poly-drug use is discussed in Chapter 8. See also Dotson, Ackerman and West 1995; Von Sydow et al. 2002.

Preparing for the rave

Southgate suggests that preparing for a drug experience is reflective of a phenomenon called 'folk pharmacology':

> Folk pharmacology she explains involves a range of knowledge and practices from how to score drugs to how to reduce harm. Strategies include having support networks around if taking a new kind of drug, injecting or taking large quantities of a substance (Southgate quoted in Haire 1999, p.19).[381]

Arranging to score

In various qualitative surveys on ecstasy use, many respondents who do take drugs at raves testified to the importance of *preparing* for a big rave or gig in terms of taking drugs. This accords with much of the international literature on 'scoring' ecstasy (see Rosenbaum, Morgan & Beck 1989; Forsyth 1995; Shewan, Dalgarno & Reith 2000). Sixty-one per cent of the sample profiled by Lenton and Davidson (1997) preferred to arrange their scoring or drug acquisition days ahead of the rave, and sometimes weeks ahead. Not to do so could result in missing out, paying excessive amounts for the drugs or risk an increased chance of being arrested for drug possession if the 'score' was done at the venue itself. Drugs may or may not be brought to the clubs depending on the security policy at the door. Those clubs which strictly 'police' entry by thoroughly searching bags or clothes may in fact encourage the consumption of drugs prior to entry. In Britain, according to one survey:

> Clubbers tend[ed] to consume their drugs before entry to a club if the club was known for either particularly zealous searches or a strict policy of passing clubbers to the police if found to be in possession of drugs for personal use. This practice raises health concerns for clubbers because it encourages the pre-club simultaneous consumption of larger quantities of different drugs by [our]

---

381 Moore's survey of ecstasy users in Perth also implicitly draws upon this notion of 'folk pharmacology', outlining a whole set of behaviours that reflect a particular culture of drug use, including the purchasing or scoring of the drugs, the relationship of buyer to seller, the distinction between a casual ecstasy user and a junkie, the process of ingesting the drug and the rituals of preparation (less complex with ecstasy which usually need only be swallowed). A full discussion of these fascinating rituals is beyond the scope of this Report. The following discussion of how ecstasy and other psychostimulant users may view 'junkies' is, however, an interesting insight into the folk culture of a particular set of drug users:

'While members of this set viewed becoming a "junkie" or dependent on drugs with some trepidation, there was also a certain degree of admiration for what was seen as a sinister yet sometimes attractive status. Being a "junkie" or at least an injecting drug user was to claim membership of a dark, esoteric, subterranean world which involved deception, risk and a certain degree of glamour. Such feelings contrasted sharply with equally strongly-felt notions of uncontrollable drug use which characterised descriptions of the "junkie".

Thus attitudes to the various adverse consequences of drug use display a marked ambivalence. Although "coming down", physical side-effects and becoming a "junkie" are recognised as drawbacks to or hazards of drug use, they may also be reinterpreted in a more favourable light in future discussions. When stories about particular events (and their negative consequences) are told and re-told, such drawbacks may become integral parts of an incident or period being remembered, in much the same way as hangovers, so often regarded in surveys as an "alcohol related problem", may become part of drinking legend amongst social networks of participating individuals. *Drug related harm and problems may become part of the folklore of drug use*' (Moore 1993, pp.64–65). (Committee emphasis)

> poly-drug using clubbers. This is particularly worrying in the case of all night dance events...because a considerable quantity of drugs might be consumed at one sitting rather than staggered [over time] (Measham, Aldridge & Parker 2001, p.167).

Buying through 'friendship networks'

It would seem that most people who score ecstasy do so from friends who in turn may purchase from an 'informal' dealer who may or may not be dealing for profit. This type of transaction is popular 'because friends won't betray you' (Ter Bogt et al. 2002, p.170). Often the purchase is made on behalf of a group of friends who then share the drug. Of particular interest, however, is a recent survey of 760 British 'clubbers' across six English nightclubs (Deehan & Saville 2003). The findings of the survey with regard to ecstasy 'dealing' were similar to previous studies inasmuch as 75% of the sample cited a friend or acquaintance as their source:

> However, 'friend in this context was often used to refer to a reliable supplier who provides a quality product, rather than someone with whom the respondent socialised' (Deehan & Saville 2003, p.3).

In any event whether such 'dealers' are characterised as friends or acquaintances, ecstasy acquisition is far less likely to be scored off the street than other illicit substances. Moreover, drug distributors, those who pass on or facilitate the deal, are less likely to do so for profit (other than cheaper or free drugs) (Lenton & Davidson 1999, p.158).[382]

Measham calls this type of dealing 'mutual societies' or 'friendship networks'. Her description of these informal dealing and distribution practices are worth quoting in full:

> There are considerable advantages to these friendship networks of user-dealers:
>
> Firstly, there are the obvious financial economies of scale of buying in bulk and missing out the middle level of drug distribution. Secondly, there is a greater security in making group drugs purchases, resulting in fewer individuals in contact with higher level drug distributors and less chance of theft of cash or buying low grade/fake drugs. And for those who were younger, less confident or less familiar with the world of drugs distribution, mutual societies might enable the less active members of the network to purchase drugs through friends without coming into direct contact with retail specialists themselves, although the more active members of the friendship network obviously would be making such contact. Thirdly, contact with other users facilitates sharing experiences and upgrading street wisdom regarding the effects of specific drugs and specific batches of drugs. Fourthly, friendship networks save time by reducing individual searches for supplies, a key issue in the hunt for the elusive 'dealer', particularly for those young adults with limited access to transport.

---

382 In Britain it has been suggested that a compromise offence for dealing between friends in a not for profit context be established. See discussion in Chapter 12.

> Respondents discussed being able to take their time over the course of the preceding week to obtain good-quality supplies from a reliable source – preferable to anonymous and unaccountable 'dealers' in clubs if the respondents did not regularly attend specific clubs with regular dealerships. Leisurely purchase in the preceding days or weeks might also facilitate the tasting or testing of drugs before purchase, if a considerable amount was being bought and they were regular customers. Fifthly, clubbers who discussed these friendship networks focussed on more than just the financial and time-saving aspects of group deals. A key feature was also the sociability and camaraderie of group drug purchases and consumption.
>
> Thus friendship networks of user-dealers could also be considered to enhance three different aspects of harm minimisation. Firstly, by collective purchases made ahead of the night out, clubbers were able to make considered purchases of potentially better-quality drugs, resulting in less chance of adverse side-effects, after effects or long-term effects resulting from variable/fake street drugs, therefore minimising those health risks specifically associated with poor-quality drugs... Secondly, their contact with regular known 'dealers' minimised the risks of violence, intimidation and exploitation by unknown organised retail drug distributors and 'gangsters' in clubland... And thirdly, the collective purchases by friendship networks ahead of the night out resulted in less chance of being caught up in the criminal justice system due to the potentially more risky purchase in clubs where, as we have seen, uniformed and plain-clothes police operate, therefore minimising the risks of being caught up in the reactive, symbolic policing of clubland (Measham, Aldridge & Parker 2001, pp.152–153).

This type of mutual societies arrangement is to be distinguished from what Measham terms 'retail specialists', that is, known dealers:

> A typical operation was of known dealers; that is known both to the customers and the staff of a club, [indeed sometimes crowd controllers or other staff may themselves be the dealers] operating an agreed distribution within that club with several employees or 'runners' working for the manager(s) based in one corner. These runners specialised in their different tasks such as smuggling drugs into the club, acting as salesmen or 'snarlers', carrying the drugs and the money, distributing individual purchases to customers and collecting money, and acting as lookouts and minders. Such an operation might be condoned or sanctioned to a greater or lesser extent by staff working in that club (Measham, Aldridge & Parker 2001, pp.143–144).[383]

383 Measham also states that the drugs issued by these types of dealers can tend to be of lesser quality:

'One of the enduring images of clubland drugs distribution is that these retail specialists or organised drug dealership "gangs" in clubs are more likely to sell poor quality or even fake drugs than if clubbers buy their drugs elsewhere before the event' (Measham, Aldridge & Parker 2001, p.144).

Whatever the source of the club drugs, it has been generally agreed that 'getting sorted' for the most part 'requires specialist knowledge of the sub-culture and pre-arrangement' (Arnold 2002, p.2) or friends or contacts who have that knowledge.

Of particular interest, however, are the findings in the most recent major survey of 'clubbers' and drug use in Britain. This survey found that many 'clubbers' were remarkably blasé about their risks of being arrested for drug possession or any other legal consequences:

> Most believed that the strategies they employed protected them from the most serious legal consequences. These included buying from trusted sources, never purchasing drugs in a club and taking their own drugs into a club. Most felt that the likelihood of being searched effectively or arrested was remote. In addition, they felt that if they were arrested, it was most likely they would receive a police caution (Deehan & Saville 2003, p.4).[384]

Financing the use

According to Moore's 1993 study of urban users in Perth, the financing of ecstasy use is much more likely to be from licit sources such as salaries, savings or unemployment benefits than illegal methods such as burglaries or stealing. This may well reflect the view that for the most part ecstasy is perceived as a non-addictive drug with planned use which does not result in the desperation surrounding scoring associated with drugs such as heroin. As Moore states: 'Funds expended on drugs [such as ecstasy] can be compared to those spent by non drug users on consumable items such as clothes, compact discs, alcohol or books' (1993, p.42). Solowij's earlier study of Sydney ecstasy users found that Friday and Saturday nights were chosen as the best times to take ecstasy '[s]upporting the notion of ecstasy as a recreational drug suited to a working lifestyle' (*Connexions* 1991, p.6).

Planning, phases and rituals around the event

More recent survey evidence of Western Australian ecstasy users shows that meticulous preparation for a 'big ecstasy night' is still common. Hansen, Maycock and Lower comment on the experiences of recreational ecstasy users in Perth:

> The whole ecstasy experience is made up of events that surround the drug. Beginning with the decision to purchase; 'scoring' (the purchase of the drug); preparations for use; 'popping the tab'; the comedown and the inevitable 'eckkie blues' (the recovery phase that often includes mild to moderate, and in some individuals, intense, feelings of depression). The phases involved specific rituals that culminated in the actual use event. Each served to heighten user anticipation and expectations, which combined to create the overall ecstasy

384 Measham's survey also found that only 1% of the sample 'said they felt the purchase of illegal drugs was in some way problematic for them' (Measham, Aldridge & Parker 2001, p.157).

experience. These rituals included purchasing chubba chubbs/lollipops (to reduce the effects of gum chewing), mints, menthol drops or nasal sprays (to heighten the experience) and marijuana (for the comedown), organising music (specific to each stage), co-ordinating consumption and monitoring the group's progress.

The phases themselves were often spread out over a period of time, sometimes weeks and even months, while for spontaneous use events the phases were completed within a very short time frame. This appeared to have some effect on the experiential outcome. The physical setting (club, pub, home, beach) also tended to affect the organisational process and the various rituals involved, and therefore significantly affected the end experience...

The participants attempted to exert control over set (expectation, risk perception, mood) and setting (physical surroundings), and although it was impossible to control for the drug, they adopted measures such as using a regular supplier and having pre-taste tests as methods of semi control. New users were initiated into the ecstasy-using experience by more experienced users who helped the new initiates to interpret the symptoms they experienced during the drug use. The data revealed evidence of user folklore and myths that served to define and influence the overall drug experience. Users came to accept certain 'norms' about the effects, benefits and harms associated with their use of ecstasy. Using this knowledge they become more expert at manipulating drug, set and setting to maximise the experience and reduce the potential risks. Thus, despite the evidence of occasions of unplanned and spontaneous use, the participants revealed highly ritualised and largely controlled behaviour in relation to their ecstasy use (Hansen, Maycock & Lower 2001, pp.194–195, 197).

Taking the drug

The phrase 'popping the tab' in the last quote refers to the actual process of taking the drug, whether at the club or prior to entry. Malbon describes this process in minute detail in his detailed study of club culture and drug use in England:

> It is probably safe to say that no two clubbers have the same method or go through the same mental processes in taking ecstasy (MDMA). While clubbers might take the same amount and even the same 'brand' of pill, each will approach the experience differently. Some may 'drop' part of what they intend to take even before the night has started – maybe at home or more commonly while waiting in the queue outside, particularly if it is already late or they are very near the front of the queue. However, it is most usual to 'drop' the first amount, of what might be just one but may also be two, three or even more amounts over the course of the night, within a short space of time after entering the club. It usually takes between twenty minutes and an hour to start experiencing the effects of the drug – to 'come up' on it. Conveniently, this leaves time for the clubbers to find a space and to have a drug, deposit coats

> and bags in the cloakroom, and wander through the club generally getting into a clubbing mood, checking out the music and perhaps meeting friends. In instances where clubbers buy the drugs ('score' them) when they get into the club, thus avoiding the risk of bringing them through the security themselves and the potential difficulties and dangers of scoring the drugs beforehand, the search for a dealer from which to 'score' may also take place in these initial stages. Occasionally, perhaps due to a later arrival, a build-up of excitement or a familiarity with the club night, clubbers will 'drop' their pills immediately on entry and go straight to the dance floor, with the nervous excitement of having just taken their pill combining with the music and their familiarity to induce an impatience to start dancing and for the night to begin (Malbon 1999, pp.122–123).

Pre and post-rave health care: Minimising adverse outcomes

Pre-planning extends not only to purchasing and taking the drug, but also getting the body ready for the 'big night out', through eating the right foods, getting plenty of sleep prior to the rave or club night and generally looking after one's health. Tony Palmer from Melbourne's Youth Substance Abuse Service (YSAS) testifies to the importance which 'clubbers' give to 'forward planning':

> We know that people who take ecstasy, for example – and we are talking here about Melbourne uni law students rather than YSAS clients – will do things like 'preload'. So they will take lots of stuff that is rich in things like tryptophan, which is a precursor for serotonin, which is the neurotransmitter released by ecstasy. So they are actually preloading their bodies to have a lot of serotonin, so that when they take the drug, it will have a really strong effect.
>
> So when you look at that sort of thing and you realise that these people know what sort of foods are tryptophan-rich, what vitamin and amino acid supplements there are out there, and they have been doing that a week before they go to a rave, I would say yes, there is a lot of preplanning.[385]

This meticulousness of preparation for use also extends to the post-rave or club experience. For example, Siokou reports that ravers regularly use drugs in planning the 'coming down' phase, most commonly marijuana. Marijuana is used predominantly to counter the depressive feelings associated with 'Blue Tuesday':

> The energy that speed and ecstasy provide is only gradually sapped from the body so many ravers do not tire until two or three days later when they experience an effect commonly known as 'Blue Tuesday'. Symptoms of Blue Tuesday include moodiness, exhaustion and/or depression. Marijuana is also used to bring back the feelings induced by ecstasy tablets when its effects are wearing off or, alternatively, for putting the person to sleep. Some interviewees also use sleeping tablets to cure their insomnia. This behaviour supports

385 Mr Tony Palmer, YSAS, evidence given to the Drugs and Crime Prevention Committee, Inquiry into Amphetamine and 'Party Drug' Use in Victoria, Public Hearings (Melbourne), 27 October 2003.

> Collin's argument that young people: '[b]ecome expert manipulators of mood, choosing exactly what to take in each situation to produce specific psychopharmaceutical responses, applying sophisticated cost benefit analyses to each substance' (Siokou 2002, pp.16–17).

A study based on the questioning of a focus group of 42 ecstasy users in Scotland tested the assumption:

> [t]hat drug users are by definition reckless with regard to drug-related risk. A common assumption made of drug use is that it is a necessarily chaotic, relatively unplanned, impulsive event (Shewan, Dalgarno & Reith 2000, p.431).

Acknowledging the dearth of information available about the social and behavioural characteristics of ecstasy users and recognising that this prevents informed policy, programme and harm reduction development, the authors explain their use of focus group methodology as follows:

> The advantage of a focus group is that it allows the researcher to interact with the participants directly, clarifying issues and also observe non verbal behaviour that may contradict verbal response... One purpose of using a focus group, as opposed to individual interviews for example, is that this method offers data which includes negotiation of meaning between participants and allows the identification of subtle differences in meaning between focus groups (Shewan, Dalgarno & Reith 2000, pp.432–433).

The following response, for example, of one of the participants was fairly typical of the focus group as a whole:

> Oh yes, the majority of times when I'm using drugs I plan it in advance, just to fit in with my lifestyle. If you're going to work on Tuesday, then at weekends you know you cannot be too many miles from home, and not have recovered fully by the time you are back in class, so pretty much it's planned (Shewan, Dalgarno & Reith 2000, p.445).

Just as with Siokou's study of Melbourne ecstasy users, so too in Scotland did this meticulous planning extend to the 'coming down' phase, as indicated by the following comments from participants in the focus groups:

> 'Planning a night, aye. Organise the evening, get hash in, get booze in for later. I like to make sure I've nothing to do the next day as well. That's a definite.'
>
> 'It's nice to have some things organized for a good night. It's good to have some hash at home and some drink maybe, even if I don't actually go home, it's good to know it's there. Also I like to know I've got the day off. I also like to have company too, when I'm coming down.'
>
> 'The next night I like to have a few joints and a few beers and chill [relax]. It just takes off the rough edges.'
>
> 'That's true, the comedown can be a bit nasty, and a wee drink can smooth it all off for you.'

> 'Yeah, it's like being prepared, you know? It's like the more you do it the more you become...'
>
> 'You know what to expect.'
>
> '...yeah, and you know what's going to make you feel *most comfortable*, 'cos that's basically what everyone wants, is to feel as comfortable as possible, before, during and after. I mean the only hassle for us is if we've got to go somewhere, who's going to drive, that's a hassle sometimes' (Shewan, Delgarno & Reith 2000, p.447). (Authors' emphasis).[386]

This fascinating exercise in ethnography is summed up in the words of one of the participants: 'Drug taking *has* to have rules' (Shewan, Dalgarno & Reith 2000, p.447). (Authors' emphasis)

Drug, set and settings

Drug

When it comes to considering the *drug* ecstasy, a Scottish survey from the mid 1990s has revealed some fascinating results. Forsyth (1995) states that the pattern of ecstasy use (in Glasgow) deviates from all other drugs in as much as the sub-culture has grown up around several brand names, designs, forms, sizes and colours of ecstasy pills, tablets and capsules. A survey of 135 users of ecstasy in the Glasgow area who were part of the rave scene were interviewed about their experiences of dance drugs. Among other findings, respondents were able to identify over 300 forms of substance being marketed as ecstasy, each with their own peculiar characteristics, shapes, colours, names etc. A physical description and an account of the subjective effects of these different types were given by each respondent. Brand names seem to be commonly ascribed to a particular feature of the drug, for example form (liquid E, bayer E); content (Saddam Hussein, madwoman); shape (snowball, rusk, brown burger); colour (pink and white, Manchester United, ie. red as per their guernseys); effect (smacky E, speedy E) and so on.[387] Forsyth argues that a definite 'consumerist' culture has been built up around ecstasy acquisition:

> There is an interesting parallel here between users' beliefs about the dance drug ecstasy and dance drug music; both are mixed. Perhaps Ecstasy can be seen as representative of a wider youth culture of conspicuous consumption, rather than simply being another drug used by drug users. From the point of view of the user, the importance of ecstasy lies in its place as part of a wider lifestyle, not merely as a drug, important for only its pharmacological effects.

---

386 Lewis and Ross' early study of the gay dance party scene also examines the 'comedown period', in the context of post-dance 'recovery parties':

'These recovery parties [are] organised within the established gay social institutions such as hotels, bars, nightclubs, saunas and private parties. Previous researchers suggested that these traditional gay venues provided patrons with a relatively safe environment to interact sexually and socially with other men' (1995, p.59).

387 For a chart classifying the various ecstasy tablets available according to particular categories, see Appendix 14 based on a table in Hammersley, Khan and Ditton 2002, p.40.

> When buying Ecstasy, the user is buying a feature of a lifestyle not a substance (Forsyth 1995, p.207).

In other words, unlike or to a lesser extent than drugs such as heroin and methamphetamines, ecstasy is part of an overall package in which the chemical properties or the rush of the drug is only one, albeit a significant, aspect. Despite some recent evidence that ecstasy may be crossing over to become an injectable street drug,[388] it is still largely inseparable from other aspects of the youth culture such as music and dance.

Set

Similar to surveys of ecstasy use in Australia, the Scottish focus groups of Shewan, Dalgarno and Reith showed that planning extended beyond the scoring of the drug to being in the right emotional mood when taking the drug; that is, the 'set' must be right. The consensus of the groups was that 'ecstasy was not a drug that should be taken when experiencing psychological difficulties of some sort' (2000, p.442). As one participant commented:

> It's [ecstasy] definitely something I wouldn't take if I was feeling down or depressed. It's definitely not something I would take to get out of that...there's only one drug I'd bother with and that's alcohol, you know, to get yourself through a bad patch (quoted in Shewan, Dalgarno & Reith 2000, p.442).[389]

Setting

When it came to a discussion of *setting*, participants were of the opinion that while ecstasy was most often taken in the context of a rave or dance club, and often to the beat of loud music, other settings had been (sometimes inappropriately) used:

> I sat in a Jacuzzi with big bags under my eyes...it was quite a scary experience, 'cos with my dilated pupils, looking around and seeing the Sunday morning hangover faces, plus the overheating effect of the water, I suddenly felt very sick and out of place on my drug [ecstasy] (quoted in Shewan, Dalgarno & Reith 2000, p.444).

---

388 A study conducted by NDARC (1998) found that 16% of a sample of young ecstasy users from Victoria, New South Wales and Queensland (n = 329) had injected ecstasy and 10% had injected ecstasy within the six months preceding the interview (NDARC 1998, p.8).

389 Shewan, Dalgarno and Reith ground their research in Zinberg's framework of drug, set and setting referred to earlier, and previous work done by Weil (1972).

'"Drug" is particularly relevant in the context of this study due to the variability in the amount of MDMA present in a tablet, and the presence of other psychoactive drugs such as MDA, ketamine or MDE.

"Set" is defined by Weil as a person's expectation of what a drug will do, considered in the context of a whole personality.

"Setting" is defined as the physical and social environment in which a drug is taken. As both Weil and Cohen have pointed out, the possible interactions of these components are equally as important as determinants of a drug experience as are the components individually' (Shewan, Dalgarno & Reith 2000, p.438).

On the other hand, participants said taking ecstasy in atypical settings such as the home could also be pleasurable:

> 'I've taken E sitting in the house, and I enjoyed it.'
>
> 'A couple of my friends took it at home just sitting in the living room and the two kids had got up during the night, and this was about two in the morning, and they said it was one of the best times they'd ever had...E'd out of their heads with two kids, playing: how relaxing can you get?' (quoted in Shewan, Dalgarno & Reith 2000, p.444).

Moore's study of ecstasy users in Perth also comments on the use of the drug in 'mellow' domestic settings. Similar feelings of 'pleasant euphoria' expressed by those in the Scottish focus studies were experienced by the Perth respondents:

> Yet, Ecstasy users also describe the experience as one of clarity. There is no fuzzying or distorting of the senses; just heightened appreciation of sensory messages and a supreme sense of well being. The experience in these quieter settings is not as intense as those where the drug user is bombarded with stimulus (like the nightclub). People report being able to drive a car, conduct conversations and generally conduct themselves without loss of control under its influence (Moore 1992, p.56).

Luckman (2000) contrasts the experience of the raves as outlined by Lenton and Davidson with the ecstasy tripping that takes place in nightclubs, particularly in the big cities of Australia. According to Luckman, the death of Anna Wood resulted in a regulatory framework for clubs that was aimed at providing information to (young) people on the dangers of ecstasy and ways in which to reduce the harms associated with it. This is compared to the relatively ad hoc raves that still take place in usually rural settings around Australia:

> [t]he release of governmental guidelines regulating the conduct of dance parties/raves has brought little joy to those for whom dance music cultures are more a personal cultural (or political) commitment than simply a money making strategy. Put together largely by police authorities, in consultation with various other governmental agencies, community groups and commercial entrepreneurs, the final documents privilege forms of organising dance party entertainment that are only possible where financial capital already exists. However...small scale operations continue, especially in places outside the eyes of the law (of which there can be many in a place as large and thinly populated as Australia). More DIY and counter hegemonically motivated corners of the scene which remain strong and active, particularly in places such as the North Coast of New South Wales [sic]. Since the sixties, this lush and climatically agreeable part of the country has been a haven for counter cultures, and with the tourist mecca of Byron Bay not too far away... While there are some suitable indoor venues, given the generally pleasant year round weather, most events in this region and in the Brisbane hinterland are conducted outdoors.
>
> It is these sites that highlight more than anything else the limits of official regulatory regimes...bush raves are frequently organised in a clandestine

> fashion with ticket holders having to follow telephone, checkpoint or online directions to get to the final – unadvertised – venue or site. A further variable in the Australian scene is the difficulty, and to an extent the pointlessness, of spending significant resources on policing raves and dance parties given the nation's vast open spaces. In the UK and Continental Europe community complaints have commonly been the impetus behind police crackdowns on events. This has also been true of events held in urban Australia, with sometimes violent police closures of free parties in Sydney an example. But in the open and relatively unpopulated spaces of rural Australia this is less of a concern (Luckman 2000, pp.221–222).

Importance of drug, set and setting

Most of the studies of ecstasy use and rave/dance culture examined in this setting have directly or indirectly referred to the importance of drug, set and setting. The following comments that apply specifically to the Scottish focus studies of Shewan, Dalgarno and Reith (2000) could no doubt be applied to all of these across the board:

> The...data indicate participants' awareness of drug, set and setting which can lead to both adverse and positive effects when using ecstasy. The general trend within these data is not only recognition of these factors, but also a pattern of use which was aimed towards minimising harm, while maximising enjoyment. The data...indicate participants' general awareness of the application of drug, set and setting in combination and particularly the benefits of planning and preparing for an ecstasy taking episode on the basis of these three principles (Shewan, Dalgarno & Reith 2000, p.445).[390]

In the context of beliefs about ecstasy use and harm reduction knowledge in the rave scene, Boys, Lenton and Norcross state that :

> Information campaigns targeted at people in the rave and dance party scene appear to have been well received. However, much of the harm reduction material targeting dance drugs has tended to focus on the effects of taking an individual drug in isolation. There seems to be little information about the possible effects of combining drugs, possibly because the research needed to support such information is scarce (1997, p.228).

Harm reduction principles and practices in the context of the culture of use will be discussed further in Chapter 19.

The culture and the local experience

A review of the academic literature on clubbing and its relationship to drug use is a valuable exercise. It can give insight to a somewhat rarefied world that may be relatively unknown to many readers, and indeed writers, of Reports such as this. It also has been an important source of material on international trends

390 See in particular Lewis and Ross 1995 for a detailed discussion of the gay dance party culture and its relationship to drug use.

with regard to the rave scene and the use of amphetamine and 'party drugs'. Nonetheless, no matter how up to date a literature review is it can only tell half the story. It can only give second-hand accounts of the experience of those for whom both clubbing and drug use may be central experiences in their lives. For this reason the Drugs and Crime Prevention Committee and its staff has endeavoured to meet with as many 'players' in the rave and club scene as practicable.

Meeting with the players

The people with whom the Committee met ranged from first aid and harm minimisation officers located at nightclubs, to club owners and 'rave' promoters, police and ambulance officers. Most importantly, the Committee has also sought to speak with 'clubbers' and 'ravers' themselves in order to note their own observations on the culture of the scene and in some instances why drug use may be integral to that culture.

In doing so, the Committee has tried to contextualise the settings of 'party drug' use and comment on the nature of the dance, party and rave scene (including the perceived positive aspects). There were a number of exercises in particular that were helpful in assisting the Committee and its staff to understand the background to the club and rave 'scene'. The first was a forum convened by the Committee attended by club, rave and venue operators, promoters and their staff and volunteers.[391] The knowledge gained from this forum, particularly with regard to harm minimisation practices, was invaluable. Secondly, Committee staff attended a training session held by RaveSafe that aims to give people who operate or work in club and rave venues best practice knowledge with regard to harm reduction measures and associated information to enable them to make their clubs and raves safe and secure environments. Much of the discussion in Chapter 19 concerning harm minimisation draws from these useful meetings. Finally, individual meetings and discussions with Mr Ben Horan, formerly safety and first aid officer with ZoS Nightclub, Ms Natalie Russell, Co-ordinator of RaveSafe and Mr Pip Darvall, Promoter of Earthcore, one of the biggest outdoor 'raves' held in this country, have proved to be of great value in informing many of the themes of this chapter.

Clearly, it is nonsensical to believe that this Committee could fully appreciate the breadth and variety of club and rave culture. For this reason, interviews with the many people involved with the 'scene' have been extremely useful.

'Club culture' and raves are not homogenous entities. There are manifest differences both between the club and the rave experiences and within them. There is also a deal of crossover. The strict boundaries between a 'traditional' rave and a commercial club night are not in all cases as strictly demarcated as they once were.[392] As stated in a Submission from RaveSafe to the Committee:

391 For a list of attendees at this forum see Appendix 4.

392 See discussion earlier in this Chapter.

> ... the culture of 'party drug' users is becoming more difficult to define. Traditionally a 'raver' was someone who attend a rave event, as defined by Nolan and Siokou, but with the increasing popularity of the dance culture, and the crossing over of party drug use into the club environment, many of the issues relating to party drug use are the same for 'ravers,' 'clubbers' or 'partygoers.' Many people who attend smaller club events, or even larger scale 'commercial' dance events do not identify themselves as 'ravers,' but are using the same types of party drugs as the traditional 'raver'. It is important that these users of party drugs in 'club' environments are not missed when we refer to the 'rave culture' or 'ravers'...and perhaps the terminology needs to be changed to partygoers or ravers/clubbers?[393]

Bearing this exhortation in mind, the Committee has drawn from the experiences of those who attend both commercial clubs and those who participated in one 'rave' in country Victoria.

A rider

The Committee wishes to state from the outset that it does not condone the use of any illicit drugs in the venues or festivities attended by the clubbers and ravers. It should be also noted that it has grave concerns about the levels of licit drugs taken in such circumstances, including alcohol.[394] Nonetheless, it would be foolhardy to ignore that for many of the young clubbers the 'vibe' of the club and rave scene, including the use of mind altering substances, is a crucial part of the experience. In all of the Committee's Inquiries, as much as possible, it has tried to include input from those most closely associated with the subject in hand. To understand or acknowledge their experiences is neither to approve nor condemn.

It should be stated at the outset that despite the topic of this Inquiry, the Committee was not interested in any individual or club having, taking, or not taking as the case may be, any licit or illicit drugs. If such information was volunteered by people, and it was, it was treated with complete confidentiality.

The world of 'clubland'

The following information is a composite picture based on the views of a number of young clubbers, promoters, club staff and club owners who regularly

---

393 Submission of RaveSafe to the Drugs and Crime Prevention Committee, Inquiry into Amphetamine and 'Party Drug' Use in Victoria, October 2003.

394 Committee Members and staff have received anecdotal reports about certain Melbourne nightclubs being used for drug distribution or at least facilitation of use. For example, one club is rumoured to supply special mirrors in toilets to allow patrons to cut lines of cocaine, although such occurrences remain speculative. These views, however, were also expressed by a police officer in Queensland with whom the Committee met:

['We saw] specific shelving placed in the cubicles so that they can do their lines of coke or they can do their lines of amphet or whatever. Because where they were doing this on the top of the cistern, these nightclubs had specifically put in glass shelving to facilitate that. So it is obvious what it is about. As part of that process we actually took some swabs, and had them tested. The swabs that we took were so powerful they wrecked the machine' (Queensland Police Officer, in conversation with the Drugs and Crime Prevention Committee, Brisbane, 27 June 2003).

attend Melbourne nightclubs and dance venues. Such clubs ranged from the more ambient and sophisticated atmosphere of Croft Alley to the relatively 'hard core' nature of Hard Kandy.

Gaining entry

One of the key aspects of the whole club experience is passing 'the door entry test':

> The door is one of the few places that clubbers sometimes have to literally prove their identity both in the simple sense of age but also in the more complex sense of passing themselves off as the 'right type of clubber' for that club – proving their 'social identity'. The door becomes a *defining moment*, the moment where you both partially take on and are partially ascribed an identification (Malbon 1999, p.63). (Committee emphasis)

This literal 'rite of passage' became evident during the club explorations of our interviewees. At one club a dress code of 'no black allowed' (except for bouncers) was used in part to distinguish between those who were and were not allowed entry.

For some of the clubbers some clubs seemed to operate more stringent search and entry policies while others seemed relatively 'lax'. Indeed, according to one interviewee at one club it was highly probable that one of the crowd controllers might have consumed some type of psychoactive substance himself. Clearly striking a balance between too little and too much or too rigid security is difficult, as summed up by a British crowd controller:

> It's a balance between not letting people deal and take drugs openly, taking the piss out of the door staff on the one hand. And on the other, to accept that people are here to have a good time, dance and take drugs. And if they weren't here we wouldn't have a job (Measham, Aldridge & Parker 2001, p.167).[395]

For those working in the clubs it is equally difficult to state whether club patrons had consumed their drugs before or during their entry to the clubs. Clearly there was drug taking in each of the clubs visited or staffed by those the Committee spoke to. The fact that lollipops were available at some clubs seems to be a practical acknowledgement that this was indeed the case.[396]

The presence of groups such as RaveSafe with the permission and in some cases encouragement of owners at various clubs is also testament to the tacit awareness

395 The role of crowd controllers with regard to intoxicated patrons of clubs, particularly intoxicated by 'party drugs', is discussed in the harm reduction sections of Chapter 19. Suffice it to state at this point that concerns have been expressed not only about how security staff may handle the 'door', but more importantly how they deal with people who they believe are ostensibly drunk but in fact may be suffering the ill effects of drugs such as GHB. The Committee has met on several occasions with Mr Ben Horan, at the time an employed first aid officer at ZoS nightclub. Indeed Mr Horan was the Committee's guide during its visit to ZoS. His views on the ways in which clubs and club owners could become better 'corporate citizens' with regard to safety and harm reduction measures in nightclubs were invaluable and will be discussed further in Chapter 19.

396 It would be naïve to think that the reason for the latter was not, at least in part, used as an adjunct to prevent or lessen the jaw grinding associated with ecstasy.

(if not acceptance) that drug use takes place in dance and club venues. The role of RaveSafe at clubs and the promotion of harm minimisation measures to reduce the likelihood of dangerous outcomes of taking 'party drugs' are discussed in detail in Chapter 19 of this Report.

The vibe

The concept of the DJ as the 'shaman' performing religious 'mantras' before the congregation as discussed in the literature was, according to clubbers, very much in evidence at Clubs such as 'Hard Kandy'.[397]

> If the DJ is visible, perhaps on a raised stage or platform at the 'front of the dance floor, then the clubbers will be more likely to face him (or less usually, her). If the dance floor is relatively small or the periphery too well lit, then the clubbers will be more inclined to face *into* the dancing crowd in an attempt to avoid eye contact with non-dancers, who it might be assumed with some confidence are not on the same motional and emotional 'wavelength' as the dancers are at that moment. If dancing within a group of friends, the clubbers may be more likely to face other members of that group. If alone, they will be more likely to face the 'front' of the club, perhaps where the main lighting rig or slide projector images are positioned... In any case, any environmental feature – physical or social – which encourages crowd interaction on the dance floor will be more likely to foster an intensive interaction as a result of the ecstatic [environment], with the reverse (withdrawal) being the case in instances where crowd interaction is difficult (Malbon 1999, p.130).

Of interest in terms of interaction, however, is that rarely is it viewed as appropriate for the clubber (or raver) to interact with the 'high priest':

> [i]t was simply out of the question to talk to the DJ, so people tried to attract their attention through their dancing...they would be the ones the conductor heeded most (Ringdal 1991, p.68, quoted in Lewis & Ross 1995 p.147).

The Committee's interviewees observed all these varying forms of interaction during their club visits. This variation of engagement was particularly noticeable in clubs such as Room 680, which had a variety of different dancing rooms.

The DJs of dance clubs are viewed as 'cultural heroes' and the sanctified 'custodians of the dance party tradition' (Lewis & Ross 1995, p.146).[398] According to one clubber with whom the Committee staff spoke, dance venue promoters will target a particular crowd by using particular DJs whose music and track selections the crowd know and can rely upon to be played.

---

397 For a discussion linking the shaman to the modern rave party and the ritualistic use of drugs, see Nencini 2002.

398 Ringdal's study of the dance party phenomenon suggests that the dance party DJ has Weberian qualities of charisma (Ringdal 1991 in Lewis & Ross 1995). Philosopher Max Weber referred to a charismatic person as one set apart from the ordinary, and endowed with exceptional powers and qualities. The role, services and 'rites' of the DJ set him or her apart from the ordinary musician or entertainer.

Malbon also writes of the importance of playing special 'anthemic' musical tracks which '[c]an trigger a very sudden shift across the dance floor from predominantly withdrawal to mostly intensity' (1999, p.130). One of the clubbers testified that indeed this was the case and that some of these anthems had already been played that night.

Technical effects which are important aspects of the presentation at both clubs and raves include lasers, strobe lighting, smoke machines, dry ice and other forms of visual, aural and even olfactory stimuli.[399] Again such effects were in evidence at many of the clubs which the Committee visited. The bigger the club, generally the more extensive the effects.

Of course one needs to be careful to not reduce the idea of clubs and clubbing to one homogenous mass, no matter how much the externals such as technical features may be similar. Clubs are diverse entities catering for different styles and musical tastes. Even within the one club there may be different club nights with different themes, such as students' night, gay and lesbian night, or 'hard core' night. This was certainly true of clubs such as ZoS and Room 680.

Club owners acknowledge that different clubs will deliberately cater to different sub-cultural groups, all of whom may prefer different types of music.

Differences with regard to musical tastes also may determine the popularity of a club or the type of clubber who attends. It may be that the type of music on offer is also associated with the types of drug that are taken or available at particular clubs. This is, at least, the view of one Melbourne based club owner:

> To clarify, my overview of the industry is that the style of music is very heavily determining where the use of illegal substances goes in terms of clubs and even the bigger parties that some of these guys run.
>
> Have a look at the history of music: it is no coincidence that there was a music style in the mid-to-late 1980s by the name of acid house. The music is very closely aligned to the travelling of that recreational drug. So, when you look at the history of dance music – and that is what we are talking about – over a long period of time it has gone through a number of changes. Towards probably the early 1990s on the music started to be of a harder style – a style of music, progressive house, was around, and some other music styles – the path of music went in a tougher direction. Therefore, I think, what happened industry-wide was that the use of recreational drugs became more prevalent. Maybe I am putting the cart before the horse when I say that, because the change in that music style could have been somewhat related to the manufacture of illegal substances – in other words, there is greater availability, the style and

399 Lewis and Ross drawing from the work of Bogoras (1979) claim that shamans in pre-literate societies:

'[u]sed similar stimuli (such as drugs, drums, music, dance, coloured objects and smoke) to facilitate an altered state of consciousness among their initiates. Both the shaman and the dance party organisers recognised the importance of set and setting in creating a consciousness-changing environment' (1995, p.50).

> nature of the drugs change, and it therefore has a very close relationship with the style of music.
>
> What has happened in the past, probably, two or three years – and I talk specifically about clubs – is, I think, that the style of music has somewhat softened and become, perhaps, a bit more cultured and easy to listen to. There seems to be a trend for some venues to follow that style of music because it is more closely related to consumption of beverages. Again, you get back to that financial agenda: you cannot make money if you do not sell any drinks, or it is very difficult to make money if you do not sell any drinks. So I think what has happened in the past few years is that the tougher styles of music, particularly in clubs, has probably softened a little bit, and therefore the abuse of recreational drugs has changed a little bit from the trend perhaps three or four or perhaps five years ago.[400 401]

The place of alcohol

As indicated in the previous quote some clubs have placed a heavier emphasis on the sales of alcohol[402] (or at least their patrons demanded or drink more alcohol) than others. The place of alcohol (or not, as the case may be) at clubs and raves has been discussed previously. However it is interesting that Natalie Russell should state in this regard:

> In the earlier years of ecstasy use in Australia, it was predominately limited to use at 'raves' where little or no alcohol was available. However as ecstasy has permeated the club environment, and is now being used by many people in settings where alcohol is served, many users are consuming both alcohol and ecstasy in these club environments.[403]

---

400 Mr Tom Walker, Seven Nightclub, evidence given to the Drugs and Crime Prevention Committee, Inquiry into Amphetamine and 'Party Drug' Use in Victoria, Public Hearings (Melbourne), November 2003.

401 Members of the Committee staff met with Jim and Angela (not real names), two clubbers and 'ravers', some days after the Earthcore festival had taken place (see below). They agreed that the type of music very much was matched to the type of drug in favour. For example, musical styles such as 'psy trance' and 'acid trance' are most often associated with MDMA and hallucinogens such as LSD. At clubs such as 'Hard Kandy' where the music tends to be hard core 'Ice, Coke and Speed is needed for energy' (Jim and Angela in conversation with the Drugs and Crime Prevention Committee staff, 8 December 2003).

402 Measham, Aldridge and Parker in the British context state that there is some evidence that some club owners fearing the loss of alcohol sales in dance clubs deliberately 'shifted their music policy to more mellow sounds such as house and garage'. They continue:

'These sub-genres of dance music were perceived to attract more stylish and sophisticated customers than hardcore customers who it was hoped would take fewer drugs, drink more alcohol, boost profit margins and reduce drug and gang related trouble in clubs. The change in music policy was an attempt to change the class base of customers and to draw back the drinking, paying employed and up-market crowd. In these instances, club policy was used directly to determine, attract or deter specific customer profiles' (2001, p.50).

403 Ms Natalie Russell, Co-ordinator of RaveSafe, cited in a Submission of RaveSafe to the Drugs and Crime Prevention Committee, Inquiry into Amphetamine and 'Party Drug' Use in Victoria, October 2003.

Conversely, Ms Russell states:

'with the increase in popularity of ecstasy and its current status as a 'mainstream' drug, users are taking the drug not only in dance environments, but at home, parties and even the pub. At all these locations alcohol is quite common; but most importantly ecstasy is being viewed as a common substance to take on a night out, not just for attending a dance event.'

In Measham's wide-ranging study of British dance clubbers in the late 1990s, alcohol was one of the primary drugs of choice of the sample. According to Measham this reflected the change in the British (and arguably Australian) dance and club scene and leisure patterns generally:

> Distinctions between pubs and bars, nightclubs and dance clubs, 'raves' and festivals are all blurring, even disintegrating and reformulating... Essentially dance clubs and night clubs are part of a broader leisure industry which not only hosts illegal drug use but provides the key features for the ideal night out. 'Time out' is about meeting with friends and going out to 'town' – drinking, socializing, listening to music, dancing, meeting new people and partners – and only perhaps taking illegal drugs (Measham, Aldridge & Parker 2001, p.4).

The clubs that 'rely' upon alcohol tend to be less about hard core raving than socialising with members of the other sex. For the younger male clubbers attending these clubs, the night is at least in part about 'picking up'. As this Report has previously mentioned, research has suggested that many women in particular have indicated that in terms of having a good time, '"drug" clubs are nicer places to be than "alcohol" clubs because of the good atmosphere and the lack of aggression' (Measham, Aldridge & Parker 2001, p.60). This was certainly the view of many of the women the Committee met with.[404]

Club nights such as 'Hard Kandy' are, according to their attendees, more closely aligned to a 'rave'. Alcohol is little in emphasis. Water is freely purchasable and lollipops are also readily available.

Communality and exstasis

The music, the dance and the vibe was everything to this crowd. People were turned to the DJ mounted on his 'altar'. Clubbers danced as a group, danced with friends or danced alone. Particularly striking was the fact that young men would dance alone or even more unusually with other young men. Yet this was not a gay venue and it is doubtful that these men were or considered themselves to be homosexual.[405]

---

404 Mr Paul Todd of the Sugar Suite club in Lonsdale Street, Melbourne, told the Committee that: 'The 'kids' in the district were simply not drinking alcohol, preferring to take 'party drugs' in conjunction with the dancing and clubbing'.

Yet it is alcohol that, at least in the past, makes money for the clubs. Mr Todd, stated that it was difficult to strike a balance of providing a club that was safe, friendly *and* profitable. He believed that that the only alternatives are to charge high prices for water or steep door entry charges to cover expensive DJs and mandatory security staff. But even then the average of two bottles of water over a whole nights clubbing could not compare with a whole night of alcohol consumption as may have occurred ten years ago. It was an unfortunate 'Catch 22' situation. The culture of 'high traffic, high volume, more "beer" and consequent profits was well and truly over, at least for smaller clubs' (Mr Paul Todd, Sugar Suite owner, in conversation with the Drugs and Crime Prevention Committee, Melbourne, 15 November 2003).

405 This seems to be an international trend. Ter Bogt's study of Dutch clubbers notes that 'although in the past boys were less inclined to dance than girls, house [music] [often in combination with drugs] succeed[ed] in drawing boys massively to the dance floor' (Ter Bogt et al. 2002, p.171).

A clear sense of empathy, of a shared ethos is said to exist between the clubbers. Non-verbal communication on the dance floor is said to be much in evidence. The experience of two British clubbers in Malbon's study 'We both grin because we don't NEED to say anything' (1999, p.131) is, according to the young people with whom the Committee spoke, apparent also at the Melbourne clubs such as 'Hard Kandy'.[406]

This type of feeling, this empathy and *exstasis* (see Malbon 1999[407]) does not necessarily need a chemical impetus. Many of the clubbers with whom Committee members spoke would agree with Malbon's comment that, '[i]t certainly appears feasible to experience music in a heightened form and as inducing an oceanic [ecstatic] experience through dancing *without* the use of drugs at all' (1999, p.133). (Author's emphasis)

According to some clubbbers, the atmosphere of clubs such as Hard Kandy could to a lesser degree be equated to that in evidence at outdoor raves such as Earthcore – the 'Rumble in the Jungle'.[408]

'Rumble in the jungle' – The outdoor 'rave'[409]

> *2 a.m. – main dance floor, chaos…*
>
> The music dominated the dance floor. Everyone was dancing – on the balcony, on the little stages that projected out onto the dance floor like catwalks (look at me, 'cos I'm looking at you!), in the bar, behind the bar, *on* the bar. I really enjoyed dancing. I felt myself slipping in and out of submission to the music. No sooner had I forgotten what I was doing, and my dancing had become almost automatic, than I was suddenly aware of myself again, conscious of moving my feet, looking at what my arms were doing. I looked at people dancing and noticed how overtly they were looking at everyone else. I don't just mean glancing either. I mean really *looking* at someone, as though that was completely normal. I could feel myself being scanned, but wasn't affronted or anything by this. We all seemed to want the music to take us over; to *become us* in some way. Okay, we each stamped our individuality on it in our own way – a neat little step here, an arm movement there – but [we] were essentially doing the same thing as each other and in the same place and at the same

406 It could also be remarked that quite apart from any feelings of empathy, the extremely high noise levels at the clubs militated against any meaningful verbal communication.

407 Malbon explains 'exstasis' as reflecting: 'The notion of the crowd as in some way superseding the individual, as enabling the widespread experience of loss of self among those within it and of it' (Malbon 1999, p.71).

408 This was the promotional name given to Earthcore 2003.

409 While Earthcore is certainly representative of one of the larger organised raves, according to Earthcore's chief organiser and promoter, Pip Darvall, there are many other types of rave taking place in Victoria each weekend:

'…[t]here's basically an outdoor event every weekend somewhere in Victoria of dance party style… It ranges from 200 people to upwards. Most of the smaller events, up to 800 to 1,000 people at the most and they tend to just "find a good spot". A good spot is picturesque and within an hour, an hour and a half of Melbourne, not too near to people that are going to be impacted with noise and attract attention, and they just bring a sound system and a generator and go for it. It's very rudimentary' (Mr Pip Darvall in conversation with the Drugs and Crime Prevention Committee, 12 December 2003).

> time. Certain tracks that were clearly club favourites were greeted rapturously by the [dancers], and I found it easy to become enthused. The atmosphere was contagious... Sweat becomes something to be proud of rather than a social stigma (Malbon 1999, p.xii).

The setting

Earthcore is a three-day open air 'rave' held each year. In 2003 it was located near Shepparton in rural northern Victoria. Earthcore, among other things, is a music and dance festival playing a variety of musical styles including trance, electro-ambient, house and tribal. In 2003 the occasion was particularly special, as it was the eagerly awaited tenth anniversary of the event. A number of local and overseas DJs and mixers were employed on a number of sound stages. The participants camped on extensive grounds by the Goulburn River.

The logistics of Earthcore are staggering. The Committee met with the chief promoter and organiser of Earthcore, Mr Pip Darvall, two weeks after the event. Mr Darvall's views and thoughts on the festival have been incorporated into much of this section.

There were no 'pass outs' and security staff enforced a strict no importation of alcohol into the grounds policy. Alcohol was available at a specially designated marquee, but drinkers had to consume it strictly within the parameters of that designated space. Nor were there, according to Mr Darvall or 'ravers' with whom the Committee subsequently met, any unpleasant or violent incidents related to alcohol over the three days. This accords with much of the literature on raves, particularly outdoor raves of this nature. Alcohol, according to promoter Pip Darvall, is simply 'not an issue'.

> Alcohol in general isn't an issue. That's my personal belief. If people are going to drink, which at previous events people have been allowed to bring in their own alcohol and people wander around with a stubby or sit in the camp and have a few drinks. Alcohol is not really a big deal, its more like you see it in the afternoons, people sitting around in the camps and so on and wandering around, its more like they're going to a Barbie or they're going camping and having a few drinks, its not really a big issue. This time, as you mentioned, we couldn't have alcohol within the public area of the event, it could only be in the licensed area and so we had the boot search at night when people came in. We got a large proportion of the alcohol, some people obviously snuck some in and there was still a few people wandering around, having a drink but not as much as normal because that was the climate but then I guess that would have been balanced off by in the bar, we had a small bar, they were drinking there instead so the same amount of alcohol was probably consumed but just a little bit more concentrated in one area. We don't have fights; we don't have drunken loutish behavior...[410]

410 Mr Pip Darvall, in conversation with the Drugs and Crime Prevention Committee, 12 December 2003.

First Aid and Ambulance Officers were always on hand as were members of RaveSafe (see Chapter 19). It would seem that most of the medical problems associated with the festival were similar to those struck in the commercial clubs, the main 'culprit' being GHB and surprisingly, given its relative rarity in Victoria, the hallucinogen LSD.[411]

The day

Earthcore to some observers gives the appearance of being a mixture of carnivale, dance party, music festival, 'agricultural show' and 'love in'. There are also a diversity of stalls and booths on site. These range from vegetarian cafes, coffee stalls where the coffee beans were hand ground by the purchaser pedalling a bicycle, stalls set up by Greenpeace and the UNHCR, to 'shops' selling colourful and exotic clothing, glow sticks and other 'raving' paraphernalia. There was apparently even a barbeque stall run by the local footy club members who, according to Mr Darvall, were getting into the 'exotic' atmosphere 'big time'.[412]

According to two young people in attendance with whom the Committee later met, during the daylight hours, although there is always music being played, some 'punters' took the opportunity to relax, 'recharge the batteries' in preparation for the night's dancing or swim in the river. 'Street' performers, jugglers, and other artists employed by the promoters freely roamed the campsites. Workshops were held in everything from yoga to reiki. Such services were not just about enjoyment but served an important harm reduction purpose:

> [w]e pay a lot of people as well to provide roving entertainment. One of the things from a management and harm minimisation perspective is that the devil makes work for idle hands to do and you can't have people there for a long period of time which we do, some people might be there for 48 to 72 hours, you need a lot of staff to keep people entertained. A lot of that is provided by the environment, they can just go to the river or have a snooze under a tree but you need a lot of staff to keep it going.[413]

The night and the vibe

For all the fair-like atmosphere these 'sideshows', while enjoyable, are very much secondary to the main attraction. According to the 'ravers', it is when the sun sets that the real fun and the raison d'etre of the festival begins – the dancing, the rave.

Men, women and (in some cases) children danced to the pulsating rhythms. They danced alone and together, their bodies and eyes fixated for the most part on the DJ. And yet this was apparently not the climax of the night. The

411 Recognising the reality of drug use at raves, if not condoning it, and therefore the need for a safety and harm reduction message, Mr Darvall has published warnings on the Earthcore web site alerting ravers and participants to the dangers associated with taking GHB. For further discussion of harm reduction measures in the context of Earthcore, see Chapter 19.

412 Mr Pip Darvall, in conversation with the Drugs and Crime Prevention Committee, 12 December 2003.

413 Ibid.

Committee representatives were informed by Natalie Russell that traditionally the period of peak activity for ravers was the coming of the dawn. Sunrise sees an almost frenzied release of energy, as the collectivity perceives that the end of the rite is not far away.[414]

Many of the observations about the role of the DJ as priest, shaman or guru were being realised on this hot dusty night. The atmosphere created at Earthcore, according to those in attendance, very much paralleled the ecstasies, altered states or trance-like states of being described in the academic literature. Malbon summarises these feelings well. His descriptions could easily be extrapolated to those rapt participants surrounding the sound stages at Earthcore:

> These experiences [are] characterised by one or more of these sensations: ecstasy, joy, euphoria, ephemerality, empathy, alterity (a sense of being beyond the everyday), release, the loss and subsequent gaining of control, and notions of escape. In her work on altered states Marghanita Laski describes... [what she calls an ecstatic experience] 'as being one in which all sense of self and time and the everyday world seem to vanish...a state of anxiety is replaced by mental tranquillity'. Pleasurable fluctuations between awareness of self and environment, between sensations of intensity and withdrawal, and between practices of interaction and reflection are foregrounded (Malbon 1999, p.107).

Safety and security

Certainly promoters, staff and 'punters' associated with Earthcore have been impressed by the relatively low-key approach taken by law enforcement officers at the venue. Safety and security at the event was a threefold responsibility of Earthcore staff, paid private security officers especially trained in non-confrontational security measures and volunteer organisations such as the Pt'chang non-violence patrols. Members of Victoria Police did occasional patrols of the site. Yet the overall impression is apparently one of good natured and harmonious co-operation between all parties. This view was confirmed when Committee staff met with Mr Pip Darvall a fortnight later:

> [o]ne of the really positive things about the whole dance music thing and I guess from the angle that we're involved in is that so many girls come because traditionally that wasn't the case and if they come and they feel safe, well fantastic. Especially to feel safe wondering around the bush, a lot of people think "gee, no one got raped". The police were amazed, it's much more of a community feel and people feel safe and that's terrific.[415]
>
> I think that here in Victoria we've got a far better approach than in NSW. Just

414 Committee staff met with Jim and Angela, two young 'ravers' who attended Earthcore 2003, a few days after the event had taken place. They confirmed that the sunrise period is where the ravers feel most 'at one.' At the break of dawn special 'sunrise anthems' are played and:

'Everyone feels the same thing at the same time, you are a ball of energy, it is a collective consciousness, almost a sun worship thing' (Jim and Angela in conversation with the staff of the Drugs and Crime Prevention Committee, 8 December 2003).

415 Mr Pip Darvall, in conversation with the Drugs and Crime Prevention Committee, 12 December 2003.

> through my contacts with events also in NSW, the police here are far more proactive; they're very happy to actually talk about things and come to the events and discuss issues that might arise. I've been impressed to be honest, at the support that we have received from the police, I guess because they see we try to do our best to try to make it a safe environment and we don't really cause them any problems but in NSW it's a very different story. The police seem to have a very combative kind of attitude and have closed down parties in the past which have caused deaths. They don't seem to have a particularly good attitude to it at all.[416]

The attitude of the police was summed up by the words of one young raver with whom the Committee staff later spoke: 'The police take a relaxed approach. They will only step in if there is blatantly obvious drug use'.[417]

Only those in the know...

One aspect of raves such as Earthcore and raving itself that continually is commented upon in the literature is the idea that if you are not part of the rave crowd, if you do not take the drugs or subscribe to the culture, you simply 'don't understand'. What ravers (and clubbers) experience 'is beyond description or translation unless you were there' (Malbon 1999, p.173). The outside world, the 'straight' world does not exist for those caught up in the 'vibe' until such time as they pack up their cars and return to the work-a-day world in Melbourne, Adelaide or Sydney.

According to the respondents, those ravers in attendance at Earthcore were all overwhelmingly friendly (whether such amity was chemically induced or not).

They were totally immersed in the colours, the music, the smells and sounds of the bush, the high-octane energy – indeed to them the 'vibe' was infectious. Communality as described earlier in the Chapter was everywhere in evidence.

Raving diversity

Just as not all dance clubs are the same so too not all 'raves' will share the same ethos. For example, some raves and ravers may have a focus that is very much in tune with environmental preservation and 'green' politics, others may not. One example of the 'green' type of rave is those held and promoted by the group Transplant.

Transplant is a volunteer organisation that delights in providing and participating in music raves after having helped revegetate the bush. The Committee met with a representative of Transplant in November 2003. He described his organisation as follows:

> I belong to a group called Transplant. Transplant organises outdoor revegetation projects in rural areas around Victoria. As a celebration at the end of a planting we hold a dance party. We have been going now for about four

416 Ibid.

417 John (pseudonym) in conversation with staff of the Drugs and Crime Prevention Committee.

> years and have planted close to 150 000 trees in various areas. We work with Parks Victoria, DNRE and Landcare in different areas. We are an incorporated not-for-profit organisation. We generally operate during the planting season, which is winter and spring. In summer we do weeding at the You Yangs, for which we receive funding from Parks Victoria.
>
> We generally do what we do because we believe very much in the revegetation of our country, and we also believe that we connect urban and rural people together. We take the ravers out from the city and connect them with rural people. We demystify what I think rural people think of us and what we think of rural people, and we provide a safe environment for artists, both performers and musicians, to perform. We are not big by any stretch of the imagination. There are only 60 or so members, and probably maybe 15 to 20 of those are active. That is pretty much what we do. I am not a clubber. I do not go out in the city, so I can only speak from my perspective of the outdoor dance party scene. That is the only position I will be able to talk from today, not from a clubbing perspective whatsoever.[418]

Some raves may be 'New Age', others may be purely about the music. Some organised raves or club nights may have a parallel aim of fostering community development, particularly in the context of youth work One such outfit is SMILE Police Productions (SPP). The Committee met with the promoter of SPP in November 2003. He explained the role of his organisation as follows:

> SMILE is an acronym that means save many individuals, let's educate and police it. I put on indoor warehouse dance parties, as opposed to clubs, where we hire out, say, a sports complex for basically the one night. We generally do about two or three events like that a year. The people we would target are aged between 18 and 22. We hold all major events as well, and we generally have a 17-plus age bracket.
>
> The type of kids that we attract are generally kids that are unemployed, kids that are on the streets, kids that are at universities and just any kids or people who are low-income earners and who have just got their first year of work or anything like that. We get as many kids involved in that as possible by getting them to create décor and helping out with the actual event itself so they can be more proactive and not just loitering around the streets but actually out there, doing something constructive. Our parties range from about 2000 to 5000-people events.[419]

Other raves such as 'Earthcore' may have aspects of all these approaches.

---

418 Mr Tim Harvey, Transplant, evidence given to the Drugs and Crime Prevention Committee, Inquiry into Amphetamine and 'Party Drug' Use in Victoria, Public Hearings (Melbourne), 10 November 2003.

Of interest is that Mr. Harvey reinforces the idea that while some people may share a love for and participation in both club culture and attending more traditional 'outdoor' raves, this is by no means always the case. In some ways, these groups are very much separate 'tribes'.

419 Mr Garth Lategan, SMILE Police Productions, evidence given to the Drugs and Crime Prevention Committee, Inquiry into Amphetamine and 'Party Drug' Use in Victoria, Public Hearings (Melbourne), 10 November 2003.

Conclusion

Raves, clubs and 'party drugs' are inextricably linked. Yet drugs are not the only part of the story or by any means the most predominant. To repeat Lenton's comment, raves are not 'drug supermarkets'. There are many positives to these venues, their energy, their colour and their life. Those who attend them revel in a sense of belonging, community and unity. The task for the policy-maker is to encourage the positive aspects of this energy without condoning the drug use associated with it. Equally they must devise realistic policies and programmes that reduce the dangers and harms associated with 'party drug' use.

The profile of the clubbers and ravers in this chapter is for the most part a profile of urban people in metropolitan contexts, notwithstanding the rural locations of raves. The problems and needs of people in country Victoria have been very much neglected. This Report seeks to at least in part redress the balance. The final chapter in this Part shifts from a focus on the city to a specific examination of amphetamine and to a lesser extent 'party drug' use in rural and regional areas of Victoria.

11. An Overlooked Problem: Amphetamine and 'Party Drug' Use in Rural and Regional Victoria

Introduction

Throughout the course of the Inquiry the Committee has become aware of the relative paucity of research and lack of attention given to drug and alcohol use and misuse in rural and regional Victoria, and specifically the use of amphetamine and 'party-drug' type substances. The Committee's *Discussion Paper* (2003) called for more information about the prevalence and concomitant cultures of amphetamine and 'party drug' use within discrete sections of the wider community, including rural and regional communities and Indigenous Victorians. The Committee also distributed a set of questions specific to rural and regional contexts with a view to eliciting focussed comment on experiences and issues peculiar to each region, town centre or organisation. There was not a strong response to this initiative, however the perspectives, research directives, opinions and evidence that *were* received from representatives, organisations, Shire and City Councils and members of various communities contacted outside the bounds of metropolitan Melbourne have been invaluable in the pursuit of greater understanding.[420] Of particular value were Public Hearings held in the regional centres of Benalla and Moe. A meeting with representatives from the Australian Rural Centre for Addictive Behaviours (ARCAB) in Warrnambool was also extremely enlightening.[421]

There are many studies, research reports and prevalence data that focus on general (state or national) or urban/metropolitan use of illicit and licit drugs. However, there is very little data that gives specific information on drug use patterns and prevalence within rural and regional Victoria.

---

420 For a list of community agencies that responded to this request see Appendix 9.

421 The Committee is grateful for the input of Ms Jeanette Powell MP (Shepparton) in forwarding the Committee relevant articles and submissions relating to amphetamine and 'party drugs' in the regional centre of Shepparton and surrounding districts.

Given that in 1996 just under 30 per cent of all Australians, or around 5.3 million people lived in non-metropolitan areas,[422] the deficit in concerted attention to illicit drug use and misuse among rural and regional populations is regrettable. Clearly the demographics of these rural and regional populations are different from those of the cities. It follows that the factors bearing on illicit drug use and communities' capacity to respond to this problem are also nuanced and often different from those encountered in metropolitan contexts. It should be stated from the outset that in both Melbourne and rural and regional areas of the state the drugs of most concern according to numerous indicia (economic, health and social costs) are the licit substances of alcohol and tobacco. This is testified to by a number of respondents to this Inquiry, as is outlined later in this chapter.

The terms 'metropolitan', 'rural' and 'regional' are used as much as possible throughout this chapter in accordance with the Rural, Remote and Metropolitan Area (RRMA) classification system.[423] 'Metropolitan' and 'urban' here refer to capitals and other large cities, and 'regional' to rural and remote towns and cities.

The Committee has appreciated particularly the input of Dr Rodger Brough and Ms Suzan Morey of ARCAB in establishing initial contacts and basic data collection.[424] Notably, Dr Rodger Brough problematised any claim to a serious 'rural perspective' and articulated perhaps the most critical point to emerge from this facet of the Inquiry:

> Rural people are best placed to gather, collate and interpret data from rural communities. Why? Because, when urban researchers have controlled the conduct of rural research – as well as the research agenda – the outcomes are predictable. Either data from all rural communities are lumped together, or one or two communities are studied only. Either way, by reducing or eliminating the community contextual information the data are rendered virtually meaningless. Little wonder that real progress on the development of solutions to rural problems and issues has been painfully slow. The consequences of this situation

---

422 *Rural, Regional and Remote Australians: An Overview of the People, their Health and Health Services*, National Rural Health Alliance (NRHA) and Department of Health and Ageing, March 1999, p.28.

423 **Metropolitan Areas**
- Capital city
- Other metropolitan centre (population of 100,000 or more)

Non-metropolitan Zones
- Rural Zone
  Large rural centre (population 25,000–99,999)
  Small rural centre (population 10,000–24,999)
  Other rural area (population less than 10,000)
- Remote Zone
  Remote centre (population of 5,000 or more)
  Other remote area (population less than 5,000)

(Department of Human Services and Health, *Rural, Remote and Metropolitan Areas Classification*, Australian Government Publishing Service, Canberra, November 1993, p.6).

424 ARCAB is an initiative of the Western Region Alcohol and Drug (WRAD) Centre with seed funding from the Department of Human Services.

> are that when major drug-related reports are undertaken, one of two outcomes occurs in respect to rural issues: they are either ignored, or a very brief sub-section is included which parrots off the well known list of general 'rural issues'... The problem with reporting 'metropolitan' vs 'rural' perspectives on issues is that it fails to appreciate the diversity of rural communities and the relative prevalence of particular alcohol or other drug problems that are unique to a particular community. Data needs to be disaggregated and reported on a Local Government Area basis to be meaningful and relevant to real people's (ie. real rural people's) circumstances.[425]

This point was echoed by numerous other members of rural communities throughout Victoria. In acknowledging such an issue as problematic from the outset, the Committee's hopes are twofold. First, that the issues and perspectives canvassed in this chapter will be taken to represent a starting point in recognising the complexities and heterogeneity of the regions that comprise 'rural and regional Victoria', and secondly, that recommendations and concerns with regard to substance use and misuse and service systems will be recognised and acted upon.

The diversity of the regions

There is a tendency to view rurality as monolithic, but the reality is very different. Inevitably, attributes of rurality and remoteness will vary in their importance with different policy issues (Department of Human Services and Health 1994, p.6). As regards illicit drug use, the distinctive characteristics of each region and rural centre must be accounted for in order to attain an accurate picture of prevalence and patterns of usage, as well as the obstacles and best means of service provision. In light of this, ARCAB has established itself as a forerunner in community-based innovative and collaborative research, training and advocacy projects. Its submission to the Committee highlights the need to recognise the heterogeneity that distinguishes towns, cities and regions throughout Victoria as well as the common and congruent factors that allow similarity. It states:

> Rural communities are not homogeneous and are not readily classifiable into groups for comparability... It is impossible to capture the essence of the impact of social issues (like addictive behaviours) in richly diverse rural communities by sampling just a handful of rural communities.[426]

Indeed, cumulated project experience has:

> ...reinforced the importance and value of collecting data from a number of rural communities to be able to comprehensively and effectively understand the impact of social issues in rural communities.[427]

425 Submission of the Australian Rural Centre for Addictive Behaviours (ARCAB) to the Drugs and Crime Prevention Committee, Inquiry into Amphetamine and 'Party Drug' Use in Victoria, 7 November 2003.

426 Ibid.

427 Ibid.

Similarly, a Turning Point Discussion Paper reflects the obvious point that factors like 'the industry base and demographic of local areas, as well as supply options…can influence drug use patterns' (Turning Point Alcohol and Drug Centre, 2003, p.6).[428] And further, that 'the strongest message heard from people in rural and regional Victoria was that the nature of the drug problem varies *within regions* and between rural and urban areas' (Turning Point Alcohol and Drug Centre, 2003, p.6). This was testified to by Dr Brough when he spoke with the Committee:

> The other thing that I think is not always appreciated is that rural Victoria is not a homogenous culture and group of people. There are different issues, cultures and mixes of population groups. There are different drug problems in different areas. The epidemiology differs from one part of Victoria to another. There are a number of factors. So when we read reports of metropolitan data and reports of rural data, they do not make a lot of sense and they do not really give you a lot of information about what is going on in rural Victoria because all the results are aggregated. There needs to be some way of disaggregating data to make it relevant and appropriate to particular areas. It is only in the last year or two that we are starting to see some reports coming out that are doing that – giving some rural data based on local government areas and that sort of thing, so it starts to become meaningful and relevant to local communities. There was a report put out by Turning Point about alcohol consumption in Victoria. That was a really good study that started to highlight the differences not only between metropolitan and rural areas, but also between different rural areas. That was an extremely useful report for a whole lot of reasons, not the least of which was that it highlighted the issue of needing to get locally relevant data into the report material…[in short]…we need some sort of a reasonable study of issues in rural and regional areas that start to pick up some of the finer issues that relate to the different cultures, the different prevalence of different drug problems in different areas, the particular reason why certain models of service delivery may not be appropriate in one area but are relevant in another area. You cannot look in rural areas at putting the same service model into exactly the same situation. You need to modify it to local conditions and the local skills of the local people in the area. There are a whole lot of things that you need to take into account. We really think that some sort of study specifically looking at rural and regional areas is overdue and very much needed.[429]

A comment from the manager of Latrobe Community Health's alcohol and drug service[430] highlights one aspect of such regional diversity and signals the imperative to understand each community in its particular context:

---

428 The Turning Point Alcohol and Drug Centre Discussion Paper is based on Service System Review workshops held throughout rural Victoria in 2003.

429 Dr Rodger Brough, ARCAB, in conversation with the Drugs and Crime Prevention Committee, Inquiry into Amphetamine and 'Party Drug' Use in Victoria, Melbourne, 6 October 2003.

430 Latrobe Community Health Service provides for the entire Latrobe region and is the largest regional community health service in the state.

> Wellington has Fulham Prison up there, so it has its own specific problems of visitors coming up and using all sorts of things... Each of the areas have different problems. Even each town can have different use patterns and different drugs.[431]

Representatives from Latrobe Valley Indigenous communities also testify to the need to recognise heterogeneity in both mainstream and Indigenous communities:

> There is a difference between urban and rural communities. Even though it is rural here, there is a difference between the Warragul community and Drouin community and Morwell community as well. I live near Echuca, in Shepparton. They are 40 minutes apart and I live on a little mission between those two called Cummeragunja. Within 45 minutes there are five different communities and those communities are entirely different.[432]

Such comments accord with some research literature that criticises the undervaluing of diverse factors that may contribute to problematic (and non-problematic) drug use in general populations. Such omissions are even more noticeable in the (relatively few) research writings on drug use in rural communities. Factors that may be noticeably omitted in addition to rurality per se may include ethnicity, social class, age and – particularly importantly – gender. Moore, for example argues:

> The authors of research reports appear to collapse even the broadest cultural categories and deny the phenomenological importance of perceived cultural differences, despite the varying cultural and social backgrounds of multicultural Australia. Underlying this tendency is the assumption of (or desire for) homogeneity in large populations. Even in the Aboriginal area where cultural and social differences are most obvious, it has only been relatively recently that public health teams...have consciously incorporated these cultural and social differences into health promotion campaigns and programmes for the prevention of drug problems (Moore 1990, p.335).

Moore argues further that Australian drug research paradigms are almost exclusively of the prevalence/epidemiological variety, assuming homogeneity or at least ignoring diversity. This is particularly true of research into drug use in rural and regional Australia.

---

431 Mr Ron Marshall, Latrobe Community Health Services, evidence given to the Drugs and Crime Prevention Committee, Inquiry into Amphetamine and 'Party Drug' Use in Victoria, Public Hearings (Moe), 23 October 2003.

432 Mr Rick Henderson, Acting Executive Officer, Central Gippsland Aboriginal Co-operative, evidence given to the Drugs and Crime Prevention Committee, Inquiry into Amphetamine and 'Party Drug' Use in Victoria, Public Hearings (Moe), 23 October 2003.

The prevalence of amphetamine use and the extent of the problem

While there is widespread acknowledgment of the special and heightened macro-environmental risk factors bearing on communities in rural and regional settings,[433] the need for more extensive, comprehensive and disaggregated data and research remains. More particularly, the dearth of relevant and accurate literature addressing the increase in illicit substance abuse in rural contexts should be rectified.

At a national level, research conducted by Paul Williams, Australian Institute of Criminology, has shown that between 1988 and 1998 the use of illicit drugs increased in regional Australia by 77 per cent for heroin, 131 per cent for amphetamines, 37 per cent for cocaine, and 47 per cent for cannabis (Willams 2001). Similarly, an Australian National Council on Drugs (ANCD) report shows the use of amphetamine and amphetamine-type substances is increasing in rural and regional areas (ANCD 2001). While such exponential increase in amphetamine use clearly warrants concern, amphetamine use must be examined in a context of both wider drug use patterns and as subject to community and regionally specific circumstances.[434] It would appear, for example, that 'party drugs' such as MDMA (ecstasy), ketamine and GBH are far less prevalent and subject to both use and abuse than methamphetamine in rural areas. This is confirmed by representatives of rural and regional communities with whom the Committee has met.[435] One possible reason for this varying pattern of drug use is that young people in country areas have far less access to the types of clubs and venues in which such drug use traditionally takes place.[436] The importance of the cultural context in which drug use occurs is developed further later in this chapter.

Paul Williams' study has utility in providing some initial general comments and contexts, although these are again reflective of a national, aggregated whole rather

---

433 For example, see National Drug and Alcohol Research Centre, 'Structural determinants of youth drug use', by Catherine Spooner, W. Hall and M. Lynskey, *ANCD Research Paper*, UNSW, 2001 p.20.

434 Such data is of course nationally based and does not give particularly detailed or rich insights into rural drug use in specific Victorian regions.

435 See for example the transcripts of evidence of rural and regional witnesses as listed in Appendix 9.

Mr Frank Coughlan of the Latrobe Valley Community Health Service believes the age of 'initiation' for younger drug users is generally lower in rural regions, particularly with regard to alcohol and cannabis. It is not unheard of for children aged 14 to be partaking of these drugs at least once or twice a week. Mr Frank Coughlan, evidence given to the Drugs and Crime Prevention Committee, Inquiry into Amphetamine and 'Party Drug' Use in Victoria, Public Hearings (Moe), 23 October 2003.

436 Indeed, although such a view is conjecture, it could be plausibly argued that the small number of young people from rural communities who *do* take 'party drugs' would travel to clubs and venues in Melbourne to do so. Other possible locales and contexts of such drug use may be at open-air raves such as 'Earthcore'. While such events take place in rural settings they are not 'organically' rural, most often being organised in and from cities such as Melbourne and with many if not most of their attendees travelling from the city and metropolitan regions to experience the event.

than addressing the circumstances of individual states or regions. However, Williams' research shows that compared to metropolitan areas there are proportionally fewer people using illicit drugs in regional Australia (Williams 2001), and that rates of 'recent use' (defined as within the previous 12 months) among respondents were generally lower in regional areas.[437] Between 1988–1998, amphetamine use increased at an average annual rate of 9.5 per cent in metropolitan Australia versus an average annual rate of 8.75 per cent in regional settings (Williams 2001). While levels of use are lower than those recorded in metropolitan areas, illicit drug use in regional Australia approximates rates observed in the cities 'just a few years ago' (Graycar quoted in Williams 2001, p.1), with accelerating rates for some substances including amphetamine and amphetamine-type substances. Summarising the results of his study, Williams predicts:

> The growing pool of regular users in regional Australia might...soon result in a critical mass and scale to support a more reliable illicit drugs market from both supply and demand perspectives than that which presently prevails. This will impact on all of the factors sufficient to encourage younger ages of initiation, higher rates of retention of users and, hence, even higher rates of growth in the use of illicit drugs (Williams 2001, p.5).

And further, that:

> There is no evidence that regional Australia's bush spirit, often promulgated as a virtue of small town, rural and remote living, is a sufficient defence against the attraction of drug experimentation by its youth. Regrettably, and despite the evidence that the vast majority will cease use without intervention, for some regional youth their use will become habitual and problematic (Williams 2001, p.5).

A hierarchy of drugs?

Evidence presented to the Committee invoked what could be termed a 'hierarchy of drug use' that seemed to apply generally to most rural and regional centres. This 'hierarchy' has problematic alcohol use as having the most widespread and adverse impact, with alcohol being the primary drug of concern of most clients presenting to health services. Even a cursory overview of the little literature pertaining to drug use in rural and regional settings reveals that, as the ANCD reported, 'without question, alcohol remains the substance of most concern' (2001, p.2). Indeed, based on the views of alcohol and drug service providers working in Victoria, Turning Point Alcohol and Drug Centre notes that:

> Alcohol, tobacco and cannabis consumption are often seen as part and parcel of the rural existence, even stereotyped in a cultural sense as marking part of the 'rural character' (Turning Point Alcohol and Drug Centre 2003, p.5).

437 The exception to this, Williams notes, are rates of recent usage of heroin, painkillers and tranquillisers within the period of study between 1988–1998, where rates grew faster in regional Australia than in metropolitan areas.

Evidence heard by the Committee accords with this analytical 'hierarchy of drug use'. For example, Mr Ron Marshall, Manager of the alcohol and drug service in the Latrobe region, confirmed amphetamine-type substance abuse was an issue among the client population but qualified his statement, emphasising that:

> [O]ur most common problem is alcohol. It washes away everything in its wake. For illicit substances, it is cannabis. For younger people, that is where they first go, of course – to alcohol. Then some will use amphetamines, but that is very small.[438]

Mr Frank Coughlan, whose primary work as an outreach clinician in the same region entails a case load of approximately 150 clients per year, ranked alcohol and cannabis as the two major drugs of concern, with some minimal heroin use. He explained:

> Three per cent or four per cent would be primary users of amphetamines. Probably somewhere around 15 per cent to 20 per cent would be as secondary [users], with alcohol or cannabis being the primary [drug].[439]

Cannabis is also a growing problem in Warrnambool and the Western District. Unlike Melbourne, it is often a 'pure drug problem'. In other words, the primary presenting problem is cannabis, whereas in Melbourne it is most often presented as part of a poly-drug problem. Dr Brough of ARCAB also states that prescription opiates are becoming a real problem in that part of rural Victoria:

> My concern is that that is going to become an entrenched part of the culture in rural Victoria. The advantage to the users is that they have a pure drug. There is no possibility of contamination. They know the colours and the dosages of the capinol and MS capsules much better than I do, and a sophisticated network of people are presenting to GPs, either threatening them, saying, 'We know where you live', which, of course, in rural areas they do know where you live, and they know what school your children go to, and all these other things, or they are just getting very smart at presenting with stories of chronic pain that justify prescribing MS-Contin or capinol, and this is a growing problem that is becoming quite an issue.[440]

Similarly, in the Latrobe Valley anecdotal evidence suggests that, partly as a result of the so-called 'heroin drought', many injecting drug users have turned to benzodiazepines as a substitute.[441] Misuse of 'dexies' (dexamphetamine) that

---

438 Mr Ron Marshall, Latrobe Community Health Services, evidence given to the Drugs and Crime Prevention Committee, Inquiry into Amphetamine and 'Party Drug' Use in Victoria, Public Hearings (Moe), 23 October 2003.

439 Mr Frank Coughlan, Drug and Alcohol Clinician, evidence given to the Drugs and Crime Prevention Committee, Inquiry into Amphetamine and 'Party Drug' Use in Victoria, Public Hearings (Moe), 23 October 2003.

440 Dr Rodger Brough, ARCAB, evidence given to the Drugs and Crime Prevention Committee, Inquiry into Amphetamine and 'Party Drug' Use in Victoria, Public Hearings (Melbourne), 6 October 2003.

441 See for example comments of Mr F. Coughlan, Outreach Clinician, Latrobe Community Health Service, evidence given to the Drugs and Crime Prevention Committee, Inquiry into Amphetamine and 'Party Drug' Use in Victoria, Public Hearings (Moe), 23 October 2003.

have been prescribed for a young person's own use or for others is not unknown in rural areas, particularly in the Latrobe Valley.[442]

There has also been anecdotal evidence from a variety of sources that the ADHD drug 'Ritalin' (methylphenidate) has been used as a drug of abuse in rural and regional communities:[443]

> ...the problem I have is that the youth tend to go out on a Friday or a Saturday night, when they purchase and seem to love those big, black cans of Woodstock bourbon. Into that they tend to mix medication, the Ritalin medication and anything else they can get on – anything to give themselves a bit of an alcohol-drug-affected sort of condition.[444]

Having acknowledged alcohol and cannabis use as relatively more problematic across the board and, at least with alcohol, almost universal in its use (and abuse), rates and prevalence of amphetamine and 'party drug' use vary considerably between regions. Indeed, submissions received by the Committee from Councils and service providers throughout Victoria used language describing the prevalence of amphetamines within their community that ranged along a continuum of 'not known'[445] or 'not prevalent'[446] through to 'rife'.[447] [448] For instance, amphetamine use in the Upper Hume region was framed as 'a significant problem',[449] fourth on a list of the eight most common drugs used by clients presenting for treatment or support from the Upper Hume Community

---

442 Evidence of Mr Ron Marshall given to the Drugs and Crime Prevention Committee, Inquiry into Amphetamine and 'Party Drug' Use in Victoria, Public Hearings (Moe), 23 October 2003.

443 One respondent to the Committee based at Benalla gave evidence that some parents in the area even took their children's Ritalin tablets to Melbourne in order to trade or sell them. Evidence of Pastor D. Marshall, Rose City Christian Life Centre, given to the Drugs and Crime Prevention Committee, Inquiry into Amphetamine and 'Party Drug' Use in Victoria, Public Hearings (Benalla), 22 October 2003. Such a claim however has not been substantiated.

444 Sergeant G. Waters, Victoria Police, evidence given to the Drugs and Crime Prevention Committee, Inquiry into Amphetamine and 'Party Drug' Use in Victoria, Public Hearings (Benalla), 22 October 2003.

445 Submission of Murrindindi Shire Council to the Drugs and Crime Prevention Committee, Inquiry into Amphetamine and 'Party Drug' Use in Victoria, 10 October 2003.

446 Submission of Moorabool Shire Council to the Drugs and Crime Prevention Committee, Inquiry into Amphetamine and 'Party Drug' Use in Victoria, 7 October 2003.

447 Submission of Goulburn Valley Community Health Service to the Drugs and Crime Prevention Committee, Inquiry into Amphetamine and 'Party Drug' Use in Victoria, 7 October 2003.

448 It should be noted that the authors of submissions received by the Committee usually prefaced their evaluations of the level of amphetamine and 'party drug' use within their community with one or two caveats. Namely, either that their evaluation was based to a higher or lesser degree on anecdotal evidence and/or that no hard data was available thereby precluding analysis at such a specific level. This lack of data and research was highlighted and is discussed further below.

449 Submission of Upper Hume Community Health Service (UHCHS) Wodonga to the Drugs and Crime Prevention Committee, Inquiry into Amphetamine and 'Party Drug' Use in Victoria, 21 October 2003.

Health Service (UHCHS).[450] Statistical data from this service indicates young people are the main group using amphetamines in the region, although long-distance transport drivers and shift workers also accessed the service when their amphetamine use became problematic. Among clients accessing the Needle Syringe Program in Wodonga, amphetamines appear as the primary drug of choice.[451] A Withdrawal Nurse from the Central Hume region cited Myrtleford as an example of a town where there is 'a very established and strong amphetamine using culture'.[452] These stand in juxtaposition to the Latrobe region, for example, where amphetamine use was categorised as 'not a major problem', 'mainly experimental' and 'almost never injected'.[453] One thing that can almost be stated with certainty is that, as in Melbourne, poly-drug use is a fact of life in rural Victoria, particularly among young people.

Access and availability

In terms of prevalence and availability, there are myriad factors within each region. One Alcohol and Other Drug (AOD) worker in the Hume region with Open Family Victoria related that most young people he came into contact with found 'amphetamines and related stimulants are easy to access and readily available...provided you have the money'.[454] The Manager of the Council's alcohol and drug service in the same region concurred:

> Anecdotal evidence...indicated that the supply of amphetamines...meets the demand – there is local supply and regular importation from some metropolitan areas. We are informed by clients that the cost and the availability have ensured that amphetamines are easily accessible in the local region.[455]

450 The submission of UHCHS supplies survey figures as follows:

'Amphetamine use is a significant problem in the Upper Hume region of Victoria.

The majority of clients accessing the Needle Syringe Program (NSP) based in Wodonga appear to be using amphetamines as their primary drug of choice. A survey of clients presenting to this NSP was conducted for a one-month period in August 2001. A total of 54 clients participated in this survey. Clients were asked what drug they were currently injecting and the response was as follows:

54% Amphetamines

27% Heroin

5 % MS Contin

5% Kapanol

5% Steroids

4% Morphine (vials).

451 Submission of Upper Hume Community Health Service (UHCHS) Wodonga to the Drugs and Crime Prevention Committee, Inquiry into Amphetamine and 'Party Drug' Use in Victoria, 21 October 2003.

452 Ms Lynda Johnson, Withdrawal Nurse, Central Hume Alcohol and Other Drugs Service, evidence given to the Drugs and Crime Prevention Committee, Inquiry into Amphetamine and 'Party Drug' Use in Victoria, Public Hearings (Benalla), 22 October 2003.

453 Mr Ron Marshall, Latrobe Community Health Services, evidence given to the Drugs and Crime Prevention Committee, Inquiry into Amphetamine and 'Party Drug' Use in Victoria, Public Hearings (Moe), 23 October 2003.

454 Submission of Open Family Victoria, Hume Region to the Drugs and Crime Prevention Committee, Inquiry into Amphetamine and 'Party Drug' Use in Victoria, 13 October 2003.

455 Submission of Upper Hume Community Health Service (UHCHS) Wodonga to the Drugs and Crime Prevention Committee, Inquiry into Amphetamine and 'Party Drug' Use in Victoria, 21 October 2003.

Even if 'readily available', however, access is probably tempered to some degree by smaller 'networks' of individuals engaged in drug use and distribution. For example, Senior Sergeant Gye, based in Morwell, said 'the networks are a bit closer here... You really have to know someone before you can source amphetamine. It is not proactively sold.'[456]

There is some, admittedly sketchy, evidence of manufacture and distribution networks in central and northern Victoria. A submission from the Goulburn Valley Community Health Service based in Shepparton states:

> Rumours exist that there are a number of clandestine laboratories in the region which may be associated with various motorbike clubs who regulate production, distribution and control of amphetamines in the area. Historically the Shepparton area has been seen by services as a high alcohol and cannabis use area. However there is also a high level of speed use and at times Shepparton has been called 'the speed capital of Victoria'. Local Police report a number of recent raids on properties finding Ecstasy, Amphetamines and Cannabis.[457]

One issue pertaining to supply that several respondents to this Inquiry have mentioned as significant is the importance of central transport routes. In the context of drug use in central Victoria the Hume Highway has been crucial, being the main conduit between Melbourne and Sydney. A police officer from the north-eastern Victorian town of Benalla states:

> We never get past the fact that most of our work – be it drugs, be it traffic; everything we seem to deal with – is to do with the main arterial route between Melbourne and Sydney. Our traffic department members are continually pulling up cars whose passengers are involved with criminals, drugs, large amounts of money, et cetera.[458]

Mr Jurgen Hemmerling, Senior Drug Outreach Worker of Open Family (Hume Region) based in Wangaratta, also states in this regard:

> One of the things that needs to be said about the availability of amphetamines and related stimulants in the country, from the kids that we see and from what they tell us, is that if you want those substances and you cannot get them within 20 minutes, then you are not trying.[459] They are available in most of

---

456 Senior Sergeant Craig Gye, Traralgon Police, evidence given to the Drugs and Crime Prevention Committee, Inquiry into Amphetamine and 'Party Drug' Use in Victoria, Public Hearings (Moe), 23 October 2003.

457 Submission of Goulburn Valley Community Health Service to the Drugs and Crime Prevention Committee, Inquiry into Amphetamine and 'Party Drugs', October 2003.

458 Sergeant Graham Waters, Benalla Police, evidence given to the Drugs and Crime Prevention Committee, Inquiry into Amphetamine and 'Party Drug' Use in Victoria, Public Hearings (Benalla), 22 October 2003.

459 The submission of Open Family Australia from its Wangaratta office states:

'Most young people report that amphetamines and related stimulants are easy to access and are readily available in a rural environment, provided you have the money. This supports Fay & Miller's 2002 research where 92% of respondents stated that these substances were easy/very easy to obtain. This of course, in an unemployed population, tends to lead to further criminal and anti-social activity, thus further exacerbating problems for both the users and the local community'.

> the towns in a rural environment. The other thing that needs to be said from my point of view is that the Hume region is a little bit unique. It has two major transport routes transversing the entire region. We have Shepparton, which goes up to Sydney and Brisbane, and we have the Hume Highway. So not only do we have recreational use for all sorts of good and bad reasons, but we have a high incidence of occupational use with the transport industry. It needs to be recognised. Given that they are the two major transport routes north and south, it is not surprising that these sorts of substances are fairly readily available – it is a given – and I think it needs to be recognised.
>
> Again from my point of view and from some of the young people we have seen, there seems to be a link-up in some areas, particularly Albury–Wodonga and I think Benalla–Wangaratta, and there is some anecdotal evidence of link-ups with some of the motorcycle gangs or clubs that are becoming more active in the area.[460]

Similar comments were made with regard to the town of Wodonga on the Victorian side of the New South Wales–Victorian border. The problem of availability of drugs is exacerbated by Wodonga being on both the main Melbourne–Canberra and Melbourne–Sydney routes.[461] There is some anecdotal evidence given of manufacture of amphetamines in the central Victorian area, with possible links to motorcycle gangs, but the Committee has not received any substantial evidence of this. There is also some evidence, again anecdotal, that amphetamine production and use can have a social cost on rural communities in terms of crime and violence. While there is a substantial amount of writing on the links between amphetamine, crime and violence in the United States, there is little if any research in this area in the Australian context.[462]

---

460 Mr Jurgen Hemmerling, Youth Outreach Worker, Open Family Victoria (Hume Region), evidence given to the Drugs and Crime Prevention Committee, Inquiry into Amphetamine and 'Party Drug' Use in Victoria, Public Hearings (Benalla), 22 October 2003.

461 See comments of Ms Jane Campbell, Rural Manager, Odyssey House, evidence given to the Drugs and Crime Prevention Committee, Inquiry into Amphetamine and 'Party Drug' Use in Victoria, Public Hearings (Benalla), 22 October 2003. See also the comments of Ms Deb Heery, Team Manager, Alcohol and other Drugs Unit, Upper Hume Community Health Service, evidence given to the Drugs and Crime Prevention Committee, Inquiry into Amphetamine and 'Party Drug' Use in Victoria, Public Hearings (Benalla), 22 October 2003.

462 There is a substantial body of American literature that testifies to the negative impacts the manufacture and trade of amphetamines has had on small-town and rural communities in the United States, particularly the mid-Western states. Wermuth, for example, writes:

'Smaller towns and rural areas may be especially vulnerable to the devastating effects of methamphetamine. Small cohorts of adolescents may be heavily influenced by the homogeneity of their peer culture and rural youth have historically shown a pattern of attraction to stimulants. When methamphetamine catches on, the overall effects, especially related to illegality, on small rural communities can be devastating. Fargo, North Dakota, had this experience when a wave of crime was brought on in the early 1990s by the spread of methamphetamine use; as the market flourished, gangs from Chicago and Minneapolis pushed in and violence increase. Small communities as well as urban areas in which methamphetamine has become popular have seen increased hospital emergency department episodes, surges in crime, and explosions and fires from the methamphetamine cooking process. In addition, clean-up of toxic laboratories is dangerous and very expensive, though the Federal government offers some assistance to communities unable to manage it by themselves...

The *economic* role of the methamphetamine trade and the employment it provides are central in understanding its spread. Especially in rural and semi-rural areas, it provides income to

In addition to the mention of motor cycle gangs, Benalla police also comment that drugs can be brought into the community by a transient or 'floating population' who may stay in the area in temporary housing while waiting for more permanent (public) housing. Similar comments have been made with regard to other areas of the state. Dr Brough from ARCAB has given evidence that people with drug problems who travel from the city to rural areas can have serious disruptive effects on those communities. Despite the anecdotal nature of the evidence, it would appear that amphetamine-type drugs in particular are mostly accessed from Melbourne, usually by those who have travelled to Melbourne, 'scored' and brought them back to their local communities.[463] This

---

many individuals who have few options in the legal job market. Young white men in rural or semi-rural areas who are unemployed or marginally employed may be especially attracted to the methamphetamine trade for income and as a way to support their own drug habit' (Wermuth 2000, pp.427, 431).

A police officer from Perth, Det Sgt Paul Steel, has witnessed first-hand the effect of methamphetamine production on small town and rural America. Det Sgt Steel based in the clandestine laboratory unit of WA Police visited a number of American states and police forces specialising in 'clan lab' investigation as part of a Churchill Fellowship. He related his findings to the Committee:

'In States such as Des Moines, Iowa – or Iowa was the State, Des Moines was the Capital – the methylamphetamine problem there has completely decimated very small rural communities.

Where you have towns – and we have them in Australia as well – with populations of under 1,000 people, 90 per cent of their children or their younger generation are using amphetamines and probably 50 per cent of those are actually manufacturing them. That is largely due to the availability of precursor chemicals. States like that have a problem that is completely out of control, both in terms of party drug use and in terms of hard core addictive drug use.

But in the time that I was in Iowa we went through quite a few of these very small, little towns. They use anhydrous ammonia as part of their farming, so available in virtually any field that you would look at there is this ammonia gas. Well, ammonia gas is the hardest thing to source in terms of manufacturing methylamphetamine via the nazi-method. The only other thing they need is a pseudoephedrine-based medication. In the US you can buy that at a hardware store or a service station, and they can use lithium metal out of lithium batteries for cameras and things like that.

That's it. That is all you need. So, because it has become so ingrained in these little communities that, you know, amphetamine use, for a start, because it's highly available and, secondly, how easy it is to manufacture. You don't need glassware; you can do it in a glass or a glass demijohn, whatever you like. They found that a very large percentage of their youth have become users and to support their own habits they've then become manufacturers of the drugs. That obviously has all the social implications that go with that, in terms of, you know, not working...

...[b]asically, all the behavioural and social issues that you would expect with large scale drug use within a community, and for the parents and the owners of the farms that, you know, want them taken over by the children it has all the family-type implications as well, so they have really noticed – well, Iowa has a population of maybe – I don't want to mislead you here but it's definitely less than 2 million people – and they have around a thousand clandestine laboratories per year, so in a population that's, I mean, that would be like, you know, you getting that many in Victoria, it's just, you know, almost unworkable' (Det. Sgt Steel, WA Police, in conversation with the Drugs and Crime Prevention Committee, Perth, 1 October 2003).

For an account of the links between amphetamine production, violence, crime and rural America, see Jenkins (1999, pp.138–142). See also Rawson, Gonzales and Brethen 2002 and Pennell 1999 for further accounts of how methamphetamine has impacted upon rural communities in the United States.

Fortunately, it would seem that, at least thus far, Australian rural communities have not been affected by drug use or drug production to quite this extent.

463 Mr Frank Coughlan, evidence given to the Drugs and Crime Prevention Committee, Inquiry into Amphetamine and 'Party Drug' Use in Victoria, Public Hearings (Moe), 23 October 2003.

is particularly true of the MDMA/ecstasy that is associated with nightclubs and other party venues in towns such as Traralgon, Warrnambool and Shepparton.[464] For example, young people residing in Gippsland or the Latrobe Valley might go to Dandenong on the fringes of the Melbourne metropolitan district to buy drugs.

From a law enforcement perspective, police officers operating within the Latrobe Valley, encompassing the regional centres of Churchill, Moe, Morwell and Traralgon, have noticed a 'slight increase' in charges resulting from the seizure of amphetamines and relating to the trafficking of amphetamines between 2000 and 2003:

> ...the 25 to 29 year old age group has been the most predominant in relation to possession of amphetamines. Trafficking of amphetamines is again fairly low numbers, but we have had 11 people charged who are 30 to 39 years of age, which would indicate that the traffickers are a bit older than the users.[465]

As regards 'party drugs' and ecstasy, the officers were aware of anecdotal evidence implying an increase in their availability and use associated with the 'nightclub precinct' based in Traralgon, but maintained the number of charges and seizures was too low to imply any trend.[466] Drug selling and buying is simply not as noticeable in country areas, or at least as 'visible' as it may be in the city.[467]

> I have worked in Melbourne and it is a much different scenario than it is down there [Gippsland]. In Melbourne you can walk down a lot of streets in some suburbs and you will find people that are selling drugs, using drugs and doing all that. It is not something that occurs on the street in a rural setting, purely and simply because it is way too exposed, more often than not. So that is not an issue that we have particularly. We get reports of people dealing drugs in the street, if you like, particularly young people, but it is not an everyday occurrence.[468]

464 See, for example, evidence given by Inspector Notman, Victoria Police, Latrobe District, to the Drugs and Crime Prevention Committee, Inquiry into Amphetamine and 'Party Drug' Use in Victoria, Public Hearings (Moe), 23 October 2003.

465 Inspector Notman, Morwell Police, evidence given to the Drugs and Crime Prevention Committee, Inquiry into Amphetamine and 'Party Drug' Use in Victoria, Public Hearings (Moe), 23 October 2003.

466 Ibid.

467 Ron Marshall from the Latrobe Community Health Service in Gippsland posits the interesting view that the fact young people may have to go to Melbourne to 'score' amphetamines and/or party drugs may act as a 'protective factor', given some young people may not have the means or the ability to travel those distances. On the other hand alcohol and cannabis being freely available in the area naturally results in them becoming frequently used drugs of abuse. Mr Ron Marshall, evidence given to the Drugs and Crime Prevention Committee, Inquiry into Amphetamine and 'Party Drug' Use in Victoria, Public Hearings (Moe), 23 October 2003.

468 Inspector Notman, Morwell Police, evidence given to the Drugs and Crime Prevention Committee, Inquiry into Amphetamine and 'Party Drug' Use in Victoria, Public Hearings (Moe), 23 October 2003.

Contexts and patterns of use

It is significant to note here that throughout the course of the Inquiry responses to questions about the use of amphetamine and/or 'party drugs' usually focussed on issues surrounding the former only, to the exclusion of substances like MDMA (ecstasy), ketamine or GHB. The higher rates of amphetamine use over and above other substances ostensibly reflects the primacy of notions of culture and context in drug-taking behaviour. Indeed, literature supports the comment by one rural alcohol and drug worker that 'most recreational drug use is meaningful for the people who partake'.[469] As with those who use drugs in Melbourne and other major cities, the profiles of users and the reasons they may use will vary greatly depending on the context.[470]

Unfortunately, there is very little information available about the drug-using patterns and cultures of discrete populations and minority groups in country Victoria. For example, despite Shepparton having a small 'gay scene' there is no same-sex attracted service and little knowledge about drug use within that community. One could plausibly posit, however, that gay men and lesbians in rural communities are even less likely to be open about both their sexuality and their drug use than their counterparts in Melbourne. Similarly, Shepparton has high concentrations of European and Middle Eastern migrants but little is known about their drug-taking behaviours 'as there is a reluctance to attend mainstream services, possibly brought about by cultural barriers, stigmas and beliefs'.[471] Despite Indigenous populations having fairly high levels of injecting drug use in their communities, there is also a paucity of information on the cultural contexts of their use.

With regard to young people generally, Mr Jurgen Hemmerling states:

> In my experience, most young people's use is situational and reflects the notion of bingeing, however; I have experience of young people using amphetamines and related stimulants on a regular and on-going basis. Some of the reasons given include, weight control in young females, self medication for undiagnosed ADHD/ADD and, in some people who are being treated with neuroleptic medications for a psychiatric condition, where they feel the medications are making them too slow.[472]

Mr Hemmerling also notes that due to the primacy of alcohol as a drug of choice, amphetamines can often be favoured due to their ability to make

469 Submission of Open Family Victoria (Hume Region) to the Drugs and Crime Prevention Committee, Inquiry into Amphetamine and 'Party Drug' Use in Victoria, 13 October 2003.

470 The context of drug use, however, within Indigenous, gay and culturally and linguistically diverse communities has been discussed in Chapter 9.

471 Submission of the Goulburn Valley Community Health Service to the Drugs and Crime Prevention Committee, Inquiry into Amphetamine and 'Party Drug' Use in Victoria, October 2003.

472 Submission of Open Family Australia to the Drugs and Crime Prevention Committee, Inquiry into Amphetamine and 'Party Drug' Use in Victoria, 13 October 2003.

consumers of alcohol feel they can drink more without becoming intoxicated.[473]

As has been previously mentioned, amphetamines may be part of a functional use profile in rural areas, particularly in areas which are linked to or close by major transport networks. Goulburn Valley Community Health Service states that this is true of Shepparton as a hub of the transport industry. Shepparton is also a centre for transient workers and backpackers:

> Unique to Shepparton is the amount of itinerant seasonal workers that pass through because of the fruit industry and factory work. Anecdotal evidence would suggest that the amount of illicit drugs that are available at this time increases significantly. The use of amphetamines and party drugs lends itself to this client group. The use of amphetamines as a way to be able to continue to work at a fast pace over long hours and then be able to enjoy themselves has seen these drugs... [preferred by] this population. Within this is also the overseas travellers/backpackers who work the season but are also in the age group that allows them to experiment and try new experiences.[474]

The Upper Hume Community Health Service based in Wodonga has also stated that long-distance transport drivers (and shift workers) have accessed their drug treatment facilities when 'their amphetamine use has been problematic for them'.[475] The submission from ARCAB discussing trends in Warrnambool and south-west Victoria notes that there are reports of young women using amphetamine as a weight loss measure. Shift workers, particularly chefs, and those working long hours 'are an identifiable sub-population who report amphetamine use'.[476]

In Warrnambool, community parks and football grounds were cited most frequently overall as places where people would use amphetamine and amphetamine-type substances such as ecstasy 'when there is no-one around'.[477] These spaces can again be contrasted with Moe or Castlemaine, for instance, where amphetamine use often occurs in private homes.[478]

The Committee heard evidence that ecstasy use in the Latrobe region was associated directly with the nightclub and entertainment precinct in Traralgon.

---

473 Ibid.

474 Submission of the Goulburn Valley Community Health Service to the Drugs and Crime Prevention Committee, Inquiry into Amphetamine and 'Party Drug' Use in Victoria, October 2003.

475 Submission of the Upper Hume Community Health Service to the Drugs and Crime Prevention Committee, Inquiry into Amphetamine and 'Party Drug' Use in Victoria, October 2003.

476 Submission of ARCAB to the Drugs and Crime Prevention Committee, Inquiry into Amphetamine and 'Party Drug' Use in Victoria, October 2003.

477 Ibid.

478 Submission of John Parkinson, Castlemaine District Community Health Centre Inc. to the Drugs and Crime Prevention Committee, Inquiry into Amphetamine and 'Party Drug' Use in Victoria, 22 October 2003.

The Macedon Ranges Shire similarly reports, 'The culture of "pill popping" and party drugs is developing within the Shire with the increase of underground "raves"'.[479]

Accessing information

A submission from the Goulburn Valley Community Health Service personnel states that there is very little information with regard to 'party drug' use in their local area:

> If this population of illicit drug users is invisible then this is more so in the regional areas of Victoria, as there is no direct scene that supports 'party drug' use. There are no great numbers of 'raves' in Shepparton therefore the harm minimisation message for those taking ecstasy or other party drugs is ad hoc, poorly delivered or simply not well targeted. Anecdotal evidence would suggest that party drug use is rife within the hotel scenes of Shepparton and home parties yet it appears that users are either supporting and educating themselves and delivering their own safe using tips, or alternatively, have little support, education and may be using unsafe practices.
>
> A lot of work is done with the younger population through early education within the school system and community settings where young people gather ie. sporting clubs, alternative education settings, youth groups. These young people are wanting to know a lot more information about party drugs which may indicate a potential to use. There has also been a high demand from other groups requesting that AOD workers come to their clubs/associations to talk about alcohol and other drug use.[480]

The community agency RaveSafe, which advises on and monitors harm reduction mechanisms at raves and commercial nightclubs, has noticed a distinct difference in the patterns of 'party drug' use among young people in rural areas compared to their counterparts in Melbourne. Ms Natalie Russell, Co-ordinator of the RaveSafe program for Victoria, told the Committee at its Public Hearing in October 2003:

> I guess one of the noticeable things from attending [country events] is that many of the party goers that were there tended to not go out as frequently as those in Melbourne and therefore possibly their knowledge about party drugs was less because of the fact that they do not have the network or friends that they regularly talk to about party drugs, whereas people in Melbourne who are going out all the time often I guess communicate a lot more about those issues. But on Saturday night these kids from Bendigo chose to go out every

479 Submission of Macedon Ranges Shire Council to the Drugs and Crime Prevention Committee, Inquiry into Amphetamine and 'Party Drug' Use in Victoria, 13 October 2003.

480 Submission of the Goulburn Valley Community Health Service to the Drugs and Crime Prevention Committee, Inquiry into Amphetamine and 'Party Drug' Use in Victoria, October 2003.

> now and then when a rave would come close to them, and I found that their knowledge was not as great as those party goers in Melbourne. The way we are sort of trying to keep them up to date with current drug information is getting them to join our email newsletter and keeping in contact via email if they cannot access a lot of raves in Melbourne.[481]

In south-west Victoria anecdotal reports suggest ecstasy use has increased, but the numbers are still quite limited. Because users of MDMA do not view their use as problematic and do not consequently present to treatment services it is hard to gauge accurate prevalence data of use, as is the case with the rest of the state, including Melbourne.[482]

Clearly disparities exist between regions and regional centres in terms of the availability of amphetamines and the patterns of use. These differences are further evidenced in the apparent contexts and cultural locales of amphetamine use. What has been represented above is a sample of frequently complimentary, though by no means homogenous, accounts of local amphetamine use and misuse. As will be discussed in the next section, far more research needs to be done that concentrates on the specificities of drug use in rural communities.

Rural service issues: Responses from the sector

A paradox appears in discussing the issue of drug use in rural and regional communities. On the one hand rural and regional communities *do* have specific local problems and issues that need disaggregating and addressing separately. On the other hand there are definite problems and issues that continually arise that would seem to be common to *all* rural and regional communities. The following section focusses principally on some of these commonalities and the capacity of disparate communities to respond to them.

Lack of research and data

The paucity of context-specific, comprehensive research and data that would enable a clearer understanding of illicit drug use in rural and regional Victoria, and amphetamine and 'party drug' use in particular, is central to understanding the issue of drug use in rural and regional Victoria. More quantitative and qualitative research that engages community contextual information, as Dr

---

481 Certainly the Internet is one way in which the 'tyranny of distance' can be somewhat ameliorated. An example of rural service delivery that creatively uses the Internet was presented to the Committee by the Drug and Alcohol Services Council (DASC) of South Australia when it visited Adelaide. DASC has published guidelines and education material for venue operators and licensees with regard to 'party drug' use on their premises. All such material is available on-line, and country hotels and the like are encouraged to link to the Internet to access it. DASC is also liaising with the Office of Liquor and Gambling (S.A) to put licensee training packages on-line in order to 'better support rural licensed premises where we have not had a significant impact to date' (Simone Cormack, DASC, in conversation with the Drugs and Crime Prevention Committee, Adelaide, 3 October 2003).

482 Submission of ARCAB to the Drugs and Crime Prevention Committee, Inquiry into Amphetamine and 'Party Drug' Use in Victoria, October 2003.

Rodger Brough has emphasised, is required.[483] Any data must be disaggregated appropriately to reflect the distinguishing characteristics and dynamics of each region and rural centre. Research agendas and reports that purport to inform drug-related policy should be set in consultation and under the purview of representatives of rural and regional communities contending with the issues on a daily basis. Moreover, wherever possible, Dr Brough suggests such research be designed and conducted by local people or people with experience of rural and regional life.

Indeed ARCAB has recommended to this Committee that:

> There is a demonstrated broad need, highlighted by ARCAB's comments to this inquiry, for a system of maintaining active links with rural communities to enhance data collection, community building and linking between rural communities such as that envisaged by ARCAB. The essential component of this recommendation is that any system is located in rural Victoria and actively maintained and supported with ongoing funding. There is no reason why this should not be a national issue with access to Federal government funding assistance – the issue is not state specific, by any means. Better rural-specific health research, and more of it, will lead to better information, better government policy, better services, and improved health outcomes. Nine out of ten 'rural' research papers are currently produced by urban-based researchers... This is not good enough.[484]

Many such representatives with whom the Committee met strongly advocated the need for further research and data collection in their region. The Goulburn Community Health Service writes of the 'circularity' of the problem with regard to researching drug use among rural and regional communities. In other words, when there are obstacles placed in the path of drug users accessing treatment or services in the country (such as distance, isolation, problems in maintaining anonymity) then clients may not access those services, even when they exist. Without a substantial base of clients, it is difficult to draw useful data pertaining to patterns of drug use in the locality:

> Whilst there is a lot of anecdotal evidence and a little research into the problems of amphetamines and party drug use, it appears there is even less research pertaining to regional/rural use. This may be directly related to the

---

483 One such project which demonstrated the importance of collecting data over a wide rural base was the *Victorian Rural Heroin and Methadone Project.* As Dr Brough of ARCAB explains: 'This project experience, over three years, reinforced the importance and value of collecting data from a number of rural communities to be able to comprehensively and effectively understand the impact of social issues in rural communities. Rural communities are not homogeneous and are not readily classifiable into groups for comparability. ARCAB passionately believes it is impossible to capture the essence of the impact of social issues (like addictive behaviours) in richly diverse rural communities by sampling just a handful of rural communities' (usually major regional centres when this "rural representation" approach is undertaken) experience' (Submission from ARCAB to the Drugs and Crime Prevention Committee, Inquiry into Amphetamine and 'Party Drug' Use in Victoria, October 2003).

484 Ibid.

> invisibility of this drug community. It appears that both research and responses are directly related to visibility and an acknowledgment that a problem or concern exists. If users of these illicit substances do not present for treatment then it is hard to collect relevant statistics for this community. Engagement with clients who use amphetamines is difficult as they often use in isolated groups and are less likely to be extrovert about their use.[485]

The *Discussion Paper* for this Inquiry detailed the paucity of research into amphetamine and 'party drug' use generally in Australia, let alone that applying to such use in the rural sector. People from the rural sector with whom the Committee met noted in particular the few treatment options and the lack of treatment research for amphetamine and amphetamine-type substance users, including the lack of knowledge around effective pharmacotherapies. This was noted on numerous occasions by withdrawal nurses, alcohol and drug clinicians, workers and counsellors operating within different facets of rural and regional community health services. As Ms Deb Heery commented:

> In a way we have felt a bit isolated as service providers in that there have not been a lot of guidelines and protocols to manage withdrawal and ongoing treatment with amphetamine users who are presenting to our service.[486]

These professionals reiterated the need for further resources and creative research both medical and social/qualitative into drug use generally in rural communities.

One research project that seems to have produced positive results for drug (methamphetamine) users in rural and remote Australia was the Queensland Health Survey on Amphetamine Usage. This was a collaborative venture through two arms of the Queensland Government. In June 2003 the Committee met with the co-ordinator of the project, Mr Robert Kemp:

> The Queensland Crime Commission in particular had a strong interest in drug markets, and quite a strong interest in amphetamines and related drug markets. Queensland Health basically put forward the idea of some kind of collaborative exercise between justice and health. It was a great idea. They had the fund and we had the expertise.
>
> We formed a collaboration at that point in time; and it has taken a long time to work it through. It has been a priority issue for both organisations. Rather than

485 Submission of the Goulburn Valley Community Health Service to the Drugs and Crime Prevention Committee, Inquiry into Amphetamine and 'Party Drug' Use in Victoria, October 2003.

486 Ms Deb Heery, Upper Hume Community Health Service, Wodonga, evidence given to the Drugs and Crime Prevention Committee, Inquiry into Amphetamine and 'Party Drug' Use in Victoria, Public Hearings (Benalla), 22 October 2003. In her written submission to this Committee Ms Heery reports that UHCHS is liaising with staff from the Greater Murray Health Service across the river in Albury, NSW on a research project being auspiced by the latter service as part of the NSW statewide drug initiative. The brief for this project is research into effective amphetamine treatment options, particularly for regional areas.

> going out to a university, which has been the standard practice, we have chosen to use our own staff and our own expertise and our own resources.[487]

Each of the 39 health districts in Queensland has an ATODS (Alcohol, Tobacco and Other Drugs Services) unit located within it. These range from the very small sole practitioner through to the large clinic services.

The research survey methodology utilised these services and the ATODS persons in 17 locations across Queensland (from the outback to the tropics) agreed to be research supervisors:

> They in turn recruited a number of peer interviewers, which were stable people with good contacts with the drug-using communities in those areas. In the end we landed up with 40 peer interviewers who went through the data collection process. Our original target was 500 questionnaires across the state. We achieved that easily, so we came back and requested more funding and at the end got 690 completed. Each survey participant was paid for his time, and each peer interviewer was paid as well. It took anywhere from about 45 minutes to an hour to complete the survey form; it was a comprehensive book, basically. Out of the 690 we landed up with 665 usable survey instruments, which is about 96 per cent, which is amazing.

The survey document was a wide-ranging questionnaire that asked amphetamine users a broad variety of questions pertaining to their drug use, as well as matters pertaining to their non-using lives. The research seems to have addressed the concerns expressed in this section in two ways. First, it used local networks to administer, conduct and supervise the research. For example the amphetamine use patterns of a miner in Mount Isa may be very different from a recreational user in Cairns. Second, it utilised a peer education methodology which instils confidence in the person being interviewed. A research 'subject' is much more likely to 'open up' to someone who is a former user or has worked with users than an academic from a university or clinical background. This project seems a good example of collaborative research that can assist disparate remote, and rural communities to address drug use within their areas.

The luxury of 'extracurricular' activity

As desirable as further and well funded research into drug use and drug treatment in rural communities is, such research is of questionable value when practitioners and workers in the field simply do not have time to read or study it. This was a common refrain that the Committee heard from overworked and under-resourced drug and alcohol specialists and general health and education workers. For example, when the Committee asked Mr Ron Marshall from Latrobe Community Health Service what research he was aware of in the area, he responded: 'We are so busy that we do not have time to catch up on reading

487 Mr Robert Kemp, Manager, Queensland Needle Availability Support Program, Queensland Health, in conversation with the Drugs and Crime Prevention Committee, Brisbane, 27 June 2003.

research'.[488] Mr Jurgen Hemmerling echoes such a plaint by expressing his frustration in not having adequate data available to him with regard to amphetamine use in his region *and* having very little time to study it if it was available: 'We do stuff like this in our "spare time"'. The same constraints apply to grant and submission writing. For example, Mr Hemmerling wryly commented that the submission he wrote for this Inquiry was 'written over two nights between the hours of 8 pm and midnight after a full day at work'.[489]

The double constraints of time and money (or lack thereof) appear also to apply to 'peripheral' areas such as health promotion and health prevention; often such projects may be done in the staff's own time. This is certainly the experience of workers at the Upper Hume Community Health Service:

> We are funded by the Department of Human Services to provide drug treatment services as opposed to health promotion and early intervention strategies. UHCHS has identified there is a gap in these areas, and at times attempt to implement health promotion and early intervention initiatives within our funding constraints. This has often been a reactive rather than proactive process which can be ad hoc, rather than planned evidence based initiatives which we believe would be a much more effective use of resources and would have more positive outcomes for the broader community.[490]

Unfortunately, these constraints and the reality of pragmatic everyday service delivery seem to express the reality of many workers in this field.

Spatial or locational disadvantages

As has been highlighted throughout this chapter, the issues and problems of rural and regional communities are often different from those experienced in metropolitan areas. A number of issues within these communities can be specifically related to degrees of geographical isolation and remoteness, but the dynamics of wider social, political and economic processes are also factors. In a helpful paper delineating the structural determinants of drug use among youth in Australia, the authors point out:

> Research has established that spatial or locational disadvantages are the outcomes of social, political and economic processes. Areas lack particular facilities because of a myriad of decisions by communities, governments and planners, rather than just the physical characteristics of location (National Drug and Alcohol Research Centre (NDARC) 2001, p.16).

A pertinent example of such a process would be the emphasis on competitive tendering in the 1990s, whereby the critical co-operation between alcohol and

488 Mr Ron Marshall, evidence given to the Drugs and Crime Prevention Committee, Inquiry into Amphetamine and 'Party Drug' Use in Victoria, Public Hearings (Moe), 23 October 2003.

489 Mr Jurgen Hemmerling, Open Family Victoria (Hume Region), evidence given to the Drugs and Crime Prevention Committee, Inquiry into Amphetamine and 'Party Drug' Use in Victoria, Public Hearings (Benalla), 22 October 2003.

490 Upper Hume Community Health Service, evidence given to the Drugs and Crime Prevention Committee, Inquiry into Amphetamine and 'Party Drug' Use in Victoria, Public Hearing (Benalla), 22 October 2003.

other drug agencies in rural and regional Victoria was diminished as larger agencies were better equipped to engage in the tendering process. The outcome was increasingly inequitable resource allocation, with rural areas consistently disadvantaged compared to larger regional centres (Turning Point Alcohol and Drug Centre 2003).

Geographical isolation clearly has flow-on consequences for accessing appropriate services. A submission from the Wodonga based Upper Hume Community Health Service states:

> A key problem for service delivery in this region is 'geographical isolation'. Specialist withdrawal and residential rehabilitation services for young people and adults are based in Melbourne – the cost and logistics of clients travelling to Melbourne can be a barrier to further treatment options. 'Geographical isolation' is also a problem *within* this region itself. Due to limited public transport, many clients have difficulty accessing our office in Wodonga or regional offices in Corryong, Yackandandah, Beechworth or Mt Beauty. This requires outreach to be offered by our staff on a regular basis – often home visits – where travel time and costs can often be a strain on resources.[491]

The Goulburn Valley Community Health Service similarly argues that providing appropriate drug services to those in the more remote parts of their catchment area is very difficult:

> Within this area there is a limited service of Alcohol and Other Drug counselling delivered from major regional centres. Outreach to smaller rural towns such as Cobram, Numurkah, Nathalia, Yarrawonga, Mooroopna and Euroa is conducted weekly and the majority of the time people want immediate help, there and then. There are limited resources to service the smaller townships and even fewer resources for consumers that live on isolated properties. Public transport from these areas to townships is non-existent.[492]

For example, Dr Brough of ARCAB gives the example of a heroin user who is receiving methadone in order to 'come clean'. If he or she lives in an outlying part of the Western District, often because of cheaper housing, it may be difficult to have regular access to the supplies of methadone:

> That is something, particularly in the outlying areas such as Mortlake and so on, where the housing prices have not escalated as much as they have in Warrnambool and along the coast, where services have been pulled out of those towns from banks to health services being downgraded, et cetera. Yet they are finding that because rental housing and even purchasing housing is so cheap they have had people moving into the areas. What has happened is that I have had a couple of patients on methadone out there, but when the pharmacy closes on Saturday the local community health centre which has been downgraded from the hospital has only one staff member on and the centre

491 Ibid. (Committee emphasis)

492 Submission of Goulburn Valley Community Health Service to the Drugs and Crime Prevention Committee, Inquiry into Amphetamine and 'Party Drug' Use in Victoria, October 2003.

> does not like the one staff member seeing the people to pick up their methadone, particularly if they have a history of violence, et cetera. So provision of service for those people when the drug and poisons unit not unreasonably runs a pretty tight ship in terms of having to pick up methadone pretty consistently and pretty regularly becomes difficult. It makes those sorts of things difficult for people to access services in an equitable sort of way.[493]

Ms Suzan Morey, also from ARCAB, adds:

> It can take them [drug users] a day. Some of our clients can spend an entire day working out how they are going to get to the pharmacy in the rurally isolated area they live in to get their methadone. Every single day that is their prime focus.

Factors pertaining to distance and location are felt not only by those who live in remote parts of the state but also by people who live in rural areas relatively close to Melbourne. Local government areas that straddle outer suburban Melbourne and rural districts face specific problems. This is exemplified in the submission from the Shire of Macedon Ranges, located in the Kyneton district:

> Macedon Ranges Shire is located between the metropolitan and rural councils, and as such has elements of both lifestyles. Access to illicit drugs, including amphetamines and 'party' drugs, is more limited than in Melbourne, although this is starting to change as development in the area increases. For workers in the area, including Council youth workers, this means keeping up with Melbourne trends is important, but being aware of their local applicability is paramount.
>
> In our region, lack of public transport is an issue that results in many tangential concerns. Whilst anecdotal, the small but increasing number of over 20s commuting to Melbourne to 'party' suggests some are likely to drive home, possibly under the influence of both alcohol and party drugs. Any campaign that combines harm minimisation and road safety would need to take into

---

493 The Committee has been given evidence that just as some drug users may move from country areas to Melbourne to have better access to the drug markets, conversely there has been some evidence of drug users moving from Melbourne to country and provincial areas partly because of cheaper accommodation options, particularly shorter waiting lists for public housing but also partly in order to 'kick their habits'.

For example, Ron Marshall from Latrobe Valley Community Health Service states:

'There appears to be a trend for city based long-term users – those people that you are talking about – to travel to regional locations and stay for short periods to escape whatever threats they may perceive, undertake a self-monitored withdrawal or cease drug use and rest their bodies. So we are getting the tired drug users as well, who sometimes relapse and then they will seek our services' (Mr Ron Marshall, evidence given to the Drugs and Crime Prevention Committee, Inquiry into Amphetamine and 'Party Drug' Use in Victoria, Public Hearings (Moe), 23 October 2003).

However there is also the corollary that for some people raised or living in rural areas the local 'scene' may encourage their drug taking:

'Reports from clients suggest that some people move to this region from Melbourne to 'get away' from the drug culture, but also some locals state that they can only see change occurring for them by moving away from this region because of their entrenchment in the local drug culture' (Submission of Upper Hume Community Health Service, to the Drugs and Crime Prevention Committee, Inquiry into Amphetamine and 'Party Drug' Use in Victoria, October 2003).

> account that options are limited – a taxi fare from Melbourne to Kyneton, for example, would be prohibitive for most people.[494]

The pressures and obstacles wrought by such macro and structural factors do not go unnoticed and are negotiated by rural and regional communities, and perhaps particularly community health workers and their clients, on a regular basis.

> Studies of young people in urban fringe suburbs and rural settings reveal that they feel disadvantaged by their location in regard to service provision (NDARC 2001, p.16).

Acknowledgment of this relative deficiency of services, which also includes recreational facilities and opportunities, has given birth to an incisive body of literature examining the social ramifications of insufficient stimulation 'leisure boredom'. The concept of 'leisure boredom' has an extensive literature. It has been conceptualised as 'a state of under stimulation, under arousal, lack of momentum or a lack of psychological involvement associated with dissatisfaction in the task situation' (Brissett & Snow 1993). For a valuable discussion of the links between leisure boredom, lack of leisure opportunities and alcohol and drug abuse among young people in Australian rural communities see Patterson and Pegg 1999. Patterson and Pegg argue that in Australian rural communities 'access to suitable entertainment, recreation and sporting facilities was severely restricted in rural areas' (p.27). This has a particularly deleterious effect on males (although females in rural areas had actually fewer leisure activities available to them if they were not interested in sport).

Research supports the hypothesis that youth (especially young males) living in rural areas experience high levels of leisure boredom and have a greater propensity to drink large quantities of alcohol, resulting in feelings of alienation and marginalisation that often render them vulnerable to depression and suicide (Patterson & Pegg 1999, p.28). Indeed, the results of a study of the relationship between 'leisure boredom' and alcohol and drug dependence among youth supported the contention that youth in rural areas are more likely to experience high levels of boredom and 'social disconnection', often translating to an increased likelihood of using large quantities of alcohol or drugs (as compared to their metropolitan peers) (NDARC 2001, p.17). This correlate was also briefly discussed in Spooner et al., where:

> ...boredom has been identified as a significant contributor to young people becoming involved in risk-taking behavior. This trend is particularly evident for young people who are spatially disadvantaged through living in urban fringe or rural locations (NDARC 2001, p.16).

Service delivery

The exigencies pressing on effective service provision in rural and regional areas of Victoria are striking. Service providers and their clients are invariably faced

---

494 Submission of the Macedon Ranges Shire to the Drugs and Crime Prevention Committee, Inquiry into Amphetamine and 'Party Drug' Use in Victoria, October 2003.

with significant issues relating specifically to the condition of rurality. These issues are best addressed from the dual perspectives of *provision* and then *access*.

Service provision

Staffing issues

A primary issue for rural and regional service providers is the relative lack of appropriately trained staff. The general statewide imperative to recruit, retain, train and educate a strong workforce is the focus of the workforce development strategy; however it is worth acknowledging that rural and regional areas of Victoria have experienced heightened problems (Turning Point Alcohol and Drug Centre 2003). In noting this, the Turning Point Service System Review states:

> In rural areas the role of the GPs, public hospitals and associated health and welfare services is even more critical than in urban locations... Rural agencies are often smaller, with less capacity to provide mentoring, training and supervision for staff (Turning Point Alcohol and Drug Centre 2003, p.7).

One issue that is raised frequently in meeting rural and regional workers in the field is the difficulty in *attracting* staff. The issue of 'enticing' medical practitioners to country practices and hospitals is well known. This is particularly the case for specialist drug staff.

Ms Tauridsky from Central Hume Alcohol and Other Drugs Service states:

> One of the things we find most difficult is that the levels of funding we get sometimes do not include the particular issues we face in a rural community about access to service. We will be funded for a position, to get an appropriately skilled experienced worker, but it will just cover their wage. It will not include something like: it is a regional position, so how will we get this worker to see people and to actually service the community?
>
> We are always struggling to find people who have not just the skills to deal with [clients] but also some really good values around making a real service available.[495]

Mr Frank Coughlan, clinician with the Latrobe Community Health Service, states:

> I have to say – this will sound like a criticism and it is – we are seriously understaffed because we cannot get the people we need. We cannot get the numbers we need. The case load is huge and the distances that have to be travelled by those staff are astronomical.[496]

Mr Jurgen Hemmerling from Open Family also comments:

495 Ms Elena Tauridsky, Central Hume Alcohol and Other Drugs Service, evidence given to the Drugs and Crime Prevention Committee, Inquiry into Amphetamine and 'Party Drug' Use in Victoria, Public Hearings (Benalla), 22 October 2003.

496 Mr Frank Coughlan, evidence given to the Drugs and Crime Prevention Committee, Inquiry into Amphetamine and 'Party Drug', Use in Victoria, Public Hearings (Moe), 23 October 2003.

> I have alluded to things like the fact that it is difficult to attract professionals if you are employing or advertising a position of 0.5 or 0.8, and I think that is true. But if those positions exist then we owe it to the communities that we live in to ensure that they are in fact filled and supported.[497]

The written submission from Open Family is even more emphatic:

> Recruitment and retention of adequately trained and experienced staff in the A&OD sector in rural Victoria is an on-going concern, with some regional agencies having had, or currently having vacant positions for in excess of six months. This seriously limits the opportunity for young people to access services. Many positions in the A&OD sector, tend to be funded at .6 or .8, or as 1 year contracts, this does not encourage professionals to take up vacancies. The other problem lies in the lack of recognition and career structure within the A&OD sector, which is a greatly limiting factor in attracting and retaining suitably skilled and qualified staff. Why would a social worker or nurse take up an A&OD position for less than $40k when they can quite easily get $60k in more mainstream career structures. This must be addressed with some urgency, or the A&OD service structure (such as it is) in rural Victoria could collapse.[498]

Recognising the difficulties in getting well trained and experienced staff, Mr Ron Marshall of the Latrobe Community Health Service stresses the importance of training on-site the staff you actually have and encouraging them to do specialist upskilling like the Certificate 1V in Drug and Alcohol Studies. Students on placement are also encouraged as one way of 'filling in the gaps':

> There is a problem in getting trained, experienced staff. What we tend to do is train our own staff by putting them with more senior, experienced workers and starting them off with very low loads—client loads, that is—and slowly building them up, letting them be exposed to all the educational programs we have or that come along. We have just found it easier than trying to attract staff from Melbourne or wherever you can get them from.[499]

Never enough time never enough money

Another issue is that of standardised service types and protocols. Turning Point states 'there is a consistent tension around the suitability of some standard service types for rural and regional settings' (2003, p.7). This was brought to the Committee's attention on numerous occasions, particularly with reference to the model of unit costing (structured in terms of 'episodes of care'). The requirement to renegotiate contracts annually was also a 'weakness' and an important issue for one Indigenous community with whom the Committee met:

---

497 Mr Jurgen Hemmerling, Open Family Victoria (Hume Region), evidence given to the Drugs and Crime Prevention Committee, Inquiry into Amphetamine and 'Party Drug' Use in Victoria, Public Hearings (Benalla), 22 October 2003.

498 Submission of the Open Family Victoria (Hume Region) to the Drugs and Crime Prevention Committee, Inquiry into Amphetamine and 'Party Drug' Use in Victoria, October 2003.

499 Mr Ron Marshall, evidence given to the Drugs and Crime Prevention Committee, Inquiry into Amphetamine and 'Party Drug' Use in Victoria, Public Hearings (Moe), 23 October 2003.

> [T]he rapport with the community has to be built all over again. Working with the Koori community... is about building up trust .[500]

Structures and levels of funding relating to the particular context of rural and regional service provision are a perennial issue arguably impacting on every aspect of service. There was a general consensus among representatives of drug and alcohol service providers that travel costs and time were not appropriately recognised by those dictating the terms. The representative for Open Family Victoria operating within the Hume region made this point well:

> There is very little recognition, I believe, from the government and the Department of Human Services in terms of what it actually costs to provide a service in the country. Our workers currently in the Hume region average 50,000 kilometres a year. Petrol costs in the country are higher. The travel time to 50,000 kilometres, if you are sitting on the speed limit, is a long time to be not as effective as you possibly could be. There is technological stuff as well. The computer systems and stuff that we are required to have to do the DHS reporting and other legal stuff has a two-year shelf life and then you have to upgrade it, and generally speaking that is not funded.[501]

Mr Frank Coughlan from the Latrobe Community Health Service in his evidence to the Committee echoed these comments:

> Where somebody in my position who works outreach can travel, in Melbourne they can go around the corner to see clients or obtain services. I will very often drive 300 kilometres a day to attend the clinics I do, so there are huge differences and we are funded on the same regime as Melbourne services...
>
> Our issues are really not recognised. There are things like travel, the kinds of services that we provide, episodes of care. Each CCCC counsellor is required to turn over 110 a year. That is the same for Melbourne as it is for rural. We do not have the capacity, as I said before, to see a client around the corner. We can travel 50 kilometres, 60 kilometres or 100 kilometres to see somebody who does not turn up. We do not get funded for the time involved with that. The Melbourne or city-centric approach does not work for country Victoria. I cannot speak for other regions, but I would say they are probably all saying the same sort of stuff.

Moreover, according to Mr Ron Marshall, funding of vehicles (which he believes to be inadequate) does not take into account times in which a worker may travel long distances into the country only to find the client has not kept his or her appointment:

---

500 Mr Rick Henderson, Acting Executive Officer, Central Gippsland Aboriginal Cooperative, evidence given to the Drugs and Crime Prevention Committee, Inquiry into Amphetamine and 'Party Drug' Use in Victoria, Public Hearings (Moe), 23 October 2003.

501 Mr Jurgen Hemmerling, Open Family Victoria (Hume Region), evidence given to the Drugs and Crime Prevention Committee, Inquiry into Amphetamine and 'Party Drug' Use in Victoria, Public Hearings (Benalla), 22 October 2003.

> [If] we travel all the way out there and all the way back and they have not been there, then it does not count. Later on you will hear me talking about the city-centric type focus; those things have never been addressed.
>
> The miles that we do, the distances, the time we waste – well, most of it is not wasted, but there can be a waste of time – are never allowed for in our funding. We receive exactly the same funding and targets as the city folk... The fact that a staff member might be asked to travel hours to see a client does not seem to be a possibility for policy makers: if a client does not show up, see the next one; but that next one is four hours away.[502]

Mr Jurgen Hemmerling argues that the 'tyranny of distance' is poorly understood by funding bodies:

> There is poor or limited recognition of the increased travel costs associated with service provision in rural Victoria. Whilst Open Family staff in Hume average 50,000km per annum, our city counterparts average 20,000km per annum. Then there is the added impost of higher fuel prices and wear and tear of motor vehicles. This is not reflected in funding allocations to rural services. Travelling time is also not factored into funding allocations. This makes the provision of services to rural Victorians more costly and generally is a limiting factor to potential and current service users.[503]

Further, a significant proportion of the drug and alcohol workers presenting to the Committee, as well as numerous submissions received by the Committee, expressed concern that services were largely 'reactive', rather than 'proactive'. More funding directed toward early intervention programs and drug and alcohol education initiatives were frequently recommended.

Service access and structural issues

Access to a comprehensive suite of drug and alcohol services, particularly to services requiring specialist and technical training and facilities, is often limited by rural and regional circumstances. Some of the structural factors mitigating against good service delivery in country areas were outlined in the submission to this Inquiry from the Goulburn Valley Community Health Service based in Shepparton:

> There are many structural or macro factors that contribute to alcohol and other drug use in this region. Currently in Shepparton there are no General Practitioners that offer a Bulk Billing service, and only two Methadone Prescribers who are actively involved in treating referred clients. This has huge implications for clients seeking withdrawal support, pharmacotherapies or

502 Mr Ron Marshall, evidence given to the Drugs and Crime Prevention Committee, Inquiry into Amphetamine and 'Party Drug' Use in Victoria, Public Hearings (Moe), 23 October 2003.

503 Submission of Open Family Victoria (Hume Region) to the Drugs and Crime Prevention Committee, Inquiry into Amphetamine and 'Party Drug' Use in Victoria, October 2003. Mr Hemmerling also comments that it is not uncommon for him to often drive young people to Melbourne in order to use withdrawal services and then pick them up and return them after this is completed (Evidence given to the Drugs and Crime Prevention Committee, Inquiry into Amphetamine and 'Party Drug' Use in Victoria, Public Hearings (Benalla), 22 October 2003).

> other treatment. A medical consultation in the Goulburn Valley can cost anywhere between $40 to $50 per visit.
>
> Currently Goulburn Valley Health A&E Department is not willing to provide an after hours NSP, and although funded for a Rural Withdrawal Support Program, have no staff member offering Withdrawal Support Services. This affects people's belief in a system where help is supposed to be readily available. Clients seeking withdrawal support are offered weekly counselling through GV Community Health or are assisted in accessing residential services in Melbourne or Wagga Wagga.
>
> There is an increased number of young people reporting to the service providers that (1) with the isolation and long distances required to attend clubs/pubs on a weekend, (2) the recent police crack down on drink driving, (3) the cost of a taxi is exorbitant for such distances, these factors combined leads young people to use alternative substances where detection from police is less likely and/or identifiable.[504]

Hours of operation

One issue precluding full client access to services as indicated in the preceding quote was restricted hours of operation. Based on feedback from a youth 'Speak Out' conference in Albury–Wodonga in September 2003, a representative related to the Committee that:

> Mainstream agencies shut at 5, they are not open on weekends, they are usually located on their own, and it becomes problematic for people to access them. People do not have problems between 9 and 5; they extend through a broader range of hours.[505]

Certainly the issue of after-hours access or lack thereof is one that comes up time and time again, in Melbourne as much as in the country. This is particularly pertinent to the issue of needle and syringe programmes. It is stated in a submission from Anex, the peak body for needle and syringe programmes in Victoria, that access to necessary preventative equipment such as clean needles and fits is severely limited after hours and on the weekends, particularly in the country.[506] According to Goulburn Valley Community Health Service, some communities such as Shepparton facilitate 'very active but unfunded Needle Syringe program[s]'.[507]

After-hours access was not the only issue that concerned young people at the Speak Out conference. Some of the reasons given as to why young people in particular can not or will not access services in rural areas include:

504 Submission of Goulburn Valley Community Health Service, Drugs and Crime Prevention Committee, Inquiry into Amphetamine and 'Party Drug' Use in Victoria, October 2003.

505 Mr Jurgen Hemmerling, Open Family Victoria (Hume Region), evidence given to the Drugs and Crime Prevention Committee, Inquiry into Amphetamine and 'Party Drug' Use in Victoria, Public Hearings (Benalla), 22 October 2003.

506 Submission of Anex to the Drugs and Crime Prevention Committee, Inquiry into Amphetamine and 'Party Drug' Use in Victoria, October 2003.

507 Submission of Goulburn Valley Community Health Service, Drugs and Crime Prevention Committee, Inquiry into Amphetamine and 'Party Drug' Use in Victoria, October 2003.

- Poor geographical location of agencies
- Unsuitable hours of operation
- No outreach services
- Too judgemental / lack youth friendliness
- Confidentiality concerns
- Lack of respect / poor attitudes to youth
- Lack of appropriate information / communication.[508]

Some of the possible solutions proposed by young people include:

- Training of reception and other agency staff
- Co-location with a non welfare agency
- Accessibility to 8pm and weekends
- More information presented to schools by agency workers
- Advertising of agency policies
- Adoption of a shared vision
- Transport provision.[509]

Some of these suggestions certainly deserve consideration.

Housing and unemployment

Another important issue that emerged at several junctures throughout the Inquiry was how housing and employment circumstances related to increased rates of substance abuse. The Research Paper from NDARC notes how:

> ...unemployment tends to cluster geographically, creating environmentally deprived neighbourhoods... [where such] concentrations of poverty and unemployment create a double burden for the poor (NDARC 2001, p.9).

And further:

> ...that people from low-SES groups, unemployed or underemployed, and the homeless are at much greater risk of substance abuse than the general population (NDARC 2001, p.9).

It was stated in a submission from the Goulburn Valley Community Health Service that:

> There is a lack of housing and a long waiting list for people wishing to access public housing. Homelessness is a common problem among problematic users, who often access Caravan Parks, Hotels and Motels as a last resort.[510]

Mr Jurgen Hemmerling from Open Family stresses what he sees as the crucial link between basic security needs or the lack thereof and problematic drug use:

---

508 Cited in the submission of Open Family Victoria (Hume Region) to the Drugs and Crime Prevention Committee, Inquiry into Amphetamine and 'Party Drug' Use in Victoria, October 2003.

509 Ibid.

510 Submission of Goulburn Valley Community Health Service to the Drugs and Crime Prevention Committee, Inquiry into Amphetamine and 'Party Drug' Use in Victoria, October 2003.

> [i]t is really hard to deal with someone's alcohol and drug issues if they have nowhere to live or if they have not eaten for three days. So there are some priority issues that obviously take place. The research will indicate that if people do not have safe and secure housing they will not do well regardless of what interventions you have. So that could be the priority issue and that might be the first thing we do: organise stable housing, get them a food voucher or take them out and get them a feed or whatever, and then look at the other stuff. Again that is part of developing a relationship and a commitment with the people that you work with.[511]

It certainly seems clear that the dynamics of service provision in rural and regional circumstances demand greater flexibility in adapting to the needs of individual and local communities.

Specialist versus generalist services

It would seem that most workers in the field (medical, youth, education, allied services) would prefer ideally to see well funded specialist drug and alcohol services in their regions. Such services should also be broken down into even more specialised areas such as youth drug services, women's drug health etc. A lack of specialist withdrawal services is particularly acute. Ms Johnson from the Central Hume Community Health Service states:

> I have been sending a lot of people to Melbourne recently. In some circumstances if people's problems are particularly complex I think they are best served in a specialist alcohol and drug facility rather than putting them in what are already stretched health services in general hospitals. So rather than putting nursing staff under undue pressure with somebody who is going to be going through what I would predict to be severe withdrawal I will send them down to Melbourne where I think they will get specialist treatment.[512]

In such cases, not only is the client is sent away from his or her family, friends and local community supports (if he or she has them) but is also put in a hospital environment, which may not be the ideal location for something as physically and emotionally draining as drug withdrawal.

> And particularly with youth. Putting a young person in a hospital to undergo withdrawal is not appropriate particularly. If there was a specialist set-up in the north-east it would need to have also a unit for older people and a unit for youth.[513]

---

511 Mr Jurgen Hemmerling, Open Family Victoria (Hume Region), evidence given to the Drugs and Crime Prevention Committee, Inquiry into Amphetamine and 'Party Drug' Use in Victoria, Public Hearings (Benella), 22 October 2003.

512 Ms Lynda Johnson, Central Hume Alcohol and other Drugs Service, evidence given to the Drugs and Crime Prevention Committee, Inquiry into Amphetamine and 'Party Drug' Use in Victoria, Public Hearings (Benalla), 22 October 2003.

513 Ms Rachael Meadows, Drug Diversion Worker, Central Hume Alcohol and Other Drugs Service, evidence given to the Drugs and Crime Prevention Committee, Inquiry into Amphetamine and 'Party Drug' Use in Victoria, Public Hearings (Benalla), 22 October 2003.

These concerns are echoed by Mr Jurgen Hemmerling:

> I think it is fair to say that within this region there are very limited services for people .... In terms of withdrawal services, no, there are not any locally. That is a concern. Last year one of our workers sent a young person from Yea to Melbourne because it is the only place to access services. Because of the escalation of risk factors – like Melbourne being a big city, having anonymity and more drugs being available – that person actually overdosed and died. So that is a concern for us.[514]

Mr Frank Coughlan, Latrobe Community Health Service, stresses the technical and highly specialised nature of much drug support work:

> I know we – and most services, to my knowledge – have trouble finding good withdrawal staff, good nurses who know toxicology and are able to engage in that particular area of medicine because it is a very specialised area. It can be very taxing on an individual. It is not like a regular ward nurse or a district nurse. They tackle a whole range of problems and it is not just the sickness side of it or the associated illnesses. There is behavioural stuff that goes with it, too. So it is difficult to find good people. When we get them, we tend to try and nail them.
>
> ...From a training aspect I would suggest that it would be a wonderful idea if we could have nurses and doctors trained at source, while they are doing their degree. This is another criticism: most of the GPs that I encounter know little about what we do, what is involved in drug treatment. Funding is always an issue, as you say. We need more money. We need more staff. We need to have Melbourne-centric ideas changed. This is not Melbourne. It is the country.

The submission from the Open Family agency, Wangaratta, also thought there was merit in 'upskilling' local doctors, and that this was sometimes the only choice available. Such an option, however, is not without its problems:

> It should be said, in the rural Victorian context, there is a lack of locally based withdrawal options, with the only residential facilities being available in Melbourne. There could be much to offer in terms of enlisting and upskilling local GPs to provide medical withdrawal interventions to their local communities. This can be a somewhat vexed issue, with rural GPs already being overworked and poorly compensated.
>
> If we mean to provide holistic services to the local population, then they need to be adequately resourced and compensated.[515]

As well as the problem of attracting staff, it is also difficult to find staff with appropriate skills, as expressed in the submission from Goulburn Valley Community Health Service:

514 Jurgen Hemmerling, Open Family Victoria (Hume Region), evidence given to the Drugs and Crime Prevention Committee, Inquiry into Amphetamine and 'Party Drug' Use in Victoria, Public Hearings (Benalla), 22 October 2003.

515 Submission of the Open Family Victoria (Hume Region) to the Drugs and Crime Prevention Committee, Inquiry into Amphetamine and 'Party Drug' Use in Victoria, October 2003.

> Habitual amphetamine users have many health problems, but often find mainstream, orthodox medical services forbidding, judgemental, inaccessible, costly or inappropriate to their needs. As well as this, many general practitioners and general health workers feel ill-equipped to deal with drug user issues, either due to a lack of sufficient support or through generally lacking the time and skills to appropriately address the complex needs of drug users.[516]

Workers from the Central Hume Alcohol and other Drugs Service state that a judgemental attitude by mainstream service providers can even extend to some hospitals refusing to admit drug-related cases who are characterised as 'time wasters'.[517] They also feel that specialists in the drug field not only have the technical skills but, for the most part, also the 'people skills' to effectively work with and understand what can often be a difficult population.

The reality of life in the country, however, is that many workers have to be specialists by default – jacks and jills of all trades by necessity if not by inclination:

> Folks who work in drug treatment in Melbourne or in very large regional cities tend to be specific in their job. They could be CCCC counsellors – that is, counselling, consultancy and continuing care. That is primarily their role. Most of us working in regions, such as I do, cover everything. For myself, I cover the one-on-one counselling, I do drug education in quite a number of schools around Wellington. I am involved with various parent support groups and codependent support groups because there is none of that. There is no funding for it. I run it my own way, just so that these people are [getting services]...
>
> We have areas where I can be covering forums with drug education with parents in schools. We cover a range of areas – involvement with admission of clients to withdrawal in hospital, which is something I do a lot of. Liaison with all the services in the region I work with is huge. It is not a specific role. It is a very generalised role but we have to know this stuff. We have to be involved with community services around the area, so we are looking at health, welfare and a whole range of other stuff that goes with it.[518]

Mr Ron Marshall agrees:

> The other major difference for our staff is that they very often have to provide a variety of other services for clients. I am thinking about CCCC workers, helping with accommodation or dealing with a relationship crisis, or even taking a baby to a doctor because there is no transport. They do all those sorts of things. I have come to the view that rural drug treatment services are really

---

516 Submission of the Goulburn Valley Community Health Service to the Drugs and Crime Prevention Committee, Inquiry into Amphetamine and 'Party Drug' Use in Victoria, October 2003.

517 Ms Lynda Johnson, Central Hume Alcohol and other Drugs Service, evidence given to the Drugs and Crime Prevention Committee, Inquiry into Amphetamine and 'Party Drug' Use in Victoria, Public Hearings (Benalla), 22 October 2003.

518 Mr Frank Coughlan, evidence given to the Drugs and Crime Prevention Committee, Inquiry into Amphetamine and 'Party Drug' Use in Victoria, Public Hearings (Moe), 23 October 2003.

> different than city based services – a different style of service. I think that has been acknowledged in the [Turning Point] service system review that has recently been done.[519]

Certainly drug workers in the regions recognise the importance of 'upskilling' general staff, particularly nurses and especially in the smaller towns and communities. However, it is thought that the training of generalist staff in drug issues should be complementary to rather than in substitution of specialist services:

> In lots of ways to skill up the general population of professional workers in hospitals and elsewhere is a really positive thing and I would continue to advocate that as a professional alcohol and other drug worker. We do a lot of work in upskilling general nurses in hospitals and in various other places in the community. I think that is a really important role we fulfil in trying to do that. This is not just an isolated alcohol and drug problem for specialist treatment services. I think this should in some ways be incorporated into generalist settings. But we are doing that when health services are quite stretched, as you probably already know. There is a significant shortfall in specialist services.[520]

One combination system that seems most promising is run through the Gippsland Withdrawal and Rehabilitation Service. Mr Ron Marshall from Latrobe Community Health Service explained the role of this programme to the Committee:

> The new Gippsland Withdrawal and Rehabilitation Service [is] a hospital based withdrawal service to overcome the problems of sending people to detox centres in Melbourne, the closest one being Dandenong, which takes them away from their family and friends. We have developed a program whereby they go to local hospitals for a short stay, four or five days. Then they are picked up by rehabilitation support workers for up to three months after that.
>
> [Withdrawal is done] in the hospital. After they come out they would go back to their homes. If that is not suitable, they might be referred to our supported accommodation program, which is our homes they are living in and intensely supported while there. We have one program at least that runs across the entire Gippsland region. That is the Mobile Drug Safety Worker project, basically an educational program relating to injecting drug users but also some practical assistance: clean supply of needles and syringes, advocating for public disposal bins and those sorts of things.[521]

Such a service is an example of innovation, creativity and adaptability being used to meet the realities of a poorly funded rural sector. A recent review of drug

519 Mr Ron Marshall, evidence given to the Drugs and Crime Prevention Committee, Inquiry into Amphetamine and 'Party Drug' Use in Victoria, Public Hearings (Moe), 23 October 2003.

520 Ms Lynda Johnson, Central Hume Alcohol and other Drugs Service, evidence given to the Drugs and Crime Prevention Committee, Inquiry into Amphetamine and 'Party Drug' Use in Victoria, Public Hearings (Benalla), 22 October 2003.

521 Mr Ron Marshall, Latrobe Community Health Service, evidence given to the Drugs and Crime Prevention Committee, Inquiry into Amphetamine and 'Party Drug' Use in Victoria, Public Hearings (Moe), 23 October 2003.

treatment and service delivery by Turning Point Alcohol and Drug Centre makes the salient point that such initiatives throughout rural Victoria need to be systematically supported, reviewed and developed where appropriate (2003, p.7). An integrated service system with cross-sectoral collaboration and co-operation between generalist services and specialist back-up is the ideal identified in the Victorian Government's Drug Policy Expert Committee Report – *Drugs: Meeting the Challenge* (2000c, see pp.109 ff.).

Anonymity and confidentiality

In addition to the necessity for long-distance travel and the lack of public transport options, the social dynamics particular to smaller communities, while often positive, could also be an obstacle in accessing services. Indeed, the 2001 'Rural and Regional Alcohol and Other Drugs Consultation Forums' noted generally:

> People in rural and regional areas tend to be reluctant to disclose their drug use… for fear of identification and stigmatisation (Australian National Council on Drugs 2001, p.7).

According to Mr Jurgen Hemmerling, the need for anonymity is particularly important for young people, especially in the drugs and mental health fields:

> The Child and Adolescent Mental Health Service does not provide an after-hours service. So what happens to young people after hours when they are suicidal or they present at accident and emergency? The adult mental health service has to see them through an initial assessment, and then they get fobbed off to someone else, someone else, and someone else. Young people do not do that. They are not socialised into accessing mainstream services. Older people are. If you want to go to the doctor, you know you have to sit in the waiting room and blah blah blah. Younger people find that too challenging. Who will walk up to a counter at age 15 – there is the counter about this high; it is all secure and all the rest of it – and say, 'I would like to see the alcohol and drugs person', or 'I would like to see the sexual health person'? It is too big an ask. Because we are also registered needle syringe exchange providers, I have also had the experience of going to a community health agency to get some Fit Packs – I am sure people know what they are. They kindly said, 'Who are you and where are you from?'. If they are going to ask an adult for their name, which they are not allowed to do, what will they do with kids and what will a kid do? Will they stay there and get clean stuff and use safely, or will they walk out and use dirty old gear or pick up whatever they can?[522]

By way of illustrating the difficulties of accessing drug services in small country towns, Mr Hemmerling refers to the case of a local community health service in the Hume Region:

522 Mr Jurgen Hemmerling, Open Family Victoria (Hume Region), evidence given to the Drugs and Crime Prevention Committee, Inquiry into Amphetamine and 'Party Drug' Use in Victoria, Public Hearings (Benalla), 22 October 2003.

> It is a beautiful purple and yellow building out in the middle of nowhere and not surrounded by anything. If you are walking up that long footpath you cannot be going anywhere else, and if you have any confidentiality concerns you will just not do it.[523]

The written submission from Open Family to this Inquiry posits a definite connection between users not accessing treatment and other services because of a perception that their anonymity will be compromised:

> [It] can be generally said that amphetamine and related stimulant users tend not to access treatment because their use, in their eyes, is largely non problematic. This is compounded in rural areas by the fear of breach of confidentiality (where the local nurse may be your neighbour) and the lack of treatment agencies to be able to effectively engage users. (Imagine, you want assistance with your problem, but you have to go to the agency down the road, where your neighbour works and then address the receptionist to state you want to see an alcohol and other drugs worker.) This in itself is daunting for most adults in rural Victoria and a nigh impossibility for young people.[524]

Workers in the country are clearly aware of the problems surrounding anonymity and confidentiality and do their utmost to safeguard their clients' identities, often going out of their way to meet clients in areas outside their local towns. Mr Frank Coughlan in Gippsland states:

> On a number of occasions I have had inquiries from clients who would like to access a service, but they may be living in a small town like Heyfield or Maffra or Yarram where they are fairly well known. These are small communities and fairly isolated. With any of the towns in this region, when you get outside the main centres you are looking at distance, so they are virtually little communities all on their own. I have had it said to me on a number of occasions by clients, 'Well, I don't want people to see me coming in here'. There is a certain amount of street cred that is going to be knocked around if they are seen walking into a drug treatment service.
>
> They are assured that confidentiality is paramount and we adhere to that all the way down the track. If I can, I will see them at another clinic and get them involved with that; if that is possible. How the youth workers go here I am not really sure because they are working in a specialised area... We will accommodate the best way we can and continue to try and bring people in, because drug use in these regions, for a number of reasons, is starting at earlier ages I think than Melbourne. That is something else that needs to be addressed.[525]

Workers from the Central Hume Alcohol and Other Drugs Service also use innovative methods to safeguard the identities of their clients:

---

523 Ibid.

524 Submission of Open Family Victoria (Hume Region) to the Drugs and Crime Prevention Committee, Inquiry into Amphetamine and 'Party Drug' Use in Victoria, October 2003.

525 Mr Frank Coughlan, evidence given to the Drugs and Crime Prevention Committee, Inquiry into Amphetamine and 'Party Drug' Use in Victoria, Public Hearings (Moe), 23 October 2003.

> ...I am particularly sensitive about [confidentiality] it. .. With the clients I always say, 'If I see you in the supermarket I will not greet you. It is not because I am being rude; it is just simply because people know that I am with the drug and alcohol service and they might ask you, "How do you know her?"'. That comes from my experience working with people around domestic violence and thinking about their safety. But I have people here who go, 'Oh, Elena, she is my welfare worker', or 'She is my drug and alcohol counsellor'. They are quite unfussed that people know they are accessing a service. People have different sensitivities about that.[526]

> We actually try to accommodate people as much as possible. Last week a lady said to me, 'I really don't want to ever see you on a Thursday because I go walking with the walking group and they meet outside the community health centre and I don't want to be seen walking into the community health centre'. So I will simply see her on another day. Sometimes it will be a matter of my saying to people, 'If you have transport would you like me to meet you in another town where people don't know you?'. We will accommodate that as much as possible, but it is not always possible.[527]

Mr Jurgen Hemmerling suggested that one way of addressing the problems associated with anonymity, or lack thereof, is to create 'one stop shops':

> I think there is a lot to be said for co-location with other services – perhaps even a one-stop shop where a range of services are provided as well as other things – like there might be a cafe in there, and things like that. That would make it not so obvious that you are going in there to get something dealt with. There have certainly been some services structured like that.

Ms Deb Heery of UHCHS cites outreach work as another important aspect of guarding privacy and confidentiality:

> We try to provide outreach as much as possible. We try to work with young people in environments that they are more comfortable with accessing. We work very closely with the Open Family street workers that are situated throughout the Hume region and with other youth-specific services – the City of Wodonga, youth services, Central Hume support services and other key youth services in our area. We work closely with them and can actually go to other services to see young people if they do not feel comfortable coming to us. That is definitely the case in the smaller towns. We do have offices in a lot of the smaller towns around the Upper Hume region, but often we do home visits or meet at local cafes or parks.[528]

---

526 Ms Elena Tauridsky, evidence given to the Drugs and Crime Prevention Committee, Inquiry into Amphetamine and 'Party Drug' Use in Victoria, Public Hearings (Benalla), 22 October 2003.

527 Ms Lynda Johnson, evidence given to the Drugs and Crime Prevention Committee, Inquiry into Amphetamine and 'Party Drug' Use in Victoria, Public Hearings (Benalla), 22 October 2003.

528 Ms Deb Heery, Upper Hume Community Health Service, evidence given to the Drugs and Crime Prevention Committee, Inquiry into Amphetamine and 'Party Drug' Use in Victoria, Public Hearings (Benalla), 22 October 2003.

Outreach models where the worker meets the client on their own 'territory' can clearly be positive ways of protecting a client's confidentiality.

Dr Brough from ARCAB, based in Warrnambool, also has some ideas about how to address the need for anonymity of his clients:

> Again, why we think an organisation like ARCAB is important relates to being able to extract the particular rural issues and look at rural solutions for them in a particular way – for example, one of the things that we are very keen to pilot is a self-help service run through a telephone conferencing system. The need for something like that grows out of the issues that are associated with rural communities, and this gets back to the sort of things you are talking about with rural young people where anonymity is a real issue. If they attend a self-help meeting even in a city the size of Warrnambool the next-door neighbour, their mum and everybody else is going to find out about it even if they have left home and are living independently. Trying to establish self-help groups for people, particularly with illicit drug problems, is a problem partly because of the issues of anonymity but it is also an issue in terms of not being able to have enough people with enough clean time to be role models, to be the infrastructure supporting the group. So we see a real place for self-help groups in supporting people in their efforts to give up drugs, but they are the sort of services that are basically denied people in rural communities by virtue of the anonymity issue and the lack of numbers in any one geographical location.
>
> They are the sorts of proposals and innovative ideas that we think are going to come from people in the bush because we live with the problems day and night, we are thinking about them and trying to solve them on an individual patient and client basis day in, day out, and they are the sort of reasons why we think an organisation like the Australian Rural Centre for Addictive Behaviours is important.[529]

Reversing Melbourne-centric policy?

> It is unfortunate that we tend not to see policy-makers coming to the rural areas. It is something that we really need... We need to have senior policy makers, the people who are actually dictating our terms, coming and talking to troops on the ground. They need to come and talk with me and my colleague in Sale, with the guys in the withdrawal service, with the home withdrawal nurses, with youth outreach workers to see what it is we do and how they can best help us to do our jobs better.[530]

While this Committee has not travelled to every rural region in the state, it has endeavoured to contact and meet with a cross-section of representatives in the

529 Dr Rodger Brough, ARCAB, evidence given to the Drugs and Crime Prevention Committee, Inquiry into Amphetamine and 'Party Drug' Use in Victoria, Public Hearings (Melbourne), 6 October 2003.

530 Mr Frank Coughlan, Drug and Alcohol Clinician, evidence given to the Drugs and Crime Prevention Committee, Inquiry into Amphetamine and 'Party Drug' Use in Victoria, Public Hearings (Moe), 23 October 2003.

major regions of Victoria. Without exception, the refrain of workers in the area of drug, alcohol, youth and health policy has been that policy which impacts upon their work and their services is 'Melbourne-centric'. A selection of quotes taken from both written submissions and verbal presentations to this Inquiry is testament to this belief:

> The 'statewide' system of service delivery does not take into account local regional needs. As stated before, it appears that drug treatment services and resources are tailored for 'what is happening in Melbourne' which doesn't necessarily reflect the local picture.
>
> Amphetamines have been a popular drug of choice for people in this region for many years, yet statewide services and resources have not identified this as an issue.
>
> Residential services have been 'cost effectively' based in metropolitan regions but this does not provide for the physical and emotional needs of rural people at very vulnerable times in their lives (Upper Hume Community Health Service – Wodonga and environs).[531]

From Shepparton:

> If regional workers want to attend training in relation to working with this clientele, they usually have to travel three hours each way to Melbourne, where Service Providers Conferences and Professional Development is located. This also means a worker is away from the agency for a full day, in contrast to Melbourne based workers (Goulburn Valley Community Health Service).[532]

Dr Brough of ARCAB, based in Warrnambool, endorses such a view:

> The particular thoughts behind the Australian Rural Centre for Addictive Behaviours were very clearly based on the issues that occur in rural Victoria. What we see is that people in the big cities understand what the issues are. They understand the tyranny of distance and isolation and all these other sorts of things but when it comes to translating those ideas into applications of policy and applications of service models and what have you, there is often a gap between the understanding of the issues and the application of the detail of the programs and services.
>
> There does not seem to be a good linking though between the people who are proposing and advocating the models on the one hand and the people at the grassroots in the local communities who are in a position to be able to implement most effectively the model or the program, and that is where I think it is not happening, certainly not in the alcohol and drug and associated areas. We see this in program delivery, we see it in research where people from

531 Submission of Upper Hume Community Health Service (UHCHS) Wodonga to the Drugs and Crime Prevention Committee, Inquiry into Amphetamine and 'Party Drug' Use in Victoria, 21 October 2003.

532 Submission of the Goulburn Valley Community Health Service to the Drugs and Crime Prevention Committee, Inquiry into Amphetamine and 'Party Drug' Use in Victoria, October 2003.

> Melbourne come into an area for a day. They will whip down, want to meet all the right people and do all the right things and then go back; and it does not work like that. You have to have local people working over time with them to develop the links. It just does not happen. It is not the way it works. It should, but it does not work that way.
>
> ...I guess the other thing we think is important is that we need some sort of a reasonable study of issues in rural and regional areas that start to pick up some of the finer issues that relate to the different cultures, the different prevalence of different drug problems in different areas, the particular reason why certain models of service delivery may not be appropriate in one area but are relevant in another area. You cannot look in rural areas at putting the same service model into exactly the same situation. You need to modify it to local conditions and the local skills of the local people in the area. There are a whole lot of things that you need to take into account. We really think that some sort of study specifically looking at rural and regional areas is overdue and very much needed.[533]

Mr Ron Marshall agrees:

> We have DHS in Melbourne designing drug policy and we agree that policy is often written in the context of city based services. That is understandable because the policy-makers are down there. There appears to be very little understanding of the context, the patterns of use and the way treatment services work in rural areas, the huge distances we cover...
>
> I would love the policy-makers to come down and actually spend a day driving around in a car. It is really interesting. Some of the policy-makers that do come down tell us how early they have had to leave and how they got lost and they could not find the place and it is such a big area, and we say, 'Well, that's what we deal with every day'.[534]

The consensus seems to be that rural based services and their workers should have more input into policy development and be closely involved at policy-making level.[535] This does not necessarily mean making a costly trip to Melbourne:

> I think having rural representatives in policy decision-making procedures, in looking at developing guidelines and other issues, is just so valuable because often I think there can be rural-centric issues that are not necessarily identified by workers and others living in Melbourne. So having a voice and being invited

533 Dr Rodger Brough, ARCAB, evidence given to the Drugs and Crime Prevention Committee, Inquiry into Amphetamine and 'Party Drug' Use in Victoria, Public Hearings (Melbourne), 6 October 2003.

534 Mr Ron Marshall, Latrobe Community Health Service, evidence given to the Drugs and Crime Prevention Committee, Inquiry into Amphetamine and 'Party Drug' Use in Victoria, Public Hearings (Moe), 23 October 2003.

535 A positive step forward is the fact that Ms Elena Tauridsky, Manager with the Central Hume Drugs and Alcohol Service, with whom the Committee met, has recently been invited to sit as the only rural member of the Department of Human Services Work Force Development Sub Committee of the Drugs and Policy Unit.

> to actively participate in groups would be valuable. The world is becoming so much smaller and smaller now with our new technology; we do not have to have the face-to-face meetings. It is really not realistic for a lot of rural workers to have to travel to Melbourne for just a 1-hour hour meeting; it is not very time effective. Teleconferencing, email and those sorts of things are now bringing us much closer together and making us more accessible, so I do not think there is any reason why rural voices should not be heard.[536]

The challenge is to think outside the square about ways in which rural organisations and rural workers can have *real* input into policy development and policy-making structures without sacrificing valuable time away from the field.

Conclusion

This chapter has not been easy to write. The lack of literature specific to illicit drug use and misuse, and particularly amphetamine use, has been discussed above. This has meant much of what has been presented here has been constituted around seasoned and incisive input from representatives of rural and regional communities throughout Victoria. There have been many references to 'anecdotal evidence' which unfortunately remain unsubstantiated by formal or comprehensive research programmes.

Some of the most relevant and enlightening information has been supplied by rural and regional community health providers. These services have frequently made the point that their records and knowledge of drug use patterns in specific regions is limited to some degree to clients who formally *access* the respective service system. The evidence, therefore, does not account for individuals too remote to access an appropriate service or who choose, even if their drug use is problematic, not to access formal treatment or support.

The variability and complexities of drug use throughout rural and regional Victorian communities clearly requires acknowledgment, further research and prevention and treatment strategies that are informed by people with appropriate training and knowledge – of both amphetamine and amphetamine-type substances as well as the diverse cultural and environmental contexts in which they are used.

The following recommendations therefore reflect the essential need to incorporate the views and participation of rural and regional based workers, users and local community members in the development of state-wide alcohol and drug policies and services. Such an approach empowers rural and regional communities to develop locally specific responses.

536 Ms Deb Heery, Upper Hume Community Health Service, evidence given to the Drugs and Crime Prevention Committee, Inquiry into Amphetamine and 'Party Drug' Use in Victoria, Public Hearings (Benalla), 22 October 2003.

Recommendations

10. The Committee recommends that a specific Rural and Regional Drug Strategy be developed and implemented by Human Services Victoria in collaboration with the Australian Rural Centre for Addictive Behaviours and other relevant rural and regional based agencies and workers.

11. The Committee recommends that such a Strategy should provide a 'continuum of response' from prevention, early intervention, treatment and rehabilitation for rural and regional Victorians.

12. The Committee recommends that consideration be given to the establishment of specialist drug withdrawal, treatment and residential rehabilitation services in major regional centres, especially for young people.

13. The Committee recognises the importance of research into rural and regional alcohol and drug use issues by local researchers. The Committee therefore recommends the establishment of a Rural and Regional Drug Research and Information Institute to be attached to the Australian Rural Centre for Addictive Behaviours based in Warrnambool, Victoria. Such an Institute should collect and disseminate rural and regional data with regard to alcohol and drug use and undertake quantitative, qualitative, social and evaluative research. Such research will inform drug policy and practice to benefit rural and regional communities.

14. The Committee recommends that the Rural and Regional Drug Strategy and the Rural and Regional Drug Research Institute be evaluated after the initial three-year period of operation.

15. The Committee recommends that the Rural and Regional Drug Strategy, the Australian Rural Centre for Addictive Behaviours (ARCAB) and the Rural and Regional Drug Research Institute be adequately funded.

16. The Committee recognises that a considerable amount of rural and regional workers' time is spent in travelling long distances between the home agency and clients or service providers within their region. Additionally, it is acknowledged that workers may need on occasion to travel to Melbourne to attend meetings, training sessions and other work-related commitments. The Committee therefore recommends that any funding of rural alcohol and drug services should provide an adequate amount of specifically allocated funding for travel and training. Staffing levels should also take into consideration the absence of workers and the lost time through travel.

17. The Committee recommends that the state Minister for Health propose to the Australian Health Ministers' Council that the federal government give consideration to providing incentives to attract and retain adequately trained and experienced staff in the alcohol and drug area in rural and regional Victoria.

18. The Committee recommends that rural and regional representatives be included in all policy and decision making procedures in relation to alcohol and drug issues in Victoria. This should include but not be restricted to membership of relevant policy making committees and decision making bodies. Wherever practicable, such participation should be facilitated via technology that enables the worker or staff person to contribute from their home base.

19. The Committee recommends that further investigation and evaluation be undertaken into the desirability and effectiveness of relocating people with drug-related problems from Melbourne to rural and regional Victoria to access services that are already over-stretched.

PART E: Law, Law Enforcement, Policing and Supply Control

> *In describing the challenges that face all who are part of the process of containment and control of Amphetamine Type Substance use, the UNDCP [use] unusually forceful language: 'it is their flexibility which makes synthetic drugs so attractive and suitable for situations of changing trends and fashion and, at the same time, a nightmare for law enforcement and forensic chemists'* (UNDCP quoted in Klee 2001c, p.170).

It is axiomatic to state that the abuse of drugs, both licit and illicit is an international phenomenon crossing geographic, economic, social and cultural boundaries. Licit drugs, however, such as alcohol and tobacco are subject to importation controls, licensing and other international regulatory mechanisms. Illicit drugs are by their very nature only subject to the informal rules of the black market or crime syndicates – the pseudo 'licensing authorities'.

Clearly the international nature of the drug trade requires responses that, at least in part, are drawn from collaborative efforts at international level and through international and national agencies. The resources of state and local police forces can then be used to deal with problems that arise at local level.

This Part examines a variety of issues that impact upon the way the legal and criminal justice systems deal with the issue of amphetamines and 'party drugs'. It has as its underlying theme the importance of all tiers of law enforcement – global, national and local – working collaboratively and constructively to address the problems associated with amphetamines and 'party drugs', whether imported from abroad or manufactured within this country's borders.

The first chapter in the Part, Chapter 12, contains a brief discussion of the law, both domestic and international, as it applies to these drugs.

Chapter 13 examines the international and domestic supply control of amphetamines and 'party drugs'. Chapter 14 looks closely at the manufacture of amphetamines and 'party drugs' at both domestic and international levels. In particular, it focusses on the dangers faced by law enforcement officers who investigate clandestine laboratories and local communities in which such laboratories may be located.

Chapter 15 discusses a particular issue that encompasses both manufacture and supply issues, namely the difficulties associated with precursor control. In doing so, it examines both the importation of precursor chemicals, their wholesale supply and, at a domestic level, the role that pharmacies and retail chemists play in curtailing the use of precursors for the manufacture of illicit drugs.

Chapter 16 moves away from the supply or manufacture of amphetamines and 'party drugs' to the issues surrounding the distribution of the drugs once they are in Australia. In particular, it concentrates on the macro distribution of amphetamines.

The local level distribution of 'party drugs' is discussed in Chapter 17. In this chapter, the emphasis moves from a discussion of 'macro' issues pertaining to law enforcement to an examination of the problems police face in policing amphetamines and 'party drugs' at a local level. In particular, it examines the issues surrounding the use of law enforcement in Victorian nightclubs.

12. The Law Pertaining to Amphetamines and 'Party Drugs'

> Modern drug laws are primarily directed against 'profit' [derived from trafficking and organized crime] while 'pathology' [the view of drug users as persons requiring treatment rather than punishment] supports strategies of harm minimisation and decriminalisation... What is strikingly absent from the debate about drugs...is the discourse of 'pleasure'. Adopting this perspective reveals that law and legal regulation, though not necessarily the criminal law, has a significant role to play in controlling the markets for these pleasurable commodities [including licit drugs] that involve risks to consumers (Bronitt & McSherry 2001, p.877).

> *Extrapolating from the current rates of escalation in drug-related crime, the next 10 years will either see measures of decriminalisation put in place or the preponderance of the resources of the criminal justice system devoted to drug offenders (Alldridge 2000, p.199).*

> Criminal lawyers, who see the human face of those caught up in the law concerning illegal drug use have an obligation to bring what they see to the notice of their fellow citizens who may have more confidence than is warranted in the capacity of criminal law and punishment to deliver results (His Honour, Justice Michael Kirby, High Court of Australia 1999, p.273).

> *It is important to recognise that the prohibition of certain drugs did not occur as a response to the perceived risk of addiction or dangers to public health. Mugford has observed that the status of a particular drug as licit or illicit has more to do with a range of economic, political and cultural factors than a rational appraisal of its potential harm. Legal discussion of drug offences, including options for reform often proceeds without appreciation of the historical forces that have shaped Australia's drug laws* (Bronitt & McSherry 2001, p.830).

Introduction

This chapter examines a variety of issues that impact upon the way the legal and criminal justice systems deal with the issue of amphetamines and 'party drugs'. As indicated in the diverse quotes that introduce this chapter, there are clearly conflicting and contradictory positions on the role the 'law' should play in addressing the use and abuse of illicit drugs.

When it comes to amphetamines and 'party drugs' and indeed drugs generally, Webb (2003) argues there is a 'legal myopia':

> Most materials relate to health, treatment and education issues. Legal analysis has been neglected, possibly because of the view that it is 'essentially uncomplicated and, in any case, traditionally set in the prohibitionist mode' (p.80).

Certainly, the framework with regard to illicit drugs in all Australian states is for the most part prohibitionist to greater or lesser degrees depending on the drug in question. However, rarely in considering drug law is:

> [a]ttention paid to broader policy questions such as: the rationale or justification for criminalisation; the historical evolution of drug laws; the relationship of criminalisation to other regulatory strategies; and options for law reform (Bronitt & McSherry 2001, p.816).

This chapter does not present a criminological thesis on the law as it applies to amphetamines and 'party drugs'. However, it does note that it is important to bear in mind the historical and social context in which current laws apply. For example, as noted in Chapter 4, MDMA was originally viewed by a substantial sector of the psychiatry profession as a legitimate therapeutic tool. Amphetamines had (and still have) multiple functional uses. It is against this background of 'purposive use' that some quite heated debates ensued with regard to the international prescription of these drugs.[537] This section will commence with a brief examination of the main international provisions that Australia has incorporated into its domestic laws by virtue of being a signatory to various treaties and global conventions.

International provisions

International law pertaining to the control of illicit drugs, including amphetamines and MDMA/ecstasy is governed by a number of conventions to which Australia is a signatory. These include:

- The United Nations Single Convention on Narcotic Drugs (1961);
- The United Nations Convention on Psychotropic Substances (1971); and
- The United Nations Convention Against Illicit Traffic in Narcotic Drugs and Psychotropic Substances (1988).[538]

---

537 For a comprehensive account of the history and development of Australia's drug laws, see Norberry 1997.

538 These various conventions are summarised by the Australian Institute of Criminology as follows:

'The Single Convention on Narcotic Drugs (1961)

This Convention aims to combat drug abuse by coordinated international action. There are two forms of intervention and control that work together. First, it seeks to limit the possession, use, trade, distribution, import, export, manufacture and production of drugs

Subject to the 1971 convention, drugs are scheduled depending on their public health risk or therapeutic potential. Four schedules classify the drugs, with those in Schedule One having the greatest public health risk and those in Schedule Four having the most therapeutic potential.

Schedule One drugs are generally outlawed for general consumption. Amphetamines and 'party drugs' are usually placed in the first schedule. Schedule Four drugs, however, because of their perceived therapeutic benefits, will often be available under licence or prescription. The proscription of MDMA provides a useful case study of how the system operates.

In 1984 the World Health Organisation sought information about a group of amphetamine type substances including MDMA in preparation for a scheduling hearing of the Convention on Psychotropic Substances. In 1985 the International Expert Committee on Drug Dependence recommended that MDMA be placed in Schedule One, arguably after much pressure from the United States. MDMA was duly placed in that schedule in February 1986 (see Holland 2001). Webb notes, however, that the then Chairperson of the Expert Committee, Professor Paul Groff, disagreed with the recommendation and the scheduling, 'noting "the substance's potential therapeutic usefulness" while maintaining that 'international control is not warranted"' (Webb 2003, p.95).

Once a drug is placed on the Convention's schedule, signatories to the convention then adopt these schedules and their content in their own domestic legislation. In Australia, MDMA first made an appearance in the mid-1980s. The first police/customs seizure of MDMA was in June 1986. However, after forensic analysis NSW Police realised that at this time MDMA was not a prohibited drug at either national or state level. Despite being a signatory to the Convention, Australia had not as yet passed domestic legislation incorporating the scheduling of MDMA. Webb outlines the process subsequent to this discovery:

> The chemical was placed on the agenda of the National Drugs and Poisons Schedule Committee (DPSC) which classifies substances for inclusion in the

---

exclusively for medical purposes. Second, it combats drug trafficking through international cooperation to deter and discourage drug traffickers. The 1975 Protocol Amending the Single Convention on Narcotic Drugs highlights the need for treatment and rehabilitation of drug addicts. As of 1999, 168 States are parties to the Single Convention or are parties to the Convention as amended by the 1972 Protocol.

The Convention on Psychotropic Substances (1971)

This Convention establishes an international control system for psychotropic substances. It responded to the diversification and expansion of the spectrum of drugs of abuse and introduced controls over a number of synthetic drugs according to their abuse potential on the one hand and their therapeutic value on the other. As of 1999, 159 States were parties to the Convention.

United Nations Convention Against Illicit Traffic in Narcotic Drugs and Psychotropic Substances (1988)

This Convention provides comprehensive measures against drug trafficking, including provisions against money laundering and the diversion of precursor chemicals. It provides for international cooperation through, for example, extradition of drug traffickers, controlled deliveries and transfer of proceedings. As of 1999, 153 States were parties to the Convention (Australian Institute of Criminology 2003, to be found at the AIC's Illicit Drug website: http://www.aic.gov.au/research/drugs/context/international.html).

> relevant Acts of each state and territory. Although not legally binding, its recommendations are 'presented with a view to promoting uniform scheduling of substances throughout Australia'. The DPSC considered MDMA at its forty-second meeting held on 14–15 August 1986. With drug data almost non existent, the decision was made on the basis of two pieces of information. First, the United States had placed MDMA in Schedule 1 of [the Federal *Controlled Substances Act 1970* US]. Second, the WHO had earlier that year added MDMA to Schedule 1 of the Convention on Psychotropic Substances. Conforming to the international trend, the DPSC recommended that the drug be prohibited in Australia (Webb 2003, p.96).

According to Mr Sandeep Chawla, Senior Research Coordinator with the United Nations Drug Control Programme (UNCDP), the international scheduling system referred to above is far from ideal:

> The present control system...is simply inadequate for controlling illicit markets...[t]he scheduling process is slow and cumbersome; individual substances rather than chemically, or pharmacologically-related classes of drugs, are put under control. New individual substances with no therapeutic potential, structurally different though pharmacologically similar (the ATS analogues) perpetually appear on illicit markets. They cannot be scheduled fast enough. The control regime is thus bound to lag behind illicit innovation (Chawla 1998, p.35).

Of particular importance in the area of amphetamines and amphetamine manufacture is the last mentioned of these United Nations conventions. Subject to the Convention Against Illicit Traffic in Narcotic Drugs and Psychotropic Substances, an international control regime has been established to prevent precursor chemicals being used to make illicit amphetamines. Such chemicals may include diversions of licit pharmaceuticals or chemicals used in industry, but Chawla is equally sceptical about the effectiveness of these measures in preventing the manufacture of illicit drugs:

> Controlling the supply of synthetic drugs is difficult, because there are neither any easily identifiable botanical raw materials to target nor any long trafficking routes linking production and consumption areas to interdict... The precursor control regime is still young... In any case, it is not feasible to put all possible precursors for amphetamine type stimulants under international control because they have a vast amount of licit industrial uses (Chawla 1998, p.35).

Similar reservations have been expressed in Australia:

> Internationally, the success or otherwise of these strategies will depend on the number of countries which participate in them and the level of control exercised. A major problem with such regulatory regimes is that they are administratively burdensome to implement. There are many companies involved in the commerce of precursors and the chemicals themselves cannot be restricted too much because they are essential to many legitimate manufacturing processes. This means that some countries will not have the

> regulatory infrastructure or the financial resources necessary to conduct an effective level of supervision. The complexity of the system also allows for numerous loopholes to be exploited. Finally, some nations are not concerned enough about the problem or convinced of the efficacy of this approach to ensure their commitment (Wardlaw 1993, pp.96–97).

Legal control through the scheduling of specifically named designer drugs is slow and cumbersome 'in a quickly changing and flexible market' (Klee 1997 p.309). A positive step forward utilised in many jurisdictions has been the listing and proscription of precursors and other substances listed in generic forms in combination with regular monitoring and updating. As Klee comments, however, 'it will take some time for less well developed countries to acquire the administrative infrastructure to apply them effectively' (Klee 1997, p.309).[539]

This form of 'fast track legal proscription' is, however, not without its critics:

> The frontiers of modern drug laws are highly sensitive to drug markets and the emergence of new 'recreational' drugs. Rather than enact specific offences to deal with particular substances, omnibus provisions such as [s.233B(1) of the [Australian *Customs Act*] criminalise prohibited *categories* of drug. These categories, such as *'prohibited import or narcotic drug'*, are then defined in schedules appended to the drug offences. The use of regulations permits drug offences to be amended rapidly without the need to redraft the Principal Act. Indeed, the [Australian] Model Criminal Code Officers Committee (MCCOC) recommended that drug tables should not be included in legislation but should be located in regulations: Chapter 6 – *Serious Drug Offence: Report* (1998), p.23. Although acknowledging that legislating new offences by regulation was undesirable in terms of criminal law principles (as they are less visible to the public and by-pass direct parliamentary scrutiny), this development was 'practically unavoidable' because of the need to amend drug laws quickly in response to emerging threats. The MCCOC stated (p.21) 'recent problems with a sudden surge in the supply of GHB or "fantasy" in Queensland and the scramble in all jurisdictions to add the drug to their tables is an example of this'.
>
> The ease with which new drugs (which share no common pharmacological characteristics) are prohibited, by-passes the opportunity for informed debate within the community about the danger of such drugs, or the positive and negative effects of prohibition (Bronitt & McSherry 2001, p.845).

Subject to the international conventions, the Commonwealth has enacted the *Crimes (Traffic in Narcotic Drugs and Psychotropic Substances) Act 1990*.[540]

539 Further discussion with regard to precursor control is found in Chapter 15.

540 This will be discussed below under the section pertaining to federal law.

Domestic law

Australian law concerning drugs is divided between state and federal jurisdictions. The relevant federal legislation is the *Customs Act 1901*. There is further scope for the Commonwealth to enact laws with regard to drugs and drug policy pursuant to its external affairs power in Section 51 (xxix) of the Australian Constitution and, as has been discussed above, its concomitant obligations under international conventions to which it is a signatory. In Victoria, most state drug provisions and penalties are found in the *Drugs, Poisons and Controlled Substances Act 1981* (as amended). Should a state enact a drug-related law that the Commonwealth considered breached its international obligations, that law could be rendered invalid under Section 109 of the Constitution.[541]

Subject to the United Nations treaties outlined above, particularly the Convention Against Illicit Traffic in Narcotic Drugs and Psychotropic Substances, amphetamine, amphetamine analogues and derivatives and most 'party drugs', including methylenedioxy-methamphetamine (MDMA or ecstasy), have been scheduled as prohibited drugs under domestic legislation.[542]

Federal law

Customs Act 1901

The most important criminal offences under federal law are those found in section 233B of the *Customs Act*. This section prohibits the importation of certain goods, including 'narcotic goods'. Narcotic goods are listed in Column A of Schedule Six and include cocaine, codeine, heroin, MDMA, LSD, methamphetamine and analogues or derivatives of these drugs.[543]

There are also offences relating to aiding and abetting importation (and exportation) of (narcotic) goods and conspiring with another person to so import (or export). It should be noted that with regard to these provisions there is a *reverse onus of proof*. Once certain matters of proof are led by the prosecution, particularly that the accused knew or was aware of the existence of the goods brought into Australia and in his or her possession, the accused then has to prove his or her innocence on the balance of probabilities.[544]

There is no specific provision for *trafficking* per se in the Customs Act. Rather, 'What it does instead is to provide heavier penalties for people convicted of being in possession of stated quantities of a drug (thus inferring trafficking)' (Smith 2002, p.614).

541 Sec 109 states:

'When a law of a State is inconsistent with a law of the Commonwealth, the latter shall prevail, and the former shall, to the extent of the inconsistency, be invalid'.

542 For Victoria, see Schedule Eleven of the *Drugs, Poisons and Controlled Substances Act 1981*.

543 Schedule Six of the *Customs Act* is reproduced as Table E in Appendix 15.

544 For a discussion of the defences available to the defendant, see Smith 2002.

Penalties for importation or putative 'trafficking' are found in Section 235. This section creates a set of 'sentencing ranges' depending on a number of variables, including the amount of the drug seized.

If both prosecution and defence agree, the matter may be heard summarily in a Magistrate's Court where the maximum penalty imposed is $2000 or two years' imprisonment (Section 235(7)). Otherwise the trial will proceed by indictment in the County Court where the penalties are much higher.

Penalties are prescribed depending on whether the amount in question is less than a *trafficable quantity*, a *trafficable quantity* or a *commercial quantity*. These quantities for each particular type of drug are listed in the Sixth Schedule of the Act.

If the amount is less than a *trafficable quantity* the maximum penalty is $2000 and/or two years' imprisonment. A *trafficable quantity* of drugs, other than cannabis, incurs maximum penalties of $100,000 or ten years' imprisonment or both, unless the defendant has prior convictions for possessing trafficable quantities in which case the penalties are greater.[545] If the defendant has no prior convictions for offences relating to trafficable quantities *and* the court is satisfied the trafficable quantity is *not* related to any *commercial dealing* then the maximum penalty shall only be $2000 and/or two years' imprisonment.

Finally, a person may be charged with importation of a *commercial quantity* as specified in the Sixth Schedule of the Act for each drug. A defendant charged with being in possession of, or any other offence concerning this quantity of drug, is liable to a maximum sentence of life imprisonment or such sentence as the court deems appropriate.

Crimes (Traffic in Narcotic Drugs and Psychotropic Substances) Act 1990

As stated above, the Commonwealth has enacted the *Crimes (Traffic in Narcotic Drugs and Psychotropic Substances) Act 1990* pursuant to its obligations under United Nations drug treaties. This Act needs to be read in conjunction with the Customs Act. This Act is wider in scope than the importation of drugs, although it does include such provisions. Its main offences concern 'dealing in drugs' (Section 6). It covers the possession of equipment (for example laboratory equipment used to synthesise drugs); the manufacture, extraction, preparation, distribution or transportation of narcotics and psychotropic substances; and the sale, supply or possession of narcotic drugs or psychotropic substances.

Different penalties apply to the act engaged in (for example, extraction, manufacture, separation etc) and the quantities involved. As with the Customs Act, penalties vary depending on whether amounts are *trafficable* or *commercial* with the latter attracting more serious penalties.

545 In such circumstances, the court may impose a penalty of life imprisonment. See Sec 235(2)(c).

Victorian law

Laws pertaining to use, possession and trafficking

The Victorian *Drugs, Poisons and Controlled Substances Act 1981* covers mostly drug offences occurring within the jurisdictional boundaries of Victoria. These include offences pertaining to:

- Use
- Possession
- Cultivation[546]
- Trafficking.

Use

The use of a drug of dependence other than cannabis provides for a maximum penalty of $3000 or imprisonment of one year or both (Section 75(b) *Drugs, Poisons and Controlled Substances Act 1981*). A variety of diversion programmes are available for people charged with non-violent drugs offences who can show that they have a 'drug problem'. These include the Court Referral and Evaluation for Drug Intervention and Treatment program (CREDIT) and Drug Treatment Orders under the new Drug Courts. A discussion of these programmes is beyond the scope of this Paper (for further information, see Smith 2002).

A representative from Anex, the peak body for needle and syringe programmes in Australia, stated in a submission to the Committee that while Section 75 does not make the possession of a syringe or needle per se illegal, such possession can be used as evidence of contravention of that section – that is, using an illegal drug:

> Fearing that they will be arrested or questioned by police, safe disposal may be problematic for users as it involves carrying incriminating evidence to a disposal point. The implications are that people using drugs were more likely to inject hurriedly and dispose of injecting equipment inappropriately, thereby contributing to the amount of syringe litter.
>
> The possession of a needle or syringe ought to be insufficient grounds on its own to establish reasonable grounds to search a person. On most occasions it may be in the greater public interest for police members to use their discretion to overlook minor use and possession offences and take no further action.[547]

Possession

Possession is an indictable offence under Section 73 of the Act. Smith explains the relevant law as follows:

> Under common law, a person is in possession of a drug if he or she has physical control or custody of the drug to the exclusion of others not acting with the

546 As cultivation is not applicable to amphetamines and 'party drugs' these laws will not be discussed.

547 Submission of Anex to the Drugs and Crime Prevention Committee, Inquiry into Amphetamine and 'Party Drug' Use in Victoria, October 2003.

person. The prosecution must prove knowledge by the person of the presence of the drug and an intention by the person to possess the drug. In many cases, custody of a drug may supply sufficient evidence of possession, including the necessary mental element. This is because the inference of knowledge may often be drawn from the surrounding circumstances.

As well as its common law meaning, possession has an extended meaning under the *Drugs, Poisons and Controlled Substances Act* 1981: section 5 states that a person is in possession of drugs if he or she is in possession of drugs that are:

- On any land or premises occupied by the person; or
- Used, enjoyed or controlled by the person in any place whatsoever, unless the person satisfies the court to the contrary (Smith 2002, p.605).

With the exception of cannabis, the penalties relating to possession of a drug that is not related to trafficking is $3000 and/or one year's imprisonment (Section 73(1)(b)).

One area that does give rise to some interesting legal considerations is the issue of pill testing. The position when a person gives another person or persons a pill purporting to be MDMA or some other illcit ('party') drug with the aim of getting it tested for safety and/or purity gives rise to interesting issues. Would it matter if the tester was doing it for profit or for free? The position of pill testing kits is also uncertain. Although there is no direct authority on the issue, it would certainly seem at the very least that while selling pill testing kits and paraphernalia such as reagents would not render the tester liable per se, once he or she receives the pill or tablet to conduct the test he or she could be liable for prosecution on grounds of possession as outlined in this section.[548]

Trafficking

The law of trafficking is complex. In simple terms, if the prosecution proves the following matters:

- the accused was in possession
- of a scheduled drug
- of a quantity that is a *trafficable quantity*,

then this will be prima facie evidence of the crime of trafficking in the particular drug. Similar to the Customs Act, a trafficable amount is determined by reference to a prescribed weight listed for that drug in the Eleventh Schedule of the *Drugs, Poisons and Controlled Substances Act 1981*. Under Section 70(1) of the Act, the definition of trafficking has been extended to include preparing or

548 This would also appear to be the view of some officers of the Victoria Police. In Public Hearings before the Committee, Superintendent Paul Ditchburn stated:

'From a criminal law perspective, the possession or trafficking in illicit drugs is an offence. Persons facilitating the testing of illicit drugs could arguably be viewed as aiding and abetting the commission of the offence, even if the user, who is already liable, actually conducts the test. Where a third person tests an illicit drug on behalf of a potential user, at the very least they commit an offence of possession of an illicit drug'.

manufacturing a drug of dependence for trafficking, in addition to sale or possession for sale of the drug. Thus the manufacture or 'cooking' of methamphetamine may constitute trafficking even though no actual trafficking has yet occurred as long as it can be proven that the manufacture was intended to be for the ultimate purpose of trafficking. Of particular importance is the fact that at state level the trafficable amount of the drug is no longer weighed as pure amounts: 'The relevant weight is now the weight of the whole mixture, including substances other than the drug' (Smith 2002, p.607). Thus, for example, the trafficable amount of MDMA, currently listed as 3.0g, could in appropriate circumstances include a compound mixed of pure MDMA and talcum powder, baking soda, or sugar. The same would apply to the trafficable amount of amphetamine (currently 6.0 grams).

In addition to trafficable quantities, as with the federal law, a person may also be convicted of the more serious crime of trafficking in a *commercial quantity*. Commercial quantities and large commercial quantities for drugs of dependence are also found in Schedule Eleven of the Act. [549]

These categories are still differentiated between pure amounts of the drug and where the drug may be mixed with other compounds or additives. The current *commercial quantity* of amphetamine is 250 gms (pure amount) and 1.25 kgs (mixed amount). The current *large commercial quantity* of amphetamine is 750 gms (pure) and 2.50 kgs (mixed amount). The current *commercial quantity* of MDMA is 100 gms (pure amount) and 500 gms (mixed amount) respectively. The *large commercial quantity* of MDMA is currently 750 gms for pure amounts and 1 kg for mixed amounts.[550] Amphetaine precursors such as pseudoephedrine and phenyl-2-propanone [P2P] do not appear in Part Three of Schedule Eleven. Nor do 'party drugs' such as Ketamine nor 3,4-Methylenedioxy-n-ethylamphetamine [MDEA]. In other words these drugs are not subject to the commercial and large commercial quantity restrictions. These drugs are, however, listed as drugs of dependence under Part One of Schedule Eleven and can therefore attract the lesser penalties associated with possession of these drugs (Section 73 DPSCA 1981).[551]

Trafficking offences of non-commercial amounts attract a maximum penalty of 15 years' imprisonment and/or a fine of $100,000. These sentences increase to 20 years' imprisonment and $250,000 when the person is convicted of trafficking to a person under the age of 18.[552]

A conviction for trafficking in a commercial quantity results in a maximum penalty of 25 years' imprisonment. If the person is convicted of trafficking in a *large commercial quantity*, the penalties are even more severe – maxima of life

549 Section 5 of the Drugs, Poisons and Controlled Substances (Amendment) Act 2001 amended the parent act to introduce aggregate quantity provisions. In other words various drugs may be combined together to achieve a commercial quantity level.

550 See Schedule Eleven, Part Three.

551 For example pseudoephedrine currently becomes subject to Part One of Schedule 11 when in excess of 20 grams. This quantity reflects the purchase of approximately 5 packets of pharmaceuticals which contain pseudoephedrine, according to Victoria Police sources.

552 See Table F in Appendix 16 for a full list of penalties.

imprisonment and *in addition* up to $500,000 fine.[553]

Trafficking also extends to manufacture. Under Section 71A of the *Drugs, Poisons and Controlled Substances Act*:

> A person who, without being authorised by or licensed under this Act or the regulations to do so, possesses a substance, material, document containing instructions relating to the preparation, cultivation or manufacture of a drug of dependence or equipment with the intention of using the substance, material, document or equipment for the purpose of trafficking in a drug of dependence is guilty of an indictable offence and liable to level 5 imprisonment (10 years maximum).

Two case law decisions have established some important precedents with regard to trafficking. First, in *R* v *Pierce*[554] the Supreme Court of Victoria found that to offer a drug for sale without any intent to produce that drug is still trafficking. In *Gauci* v *Driscoll* [555] the Court held that a mistaken belief by the vendor that a substance is a drug when it is offered for sale is still evidence of trafficking (for example believing you are selling speed when the substance is actually baking powder).

Victoria Police proposals for legislative changes

In a submission to this Inquiry, representatives of Victoria Police have expressed reservations about the Victorian legislative framework pertaining to amphetamines and 'party drugs'. In particular, they have concerns about the operation of Section 71A of the *Drugs, Poisons and Controlled Substances Act* as outlined above:

> The definition of trafficking under the Act includes manufacture. The issue with this section of legislation is proving the intent of the person possessing the materials to traffick (manufacture). Investigators have found this problematic in prosecutions. For a prosecution to succeed under the current legislation police must first prove that a defendant found in possession of certain materials has done so in the knowledge that the materials are for the illicit manufacture of drugs. Under this section usually prosecutions only succeed where the accused makes admissions as to their intent. It is suggested to overcome the issue of proving intent that a person found in possession of any items listed in section 71A has a reverse onus applied to them.[556]

As such, Victoria Police have made the following recommendation to the Committee:

---

553 For figures of arrests and prosecutions for a variety of federal drug-related crimes, including amphetamines, MDMA and other 'designer drugs' for the period 2000–2001, see the *Australian Illicit Drug Report 2000–2001* (ABCI 2002). For an interesting analysis of criminal investigation pertaining to amphetamine and ecstasy control in Queensland, see Queensland Crime Commission 2000, 2001.

554 1996 2 VR 215.

555 1985 VR 428.

556 Excerpt from the confidential submission of Victoria Police (Drugs Policy and Services Branch) to the Drugs and Crime Prevention Committee, Inquiry into the Use of Amphetamine and 'Party Drug' Use in Victoria, August 2002. Quoted with the kind permission of Victoria Police.

> The amendment of Section 71A of the Drugs, Poisons and Controlled Substances Act 1981 to create a reverse onus provision on persons possessing certain materials with the intent to traffick (manufacture).[557]

A more recent submission to this Inquiry in response to the Committee's earlier published *Discussion Paper* expands on the problems of proving intent:

> The criminal response to legislation to prove 'intent to manufacture' gives organised crime syndicates, mainstream criminals and 'Internet cooks' a high degree of insulation or protection from the impacts of the law. As Amphetamine Type Substances become more mainstream in social settings, the law needs to be targeted toward those groups of criminals who exploit young people and cause major harms...
>
> It is rare for a single individual in a criminal syndicate to possess all the precursors and equipment used in the manufacturing process. Usually the chemicals and other materials required in the process are deliberately stored separately. It is only when the actual manufacturing process is in progress and all the chemicals and materials are present that the difficulty of proving intent is lessened.[558]

Victoria Police have put forward a number of options to the Committee that they are considering to ameliorate the problems associated with proving intent. The first is an amendment to Sec 71A to create a reverse onus of proof provision as discussed above. This could be modelled on a reverse onus provision already in the *Crimes Act* dealing with the possession of explosive substances (s.317).[559]

The second option is to create a new offence that would target the possession of precursor chemicals and scientific equipment without lawful excuse. Victoria Police argue that:

> This amendment would allow police to interrupt the chain of supply and/or manufacture thus significantly reducing the risks of explosion, contamination and environmental hazards for police, emergency services and the wider community.

Responses to Victoria Police proposals

A variety of legal bodies have commented on the desirability or otherwise of such proposals. These have included the Law Institute of Victoria (LIV), Victoria Legal Aid and the Criminal Bar Association. Each of these three organisations has serious reservations about the Victoria Police proposals, particularly the reverse onus provision. With regard to such a reverse onus the common themes of the objections are based on a:

---

557 Ibid.

558 Confidential submission of Victoria Police (Drug and Alcohol Strategy Unit) to the Drugs and Crime Prevention Committee, Inquiry into Amphetamine and 'Party Drug' Use in Victoria, November 2003. In confidence.

559 Sec.317 (4):

'Any person who makes or knowingly has in his possession or under his control any explosive substance, under such circumstances as to give rise to a reasonable suspicion that he is not making it or does not have it in his possession or under his control for a lawful object shall, unless he can show that he made it or had it in his possession or under his control for a lawful object, be guilty of an indictable offence, and shall be liable to level 6 imprisonment (5 years maximum)'.

> [l]ong recognised democratic ideal that the State should bear the burden of proof of criminal conduct when the ultimate and terrible sanction is at stake, namely the exercise by the State of its power to remove the liberty of the individual citizen.[560]

The Law Institute continues:

> Proof of mens rea [intention to commit the crime] has always been pivotal in establishing a criminal offence. To suggest that a reverse onus provision similar to that contained in s317 of the *Crimes Act* be enacted, would in our view be problematical. That section creates a need for a reasonable suspicion to exist without testing the reasonableness of the suspicion and prior to the need for an explanation.
>
> ... Reverse onus provisions are inappropriate as they create a situation where a citizen is called upon to answer a suspicion before it is tested as reasonable. The current interpretation of the law is that a suspicion of guilt is tested objectively before a Court of law rather than the suspicion being tested by the police at the time of apprehension.
>
> ... The LIV is extremely concerned to protect citizen's rights and ensure that there is no serious interference to the presumption of innocence. We are deeply troubled by the view that the law should be altered and citizens' rights to the presumption of innocence be removed simply because the police find it difficult to gather sufficient evidence of the requisite quality to establish a conviction.
>
> ... There are good reasons to adhere to the principle that the burden of proof remain with the prosecution. It should also be remembered that the State has more resources that the individual citizen. This imbalance of resources creates a power imbalance in favour of the State. The police proposal to reverse onus of proof in respect of the manufacturing and trafficking offence fails to recognise the fundamental imbalance of resources and power. It also raises the real possibility of defendants being compelled to take part in court proceedings without having the resources to establish their innocence. These defendants may not have the funding resources to afford representation and will be subjected to gross injustice caused by the power imbalance.
>
> Our system has always recognised that citizens should be protected from oppression and as a consequence from time to time a guilty person may avoid conviction.
>
> If it is true that the materials and manufacturing equipment of amphetamine manufacturers are obvious then the police should not be in fear of a provision which places the reasonableness of the suspicion clearly upon them. To argue otherwise would be to support unnecessary intrusion into citizen's civil rights and liberties...[561]

---

560 Submission of the Law Institute of Victoria to the Drugs and Crime Prevention Committee, Inquiry into Amphetamine and 'Party Drug' Use in Victoria, February 2004.

561 Ibid.

The objections of Victoria Legal Aid (VLA) are also based on the liberty of the subject:

> VLA is deeply troubled by the view that the law should be altered and citizens' rights to the presumption of innocence should be removed simply because the police find it difficult to gather sufficient evidence of the requisite quality to establish a conviction. As you are aware, our criminal justice system squarely places the burden on the prosecution to prove both the mens rea and the actus reus of a criminal offence. This circumstance is not an arbitrary mistake of history but is founded upon the long recognised democratic principle that the State, with its infinite resources when compared to those of the individual citizen, should bear the full burden of proof of criminal conduct when the ultimate and terrible sanction at stake is the exercise by the State of its power to remove the liberty of the individual citizen.
>
> The police proposal to reverse this onus of proof in respect of the manufacturing offence fails to recognise this fundamental imbalance of resources and power and raises the real possibility of innocent persons who, unable to establish their innocence, may be wrongly convicted of serious criminal offences. If the cost of preventing such an obnoxious situation is that from time to time a guilty person may avoid conviction, it is a cost that our system has been traditionally willing to bear. It should continue to do so. To do otherwise compromises a fundamental principle which safeguards the rights and liberty of all citizens.[562]

Similarly, the Criminal Bar Association argues:

> The suggested reform (favoured by Victoria Police) of a reverse onus applying to anyone found in possession of items listed in s.71A shifts the burden to an Accused. The Association does not support amending the section in such a way that requires an Accused to offer an explanation or to "disprove" his or her intention. A reverse onus situation has the potential to cause unfairness to many accused who may fall within the ambit of s.71A as it presently operates but who neither have an intention to manufacture or traffick but equally cannot and should not have to offer an explanation. An accused's right to silence is paramount to his or her right to due process and a fair trial. Put simply, a reverse onus provision in the way suggested will mean that anyone falling within the section will be assumed guilty unless he or she proves otherwise.[563]

The second alternative option put forward by Victoria Police – the creation of a separate crime of possessing precursor chemicals and/or scientific apparatus without lawful excuse – is seen as a less dangerous alternative by the legal bodies. The Law Institute of Victoria states in this regard:

562 Submission of Victoria Legal Aid to the Drugs and Crime Prevention Committee, Inquiry into Amphetamine and 'Party Drug' Use in Victoria, February 2002.

563 Submission of the Criminal Bar Association of Victoria to the Drugs and Crime Prevention Committee, Inquiry into Amphetamine and 'Party Drug' Use in Victoria, February 2002.

> There is a second proposal that a new offence be created that would target the possession of precursor chemicals without lawful excuse. This in itself would be more than adequate. Once the precursor chemicals are identified and scheduled it is difficult to imagine a defendant escaping prosecution as there would rarely be any lawful excuse that would suffice.[564]

Similarly, the Criminal Bar Association responds:

> The second option of amending the section by creating a new offence of possession without lawful excuse is a much fairer reform.
>
> It does not offend the notion that a person is presumed innocent until proven guilty (as reverse onus provisions do) and is potentially much simpler to prosecute without the "intention to traffick (manufacture)" difficulty encountered by Victoria Police. The Association also agrees that if it is necessary to amend the section then creating a new offence (of without lawful excuse) will allow Police to interrupt the chain of manufacture and therefore reduce the risks of contamination and environmental hazards to the community.[565]

The Committee expresses its thanks to Victoria Police, Victoria Legal Aid, the Law Institute of Victoria and the Criminal Bar Association. It appreciates their advice and suggestions with regard to this somewhat problematic area of legal regulation. However, for the reasons enunciated in the submissions of the three legal bodies it believes that the second option of a creation of a new offence of possession of precursor chemicals and/or scientific equipment is a preferable alternative and is the subject of the following recommendation.

Recommendation

20. The Committee recommends that the Drugs, Poisons and Controlled Substances Act 1981 be amended to insert a new offence of possession without lawful excuse of an amount to be specified of precursor chemicals and associated apparatus/equipment used for the manufacture of illicit drugs.

Quantity of drug constituting an offence

Victoria Police has also expressed reservations about the current amounts of drug (by weight) that constitute the various drug offences in the Act. In a submission to this Inquiry a representative states:

> The current amounts (by weight) of drugs deemed to constitute sufficient quantities for various types of offences under Schedule Eleven of the Drugs, Poisons and Controlled Substances Act 1981 were appropriate when

564 Submission of the Law Institute of Victoria to the Drugs and Crime Prevention Committee, Inquiry into Amphetamine and 'Party Drug' Use in Victoria, February 2004.

565 Submission of the Criminal Bar Association of Victoria to the Drugs and Crime Prevention Committee, Inquiry into Amphetamine and 'Party Drug' Use in Victoria, February 2002.

> introduced. However, the dynamics of the illicit drug manufacturing trade have changed so the law needs to reflect these changes.
>
> Serious consideration needs to be given to the Model Criminal Code Serious Drug Offences Report due to commerciality of the drug enterprises. The Model Criminal Code Serious Drug Offences is an attempt to bring a uniform approach to drug legislation in all jurisdictions. The Victoria Forensic Services Centre in consultation with the Major Drug Investigation Division have compiled a list of recommended quantities for Part 1 of Schedule 11 to bring these in line with those quantities in Part 3 of the Drugs, Poisons and Controlled Substances Act 1981. Realistic quantities of MDMA and methylamphetamine (that can be manufactured by pseudoephedrine) need close attention. The Victoria Police Drug Legislation Working Party has been convened to examine these issues.[566]

The Committee acknowledges and supports the work of the Victoria Police Drug Legislation Party to bring recommended quantities of drugs in Part One of Schedule 11 of the of the Drugs, Poisons and Controlled Substances Act 1981 into line with those quantities in Part Three of Schedule 11 of that Act. The Committee encourages further work in this area.

The Committee makes the following recommendations with regard to the quantities constituting the relevant drug offence:

Recommendations

21. The Committee recommends the amendment of Part 3 of Schedule 11 of the Drugs, Poisons and Controlled Substances Act 1981 to reduce the pure and dilute quantities for amphetamine and methylamphetamine to be in line with methylenedioxymethamphetamine (ecstasy) in order to control trafficking of MDMA. This would reflect the fact that amphetamine is now more commonly sold in tablet form.

22. The Committee recommends the amendment of Part 3 of Schedule 11 of the Drugs, Poisons and Controlled Substances Act 1981 to reduce the dilute quantities for pseudoephedrine to be in line with the current amphetamine and methylamphetamine commercial quantities. This would assist in combating pseudoephedrine diversion from pharmacies.

23. The Committee recommends that the existing offence for the possession of pseudoephedrine without lawful excuse in Part One of Schedule Eleven of the Drugs, Poisons and Controlled Substances Act 1981 be publicised and enforced.

566 Confidential submission of Victoria Police (Drug and Alcohol Strategy Unit) to the Drugs and Crime Prevention Committee, Inquiry into Amphetamine and 'Party Drug' Use in Victoria, November 2003.

Suggested changes in other states

Both South Australia and Western Australia are currently considering amending their drugs legislation to strengthen provisions with regard to the manufacture of amphetamines and the use of precursor chemicals.[567] For example, the South Australian parliament is considering whether the possession of industrial and scientific glassware without valid excuse should be subject to criminal charge if there is good reason to believe they may be used in the production of illicit drugs.[568] Victoria Police also believes there should be more stringent controls on the supply and control of precursor chemicals and manufacturing equipment:

> Victoria Police believes an appropriate legislative option to restrict certain amounts of drugs and precursor chemicals are absolutely essential. The legitimate possession of substances, material, document containing instructions relating to the preparation, cultivation or manufacture of a drug of dependence or equipment is restricted to authorised pharmacies, scientific and chemical companies and drug manufacturing companies including laboratories. There is no legal reason for any other group or person to possess precursor chemicals. Legitimate businesses have permits and security control systems to prevent illicit diversion of precursor chemicals.[569]

Detective Inspector Paul Steel from the Western Australia Police Service's Clandestine Laboratory visited the United States in 2003 on a Churchill Fellowship. His trip included visiting a variety of state police units dealing with the problems associated with policing manufacture of amphetamines and designer drugs. As a result of his experiences and knowledge gained in the United States he has recommended to the Committee the following proposals to deal with illicit drug manufacture:

> Legislation be drafted to create an offence for possession of precursor chemicals or apparatus [including glassware] with intent to manufacture. Enshrined in the body of legislation [would be] that intent would be proved if the offender is in possession of two or more specified items;
>
> Legislation be drafted to create an offence for possession of 5 or more boxes of pseudoephedrine based medications (or specified gram weight) (Steel 2003, p.28).

The American model combines strong federal legislation supplemented by co-operative agreements and collaborative legislative frameworks between states.

567 For example, Western Australia Police Service is seeking amendments to the Misuse of Drugs Amendment Bill 2003 to create an offence for possession of precursor chemicals and equipment without lawful excuse. The Victoria Police Drug Legislation Working Party is currently examining these options with relevant stakeholders such as chemical manufacturers etc.

568 As communicated to the Committee by Commissioner Mal Hyde South Australia Police, Adelaide, 3 October 2003.

569 Confidential submission from Victoria Police (Drug and Alcohol Strategy Unit) to the Drugs and Crime Prevention Committee Inquiry into Amphetamine and 'Party Drug' Use in Victoria, November 2003.

Detective Steel believes that this is an excellent method of combating the illicit amphetamine and designer drug trade on a national level.[570]

> In particular, similar lessons can be learnt in Australia with the agreement of law enforcement agencies so that the problems with clandestine drug laboratories can be alleviated and not merely transferred to another jurisdiction (Steel 2003, p.24).

Laws pertaining to other matters

Issues pertaining to driving under the influence of a drug are discussed in Chapter 7. Laws with regard to the manufacture of amphetamines/pharmacy issues are discussed below and in Chapter 14.

Existing provisions in other state jurisdictions

The following section gives a brief overview of the comparative legal provisions in each Australian state and territory.

New South Wales – Drug Misuse and Trafficking Act 1985

This Act divides offences into those of summary and indictable jurisdiction. Prohibited drug is defined as a reference to any 'preparation, admixture, extract or other substance containing *any* proportion of the prohibited drug' (s.4).

A reference to the use or administration of a prohibited drug includes a reference to the ingestion, injection and inhalation of a prohibited drug, the smoking of a prohibited drug, the inhalation of fumes caused by the heating or burning of a prohibited drug and any other means of introducing a prohibited drug into any part of the body of a person (s.5).

Self-administration of prohibited drugs (s.12)

(1) A person who administers or attempts to administer a prohibited drug to himself or herself is guilty of an offence.

(2) Nothing in this section renders unlawful the administration or attempted administration by a person to himself or herself of a prohibited drug which has been lawfully prescribed for or supplied to the person.

This is the equivalent of the Victorian use offence.

There are other miscellaneous summary offences under Division One of the Act that include administering a prohibited drug to another (s.13), possession of equipment for administration of prohibited drugs (s.11), forging and

570 For example, the states of Arizona, Nevada and New Mexico have joined forces to form a Tri-State Precursor Committee. Legislation targeting precursor control was enacted exactly the same in the three states. In addition the police, health and education departments of each state work in collaboration to investigate clandestine laboratories and educate members of the public including targeted groups such as hotel owners as to the signs of clandestine amphetamine production.

obtaining prescriptions by false representation (ss15–17) and aiding and abetting drug administration (ss19 and 20). This latter offence could arguably cover the case of pill testers referred to above.

All summary offences attract the penalty of 20 penalty units ($2000) or 2 years' imprisonment or both.

Indictable offences

MANUFACTURE AND PRODUCTION OF PROHIBITED DRUG (S.24)

1) A person who manufactures or produces, or who knowingly takes part in the manufacture or production of, a prohibited drug is guilty of an offence.

(2) A person who manufactures or produces, or who knowingly takes part in the manufacture or production of, an amount of a prohibited drug which is not less than the commercial quantity applicable to the prohibited drug is guilty of an offence.

(3) Where, on the trial of a person for an offence under subsection (2), the jury are not satisfied that the amount of prohibited drug involved is equal to or more than the commercial quantity applicable to the prohibited drug, they may acquit the person of the offence charged and find the person guilty of an offence under subsection (1), and the person shall be liable to punishment accordingly.

(4) Nothing in this section renders unlawful the manufacture or production of a prohibited drug by:

(a) a person licensed or authorised to do so under the *Poisons Act 1966*, or

(b) a person acting in accordance with an authority granted by the Secretary of the Department of Health where the Secretary is satisfied that the manufacture or production of the prohibited drug is for the purpose of scientific research, instruction, analysis or study,

or renders unlawful the taking part by any other person in the manufacture or production of a prohibited drug by a person to whom paragraph (a) or (b) applies.

POSSESSION OF PRECURSORS FOR MANUFACTURE OR PRODUCTION OF PROHIBITED DRUGS (S.24A)

(1) A person who has possession of a precursor intended by the person for use in the manufacture or production, by that person or another person, of a prohibited drug is guilty of an offence.

(2) Nothing in this section renders unlawful the manufacture or production of a prohibited drug by:

(a) a person licensed or authorised to do so under the *Poisons and Therapeutic Goods Act 1966* , or

(b) a person acting in accordance with an authority granted by the Director-General of the Department of Health where the Director-General is satisfied that the manufacture or production of the prohibited drug is for the purpose of scientific research, instruction, analysis or study,

or renders unlawful the taking part by any other person in the manufacture or production of a prohibited drug by a person to whom paragraph (a) or (b) applies.

(2A) The regulations may make provision for or with respect to prohibiting or regulating the cash sale of precursors.

(3) In this section, 'precursor' means a substance specified or described in the regulations as a precursor for the purposes of this section.

SUPPLY (TRAFFICKING) – (S.25)

(1) A person who supplies, or who knowingly takes part in the supply of, a prohibited drug is guilty of an offence.

(1A) A person of or above the age of 18 years who supplies, or who knowingly takes part in the supply of, a prohibited drug (other than cannabis leaf) to a person under the age of 16 years is guilty of an offence.

(2) A person who supplies, or who knowingly takes part in the supply of, an amount of a prohibited drug which is not less than the commercial quantity applicable to the prohibited drug is guilty of an offence.

(2A) A person of or above the age of 18 years who supplies, or who knowingly takes part in the supply of, an amount of a prohibited drug (other than cannabis leaf) which is not less than the commercial quantity applicable to the prohibited drug to a person under the age of 16 years is guilty of an offence.

(2B) Where, on the trial of a person for an offence under subsection (1A) or (2A), the jury are satisfied that the person charged had, at the time the offence is alleged to have been committed, reasonable cause to believe, and did in fact believe, that the person to whom the prohibited drug was supplied was of or above the age of 16 years, they may acquit the person of the offence charged and find the person guilty of an offence under subsection (1) or (2), respectively, and the person is liable to punishment accordingly.

(3) Where, on the trial of a person for an offence under subsection (2), the jury are not satisfied that the amount of prohibited drug involved is equal to or more than the commercial quantity applicable to the prohibited drug, they may acquit the person of the offence charged and find the person guilty of an offence under subsection (1), and the person shall be liable to punishment accordingly.

(4) Nothing in this section renders unlawful the supply of a prohibited drug by:

  (a) a person licensed or authorised to do so under the *Poisons Act 1966*, or

  (b) a person acting in accordance with an authority granted by the Secretary of the Department of Health where the Secretary is satisfied that the supply of the prohibited drug is for the purpose of scientific research, instruction, analysis or study, or

  (c) a person acting in accordance with a direction given by the Commissioner of Police under section 39RA,

or renders unlawful the taking part by any other person in the supply of a prohibited drug by a person to whom paragraph (a), (b) or (c) applies.

(5) Nothing in this section renders unlawful the administration of a prohibited drug to a person being cared for by another person in the circumstances described in section 10 (2) (d).

SUPPLYING PROHIBITED DRUGS ON AN ONGOING BASIS (S.25A)

(1) A person who, on 3 or more separate occasions during any period of 30 consecutive days, supplies a prohibited drug (other than cannabis) for financial or material reward is guilty of an offence.

(2) A person is liable to be convicted of an offence under this section whether or not the same prohibited drug is supplied on each of the occasions relied on as evidence of commission of the offence.

(3) If, on the trial of a person for an offence under this section, more than 3 occasions of supplying a prohibited drug are relied on as evidence of commission of the offence, all the members of the jury must be satisfied as to the same 3 occasions in order to find the person guilty of the offence.

(4) If, on the trial of a person for an offence under this section, the jury is not satisfied that the offence is proven but is satisfied that the person has, in respect of any of the occasions relied on as evidence of commission of the offence under this section, committed a relevant supply offence, the jury may acquit the person of the offence charged and find the person guilty of the relevant supply offence, and the person is liable to punishment accordingly.

As in Victoria, the possession of a trafficable quantity of the relevant drug will be prima facie evidence of trafficking or supplying a prohibited drug unless the defendant can prove otherwise. In the case of amphetamines this will be 3 grams. For MDMA, 0.75gs will suffice (s.29). There is an escalating series of penalties for supply offences depending on the amount of the drug in question. This ranges from $500 and/or 2 years' imprisonment for a 'small quantity' to $500,000 and/or life imprisonment for a large commercial quantity (see section 33ff.). Penalties for possession of chemical precursors for illicit manufacture of prohibited drugs is $200,000 or 10 years' imprisonment or both.

Queensland – Drugs Misuse Act 1986

The Queensland legislation refers to 'dangerous' rather than prohibited drugs. Under section 4 a dangerous drug is defined as including a number of substances listed in Schedules 1 and 2 (Schedule 2 includes the amphetamines and the main forms of 'party' drugs) and includes salts, derivatives or stereo-isomers in addition to anything that is contained within a natural substance or 'any solution or admixture'.

Serious drug offences in Queensland include *trafficking* (s.5) (for Schedule 2 drugs a maximum penalty of 20 years), *supply* (s.6) (for Schedule 2 drugs a maximum penalty of 15 years), *possession* (various penalties depending on the amount of the drug, but an average maximum of 15 years), *producing,* (also various penalties depending on the amount in question). The distinction between trafficking and supply is not clear on the face of the Act. However, the use of the term 'business' in the trafficking offence suggests trafficking is always construed as a commercial enterprise whereas the offence of supply may include cases where the offender has given or distributed the drug to another not expecting payment.[571]

A novel offence in the Queensland legislation is found in Section 8A – Publishing or possessing instructions for producing.

(1) A person who unlawfully publishes instructions, or unlawfully has possession of a document containing instructions, about the way to produce a dangerous drug commits a crime.

(3) In this section –

'document' containing instructions about the way to produce a dangerous drug includes anything designed to enable electronic access specifically to the instructions.

'publish' includes publish to any person and supply, exhibit and display to any person, whether the publication is made orally or in written, electronic or another form.

Clearly, such an offence would cover such manuals as Uncle Fester's published on the Internet and discussed in Chapter 14.

---

571 Sec.5 – Trafficking in dangerous drugs:

'A person who carries on the business of unlawfully trafficking in a dangerous drug is guilty of a crime.

Sec.4 – "supply" means:

(a) give, distribute, sell, administer, transport or supply;

(b) offering to do any act specified in paragraph (a);

(c) doing or offering to do any act preparatory to, in furtherance of, or for the purpose of, any act specified in paragraph (a)'.

South Australia – Controlled Substances Act 1984

This act needs to be read in conjunction with the Controlled Substances Act (Declared Drugs of Dependence) Regulations and the Controlled Substances (Declared Prohibited Substances) Regulations. Both sets of regulations define prohibited substances and drugs of dependence as including admixtures.

Possession – Section 31

A person must not:

a) knowingly have in his or her possession a drug of dependence or a prohibited substance; or

b) smoke, consume or administer to himself or herself, or permit another person to administer to him or her, a drug of dependence or a prohibited substance; or

c) have in his or her possession any piece of equipment for use in connection with the smoking, consumption or administration of such a drug or substance, or the preparation of such a drug or substance for smoking, consumption or administration.

(2) A person who contravenes this section is guilty of an offence and liable to a penalty as follows:

(a) [cannabis provision]

(b) in any other case – a penalty not exceeding $2000 or imprisonment for 2 years, or both.

(3) Nothing in this section renders unlawful the possession of a drug of dependence or any equipment by –

(a) a medical practitioner, dentist, veterinary surgeon, pharmacist or nurse acting in the ordinary course of his or her profession; or

(b) a member of any other prescribed profession acting in the ordinary course of that profession; or

(c) a person for or to whom the drug has been lawfully prescribed or supplied; or

(d) a person licensed to have the drug or equipment in his or her possession by the Minister.

(4) Nothing in this section renders unlawful the consumption or administration to himself or herself of a drug of dependence, or the giving of permission for the administration to himself or herself of a drug of dependence, by a person for whom the drug has been lawfully prescribed or supplied.

Manufacture. Supply and Trafficking – Sec 32

(1) A person must not knowingly –

(a) manufacture or produce a drug of dependence or a prohibited substance; or

(b) take part in the manufacture or production of such a drug or substance; or

(c) sell, supply or administer such a drug or substance to another person; or

(d) take part in the sale, supply or administration of such a drug or substance to another person; or

(e) have such a drug or substance in his or her possession for the purpose of the sale, supply or administration of that drug or substance to another person.

(4) Without limiting the generality of this section, a person takes part in the manufacture, production, sale, supply or administration of a drug of dependence or prohibited substance if the person –

(a) takes, or participates in, any step, or causes any step to be taken, in the process of that manufacture, production, sale, supply or administration; or

(b) provides or arranges finance for any such step in that process; or

(c) provides the premises in which any such step in that process is taken, or suffers or permits any such step in that process to be taken in premises of which he or she is the owner, or in the management of which he or she participates.

Contravention of these sections is subject to an ascending scale of penalties detailed in sub-section 5. Special provisions apply to the supply of drugs to minors or within school zones.

Western Australia – Misuse of Drugs Act 1981

Drugs subject to this Act are either 'drugs of addiction' or drugs listed in Schedule 1. Section 6 of the Act is a general offences prescription that applies to all drugs but has different penalties for cannabis and varying amounts of other drugs.

Sec 6. Offences concerned with prohibited drugs generally

(1) Subject to subsection (3), a person who —

(a) with intent to sell or supply it to another, has in his possession;

(b) manufactures or prepares; or

(c) sells or supplies, or offers to sell or supply, to another

a prohibited drug commits an indictable offence, except when he is authorised by or under this Act or by or under the *Poisons Act 1964* to do so and does so in accordance with that authority.

(2) Subject to subsection (3) and to section 36A of the *Poisons Act 1964*, a person who has in his possession or uses a prohibited drug commits a simple offence, except when, in the case of a person who has the prohibited drug in his possession –

(a) he is authorised by or under this Act or by or under the *Poisons Act 1964* to do so and does so in accordance with that authority; or

(b) the prohibited drug was sold or supplied, or requested to be sold or supplied, to him –

(i) by a medical practitioner or veterinary surgeon in the lawful practice of his profession; or

(ii) on and in accordance with an authorised prescription.

Indictable offences under section 6(1) are classified as 'serious drug offences'. These in turn form the basis for the more serious offence of trafficking under Section 32 as follows:

(1) If a person is convicted of –

(a) a serious drug offence and has, during the period of 10 years ending on the day, or the first of the days, as the case requires, on which the serious drug offence was committed, been convicted of 2 or more –

(i) serious drug offences;

(ii) external serious drug offences; or

(iii) offences, one or more of which are serious drug offences and one or more of which are external serious drug offences;

or

(b) a serious drug offence in respect of –

(i) a prohibited drug in a quantity which is not less than the quantity specified in Schedule VII in relation to the prohibited drug; or

(ii) prohibited plants in a number which is not less than the number specified in Schedule VIII in relation to the particular species or genus to which those prohibited plants belong,

the court convicting the person of the serious drug offence first referred to in paragraph (a), or the serious drug offence referred to in paragraph (b), as the case requires, shall on the application of the Director of Public Prosecutions or a police prosecutor declare the person to be a drug trafficker.

Tasmania – Poisons Act 1971

Part Five of the Poisons Act outlines the penalties for the importation, manufacture, refinement, possession, sale, supply and trafficking of raw narcotics, narcotic substances and prohibited substances. Under the schedules to the Act, amphetamines and MDMA/MDA or admixtures are classified as narcotics, the possession of 0.5gms of either substance gives rise to a presumption of sale or supply. The standard qualifications with regard to legitimate use by doctors, chemists, veterinarians and other appropriate people apply.

Australian Capital Territory – Drugs of Dependence Act 1989

This Act divides drugs into *drugs of dependence* and *prohibited substances.* Amphetamines fall in the former categories with most 'party drugs' belonging in the latter group.

The offences associated with amphetamine and other drug use, supply or manufacture in the Capital Territory are to be found in Part Ten of the above Act read in conjunction with the Drugs of Dependence Regulations.

Illegitimate manufacture of amphetamine and associated drugs is prohibited by Section 161 of the Act in association with Schedule Three of the regulations. Manufacture is interpreted widely and includes a person who:

(a) participates in any step or process, or causes or permits any step or process to be undertaken, in the course of that manufacture;

(b) provides finance, or arranges for the provision of finance, for such a step or process; or

(c) being an owner, occupier or lessee of any premises, or concerned in the management of any premises, causes or permits those premises to be used for such a step or process [Section 161 (4)].

The maximum penalty for such manufacture is $20,000, imprisonment for ten years or both.

The sale or supply of a drug of dependence which under Schedule One of the Regulations includes amphetamine and methamphetamine is an offence under Section 164 as follows:

A person shall not-

(a) sell or supply a drug of dependence to any person;

(b) participate in the sale or supply of a drug of dependence to any person; or

(c) possess a drug of dependence for the purpose of sale or supply to any person. Penalty:

  (a) where the quantity of the drug to which the offence relates is a commercial quantity – imprisonment for life;

  (b) where the quantity of the drug to which the offence relates is a trafficable quantity but not a commercial quantity – $100,000 or imprisonment for 25 years, or both;

  (c) where the quantity of the drug to which the offence relates is less than a trafficable quantity, and is sold or supplied to a person who has not attained the age of 18 years – $100,000 or imprisonment for 25 years, or both; and

  (d) in any other case – $10,000 or imprisonment for 5 years, or both.

Commercial and trafficable quantities are listed in Schedule One of the regulations for amphetamine and methamphetamine as 2 kilograms and 2 grams respectively.

The sale and supply of prohibited substances which include MDMA/MDA/PMA and analogues are also proscribed under Section 164 as follows:

A person shall not –

(a) sell or supply a prohibited substance to any person;

(b) participate in the sale or supply of a prohibited substance to any person; or

(c) possess a prohibited substance for the purpose of sale or supply to any person. Penalty:

 (a) where the quantity of the substance to which the offence relates is a commercial quantity – imprisonment for life;

 b) where the quantity of the substance to which the offence relates is a trafficable quantity but not a commercial quantity – $100,000 or imprisonment for 25 years, or both;

 (c) where the quantity of the substance to which the offence relates is less than a trafficable quantity, and is sold or supplied to a person who has not attained the age of 18 years – $100,000 or imprisonment for 25 years, or both; and

 (d) in any other case – $10,000 or imprisonment for 5 years, or both.

The amounts for commercial and trafficable quantities for these 'party drugs' are 0.50 kilograms and 0.50 grams respectively (Schedule Two, Regulations).

Possession and administration offences for both drugs of dependence and prohibited substances are covered under Section 169 and generally attract a penalty of $5000, 2 years' imprisonment or both, with the exception of cannabis which attracts a lesser penalty.

Northern Territory – Misuse of Drugs Act

In the Northern Territory most illicit drugs for the purposes of proscription and penalties are classified as *dangerous drugs*. Dangerous drugs are listed in a variety of schedules to the Act. Schedule 1 contains major drugs and drug groups such as heroin, cocaine and LSD but interestingly not amphetamines and most 'party drugs'. These latter drugs are listed along with their commercial and trafficable quantities in Schedule Two. Schedule Two drugs attract lesser penalties than those in Schedule One. Such a taxonomy points to the very real anomalies and inconsistencies between different Australian states and their application of drugs penalties. In many states for example, LSD might appear in a Schedule Two listing or equivalent. Conversely, in many states amphetamines and methamphetamines would usually attract the higher penalties than is the case by having them listed in Schedule Two. The only consistency between the states and territories is that for the most part cannabis offences receive a lesser penalty than other drugs, at least with regard to possession and personal use.

Possession of dangerous drugs is covered in Section 9 of the Act. For Schedule Two Drugs such as amphetamines a commercial quantity attracts 14 years' imprisonment, a trafficable quantity $10,000 or 5 years' imprisonment. The Northern Territory also distinguishes between possession in a *public* and *private* place for those amounts which are less than trafficable. Possession in a public place of less than a trafficable quantity may result in $5000 penalty or 2 years' imprisonment. Possession in a non-public place attracts a fine of $2000.

Supply is covered under Section 5 of the Act as follows (penalties are given for Schedule Two drugs only):

(1) A person who unlawfully supplies, or takes part in the supply of, a dangerous drug to another person, whether or not –

(a) that other person is in the Territory; and

(b) where the dangerous drug is supplied to a person at a place outside the Territory, the supply of that dangerous drug to the person constitutes an offence in that place,

is guilty of a crime.

(2) A person guilty of a crime under subsection (1) is, subject to section 22, punishable on being found guilty by a penalty not exceeding:

(a) Where the amount of the dangerous drug supplied is not a commercial quantity –

(iii) where the dangerous drug is a dangerous drug specified in Schedule 2, the offender is an adult and the person to whom it is supplied is a child – imprisonment for 14 years; and

(iv) where the dangerous drug is a dangerous drug specified in Schedule 2 and subparagraph (iii) does not apply – $10,000 or imprisonment for 5 years.

(b) Where the amount of the dangerous drug supplied is a commercial quantity –

(ii) where the dangerous drug is a dangerous drug specified in Schedule 2, the offender is an adult and the person to whom it is supplied is a child – imprisonment for 25 years; and

(iii) in any other case where the dangerous drug is a dangerous drug specified in Schedule 2 – imprisonment for 14 years.

Provisions against the illicit manufacture and production of dangerous drugs are listed in Section 8 of the Act. For Schedule Two drugs, production of a commercial quantity (100gms amphetamine, 25gms MDMA/MDA etc) may result in a sentence of 25 years' imprisonment. Production of a trafficable quantity (2gms amphetamine, 0.50gms MDMA) attracts a penalty of 7 years' imprisonment. Manufacture is interpreted to include the extraction and the refinement of the drug under Section Three of the Act.

Having briefly examined the main features of drug penalties, offences and regulations as they apply to amphetamines and 'party drugs' across the country, this chapter will conclude by briefly looking at some legal issues with regard to these drugs as they have arisen recently in other jurisdictions, namely the United Kingdom and the United States, both countries with big amphetamine and 'party drug' problems.

Law Reform: Some interesting developments in the United States and the United Kingdom

Like Australia, the American and British legal frameworks for illicit drugs including the amphetamines, their analogues and amphetamine-type substances such as MDMA are generally prohibitive. This is particularly the case in the United States. Some interesting legislative developments in some American states and a proposal for law reform in England warrant brief attention.

United States of America

As with Australia, the American legal system is divided between federal and (50) state jurisdictions. Similarly, there are both federal, state and in some cases local or county drugs laws on the statute books. American law generally mirrors a 'tough on drugs' drug enforcement policy that leaves very little room for harm minimisation principles or programmes (for a discussion of the American policy approach and the philosophy behind it see Chapter 19).

The key federal law is the *Controlled Substances Act* which created five escalating schedules into which drugs could be categorised. Similar to Australia, Schedule 1 contains the drugs which are considered most abusive, dangerous or with no or very little therapeutic benefit. Drugs with more benefits and fewer dangers are placed in the less stringent schedules, with Schedule 5 having the least amount of restriction.

To circumvent the problems alluded to earlier in this chapter whereby minor modifications to a drug's chemical or molecular structure would result in it having to be rescheduled as a differently named drug (a slow and laborious process) Congress passed the *Controlled Substance Analogue Enforcement Act,* commonly called the *Designer Drug Act.* As Jenkins states, this Act:

> [w]as intended to end the legal immunity of synthetic drugs closely related to some better-known chemical, such as any new variant of the fentanyl family. It did this by a sweeping prohibition of analogues 'substantially similar' to existing substances, a dramatic curtailment of legal experimentation. Specifically, the law allowed the prosecution of anyone involved with a substance '(1) the chemical structure of which is substantially similar to the chemical structure of a controlled substance in Schedule I or II (ii) which has a stimulant, depressant or hallucinogenic effect on the central nervous system of a controlled substance in Schedule I or II'.
>
> Though not officially declared scheduled drugs, analogues were treated for legal purposes as if they had been officially scheduled. The principle of similarity was extended further by the 1988 Chemical Diversion and Trafficking Act (CDTA), which regulated the precursors and essential chemicals needed for

> synthesizing illegal drugs. The new range of listed chemicals made the federal register resemble a college textbook, with notations concerning 'ephedrine, its salts, optical isomers and salts of optical isomers... Any salt, optical isomer or salt of an optical isomer of the chemicals listed above in subparagraphs M through U of this paragraph'. Within five years, the CDTA listed twenty-seven precursors and seven essential chemicals. The measure seemed comprehensive and was far-reaching enough to cause difficulties for serious researchers, yet at the same time it could scarcely succeed, because chemists could evolve still newer psychedelics and stimulants from chemical families yet unknown to the legislators. These would in turn be added to the list of analogues in an ever-spreading net of prohibition (Jenkins 1999, pp.84–85).[572]

In 1993 a federal *Domestic Chemical Diversion Control Act* enabled the federal government to have tighter control over the diversion of chemicals used in the production of illicit drugs. Hitherto, much precursor control was in the hands of state legislators giving rise to inconsistent, contradictory and unworkable regulations both within and between states. In 1996, recognising the growing menace of the methamphetamine trade and manufacture, a specific form of precursor control – the *Methamphetamine Control Act 1996* – was enacted. The Act's main objective was to forbid the sale and purchase of large amounts of pseudoephedrine. Unfortunately, as is often the case with drug supply control, when one avenue is closed another will quickly appear. One of the unintended consequences of the legislation is the large amount of ephedrine being smuggled into the USA through Mexico and Guatemala (see Wermuth 2000).

At state level, laws and particularly those concerned with drugs offences and punishment are varied and inconsistent between the states and far too numerous to enumerate here. The following discussion profiles some state laws that are of particular interest due to their uniqueness.

In most Western jurisdictions problems arise not so much with the criminal charges applicable to the possession and trafficking of amphetamines and 'party drugs' as much as the criminal activities associated with the manufacture of these drugs and the illicit use of precursors associated with them. As has been discussed above, in Victoria the definition of trafficking will extend to the manufacture of these drugs; however, it has been noted there are clear problems in proving intent. American laws for the most part circumvent these problems with reverse onus or similar provisions. Some of the best American legislation in this area, according to Australian police sources, comes from the state of Arizona.

572 Thus new drugs can be prohibited in the United States relatively quickly and in response to particular circumstances as they arise or as some critics would argue in response to a media driven agenda less concerned with thoughtful policy than political pandering. See for example Jenkins (1999), particularly in the context of the scheduling of GHB. He argues that the scheduling process was largely in response to a media driven frenzy as a result of the death of a young woman called Hillary Farias. Indeed in the curious American tradition of naming acts of the Congress after specified people (in the context of drugs – usually victims) the drug was not only scheduled but in 1998 the Hillary J. Farias Date Rape Prevention Act was enacted.

Detective Inspector Paul Steel outlined these provisions in his Churchill Fellowship Report as follows:

- An offence to manufacture a prohibited drug.
- An offence to be in possession of chemicals or equipment to manufacture a prohibited drug. Importantly it is not necessary to prove the offender's intent to manufacture the prohibited drug, merely the possession of the items.
- An offence for being in possession of more than 24 grams of pseudoephedrine. There is currently an amendment pending which will lower this limit to 9 grams. Again no intent is necessary.
- An offence for selling or supplying more than 24 grams of pseudoephedrine without a valid permit. This also is being lowered to 9 grams.
- An offence for anyone who sells or supplies a precursor, regulated chemical or other substance or equipment with the knowledge that it will be used to manufacture any dangerous drug.
- A child abuse offence for anyone who manufactures, keeps or transports any equipment or chemicals to manufacture in the presence of a child (Steel 2003, p.22).

Similar and even more stringent child endangerment laws have been passed in California:

> As with Phoenix legislation, California has implemented child abuse laws specifically relating to children being located at or in clandestine drug laboratory sites. These are not only enhancements or circumstances of aggravation but also create an offence of felony child abuse charges in their own right. This legislation has far reaching effects as it not only relates to clandestine drug laboratories, but any area where children are around drug use or drug dealing.
>
> The thrust of the legislation started as a result of a laboratory explosion in northern California. On this occasion a mother established a clandestine drug laboratory manufacturing methylamphetamine where she was living with her children. When her laboratory exploded it killed three of her children and as a result she was charged with three counts of Felony murder. The resulting case law decision concluded that clandestine drug laboratories are *inherently dangerous.* Therefore for the purposes of these charges or those of felony child abuse it is not necessary for the prosecution to prove that a laboratory was dangerous, only that the laboratory existed.
>
> As part of this program, any time a child is located in the presence of a clandestine drug laboratory, specialist child abuse investigators in company with the Child Protection Services attend the scene and conduct interviews with the child and adults. A protocol exists where the child undergoes a urine test to monitor exposure and appropriate action in respect to their health are undertaken. Results from this program have shown that in at least 35% of cases

> the children have tested positive to methylamphetamine. In addition many others have been exposed to other dangerous toxic chemicals. The actions taken in relation to the placement of the child will vary but the key solutions include removing them from the drug-endangered environment and providing medical treatment where it is required (Steel 2003, p.24).

The Committee was fortunate enough to meet with Detective Paul Steel in Perth in October 2003 and was very interested to hear him discuss the provisions outlined above. With regard to the child endangerment provisions he states:

> They [California Police] now have dedicated teams of investigators, whereby first of all they have brought in legislation saying that if you transport chemicals used to manufacture prohibited drugs in the company of a child you commit a felony. If you manufacture or have a child living with you while you are manufacturing prohibited drugs you commit a felony, but perhaps more importantly to what we deal with, if you deal drugs and you have children living at the place that you're dealing drugs or with you at the time you also commit a felony.
>
> So in any of those cases a dedicated team, consisting of child abuse investigators and a welfare worker...will attend the scene. The investigators will take photographs of where the child slept, ate, etcetera, in relation to where the chemicals or the drugs were being dealt.
>
> The welfare worker will then deal with the welfare of the child and that doesn't always require a placement, it may be that the child can go with relatives. However, they will take them to hospital where a dedicated team of medical officers will initiate a set of medical protocols and they will basically test the child's urinalysis, not generally blood, to make sure that they haven't been affected by the chemicals. Now, they have found that in 34 per cent of cases where children have been present at clandestine drug laboratories they have tested positive to toxic by-products.
>
> Interestingly, over 50 per cent of cases where drugs are being dealt the children have tested positive to the actual drugs themselves. So what they will do first off is obtain the needed medical treatment for the child, they will then move on and deal with any placement issues. [They] have a set of prosecutors who are actually trained in this type of field, so therefore when the brief comes before the Courts we are not having people who aren't aware of what is going on prosecuting them and those prosecutors deal with the same briefs all the way through, establish some parity between them.[573]

Detective Steel informed the Committee that many of the American initiatives will be presented by the Western Australian Police Minister to the National Ministerial Council on Drug Strategy with the idea of eventually adopting these measures in Australian jurisdictions.

---

573 Detective Sergeant Paul Steel, Western Australian Police Service, in conversation with the Drugs and Crime Prevention Committee, Perth, 1 October 2003.

The Committee has taken note of Detective Steel's suggestions and advice and makes the following recommendation:

Recommendation

24. The Committee recommends that legislation be drafted to protect endangered children, in particular making it a crime of child abuse, as well as a circumstance of aggravation to a drug offence, if a person manufactures, stores or transports chemicals and/or apparatus used to manufacture, prohibited drugs in the presence of children.

United Kingdom

While British law imposes relatively heavy penalties for trafficking in 'Class A' drugs, under which amphetamines and most 'party drugs' such as MDMA are classified, it is generally not as punitive as American law. Harm minimisation programmes such as needle and syringe exchanges generally operate within an approved legal framework. The key British legislation is the *Misuse of Drugs Act 1971*. In recent years this Act has been the subject of a number of inquiries, the most important being the independent Police Foundation Inquiry (Police Foundation 2000). Klee comments on the Report (known as the Runciman Report) published as a consequence of this inquiry as follows:

> Distinctions between actions based on relative risk should be reflected more accurately in law. The [Police Foundation] Inquiry acknowledged the fault lines in current legislation on drug use and the consequent damage to its credibility among young people. [Its] first conclusion was that 'it has become inescapably clear that the eradication of drug use is not achievable and is not therefore either a realistic or a sensible goal of public policy'.
>
> Among the principles identified as the bases of a law on drugs are:
>
> 1. It should infringe personal freedom only to the degree necessary to restrain serious levels of harm to users or others
> 2. It should target the drugs that cause the most harm
> 3. It should reflect the relative harmfulness of activities connected with each illicit drug or category of drugs and provide sanctions proportionate to that harm (Klee 2001b, p.89).

Yet even before the publication of this Report there were signs of a change in policing practice, if not the law, in some areas of Britain. Measham et al., for example, explains that:

> The focus of police enforcement of drugs legislation in Britain is now moving from possession to supply with the targeting of resources. Many police chiefs have said they will no longer target possession and people will only be arrested for possession if it comes to the police attention in the course of their duties.

> However...for low level recreational drug use by clubbers these distinctions do not fit with young people's experiences. For a range of reasons...there are real incentives, financial and otherwise, for people to buy their drugs in friendship networks, to buy in bulk and redistribute them, whether or not they plan to make any extra profit from such transactions (Measham, Aldridge & Parker 2001, p.178).[574]

For this reason the Runciman Report has called for the creation of a new hybrid or 'halfway' offence that recognises the 'mutual societies' that exist when it comes to selling club drugs:

> Located somewhere between possession and supply this would recognize the act of clubbing together to buy drugs where one person may be caught in possession of substantial amounts, more than for personal use, but not for commercial sale for profit.
>
> One drawback, however, would be the definition of profit in such legislation. Whilst profit is not the over-riding priority for these friendship networks, users can and do make profits in cash or kind from economies of scale (Measham, Aldridge & Parker 2001, p.179).

Another drawback with this proposal is that it may become a fall-back position for a person who *is* commercially trafficking to use as a defence. This is certainly the view of at least one Victoria Police officer when an opinion on the English proposal was sought at public hearings in October 2003.

While the above proposals are certainly in the liberal tradition of drug law reform, there have also been other more traditional counter-measures enacted for policing, particularly for policing the use of 'party drugs'. The *Criminal Justice and Public Order Act 1994* has effectively banned open-air unlicensed raves and dance parties. More recently the *Public Entertainment Licenses (Drug Misuse) Act* enables both local government officers and police to close down clubs and other venues by refusing licences or permits in cases where the club is regarded as having a 'serious drug problem' on the premises or nearby land.[575]

Conclusion

Law and law reform does not consist solely of the written law, regulations, offences or proscriptions. An essential aspect of the administration of the criminal law is the investigation and the policing of those offences. This is especially true of drugs law and policy. The problems associated with policing amphetamines and 'party drugs' is the subject of the next chapter.

---

574 Measham's survey research found that a staggering 91% of the interview sample of clubbers reported having received their illicit drugs from friends either for free or as part of a not-for-profit sale. Seventy-eight per cent of the sample reported giving or selling illegal drugs to friends.

575 Interestingly, the City of Stonnington at the time of writing was endeavouring to have a dance club within the nightclub precinct of Prahran/South Yarra closed down due to violence, weapons and drug-related incidents. Committee note: Since writing the draft of this chapter an interim order closing the nightclub was issued by the Victorian Civil and Administrative Tribunal.

13. International and Domestic Supply Control

International control of psychostimulants

From an international perspective, the United Nations Drug Control Programme has estimated that profits are higher for amphetamine-type stimulant producers, suppliers and distributors compared to heroin and cocaine 'since production is easier, supply routes shorter and a wide range of drugs can be manufactured from a number of precursors' (in Klee 2001b, p.81).

International law and policy play a large part in determining domestic drug policy. The actual legal frameworks and conventions governing drugs have already been discussed in Chapter 12. This brief section is more concerned with how the politics and administration of international drug control has a bearing on supply and policing issues in individual countries such as Australia.

Drug policy, as in any area of social or legal policy, is subject to philosophical, political and legal difference between member states of the United Nations. Many European nations, for example, have called for the United States to move beyond a 'War on Drugs' policy:[576]

> [a]nd adopt a public health approach that would require a redirection to treatment of many of the resources currently devoted to law enforcement (Lenton 2003, p.271).[577]

As Lenton suggests, criticism has been levelled in particular at the weight given to supply control and law enforcement by the American drug administration, with its emphasis on strict prohibition, despite the fact that '[s]uch policies, especially those that focus on drug law enforcement are rarely evaluated' (Lenton 2003, p.272). Moreover:

---

576 See, for example, the Editorial 'Rethinking America's "War on Drugs" as a public health issue', *Lancet*, 2001, no. 357, p.971. See also Bollinger 2002.

577 It has been argued that in some instances the United States has had a disproportionate influence on international drug policy. An example cited in Chapter 4 of this Report was the alleged pressure put on the Drug Expert Committee of the World Health Organisation to proscribe the therapeutic use of MDMA. See Van Laar and Spruit 1997 on the criminalisation of MDMA, and see generally Webb 2003; Lenton 2003.

> [in] countries outside the USA, particularly the 'supply countries of Latin America where the impact of US drug policy is probably greatest, there are the accounts of the collateral damage of this policy on social, economic and political life and civil society (Lenton 2003, p.271. See also Astorga 2001).

The main international agencies that are involved in the formation and implementation of drug policy are:

- The United Nations Drug Control Programme (UNDCP)
- The European Union (The Pompidou Group)
- The World Health Organisation (WHO)
- Interpol
- International Narcotics Control Board.

When it comes to international strategies for the containment of amphetamines' manufacture and distribution, the United Nations and its agencies have had both successes and failures due to the complex array of social, legal and political factors that arise from mediating between a mix of poor and wealthy countries with a variety of different political and ideological systems.[578]

> Closely connected to such control is the degree of power held by government. In established democracies, government credibility can be undermined if policy does not address the issues of concern to the electorate. In non-democratic countries the consequences of exploitative power are often oppressive and policies imposed rather than agreed. The success of drug control measures, agreed internationally and adopted by participating nations, will inevitably be influenced by their political profile. Any breakdown of international collaboration in an exercise that has to close the loopholes in the overall system with legislation, education, training and better lines of communication, is serious since it will be the weak points that are targeted by crime syndicates. These developments are in their infancy and there is a long way to go before the necessary infrastructures are in place, both within and between nations (Klee 2001b, p.81).

Klee argues that effective international drug collaboration is also weakened by a 'culture of blame':

---

578 And even between countries which might be said to share the same structures, political outlook, economic base or ideological worldview, for example Sweden (conservative drug policy) and Denmark (liberal drug policy). An illustrative example of the divide between an approach that could be broadly termed public health/harm reduction and one that is based on zero tolerance/law enforcement can be seen in the diametrically opposed approaches between the European Cities Against Drugs [ECAD] based in Stockholm and strongly opposed to decriminalisation and harm reduction policies and the pro harm reduction philosophies of the European Cities on Drug Policy [ECDP]. The latter group was in part formed in reaction to the hardline approach of the ECAD. Its members come from cities and countries which have been 'severely affected by drugs and drug trafficking' (Klee 2001c, p.169).

Klee argues that these differences in policy and philosophy are one of the main reasons it is so difficult for the UNDCP to achieve unanimity in cross-border law enforcement (2001c, p.169).

> [w]here the source of a nation's drug problems are attributed to lack of appropriate action elsewhere. The widespread adoption of harm reduction in Western Europe and Australia is regarded as setting a poor example by the more punitive cultures of Southeast Asia and the United States (Klee 2001c, p.159).

Despite such constraints and 'buck passing' there are a number of ways in which international agencies have been able to collaborate to contain the proliferation of drugs in general and amphetamines and 'party drugs' in particular:

- The development of subregional action plans suitable to a particular state or group of states;
- The development of international data collection, trend monitoring and early warning systems through the United Nations' Global Assessment Programme (GAP);
- Information sharing procedures between states, particularly through use of the Internet;
- Cross-border monitoring programmes;
- Collaboration between state, national and international police forces and other law enforcement agencies;
- Precursor controls, including greater monitoring of pharmaceutical companies;
- Working towards common legislation on control of drugs manufacture and trafficking;
- Education and training initiatives, particularly for police, customs and pharmacists; and
- Collaborating with non-government organisations with regard to prevention, education and treatment.[579]

It is against the background of these international initiatives that Australia's efforts to contain the manufacture, distribution and supply of amphetamines and 'party drugs' needs to be examined.

Amphetamines and supply control in Australia

Australian drug control policies are based on a three-tiered approach that equally emphasises (in theory) supply, demand and harm reduction policies. As was stated in the previous section, different emphases will be apparent in other jurisdictions:

> In countries such as the Netherlands, for example, relatively more emphasis is placed on demand reduction measures. In the United States, supply reduction strategies attract the majority of funding, public and media attention, and political support. Australia, through its National Campaign Against Drug Abuse (NCADA), has consciously attempted to integrate demand and supply

579 For an account of these programmes, see Klee 2001c.

> reduction philosophies, seeking to find a balance which is appropriate for its circumstances (Wardlaw 1993, p.91).

Demand and harm reduction policies will be discussed in more detail in Chapter 19. The focus for the rest of this section is on supply control.

Wardlaw states that amphetamines and other psychostimulants pose particular problems for law enforcement and supply control in Australia as well. One reason for this, of course, is the fact that much amphetamine is manufactured in Australia. Source control measures that take place overseas, for example crop substitution, are for the most part irrelevant in this case. The most obvious methods of supply control with regard to amphetamine are border interdiction, targeting distributors, the destruction of clandestine laboratories and the restriction of the supply of essential ingredients – precursor control.

Border interdiction

While much, if not most, of the amphetamine available in Australia is manufactured locally, significant amounts are imported from overseas. However ecstasy, as will be discussed, is mainly imported into the country, particularly from the Netherlands and other European countries. Border interdiction is therefore still important.

Detection of illicit drug imports and exports is primarily the joint responsibility of the Australian Federal Police and the Australian Customs Service. After initial detection of illicit drugs, Customs will usually notify the Federal Police for follow-up investigation.

According to the Australian Bureau of Criminal Intelligence (ABCI) the principal amphetamine-type stimulant imported into Australia during 2000–2001 was methamphetamine. The Bureau states:

> Concerns that East Asian methylamphetamine would become a greater threat to Australia appear to have been well founded. The year saw a typical background level of small seizures from parcel-post and air passengers. Superimposed on this background was a 79.1 kilogram seizure of high purity crystalline methylamphetamine in November 2000 from a shipping container which arrived in Sydney from China. The seizure fits a pattern increasingly being seen around the world in which large quantities of multiple illicit drug commodities are shipped together. In addition to the 79.1 kilograms of methylamphetamine, approximately 184 kilograms of heroin also were detected.
>
> In January 2001, Thai naval forces intercepted a fishing vessel in the Andaman Sea carrying 116 kilograms of heroin and 7.8 million methylamphetamine tablets. A route has been established for Golden Triangle drugs to be taken overland south through Myanmar, by sea to ports in Thailand or further south and east, then to consumer markets. Particularly threatening to Australia is the production of heroin and methylamphetamine as tablets and high purity powder occurring in this nearby region.

> The seizure in early January 2001 of 142 kilograms of crystal methylamphetamine in Port Klang, Malaysia, illustrates the significant place of China in the amphetamine-type stimulant trade in the region. The drug had been smuggled from China by a group with connections in Hong Kong, Singapore, Malaysia and Australia. This seizure was a result of international cooperation in an investigation of a group using Malaysia as a transit area for trafficking methylamphetamine and ecstasy in the Asia-Pacific region. Other phases of the operation included the seizure of 37 kilograms of precursors and 113 kilograms of other methylamphetamine; the activities of drug traffickers who had been of long-term interest to law enforcement agencies in Australia and Southeast Asia were disrupted. This operation was enabled by the Australian Federal Police Law Enforcement Cooperation Programs assistance with training and equipment (ABCI 2002, p.39).

In 2001–2002 the Australian Crime Commission (ACC) reported that:

> During 2001–02, the Australian Customs Service (Customs) detected a record quantity of 428.3 kilograms of amphetamine-type stimulants excluding MDMA. This included the largest detection of amphetamine-type stimulants at the border to date: 168.5 kilograms of methylamphetamine, 152.2 kilograms of crystalline methylamphetamine and 90.7 kilograms of mixed amphetamine-type stimulant tablets (as well as 1.6 kilograms of MDMA) on a small craft in Queensland in July 2001.
>
> The total weight of methylamphetamine (including crystalline methylamphetamine) detected increased from 83.4 kilograms in 2000–01 to a record 324.1 kilograms in 2001–02. There were 203 detections, a significant increase on the 49 in 2000–01. The average weight of detections rose from 1.7 kilograms in 2000–01 to 2.1 kilograms in 2001–02. All but one of the 203 detections involved importation. The single export detection was 8.7 grams of amphetamine tablets in a mail article destined for Japan.
>
> In 2001–02 crystalline methylamphetamine accounted for 154.3 kilograms in 30 detections. Between 1997–98 and 2001–02, detections of crystalline methylamphetamine increased from less than one kilogram to more than 154 kilograms (ACC 2003, pp.52–53).

Importation of illicit drugs is most commonly done by one of three ways – through the post, by sea cargo and shipment or through air passengers:

> The most commonly detected method of importing amphetamine-type stimulants was through the post. Of the 202 amphetamine-type stimulant import detections made by Customs in 2001–02, 161 (79.7 per cent) used this method. Detections in air cargo accounted for 7.9 per cent of amphetamine-type stimulant detections, with a total weight of 10.5 kilograms.
>
> In 2001–02, small watercraft accounted for 96.1 per cent of imported amphetamine-type stimulants by weight due to the record detection of amphetamine-type stimulants in July 2001.

> During 2001–02 there were 44 detected importations from the United States (21.8 per cent of detections), 32 from the United Kingdom (15.8 per cent) and 23 from the Philippines (11.4 per cent).
>
> Of the 203 detections of amphetamine-type stimulants at the border in 2001–02, 105 were in New South Wales, 60 in Victoria, 18 in Western Australia, 17 in Queensland and three in South Australia. Although Queensland accounted for 8.4 per cent of the number of detections, it accounted for 96.2 per cent of the weight of amphetamine-type stimulants detected because of the significant small craft detection (ACC 2003, p.53).

Despite the relative success of these methods there are obvious limitations to curtailing the importation of illicit drugs:

> The obvious difficulty facing Customs is in identifying likely drug shipments or couriers in the huge flow of cargo and people entering Australia each year. The majority of drug seizures (although not the majority of the bulk by weight) take place during examination of mail items. Items are diverted for examination following alerts by drug detector dogs and according to the system of indicators based on the characteristics of items previously found to include drugs, but the task of finding all the contraband among the hundreds of millions of pieces of mail coming through the system each year is too large to expect great success.
>
> Similar problems are posed by other means of entry. An increasing trend is for large importations of drugs to be made concealed in cargo inside shipping containers... With nearly three-quarters of a million containers entering Australia each year and the fact that it takes a team of officers a number of hours to search each one thoroughly, it is obvious that it is impossible to screen containers generally...
>
> As with other supply reduction strategies, border interdiction cannot be expected to stop the flow of illegal drugs. Even with more resources, the size of the problem, the opportunities for evasion and the realities of commerce and human rights which limit the application of many possible tactics (such as strip searching every passenger) all conspire to ensure that Customs can only limit some supplies and make the jobs of the criminals more difficult (and the drugs, consequently, more expensive). Even if Customs could substantially strangle importation the fact is that most stimulants (with the exception of cocaine) are produced locally and even those that are imported could be manufactured domestically (Wardlaw 1993, pp.98–99).

While there have been definite improvements in the intervening period since the above statement was written, the basic problem regarding the searching of both cargo and individuals still remains – resources are arguably, and understandably given budget constraints, never as ample as they ideally could be.

However it should be noted that the Australian Customs Service commented in its Annual Report 2002-03 that drug-supply reduction and border-protection efforts were bolstered through a range of initiatives. These included:

- enhanced examination and response capabilities (such as the introdution of the container Examination Facilities).[580]

One aspect of modern detection of illicitly imported or locally manufactured drugs that requires separate discussion is the use of drug detection dogs. This issue will be discussed in the context of local policing initiatives in Chapter 17.

Particular law enforcement issues pertaining to ecstasy

Many of the general comments pertaining to supply control of amphetamines will apply equally to ecstasy and therefore are not repeated here. This section comments solely on those issues unique to ecstasy importation and control.

In a recent comprehensive survey of the global proliferation of ecstasy, Yacoubian (2001) notes that the international community has not tackled the problem of MDMA, its analogues or other 'party drugs' anywhere near as systemically as they have approached heroin, (meth)amphetamines, cocaine or even marijuana:

> While a comprehensive understanding of the drug phenomenon has been developed based on the concept of shared responsibility and respect for the fundamental principles in international law, as evidenced by successful interdiction efforts against cocaine, marijuana, and heroin...the focus should now turn to ecstasy. The global magnitude of the ecstasy problem makes it imperative that international co-operation be strengthened so as to respond adequately to new trends and modalities confronted by the countries in their anti-ecstasy efforts (Yacoubian 2001, p.133).

It is certainly true that distribution and subsequent control of ecstasy in Australia lagged somewhat behind other Western countries, particularly the United States. MDMA/ecstasy was first noticed in Australia in approximately 1984, but it would seem that until the late 1980s few law enforcement officials, including Customs Officers and various state and federal police forces, were aware of its existence or the networks used to manufacture or distribute it (Leser 1988).

The most recent analysis of illicit drugs by the ACC makes the following general observations regarding the phenethylamine group of drugs, of which MDMA/ecstasy is part:

- Although little evidence of MDMA ('ecstasy') production in Australia was found during 2001–02, the production of 'fake ecstasy' continued.

580 This programme is part of a $190 million strategy which aims to increase inspection rates of sea cargo by using container X-ray technology. As the Australian Customs Service explains:

All sea cargo arriving in Australia is risk assessed by customs and around 80,000 containers will be inspected each year once the new facilities are fully operational. This represents approximately five percent of the total loaded import containers across these ports, resulting in considerably enhanced border protection and savings in customs processing times for selected containers (Australian Customs Service at http//:www.customers.gov.au/resources accessed 18 March 2004).

- While MDMA production remains focused in Western and Eastern Europe, there was a significant increase in detections of phenethylamines transhipped via Asian countries.
- The total weight of seized phenethylamine importations increased from 338.4 kilograms in 2000–01 to 445 kilograms in 2001–02.
- The popularity of MDMA among users continued to increase in 2001–02. Availability of MDMA also increased during the period, specifically sourced from friends, acquaintances and lower level dealers (ACC 2003, p.69).

There were no confirmed detections of MDMA-producing clandestine laboratories in 2001–2002. This is the same as for previous reporting years.

However, while there is little evidence of clandestine manufacture of MDMA similar to that of methamphetamine, as indicated by the ABCI, tablets are being produced locally with a variety of drugs and chemicals being on-sold as ecstasy.[581] The great dangers associated with these tablets have already been discussed. It remains the case, however, that manufacture of MDMA takes place predominantly offshore. Issues with regard to the manufacture and distribution of MDMA will be discussed in Chapters 14 and 16 respectively.

Recent initiatives in MDMA control

As MDMA, mixtures of MDMA and other chemicals, and other 'party drugs' have become increasingly perceived as problematic, new initiatives, particularly through the Australian Federal Police, have been instigated to curtail their availability. Many of these initiatives have been co-operative ventures with the Netherlands. This is an acknowledgment of that country's primary role as a source of MDMA production. To this end the Australian Federal Police have opened a liaison office in The Hague as part of the Australian Federal Police Law Enforcement Cooperation Program (AFPLECP):

> The value of having immediate contact with authorities in the Netherlands was quickly demonstrated. In a joint operation with the Australian Federal Police in early December 2000, Dutch drug law enforcement authorities arrested high-level traffickers and seized 200 000 MDMA tablets – some intended for Australia – and large quantities of cannabis products. The operation was developed from intelligence surrounding the seizure of 50.75 kilograms of MDMA in Australia on 15 January 2000 (ABCI 2002, p.53).

Other initiatives through the AFPLECP have included:

---

581 The ACC comments that the majority of fake MDMA is most probably produced in Australia: 'Fake MDMA is likely to be cheaper to supply than real MDMA and gives dealers a greater profit margin. New South Wales Police report that precursors used for the manufacture of MDMA and MDA are scarce and extremely difficult to obtain, primarily due to their limited legitimate use. As a consequence, the production of substances such as MDMA in Australia is difficult' (ACC 2003, p.72).

- Seminars presented in Perth, Melbourne, Brisbane, Sydney and Canberra by a team of representatives from the Dutch Synthetic Drugs Unit, the German Bundeskriminalamt, Europol and Interpol;
- An Israel–Middle East regional synthetic drug trafficking seminar;
- Short-term attachments of Australian Federal Police agents to Europol headquarters in The Hague, the Bundeskriminalamt in Wiesbaden and the Dutch Synthetic Drugs Unit in Eindhove, focused on disrupting MDMA trafficking; and
- Inquiries in Europe following the seizure in Australia of 105 kilograms of MDMA concealed in wine cartons in a shipping container from France (ABCI 2002, p.58).

The most recent Illicit Drugs Report notes that the Australian Customs Service:

> [p]articipated in Operation Mercure, hosted by the Dutch Customs Service in March 2002. The operation was an exercise in the surveillance and control of air passengers from European participating countries to America, Canada and Australia, aimed at detecting passengers carrying synthetic drugs (ACC 2003, p.82).

Conclusion

Clearly the policing of any illicit drugs, let alone such a diverse range of substances known under the broad rubric of psychostimulants, amphetamines or 'party drugs' – each with their own user profiles, effects, source background and methods of distribution – is difficult and fraught with problems. Such policies are 'limited in [their] effectiveness by the reasonable restrictions which must be placed on law enforcement in a democratic society' (Wardlaw 1993, p.102. See also Henry-Edwards 2000; Henry-Edwards & Ali 2003).

Nonetheless, law enforcement clearly has its place. And the efforts of under-resourced law enforcement officials, whether they are state police forces, Customs or other national authorities, are commendable in difficult circumstances. However, supply reduction cannot, as Wardlaw states, be seen as a 'quick fix' solution. This is arguably the way the problem is viewed in the United States. Supply reduction measures, whether internal as in the destruction of clandestine laboratories or external with the greater patrolling of our borders, needs to be but one of a series of measures. Such strategies must also examine ways to reduce the demand for psychostimulants and/or reduce the harms associated with taking these drugs. There is no longer a strict demarcation between supply and demand. As the Commissioner of the South Australian Police has very eloquently stated:

> One of the problems that has occurred over the last decade is that the agencies responsible for dealing with drugs have been polarised. It is not as prevalent today, but it was so some time ago. Essentially, the view was taken that police were responsible for dealing with the supply side of illicit drug use and the

> health sector was responsible for dealing with the demand or use side. I think that polarisation was really unfortunate.
>
> The reality is that police have a lot to contribute by taking a fairly high focus on demand and use as well. We are on the front-line...
>
> Police are also in a position to be able to act as a catalyst, to do something constructive and positive, at a point when it might make a difference; when somebody has been detected in possession of or using drugs, taking action quickly to deal with that. Whether it is referral to treatment, information, or other forms of intervention, I think there is a role there for police. Going to court should be the last consideration in all of this. There is certainly a role for courts, but there are many other mechanisms that we should be looking at using.[582]

These areas of demand and harm reduction are part of the focus of Chapter 19. The next chapter, however, will examine more closely the actual process of manufacturing amphetamines and 'party drugs', with particular focus on the dangers facing law enforcement officers who investigate such manufacture.

Much supply control of amphetamines and 'party drugs' will necessarily involve border interdiction and the importation of these drugs. Nonetheless the position of amphetamines in particular is a unique one in that unlike heroin or cocaine they are drugs that can be produced synthetically in local environments. The local manufacture of amphetamines is a complex issue that demands separate discussion. It is the therefore the subject of the following Chapter.

582 Mr Mal Hyde, Commissioner, South Australia Police, in conversation with the Drugs and Crime Prevention Committee, Adelaide, 3 October 2003.

14. The Manufacture of Psychostimulants

When discussing the control of illicit drugs in Australia it is natural to think of the patrolling of our borders as being the major way in which law enforcement agencies attempt to deal with the 'drug menace'. For the most part this reflects the reality of supply control and law enforcement, at least with regard to drugs such as heroin, cocaine and the sophisticated and complex 'designer drugs' such as (pure) MDMA. When it comes to drugs such as amphetamine and methamphetamine the picture is quite different. Much of the production of these drugs is done within our borders.[583] This poses different and unique problems for law enforcement agencies, particularly local police forces and state law enforcement agencies. It is the problems associated with the local manufacture of amphetamines and to a lesser extent 'party drugs' which is the focus of this chapter.

The attraction of psychostimulants

> The drug 'barons' can keep ahead of the law by moving to a new [drug] formulation if an existing one is placed on lists of controlled substances. As a result, access to precursors is a key issue. Without them, any development of new markets by criminal organisations would be unprofitable and hence pointless. Legislation is needed that allows for inclusion of new formulations in lists of controlled substances if the designer drug market grows (Klee 2001b, pp.81–882).

When the Committee met with Detective Sergeant Paul Steel of the Western Australian Police Service he highlighted the huge profit margin that can be achieved from turning preparations such as Sudafed into amphetamine drugs:

> By way of example, one box of 30 Sudafed tablets contains 1.8 grams of pseudoephedrine which would equate to about 1.8 grams of final product methylamphetaminehydrochloride at about 80 per cent. If you take that to a street level purity of 5 per cent you will end up with 24 grams of final product from one $11 box of pseudoephedrine which would equate, even at that

---

583 A discussion of the sourcing of amphetamines from outside Australia has already been given in Chapter 13.

> purity, to somewhere around the $4000 mark worth of methylamphetamine from one box, so it is very easy.[584]

Commissioner Mick Keelty of the Australian Federal Police has posited seven reasons why (predominantly Asian) crime syndicates in recent years seem to have moved from heroin production to amphetamine manufacture. These include:

- higher potential market for amphetamines in comparison to heroin
- the vulnerability of opium crops to location by satellite or other aerial surveillance
- opium growing is subject to the vagaries of weather
- ready availability of precursor chemicals in Asia
- there is a shorter, less intensive production and distribution chain for synthetics
- higher profit margins – methamphetamine enjoys a considerably higher mark than opiates
- impending world shortage of opium due initially to Taliban; and more recently a drought in Burma.[585]

Wilkins expands on these reasons in more detail:

- Production of synthetic drugs is not limited to any specific geographical region or affected by seasonal cycles or weather conditions. The chemicals required to produce synthetic drugs are usually cheap, and manufacture is relatively simple for anyone with low-level chemistry skills. The synthesis of methamphetamine can usually be completed in one or two days. In contrast, plant-based drugs require lengthy and labour-intensive cultivation, harvesting and extraction processes. For example, marijuana grown outdoors takes four to five months to mature.
- The scale of the production of synthetic drugs is very flexible, and can be set up in a household kitchen, small enough to fit in a car boot, and quickly dismantled to prevent detection (they are often referred to as "boxed labs" as all the necessary tools and chemicals can be stored inside a box the size of a briefcase or electric-drill case) (Australian Bureau of Criminal Intelligence 1997, 1999).
- While plant-based drugs can only produce one type of drug, clandestine laboratories can produce a number of different types of drugs, using a number of synthesis routes and alternative precursor chemicals (Australian Bureau of Criminal Intelligence 1997). There are currently four different

584 Detective Sergeant Paul Steel, Western Australian Police Service in conversation with the Drugs and Crime Prevention Committee, Perth, 1 October 2003.

585 Quoted in the submission from Youth Substance Abuse Service to the Drugs and Crime Prevention Committee, Inquiry into Amphetamine and 'Party Drug' Use in Victoria, October 2003.

"recipes" commonly used to manufacture methamphetamine (Australian Bureau of Criminal Intelligence 1997, 1999, 2001).

- While both the plant and its extraction are equally illegal in plant-based drugs (for example, cannabis plant and hash oil), many of the precursors to produce synthetic drugs are everyday legal chemicals (for example, red phosphorous) or can be found in over-the-counter drugs (for example, pseudoephedrine in cold remedies). With synthetic drugs it is only the end product that is illegal, which means action by enforcement agencies requires precise timing to be effective (that is, not before the end product is made or after it has been distributed) (Australian Bureau of Criminal Intelligence 1997).
- Structural modifications can be made to a synthetic drug to circumvent existing laws by producing a substance that is not specified in control legislation or carries a lower penalty while retaining similar effects (known as a drug analogue).
- On the demand side several features of synthetic drugs make them more attractive to drug users than the traditional plant-based drugs (United Nations Drug Control Programme 2001) (Wilkins 2002, pp.18–19).

Manufacturing psychostimulants

A recent report on illicit drug trends across Australia published by the Australian Bureau of Criminal Intelligence (ABCI)[586] stated:

> The majority of amphetamine-type stimulants available on the Australian market during 2000–01 continued to be the result of domestic production in clandestine laboratories involving both sophisticated and rudimentary techniques and equipment. Illegal methylamphetamine producers, known as 'cooks', often contract their services out to various groups, though certain groups have their own resident 'cook'. While there have been instances of qualified chemists taking part in the illegal production of methylamphetamine, the majority of 'cooks' are largely self-taught with little to no formal training in chemistry. A sharing of skills and an exchange of information on methods of extraction and manufacture take place, especially on the Internet (ABCI 2002, p.35).

There has also been a proliferation of laboratories, predominantly methamphetamine producing, established in the United States:

> In 1999, the DEA [Drug Enforcement Administration] participated in the seizure of a record high 1,948 clan labs, the vast majority (99 percent) of which were meth labs. For comparison purposes this number was 306 in 1994 – representing a 537 percent increase in just five years. In addition, state and local law enforcement officers raided more than 4,400 such labs in 1999. In fiscal year 1999, DEA arrested 8,600 people for meth trafficking – a 113 percent increase over fiscal year 1996 arrests (Hargreaves 2000, p.2).

586 Now the Australian Crime Commission (ACC), see Chapter 13.

Where and how manufacture takes place

In Australia, amphetamine, and particularly methamphetamine, is widely manufactured illegally in these clandestine or underground 'laboratories' (often referred to as 'clan labs').

Recent figures compiled by the Australian Crime Commission (ACC) show that:

> During 2001–02, 240 clandestine laboratories were located in Australia...[a] steadily increasing number discovered each year. The number of laboratories discovered in Queensland almost doubled in the reporting period (77 to 138). New South Wales recorded the next highest number (32). While no laboratories were detected in the Australian Capital Territory, the Australian Federal Police report indications of small scale production occurring but insufficient to significantly impact the Canberra market (ACC 2003, p.47).

Figures for the other states and territories can be seen in Table 14.1 below. Of particular note is the fact that in Victoria during the reporting period 24 laboratories were discovered.

Table 14.1: Clandestine laboratory detections, by state and territory, per quarter, 2001–2002

State/Territory	July-Sep 2001	Oct-Dec 2001	Jan-Mar 2002	Apr-June 2002	Total
New South Wales	9	7	4	12	32
Victoria	7	3	9	5	24
Queensland	42	28	29	39	138
South Australia	-	-	14	6	20
Western Australia	5	5	3	9	22
Tasmania	-	1	2	-	3
Northern Territory	1	-	-	-	1
Total	**64**	**44**	**61**	**71**	**240**

Note: 1. No clandestine laboratories were found in the Australian Capital Territory.
2. – signifies zero

Source: Taken from Table 4.2, Australian Crime Commission 2003, *Australian Illicit Drug Report 2001–2002*, Commonwealth of Australia, Canberra, p.47.

Ecstasy, while mostly imported from countries in Europe, has also been known to be manufactured in 'backyard labs', although these are few in number, unlike amphetamines and methamphetamines labs. According to the *Australian Illicit Drug Report 2001–2002*, there have been no confirmed detection of MDMA producing laboratories in 2001–2002 (ACC 2003) and only two possible MDMA laboratories were detected in 2000–2001 (ABCI 2002). No clandestine MDMA laboratories have been located in Victoria according to Victoria Police sources.[587] However, '[d]ue to the presence of MDMA precursors, Victoria Police

587 Confidential Submission of Victoria Police to the Drugs and Crime Prevention Committee, Inquiry into Amphetamine and 'Party Drug' Use in Victoria, August 2002. Referred to with the kind permission of Victoria Police. It should be noted, however, that late in 2003 media reports have noted that there has been at least one MDMA laboratory discovered by Victoria Police during that year.

identified a laboratory that may have been used to produce MDMA [in 2001–2002]' (ACC 2003, p.72).

While the production of pure MDMA is rare in Australia, largely because MDMA precursors are scarce and difficult to obtain, the production of fake MDMA tablets does take place in Australia. The production of fake MDMA is reputedly rising in Victoria (ACC 2003). It most often consists of methylamphetamine with adulterants of paracetamol, caffeine, ketamine or other unspecified additives.

A problem for law enforcement is the fact that these amphetamine-type stimulants, other than pure MDMA, are relatively inexpensive and easy to make:

> All that is needed to manufacture it is a basic knowledge of chemistry, a recipe, and access to precursor chemicals, predominantly ephedrine and pseudoephedrine. Large scale production is dependent on ready access to bulk quantities of these chemicals. Being controlled substances, ephedrine and pseudoephedrine are difficult to obtain on their own. However, it is easy to obtain pseudoephedrine from pharmacies where it is sold in many over the counter medicines such as the cold remedy, Sudafed. Boxes of 60 and 90 Sudafed tablets are no longer available over the counter in at least one jurisdiction (NSW), while in Queensland it is necessary to have photo ID before purchasing over the counter. But despite these regulations it is still a relatively easy matter for organised rackets in all jurisdictions to do the rounds of the pharmacies (Mundy 2001, p.3).

The 'finished product' of the (meth)amphetamine may vary in appearance depending on the quality of the precursor chemicals and the skill of the 'cook' or chemist:[588]

> Methamphetamine in its pure hydrochloride salt form is colourless, however substances on the market often have different colouration, indicating different ingredients and manufacturing processes... 'Inexperienced' manufacturers may produce a substance that is wet or even gluggy – this is unpleasant to taste, is very toxic and burns the nose, so [it] is either wrapped in a cigarette paper and swallowed with water 'bombing' or mixed and injected (Mundy 2001, pp.3–4).

Illicit manufacture of (meth)amphetamines and to a lesser extent ecstasy may be done by large underworld outfits in relatively sophisticated clandestine laboratories, as well as by individuals 'cooking' their recipes with little more than high school chemistry sets.[589] The information needed to cook the drugs,

588 Although many of the amphetamine cooks are 'amateurs' to say the least, a senior officer of the Victoria Police has commented that increasingly the criminals they are investigating and prosecuting have tertiary degrees and professional chemistry backgrounds. (Detective Senior Sergeant J. O' Brien, Major Drug Investigation Division, Victoria Police, evidence given to the Drugs and Crime Prevention Committee, Inquiry into Amphetamine and 'Party Drug' Use in Victoria, Public Hearings (Melbourne), 10 November 2003).

589 For an excellent discussion of the various methods used to produce and manufacture amphetamines (for example, Birch, Nazi, Red Phosphorous, Hydro Phosphorous methods), see Steel 2003, *Report*, pp.9ff.

however unsafely, is available from a wide range of publications over the Internet. The Committee was surprised by the ease with which these formulae could be obtained. Type 'ecstasy' or 'amphetamine' (manufacture) into any web site and numerous responses arise. For example, a search of the amazon.com on line books and music store website came up with a reference to, among numerous others, *Secrets of Methamphetamine Manufacture: Including Recipes for MDA, Ecstasy, and other Psychedelic Amphetamines. Revised and Expanded Fifth Edition* by 'Uncle Fester'.[590]

In the United States, the 'recipes' for methamphetamine are relatively simple, relying on reduction of ephedrine/pseudoephedrine, which in turn are produced from basic cold remedies:

> Although the complete list of formulas, hazards and chemicals employed to produce meth remains extensive, the vast majority of meth laboratories seized today use a common ephedrine/pseudoephedrine reduction method of manufacturing. This method requires a chemical not produced in the United States; however, laboratory operators can find the precursor chemicals needed in many over the counter cold medicines. Some clan operators purchase dozens of bottles of these cold remedies in order to extract the ephedrine or pseudoephedrine from the tablets.
>
> Meth cooks sometimes use a formula for production that uses two extremely dangerous and highly volatile chemicals – sodium metal and anhydrous ammonia. Sodium metal can ignite when it comes into contact with water and anhydrous ammonia is a deadly respiratory hazard. Some clan labs may even contain chemicals such as sodium cyanide, which if accidentally mixed with another type of chemical found in the same lab can produce a deadly hydrogen gas (Hargreaves 2000, p.4).

A report by the United Nations Drug Control Programme (UNDCP) explains the process of amphetamine and amphetamine-type stimulant synthesis in more sophisticated detail, as follows:

> One of the essential conditions for the clandestine manufacture of any synthetic substance is access to a chemical that serves as the key building block for the synthesis. This starting material – the precursor – has to fulfill a few basic conditions:
>
> - It has to have in its chemical structure some essential parts of the final molecule, so that it is possible to build the amphetamine-type substance

590 The entry comes complete with a set of reviews by satisfied (and unsatisfied) readers. Take for example, the following:

'I strongly recommend the purchase of this book. Geared towards the production of methamphetamine, the Uncle believes in hit and run tactics to avoid getting caught with a smoking gun in your hands...he also offers a range of psychedelic amphetamines that will no doubt appeal to the reader. The author was correct in saying that this is the best book in its genera [sic]; no other book in this field matches up to it in its clarity and directness. This book was the pinnacle of the underground scene in the 20th century... Filled with hardcore synthesis Fester offers a diverse range of tactics to counteract the heat and thence avoid detection' (Source and date of review withheld).

through a relatively simple process, in a few steps, requiring few and easily available additional chemicals and relatively simple technology;[591]

- The starting material should be cheap and easily available. While the preceding criterion does have some technological limits in terms of convertibility and feasibility, price and accessibility seem to be very elastic;
- The chemical structure of the precursor should provide for some flexibility in the synthesis. The number of alternates that are available on legitimate chemical markets for a given precursor, the number of end-products that can easily be made from that precursor, as well as the number of synthetic pathways that exist, or are possible, from a given precursor to a given amphetamine-type substance, all contribute to the attraction of a starting material to clandestine operators (UNDCP 1996, p.50).[592]

The manufacturing of amphetamines and amphetamine-type stimulants is attractive to backyard chemists from an economic perspective, as they are cheaper to produce than heroin or cocaine. The UNDCP states:

- The amphetamine-type end-products have a simple chemical structure, which makes them ideal for clandestine experimentation;
- Many simple chemicals can serve in the various synthesis processes, either as building blocks or as facilitators, and are cheap and widely available in most countries;
- A great number of simple synthesis methods and pathways have been developed, patented and/or published in the scientific literature, usually consisting of very few steps leading from a starting material (precursor) to the desired end-product;
- This information, and its availability, have been growing since the first quarter of the century;
- Ever-increasing technological awareness means that simple chemical conversion processes can today be performed by any amateur;
- Since ATS are very similar in chemical structure, they are ideal targets for minor structural modifications to obtain a different end-product;
- These modifications may be determined by the availability of the precursors or may be the result of a deliberate effort to circumvent legislation by manufacturing an ATS not covered by national law or international convention;
- The latter approach is similar to the molecular designing strategy in chemical and pharmaceutical research. This strategy is transposed, via the grey area between the licit and the illicit, into the manufacture of

591 As the UNDCP points out 'The relative quantities of chemical precursors required to produce a synthetic drug tend to be considerably less than the quantities of botanical raw material needed to produce a comparable amount of plant based narcotic drug' (UNDCP 1996, p.50).

592 For flow charts and diagrams outlining the synthesis of amphetamines and amphetamine-type stimulants, see UNCDP 1996.

what are called 'designer drugs', 'designer amphetamines, or more accurately, controlled drug analogues;

- It is particularly revealing that over the last decade, at least 30 amphetamine-type substances of clandestine origin have appeared in different countries; most of them have never been tested clinically;
- Finally, from the perspective of the drug user, or abuser, the *substitutive* nature of the whole group of substances should be noted; though with individual differences, they all provide pharmacological assistance in achieving very similar ends or effects (UNDCP 1996, p.126).

Chemical diversion or the use of precursors is relatively common in Australia with pseudoephedrine being the most popular of the compounds used:

> Domestic sourcing of the pseudoephedrine required for methylamphetamine production can occur through a variety of means – one of the more popular being organised runs to purchase individual packets of pseudoephedrine-based preparations (such as Sudafed) from all pharmacies in a particular geographical location.[593] Other means include the purchase of chemicals from hardware stores, armed robberies of chemical companies, theft from warehouses and establishing false companies to provide a legitimate cover for the acquisition of pseudoephedrine. The increasing incidence of theft from pharmaceutical companies, particularly in New South Wales and Victoria, is of concern to law enforcement.
>
> Methylamphetamine producers also sometimes assume the role of brokers of precursor chemicals. Groups based in Queensland's Gold Coast are known to have sourced precursors from associates in Melbourne before sending the finished product back to the same associate. In some cases, there is a division of labour occurring; associates in one jurisdiction are responsible for acquiring the precursors, while others are involved in some or all parts of the production and distribution process.
>
> The use of 'extraction houses' for the conversion of tablets to pseudoephedrine continued to be reported in New South Wales. The National Crime Authority reports that the product of a number of these houses has been used by groups for large-scale methylamphetamine production. In the Northern Territory, precursor chemicals are primarily sourced from interstate suppliers, though smaller manufacturers who are not affiliated with outlaw motor cycle gangs tend to source precursors from local chemical companies.
>
> The 2000–01 period has seen a move away from the sole use of Sudafed as a precursor to wider sourcing of pseudoephedrine-based products such as Logicin, Demazin, Actifed and generic brand decongestants. This has been a direct result of the increased restrictions on the sale of Sudafed as well as greater national awareness of its potential for use in the manufacture of methylamphetamine (ABCI 2002, pp.37–38).

593 For a detailed discussion of the role of pharmacists with regard to amphetamine manufacture, see Chapter 15.

Distribution and distribution networks are discussed separately later in this chapter, although with regard to amphetamines these are often part of the same groups or syndicates as the manufacturer. According to the ABCI:

> Most jurisdictions reported outlaw motor cycle gangs continue to play a dominant role in methylamphetamine manufacture and distribution, although Victoria Police and the Queensland Crime Commission reported that the level of involvement is not as significant as it has been in the past. There is also increasing evidence of outlaw motor cycle gangs aligning with Southeast Asian organised crime groups and other established criminal networks to produce methylamphetamine. Some Southeast Asian groups were actively supplying and distributing methylamphetamine on their own or in association with other Southeast Asian or other ethnic groups.
>
> All jurisdictions reported either direct or indirect links between outlaw motor cycle gangs and methylamphetamine manufacture (ABCI 2002, p.36).

The gangs and syndicates are most often associated with the large-scale laboratories, particularly in the Logan area of south-east Queensland. A newer phenomenon is the 'boxed lab', a relatively inexpensive way for producers to manufacture amphetamines:[594]

> A number of jurisdictions also identified an increased involvement of independent manufacturers operating small-scale, often mobile and decentralised laboratories. These laboratories are also referred to as 'boxed labs' because they can be easily packaged and moved. They present particular challenges and risks to law enforcement because they can be relocated quickly to avoid detection, collectively are capable of producing large amounts of methylamphetamine, and often contain highly flammable and explosive materials (ABCI 2002, p.36).

Although the majority of clandestine laboratories are located at the residence of the producer, following overseas trends mobile laboratories are increasingly being detected in hotel rooms, rented premises including high-rise apartments, self-storage units and vehicles.[595] Often units or flats are only rented for the duration of the manufacture process. Clandestine laboratories are also located on rural and semi-rural properties – Western Australia Police report the majority of detected production sites in that state have been in regional areas (ABCI 2002, p.36).

---

594 A senior officer of the Victoria Police Major Drug Investigation Unit estimates that 'for $10,000 you have a fully operating mini lab' (Detective Senior Sergeant J. O' Brien, Major Drug Investigation Division, Victoria Police, evidence given to the Drugs and Crime Prevention Committee, Inquiry into Amphetamine and 'Party Drug' Use in Victoria, Public Hearings (Melbourne), 10 November 2003.

595 The ACC notes that for the most recent reporting period:

'Queensland was the only jurisdiction to report the use of hotels for the production of methylamphetamine. Offenders will stay for several days to do the cooking and often use the premises as a base from which to distribute the drug' (ACC 2003, p.48).

Policing manufacture

As this chapter has already outlined, one of the difficulties associated with the manufacture of amphetamines is the ease with which they are produced:

> Would be chemists now make methamphetamine entirely from domestic legal materials. Laboratories require no elaborate facilities or natural resources, and distribution demand[s] little more than convenient access to the interstate highway network.[596] Speed manufacture [is] attractive because the process require[s] little expertise, and detailed instructions [can] be found in cheap, hands on manuals...[or the Internet] (Jenkins 1999, p.101).

When it comes to controlling the manufacture/supply of amphetamines and to a lesser extent ecstasy, a number of specialist initiatives have been put in place across Australia. In Queensland, where most of the synthetic laboratories are now located,[597] the Queensland Police has set up an Illicit Laboratory Investigation Task Force (ILITF) (now known as Illicit Laboratory Investigation Team (ILIT)) which has the specific task of investigating 'clan labs' (clandestine laboratories):

> This Task Force is contained within the State Drug Investigation Squad and is headed by a Detective Senior Sergeant, with 11 other officers. Each of these officers has undergone an intensive training course relating to the latest methods used in the manufacture of drugs such as 'speed', 'ecstasy', 'home bake heroin' and other drugs. A large part of the course is also dedicated to instruction on the safe handling of chemicals, Workplace Health and Safety Issues, and the use of self-contained breathing apparatuses (Sheldon 1997, p.17).

While many of the laboratories 'processed' by the ILITF have been the result of planned raids and intelligence, a growing number have also been located through non-specialist police officers performing routine duties:

> By way of example, 'clan lab' seizures have often been a result of such things as: police searching premises, attending normal complaints, attending fire scenes and on at least three occasions, have even been as a result of attending the scenes of traffic accidents.
>
> If recent trends are any indication of the general increase in the number of 'clan labs' in [Queensland], it has now reached the stage where *operational police officers are more likely than not to come into contact with a 'clan lab' in the course of their duties* (Sheldon 1997, p.17). (Author's emphasis)

---

596 For a discussion of the importance of the (Hume) highway for the distribution of drugs in country Victoria, see the discussion in Chapter 11.

597 This differs from the position a decade ago when it was claimed that Victoria had the highest number of manufacturing laboratories (Australian Federal Police 1991; Wardlaw 1993). Recent figures for the period 2000–2001 show that 138 laboratories were located in Queensland and 32 in New South Wales. Victoria had the third highest total with 24 laboratories, not much more than South Australia and Western Australia (20 and 22 respectively) (ACC 2003, p.47).

See Table 14.1 reproduced earlier in this Chapter.

The former ABCI has also stated that, at least in south-eastern Queensland:

> [m]any clandestine laboratories are detected as a result of calls for service or through information received from hotel/motel proprietors. In Brisbane, the Wynnum District of the Queensland Hoteliers Association has established an information exchange mechanism for the reporting of unusual odours or suspect persons staying in accommodation. Police in the Metropolitan North Region of Queensland are trying to establish a similar network with other hoteliers in Brisbane (ABCI 2002, p.47).

One of the important roles of the ILITF is with regard to the education and training of other personnel both within law enforcement agencies and in the community. ILITF for example, gives presentations and training to:

- Australian Customs Service
- Ambulance Service
- Fire Service
- Environmental Protection Agency
- Pharmacists
- Pharmaceutical Companies
- Chemical Companies
- Glassware Companies
- Hotels and Motel Associations.[598]

Detective Paul Steel of the Western Australia Police Service has studied the detection of clandestine laboratories in the United States. Various jurisdictions have gone to great lengths to establish community education programmes warning of the dangers of illicit drug manufacture. For example, a campaign titled 'What's Cookin in Your Neighbourhood' produced by the City of Phoenix, Arizona, Drug Enforcement Bureau, included a massive advertising and media campaign outlining the dangers of clandestine laboratories. The campaign also included a video titled 'Meth – Unsafe At Any Speed'.

Steel states that this successful, well resourced campaign was targeted at 'anyone who could ever conceivably stumble into a clandestine laboratory' This included:

- Community Groups
- Neighborhood Watch Committees
- Hotel/Motel Organisations
- Real Estate Agents
- Police and other law enforcement
- Fire and Rescue

598 Information provided by Sergeant Scott Feeney, Chemical Diversion Desk, Queensland Police Service in a presentation to the Drugs and Crime Prevention Committee, Brisbane, 27 June 2003.

For more information on the ILITF, see also Crook 2002.

- Ambulance
- Hospitals
- Garbage and Sanitation workers
- Social Workers
- Probation and Parole officers.[599]

In Victoria, the Major Drug Investigation Division of the Victoria Police has been active in investigating clandestine laboratories:

> Specifically, MDID operates a clandestine laboratory investigation unit, which has training for police members in the detection and safety management of clandestine laboratory sites. All investigators attending a clandestine laboratory site must wear protective clothing and abide by strict policy and procedures.
>
> MDID also operates a chemical diversion desk which is a liaison point for the chemical and pharmaceutical industry to report suspect chemical purchases or potential purchases. Advice is also given regarding security.[600]

Dangers associated with manufacture

As indicated, there are serious dangers associated with the manufacture of amphetamines. These affect the 'chemist' or manufacturer and his or her associates, the police and investigative officials who raid the laboratories, and the ultimate consumer.

> The manufacturing process is potentially dangerous, with the chemicals involved being extremely volatile. The major risks are from exposure to toxic fumes and explosions during processing. Indeed, law enforcement discovery of a number of clandestine laboratories has been occasioned by explosion or fire and by the characteristic odours which accompany the manufacture of amphetamines (Wardlaw 1993, p.96).

The dangers faced by law enforcement officials have been well documented (Sheldon 1997; Macdonald, Wilkins & Sheldon 1998; Hargreaves 2000; *Journal of the American Medical Association* 2000). Such dangers faced by 'first responders' (police, firefighters, specialist investigators) can range from inhalation of toxic fumes, frostbite through contact with anhydrous ammonia to death or injuries sustained by booby-trapped laboratories (for example, bombs set to go off should a raid take place). The latter have occurred predominantly in the United States (Sheldon 1997).

The American Hazardous Substances Emergency Events Surveillance system (HSEES) has investigated injuries sustained by first responders caused by exposure to chemicals while investigating clandestine methamphetamine laboratories:

599 Steel 2003, *Report*, p.20.

600 Excerpt from the confidential submission of Victoria Police (Drugs Policy and Services Branch) to the Drugs and Crime Prevention Committee, Inquiry into Amphetamine and 'Party Drug' Use in Victoria, August 2002. Quoted with the kind permission of Victoria Police.

> Hazardous substances released during and after an event usually enter the body by inhalation and skin absorption; acute exposures may result in cough, headache, chest pain, burns, pulmonary oedema, respiratory failure, coma and death. Of the types of responders usually on site first, police officers had the greatest number of injuries because they were present during and immediately after a release. Emergency medical technicians sustained most injuries through onsite exposure or direct contact with the clothing or skin of contaminated persons. Firefighters, the least often injured on site first responders, were likely to be wearing personal protective equipment during events... Standard uniforms worn by police officers, emergency medical technicians, and hospital personnel provided little or no chemical/respiratory protection. During some events, turn out gear worn by firefighters offered only limited protection (*Journal of the American Medical Association* 2000, p.2716).

In Australia these dangers have also been highlighted. Macdonald, Wilkins and Sheldon (1998) state that the instability of both the environment in which the drugs are manufactured and the manufacturers themselves add to the dangers:

> The reasons for stringent safety procedures become evident when the methods of making amphetamine, and the people involved in this lucrative industry, are examined.
>
> Virtually all methods of clandestine amphetamine production involve the heating of different types of chemicals, such as acetone and other solvents. The danger of this activity is increased when primitive items like camp stoves with open flames are used.[601]
>
> This creates enormous potential for an explosion of stored chemicals and glass equipment – a highly hazardous scenario.
>
> If this is not dangerous enough, the process of heating some chemicals gives off explosive and/or poisonous gases, such as hydrogen iodide or phosphene gas. Some of these poisonous gases are odourless but will cause death in a matter of minutes.
>
> Add to this that the offender is often an addicted, intravenous drug user who, as part of the symptoms of amphetamine addiction, suffers from paranoia.
>
> When the paranoia of discovery by police is realised, this person is located in his or her clan lab, surrounded by dangerous chemicals and pieces of apparatus that could easily become weapons and be used against, or thrown at, investigating police (Macdonald, Wilkins & Sheldon 1998, p.24).

Detective Paul Steel of the Western Australia Police Service has done specialist training with American clandestine laboratory detection teams. He has also testified to the great dangers of this type of work:

> In general terms, one of the largest hazards is the use of extremely flammable solvents. Several of these are so flammable that even the spark from a light

601 The dangers associated with 'home manufacture' is one of the reasons the Endangered Children laws discussed in Chapter 12 were enacted in California.

> switch or the use of a mobile telephone is enough to ignite vapours and cause an explosion. The dangers to innocent persons entering this type of atmosphere are obvious (Steel 2003, p.8).[602]

In Victoria there are stringent provisions applying to the investigation and clean up of clandestine illicit drug laboratories and the training of 'clan lab' investigators. Victoria Police advise:

> The clandestine laboratory unit staff complete the Clandestine Laboratory Safety Certification Course conducted jointly by forensic chemists and experienced investigators. Personnel attend regular interstate Clandestine Laboratory Safety Certification courses and they also attend the Australian Crime Commission National Chemical Diversion Desk Congress which is held annually. There is national liaison with all clandestine laboratory investigators where best practice has been identified and implemented. Every three years there is a National Clandestine Laboratory Course which includes international representation allowing overseas trends in this area to be shared with domestic investigators.
>
> The clandestine laboratory unit is equipped with all necessary safety equipment including fire retardant clothing and air monitoring equipment. Each time staff attend the scene of a clandestine laboratory data is recorded on a *'Laboratory Exposure'* form which every attending member is required to complete. Each member of the unit is subject to 12 monthly medical monitoring which includes, in particular, full kidney and liver function testing. There is ongoing evaluation of safety procedures and the upgrade of equipment as identified or required.[603]

Amphetamine manufacture also has clear dangers for the ultimate consumer of the drug. Prescription drugs are usually produced under strict quality controls. Consumers of ecstasy or methamphetamine may be taking a pill produced in unhygienic circumstances and with possible toxic adulterations.

It is little wonder, given the above facts, that Hargreaves states: 'Raiding a clandestine drug laboratory...has become one of the most dangerous operations a law enforcement officer can undertake' (Hargreaves 2000, p.1).[604]

---

602 While Paul Steel claims that Australian clandestine laboratory detection units are of 'best practice' standards by world comparison, few states require ongoing training and certification for their clandestine laboratory detection officers. This is something that Detective Steel believes should be mandatory (see Steel 2003, p.18).

603 Correspondence from Acting Commander Paul Ditchburn, Organisational Development Department, Victoria Police to the Drugs and Crime Prevention Committee, 23 March 2004.

604 Hargreaves also notes the risks posed to the environment from illicit amphetamine manufacture, particularly chemical contamination from the lab's hazardous wastes:

'Each pound of meth manufactured in a clan lab generates up to 5 or more pounds of toxic waste. Clan lab operators routinely dump such waste into local streams, rivers and sewage systems in order to cover up evidence of their illegal operations... The average clan lab costs $3000 to clean up. However, large production labs, because of the significant quantities of toxic chemicals and higher hazardous waste disposal charges can result in clean up costs exceeding $100,000. Annually, the overall cleanup of these labs costs the DEA and other government agencies millions of dollars' (Hargreaves 2000, p.4).

Recommendation

25. The Committee believes that both specialist and general police officers and emergency workers should be aware of the dangers associated with clandestine drug laboratories. To this end the Committee recommends the following provisions with regard to police and community education and training:

    a) Police education should ensure that all officers are suitably trained in clandestine drug laboratory awareness and safety procedures.

    b) Emergency service personnel should receive appropriate training with regard to clandestine drug laboratories.

    c) Existing certification courses for clandestine drug laboratory investigators should be regularly updated to reflect current trends in keeping with the world's best practices.

A note on the manufacture of MDMA/ecstasy

As has been mentioned throughout this Chapter, Australian chemists, particularly 'amateurs' or home 'cooks', rarely have the expertise or the access to raw materials to successfully make 'pure' MDMA. The decreasing amounts of the pure product that are found in the country tend to be 'imports':

> Western and Eastern Europe continue to be the main centres of MDMA manufacture, with a large amount of ecstasy produced in clandestine laboratories in the Netherlands (BINLEA 2001; INCB 2002; UNODCCP 2001). The Netherlands, as a central player in the international chemical industry, is an ideal location for the acquisition of precursor chemicals vital to the production of MDMA and other drugs (BINLEA 2001). The Australian Federal Police regard the Netherlands as the most significant MDMA production country, although they report that less MDMA was seized in 2001–02 than 2000–01. The quantities of MDMA seized in countries with established production links to the Netherlands continued to increase.
>
> MDMA manufacturing sites have been discovered in Belgium, Germany, Poland and the Czech Republic. The majority of countries identify the Netherlands and Belgium as the main sources of their ecstasy imports (UNODCCP 2001). The under-employment of chemists and chemical engineers in Central and Eastern European countries, particularly Poland and the former Czechoslovakia, may be linked to the increase in production of

---

The ACC has noted that the manufacture of methylamphetamine in Australia:

'[p]roduces toxic waste in a ration of ten to one – for every 100 grams of methylamphetamine illegally produced, a kilogram of of highly dangerous waste is produced and illegally buried or dumped in waterways' (ACC 2003, p.67).

According to the (former) ABCI, spoliation of the environment through illicit drug manufacturing waste is particularly noticeable in Queensland. In an effort to address this:

'The Queensland Health Scientific Services has sought to minimise the amount of chemical waste and enhance workplace health and safety by the on-site destruction of chemicals and equipment discovered at clandestine laboratory sites' (ABCI 2002, p.47).

MDMA and other amphetamine-type stimulants in these countries. Due to differences in how jurisdictions report drug seizures, it is difficult to produce a reliable estimation of global data figures. United Nations figures for hallucinogens seized globally – excluding LSD but including ecstasy – show an increasing trend since 1998.

The use of MDMA has only recently become popular in China's growing urban areas (USDEA 2002b). China's industrialised southeast has also seen the addition of MDMA to the well-established high purity methylamphetamine trade. There are reports that clandestine manufacturers in Southeast Asia may soon be producing MDMA comparable to the quality presently being imported from Europe (UNODCCP 2001). The Australian Federal Police reported high purity MDMA is being sent north from Malaysia to Thailand in exchange for heroin. And in a further example of the convergence of drug markets, an MDMA laboratory was detected in May 2002 in Cali, Columbia (ACC 2003, pp.72–73).

There are particular dangers in synthesising what purports to be MDMA. The most common starter chemicals used to manufacture 'pure' MDMA are piperonal, isoafrole, safrole and piperonylacetone (Gowing et al. 2001, p.3). However, accessing these chemicals, particularly since greater restrictions have been placed on their availability in recent years, has sometimes proven difficult. This results in the final product frequently containing a toxic or non-toxic mixture of chemical compounds that are often not related to each other (2001, p.3). As was noted in Chapter 6, these admixtures can often result in serious medical complications, including death. Pure MDMA is therefore mostly imported, partly as it takes more chemical expertise to synthesise.[605] MDMA is also more expensive to produce in its pure form. Therefore the labs that do purport to be making ecstasy are often manufacturing dangerous compound mixtures:

According to the [Australian Bureau of Criminal Intelligence's] intelligence officer Troy Kaizik, the reasons for this practice are largely economical:

"There is a fair difference in price between an amphetamine tablet and an ecstasy tablet... So what people are doing is they are producing amphetamine and basically pressing it into tablet form and selling it off as ecstasy, so they are making that much more profit."

Put $10.00 worth of amphetamine through a pill press and you have $50.00 worth of ecstasy.

Throughout the 1990s, most of the ecstasy available on the Australian market was manufactured overseas. The imported product was generally inexpensive and of high quality so demand for domestic product was minimal. But in

605 Klee notes that in Eastern Europe the production of amphetamine-type stimulants has become a lucrative business for the many unemployed chemists in the region and 'the economic and political crises that persist there make this work attractive' (Klee 2001, p.86).

recent years, as demand for ecstasy has increased, so too has the circulation of the fabricated pills.

It's a bit like moc-croc manufacturers cashing in on the popularity of real crocodile leather. Like fake fur. Like fake Rolexes. The culture of cheap imitations is universal – even in the drug world.

The analysis of ecstasy tablets seized by police in the last few years has reflected this evolution from real to fabricated ecstasy:

"In 1999 almost everything was MDMA and then there was a consistent introduction of other materials to the point now where something like maybe two in three pills aren't ecstasy. We've only had probably two, three or four serious attempts...of making MDMA as opposed to methamphetamine..." (Peter Vallely, Queensland Government Chief Chemical Analyst).

This assertion is backed up by official statistics...[606] And according to Mr Kaizik it's not just a case of the police not finding the labs. The fact is that most of the drugs marketed as ecstasy come out of ordinary amphetamine laboratories. Real ecstasy labs are few and far between.

And with so much fabricated ecstasy on the market, there appears to be more at stake for users than just fifty bucks. According to Mr Vallely, the stakes can be as high as human life:

"There are a couple of extremely toxic substances that appear in tablets from time to time, PMA being the one that springs to mind. If you take one of these other materials thinking it is MDMA, and you're familiar with the onset and the effect of MDMA, and these other materials have a slower onset, the tendency would be to think 'Well the tablet I bought had a particularly low level (of MDMA) I'll just drop another one'.

And suddenly you're in a situation where you've taken what is well within the toxic range and by the time the problems start to manifest themselves, it's far too late to really do anything about it" (all quotes in Moriarty 2001, p.9).

Conclusion

Dangers associated with the manufacture of amphetamines and 'party drugs' are serious, although not insurmountable. Some of the difficulties for law enforcement agencies stem from the fact that the various drugs subject of this Inquiry come from different sources. MDMA/ecstasy is usually imported from Europe, particularly the Netherlands, but 'fake' MDMA can be produced in clandestine Australian laboratories. Amphetamines and methamphetamines are both imported into the country and manufactured locally. Legitimate users and producers of precursor chemicals such as pseudoephedrine may feel aggrieved at

606 This is indeed the case. For example, the ABCI note:

'The trend, noted over the past two to three years, for methylamphetamine produced in clandestine laboratories in Australia to be incorporated into tablets continued during 2000–01. There have been instances of methylamphetamine being mixed with ephedrine, ketamine, caffeine, LSD or heroin, then made into tablets and imprinted with logos matching imported product and passed as ecstasy; thus attracting a higher price' (ABCI 2002, pp.36–37).

tighter controls on the production of these substances. Therefore different strategies and more resources are required to tackle the control and eradication of these drugs.

While the proactive measures used by international and domestic law enforcement agencies highlighted in this chapter are obviously to be encouraged, one of the most effective ways of curtailing the work of clandestine laboratories is to stop, restrict or reduce the amounts of essential ingredients available to the 'cooks' – that is, limit the precursor chemicals in circulation. Initiatives with regard to precursor control at both a wholesale and retail level are the subject of the following chapter.

15. International and Domestic Precursor Control

Precursors are the legitimate chemicals that can be illegitimately used by skilled and unskilled or amateur chemists to produce drugs such as amphetamines for illicit purposes. The previous chapter examined the actual processes and accompanying dangers associated with the manufacturing of amphetamines and 'party drugs'. This chapter focusses on the controls, measures and initiatives that have been put in place to curtail the manufacture of illict drugs. These include importation controls of precursors, wholesale restrictions and measures developed by pharmaceutical and pharmacy organisations to prevent the misuse of these chemicals at retail level.

International controls

Control of precursor chemicals as a law enforcement measure was first systematically used comprehensively by the United States:

> In extending the reach of earlier attempts at precursor control, the *Chemical Diversion and Trafficking Act* of 1988 included provisions to regulate the distribution of chemicals used to produce illicit drugs. The Act requires chemical companies to keep records of sales and purchases of regulated chemicals, to report any transactions of an extraordinary quantity, and to give notice to the Drug Enforcement Administration (DEA) of uncommon methods of payment and any excessive loss or disappearance of a listed chemical. By analysing these records, the DEA identifies suspicious buyers and thus locates illicit manufacturers.
>
> The precursor monitoring or restricting approach has attracted international interest and action. The 1988 United Nations Convention Against Illicit Traffic in Narcotic Drugs and Psychotropic Substances provides (in article 12) for measures to monitor and control the international movement of precursor chemicals, including those used in the manufacture of amphetamines and cocaine. In 1990, the United States was instrumental in establishing a Chemical Action Task Force, of which Australia is a member, to further examine strategies for precursor control (Wardlaw 1993, p.96).

Detective Steel of the Western Australian Police Service, a specialist clandestine laboratory detection officer, visited the United States in 2002 to examine amphetamine manufacture and control enforcement in a number of American states. He outlined how precursor monitoring works at one local level jurisdiction – San Diego, California.

> [Chemical diversion officers] attend all clandestine laboratories and record details about the chemicals, ingredients and apparatus located. They monitor and record brands, batch numbers and, where applicable, details of the retailer. The chemical diversion officer then tracks down the retail store details for these items where possible and attends the store to speak with the staff. They are advised that their products have been located at a clandestine drug laboratory and educated about their responsibilities in relation to the sale of these items. This may involve the serving of letters warning the business. If an individual retailer's products are repeatedly located at clandestine drug laboratory sites the retailers themselves may become a target of investigation and these warning letters can be used to show knowledge or reckless disregard (the Steel Report 2003, p.24).

Precursor control in Australia has taken two main forms; first, increased efforts over the last five years to target illicit importation of precursor chemicals into Australia; and second, increased domestic controls over the availability of substances such as ephedrine and pseudoephedrine, both at wholesale and retail level.

Importation control

It should be noted that tougher restrictions on controlling precursors in the United States (and other countries) has meant that in some cases clandestine production has simply been driven further underground. Such laboratories rely on the smuggling of the necessary chemicals from organised crime groups in Mexico where precursor controls are less stringent (Mundy 2001; Australian Bureau of Criminal Investigation (ABCI) 2002).

There is a risk of similar developments occurring in Australia:

> Customs and the National Crime Authority have highlighted the possibility that increasing volumes of chemicals required for amphetamine-type stimulant [ATS] manufacture may be imported by organised crime networks. Large precursor-producing industries already exist in China and India. Furthermore, due to regional instability, vulnerable states may become conduits in the future for the illicit supply of precursors for the Australian amphetamine-type stimulant market (ABCI 2002, p.38).

Federal law enforcement agencies have noticed a distinct relationship between the tightening up of domestic precursor controls and the attempted importation of large amounts of precursor chemicals:

> During 2000–01 Customs detected 1159 attempted importations of amphetamine-type stimulant precursors: pseudoephedrine/ephedrine (1025) and ephedra (134). In the majority of cases, these imports involved small

> quantities of health-and-fitness, weight-loss or cold-and-flu preparations licitly available over-the-counter in the country of origin. While in most cases these products are not intended for use in amphetamine-type stimulant production, their diversion into such production remains a potential risk.
>
> The sea-cargo seizure of 42 kilograms of pseudoephedrine-based cold-and-flu tablets concealed in furniture from Vietnam in November 2000 signified a major change in precursor importation. This sea cargo seizure indicates traffickers consider the importation of such tablets to be a viable strategy for sourcing precursors, given increased domestic precursor controls. In the same month Customs seized 12,000 tablets (approximately 11 kilograms) of ephedrine imported in an air cargo item from the United States.
>
> On 12 September 2000, a Customs detection of 100 kilograms of ephedra (containing 4.6 per cent pseudoephedrine and 1.6 per cent ephedrine) in air cargo from the United States led to the detection of a clandestine methylamphetamine laboratory in Manjimup, Western Australia, during a joint Customs, Australian Federal Police and Western Australian Police Service operation. This amount of ephedra could produce approximately four kilograms of methylamphetamine or around 47 kilograms of five per cent pure methylamphetamine tablets.
>
> Reflecting the wide-scale licit availability of these substances over-the-counter, the United States was the embarkation point for 885 detections of amphetamine-type stimulant precursors in 2000–01, accounting for 76 per cent of the number of detections. Other significant embarkation points included Indonesia (52), China and Canada (34 each).
>
> The most commonly detected method of importing amphetamine-type stimulant precursors during 2000–01 was the postal stream with 84 per cent of detections (978), which accounted for 4.2 per cent of the total weight. Air passengers accounted for a further 10.7 per cent of precursor detections and 28 per cent of the total weight.
>
> There were several significant passenger detections of amphetamine-type stimulant precursors, including the seizure of over 13,000 cold-and-flu tablets from the baggage of a passenger from Vietnam.
>
> The forms of amphetamine-type stimulant precursors detected by Customs in 2000–01 included capsules, caplets, tablets, powder, plasters, tea bags, injections, ampoules and soft gel (ABCI 2002, pp.41–42).

This trend has continued in 2001–2002, as noted in the most recent Illicit Drug Report (Australian Crime Commission (ACC) 2003).

Both domestic controls on the use of precursor chemicals and more stringent detection of their importation have led to some major supply control 'successes'. Paradoxically however, as has been discussed, increased control over the first may result in greater importation. This is not the only problem associated with such control. In some cases the chemicals used by illicit manufacturers are also used by legitimate industries, businesses and consumers:

> A major problem with such [precursor control] regulatory regimes is that they are administratively burdensome to implement. There are many companies involved in the commerce of precursors and the chemicals themselves cannot be restricted too much because they are essential to many legitimate manufacturing processes...
>
> The most obvious difficulty for any precursor control regime is that the precursors themselves may often be manufactured from yet other widely available and unmonitored chemicals. Regulations such as those passed in New South Wales allow for the list of monitored substances to be varied as needed. Obviously there is a point, however, beyond which additions cannot be made without the scheme becoming too cumbersome for police to administer and too onerous on the chemical sellers... This is particularly so because of the very wide range of drugs which could be manufactured. If amphetamine production is restricted by this scheme, there is a likelihood of illicit manufacturers simply turning to new sorts of drugs involving entirely different sets of precursors. Indeed this is likely to occur anyway as trends and fashions of drug use change over time. Further, a successful monitoring scheme could encourage an increase in theft of precursors and in importation either of precursors or, more likely, of finished drugs (Wardlaw 1993, p.97).

Moreover, strong precursor control, if it is to work properly, requires uniform co-operation at an international level. If one country has a strict regime but another does not, illicit producers will simply turn to the countries with the lax control systems. The importation of precursors from Mexico to the United States and beyond is a salutary case in point.

Domestic controls: Chemical diversion desks and precursor monitoring

Precursor monitoring became part of the national drug agenda in 1990. A Working Party on Amphetamine Control established by the Australian Police Ministers Council recommended that ways should be examined to schedule and monitor certain amphetamine precursors under state and federal legislation. In November 2001, a number of disparate national drug supply reduction strategies were combined into one National Supply Reduction Strategy for Illicit Drugs. This strategy has strongly supported the establishment of chemical diversion desks in each state and territory. Regulations implemented in most state legislation have resulted in certain substances being restricted or in transactions over a certain amount being notified to police authorities.[607] Victoria has been at the forefront of many of these initiatives:[608]

607 See for example, *Poisons and Therapeutic Goods Act 1966* (NSW). In Victoria, pseudoephedrine is a scheduled substance under schedule two of the *Drugs, Poisons and Controlled Substances Act 1981*.

608 As discussed in Chapter 12, Victoria Police have put forward a number of proposals for legislative change with regard to precursor control and manufacture. These have included reverse onus provisions and offences for having precursor chemicals in possession without lawful excuse.

> The Victoria Police Chemical Diversion Desk is involved in identifying potential alternative sources of chemicals for inclusion in the national precursors Code of Conduct and providing education on suspect purchase reporting, to identify illicit drug manufacturers. Overseas sourcing of precursor chemicals for illicit drug manufacture, particularly from China, has been identified as a particular concern requiring increased cooperation between law enforcement agencies.
>
> Victoria Police Crime Prevention Officers are working closely with the Victorian Department of Human Services (Public Health Division) and the Pharmacy Society on an initiative called Pharmacy Watch. Pharmacy Watch aims to provide advice to pharmacies on issues such as security, to reduce the incidence of burglaries and thefts of cold-and-flu preparations – for use in illicit drug manufacture – and other prescription drugs such as benzodiazepines. The program works with the Victoria Police Chemical Diversion Desk to develop ongoing strategies and training (ABCI 2002, p.47).[609]

The role and function of a chemical diversion desk can be summed up in the role statement of the Queensland Diversion Desk:

> The role of the Chemical Diversion Desk is to establish and maintain liaison with chemical, pharmaceutical and glassware companies for the purpose of collating information regarding suspicious purchases and inquiries on steroids; illicit and licit substances; chemicals and associated products.
>
> The Chemical Diversion Desk receives an abundance of information that essentially involves those persons suspiciously purchasing pseudoephedrine based products from pharmacies. This information is collated and placed on a database... For those persons who are identified as having multiple purchases or are known offenders, a report is generated and forwarded to the ILIT team for investigation. These reports are generated when the suspect has been positively identified and their current residential address has been confirmed.
>
> Feedback is provided by the Chemical Diversion Desk to chemical, pharmaceutical and glassware companies for the purpose of chemical security and increased awareness.[610]
>
> Priority areas for this Desk are both of a tactical and strategic nature. Tactically the Desk seeks to identify those persons making suspicious purchases or inquiries regarding precursor chemicals and or equipment. As a result of the

---

609 This Working Party consists of representatives from Victoria Police, Department of Human Services, Pharmacy Board (Victoria), Pharmacy Guild (Victoria) and the Pharmaceutical Society (Victoria). It has been meeting since approximately the start of 2002 to address the illegal diversion of pharmaceuticals containing pseudoephedrine:

'The working party has developed two posters: one for display in the rear of the pharmacy which advises the pharmacist and staff of the problem of pseudoephedrine sales and provides contact details to the MDID, and the other for public display advising that, due to the issue of illegal diversion, only one packet of pseudoephedrine based tablets will be sold per customer' (excerpt from the confidential submission of Victoria Police (Drugs Policy and Services Branch) to the Drugs and Crime Prevention Committee, Inquiry into Amphetamine and 'Party Drug' Use in Victoria, August 2002).

610 Officers of the Chemical Diversion Desk may also give advice to the relevant government department officers as to whether a wholesaler or chemical manufacturer should be granted or renewed a licence to produce precursors.

> information being received an assessment may be made as to shifts in the precursor chemicals sought and/or methods of production. This information is utilized to ensure current strategies capture the required information together with legislation being appropriate to address these new trends.
>
> The Chemical Diversion Desk contributes at a national level in the formulation of strategic direction of Chemical Diversion Desks.
>
> This is performed by continual liaison with the Australian Crime Commission in Canberra outlining trends or shifts in the illicit market for drugs, precursors and methods of manufacture. This information is also disseminated to the other chemical diversion desks around the country together with the appropriate law enforcement agencies.[611]

The Committee met with representatives of the Queensland Illicit Laboratory Investigation Team who expanded upon the role and duties of the ILIT and the associated chemical diversion desks at length:

> ILIT's approach to combating the synthetic manufacture of drugs is in four stages: reactive, intelligence-led, training, and pro-active. We have found that these all need to be linked together and feed back on one another so that we can get a full approach to the problem. It involves participation by members of the community as much as a policing issue.
>
> Our pro-active initiatives are recidivist offenders. We have quite a large profile of recidivists, and we actively target our recidivist offenders. We use the thinking that once you know how to make amphetamines we don't think you are going to stop, so you are going to continue on making amphetamines. We have a chemical diversion desk that maintains liaison with chemical and pharmaceutical companies. That desk is our link with all the industry people associated with the supply of precursor chemicals, glassware and some pharmaceutical issues.
>
> We also have an investigative chemistry unit – so together with members of the ILIT team and our forensic chemists, we go out and identify new methodologies that people are using to manufacture amphetamines and we try them under chemical conditions and see what they are trying to do and how they are attempting to evade detection so that we can bring up new methodologies. We also publish our findings of the methodologies internally within the state to other people who are ILIT-trained and to our investigators so they can be aware of current dangers or current modus operandi that are being used by the offenders.
>
> Reactive: ILIT is responsible for the processing and dismantling of all labs found within Queensland. We also assist regional police in the identification and sourcing of chemicals and apparatus that they may have found as a result of their investigations, and we provide support and operational advice to police

611 Background notes for a presentation to the Drugs and Crime Prevention Committee, by Sergeant Scott Feeny and colleagues, Chemical Diversion Desk, Queensland Police Service, Brisbane, 27 June 2003.

> on the front line. We also conduct controlled operations. We participate in a multidisciplinary team in covert operations, liaising with the controllers, the covert operatives, assisting them with their identification – if they walk into a planned lab we tell them what's going on. We also provide them with terminology and the necessary background to understand within a covert field what's going on.[612]

But the approach taken by Queensland Police is not necessarily a uniform one across jurisdictions, and despite the establishment of a National Chemical Diversion Database to collate local and national intelligence, a more tightly collaborative and uniform approach is needed:

> Australian jurisdictions are also working towards a unified response to criminalising precursor possession or establishing national systems to identify suspicious precursor purchases... [a]ll States and Territories have adopted a National Code of Conduct that places voluntary restrictions on the sale of chemicals used for manufacturing methylamphetamine and other psychostimulants. The Code has existed since 1994 and is also a means of monitoring suspicious sales of precursors, essential chemicals and reagents as well as laboratory equipment (ABCI 2002, p.38).

Moreover, despite the Victorian initiatives outlined above, this state does not compel pharmacists to record details of the purchasers of pseudoephedrine, unlike New South Wales. In a submission to this Inquiry, Victoria Police stated that:

> A working party consisting of Victoria Police, Department of Human Services and key stakeholders in the pharmacy retail profession has agreed that the rescheduling of pseudoephedrine based products would unduly hamper legitimate sales of these products without reducing their diversion into the illicit drug market. At this time there are no plans in Victoria to reschedule these products to bring them into line with New South Wales legislation.[613]

There have also been some co-operative and voluntary accords struck between the private sector and law enforcement agencies such as the Industry Code of Conduct:

> In 1996 the then Drug Squad in partnership with the Plastics and Chemicals Industries Association and the Scientific Suppliers Association of Australia developed and published a 'Code of Conduct' for Australian chemical manufacturers, importers and distributors. This document was developed in an attempt to prevent the diversion of precursor chemicals used in the illicit manufacture of ATS.

---

612 Detective Sergeant Jason Renwick, Illicit Laboratory Investigation Team, Queensland Police Service, in conversation with the Drugs and Crime Prevention Committee, Brisbane, 27 October 2003.

613 Excerpt from the confidential submission of Victoria Police (Drugs Policy and Services Branch) to the Drugs and Crime Prevention Committee, Inquiry into Amphetamine and 'Party Drug' Use in Victoria, August 2002. Quoted with the kind permission of Victoria Police.

> The document includes categories of drugs and materials that have been used in the illicit manufacture of ATS and requires industry stakeholders to sell these chemicals to account customers only and complete an end user declaration. The document also includes a requirement to notify law enforcement agencies of suspicious orders or enquiries.
>
> This document is a voluntary code of conduct only and there is nothing binding the industry stakeholders to adhere to it.[614]

Indeed, when the Committee met with officers of Victoria Police's Major Drug Investigation Division they stated that only approximately 50 per cent of chemical producers in the state are members of the bodies that are the key partners of the Voluntary Code of Practice (the Plastic and Chemicals Industries Association and Science Industry Australia) and of those very few would actually comply with the protocol.[615]

As well as such voluntary and regulatory measures, Customs and federal and state police are working co-operatively with science and industry to 'develop more effective blocking agents, or reformulation of the product, to prevent the extraction of pseudoephedrine by illicit operators' (ABCI 2002, p.38).

This co-operation has been even more noticeable in the last reporting year of the ACC:

> The diversion of single entity pseudophedrine-based tablets has become more difficult due to a number of law enforcement and industry initiatives. In November 2001, the New South Wales Government rescheduled single entity products from Schedule 2 to Schedule 3a (behind the counter) and introduced mandatory recording of these sales. However, there are limited legislative requirements placed upon pharmacies in most jurisdictions and the industry is largely self-regulating. For example, in Queensland and Western Australia most pharmacies treat the sale of such products as a Health (Drugs and Poisons) Regulation Schedule 3 substance requiring the customer to produce photographic identification and recording the individual's details. A relatively

---

614 Ibid. The new Code was officially launched in June 2002:

'The Code provides guidelines for a voluntary "system of practice for Australian chemical manufacturers, importers and distributors and scientific equipment and instrument suppliers" to guard against the diversion of essential chemicals and scientific equipment (New South Wales Police 2002). Parties to the Code agree to report all suspicious enquiries or orders relating to:

"all Category I chemical substances, Category II chemical substances and scientific apparatus when sold to non account customers"

"Category III chemical substances and scientific apparatus when suspicious circumstances are indicated"

"mixtures and compounds which contain Category I substances that can be extracted for the illicit manufacture of drugs"' (Australian Crime Commission 2003, p.49).

For further information with regard to the Code, see the Plastics and Chemicals Industries Association website: www.pacia.org.au/Health/IllicitDrug Code.pdf.

615 Detective Senior Sergeant J. O'Brien, Major Drug Investigation Division, Victoria Police, evidence given to the Drugs and Crime Prevention Committee, Inquiry into Amphetamine and 'Party Drug' Use in Victoria, Public Hearings (Melbourne), 10 November 2003.

> new initiative in Western Australia, it has been practised by pharmacies for a number of years in Queensland.
>
> Another example of industry self-regulating is the introduction of a national *Code of Practice for Supply Diversion into Illicit Manufacture* which was prepared jointly by Australian law enforcement agencies, the Plastics and Chemicals Industries Association, and Science Industry Australia (New South Wales Police 2002 cited in ACC 2003, p.49).

However, as the ACC itself has noted:

> There have been consequences from these initiatives. Several jurisdictions reported increasing thefts of precursor chemicals from warehouses, chemical companies, doctors' surgeries, chemists and factory yards, as well as the theft of laboratory equipment from schools. The establishment of false companies to provide a legitimate cover for the acquisition of pseudoephedrine continued to be a means of acquiring precursors during the reporting period. There was also a greater move towards Schedule 2 combination tablets for the production of methylamphetamine.
>
> Another consequence of restricting the availability of single entity pseudoephedrine-base products in Australia has been attempts to source these or similar products overseas. Outlaw motor cycle gangs are establishing connections in Southeast Asia and are believed to be increasingly sourcing amphetamine-type stimulant precursors from Thailand and Vietnam. Southeast Asian groups have also emerged as illicit importers of pseudoephedrine from Asian countries. New South Wales Police reported at least two instances where offenders were caught attempting to bring Actifed® and Rambaxi® tablets into Australia from Vietnam. There have also been several reported instances of purchases of cold and flu preparations from overseas sources via the Internet (ACC 2003, p.50).

Domestic controls: Diversion of wholesale precursors

Pseudoephedrine as a raw material and products containing pseudoephedrine are sold by wholesale. Wholesalers and legitimate manufacturers of the product are required to be licensed under the *Drugs, Poisons and Controlled Substances Act 1981*. The protocols governing the appropriate storage and control of wholesale pseudoephedrine have been outlined in the submission of the Department of Human Services Victoria to this Inquiry:

> Wholesalers are required to provide security commensurate with the risk and store pseudoephedrine and pseudoephedrine-containing products in such a way as to ensure their integrity. They are required to maintain records of transactions in a way that will enable reconciliation of quantities supplied with quantities purchased. They are required to ensure that supply is made only to persons who are authorised, licensed or permitted under the Act.

> Recognising the potential for diversion of pseudoephedrine-containing products from wholesalers and manufacturers, in September 2001 the Department wrote to all relevant licence holders to seek their cooperation in reviewing and, where necessary, upgrading security over pseudoephedrine and pseudoephedrine-containing products with respect to external (theft) and internal (pilferage) diversion threats. By March 2002, all licence holders had responded. Most responses received were considered satisfactory and the rest were followed up by Department officers to ensure that arrangements were of an adequate standard. Additionally, during 2002, Major Drug Investigation Division officers conducted audits of the two Victorian manufacturers which use pseudoephedrine raw material to ensure that, given the large quantities that they transport and hold from time to manufacture pharmaceutical products, security arrangements there were of an appropriate standard.[616]

In addition to these protocols, a voluntary Code of Conduct for Australian chemical manufacturers has been established. The weaknesses of this Code have been referred to earlier in this chapter.[617] Unlike the codes and practices of the retail sector, Victoria Police have serious misgivings about the efficacy of the Code:

> In 1996 the then Drug Squad in partnership with the Plastics and Chemicals Industries Association and the Scientific Suppliers Association of Australia developed and published, a "Code of Conduct" for Australian chemical manufacturers, importers and distributors. This document was developed in an attempt to prevent the diversion of precursor chemicals used in the illicit manufacture of ATS.
>
> The document includes categories of drugs and material that have been used in the illicit manufacture of ATS and requires industry stakeholders to sell these chemicals to account customers only and complete an End User Declaration (EUD). The document also includes a voluntary requirement to notify police of suspicious orders or enquiries.
>
> This document is a voluntary code of conduct only and there is nothing binding the industry stakeholders to adhere to it. The reality is that a minority of Victorian based chemical manufacturers, importers and distributors comply with the voluntary reporting conditions by completing EUDs and forwarding them to the MDID. A larger number of smaller chemical distributors do not comply. Clearly voluntary cooperation and compliance has failed.
>
> Victoria Police is impressed by the option of the Western Australia Misuse of Drugs Amendment Bill 2003 but requires time to consult with all stakeholders. The major purpose of the Bill is to place legislative controls on the sale and supply of chemicals and apparatus used in illicit manufacture of amphetamines

---

616 Submission of Human Services Victoria, Drugs Policy and Services Branch to the Drugs and Crime Prevention Committee, Inquiry into Amphetamine and 'Party Drug' Use in Victoria, November 2003.

617 For example, unlike Western Australia, the Code does not make it mandatory for chemical companies to report unusual or large precursor sales.

> and other drugs. Effectively this will allow two categories of precursor chemicals and associated apparatus (including pill presses) to be prescribed in Regulations and mandates other requirements relating to their supply. Principally, suppliers will be required to advise police of certain transactions. Offences are provided for non-compliance. The Bill also provides police with the ability to examine the records and premises of chemical and scientific equipment suppliers in relation to transactions and storage or these precursor chemicals and apparatus. The Bill also ensures the legitimate medical and veterinarian uses of substances, compounds and preparations are exempt. The Bill does not apply to people such as pharmacists, veterinarians and doctors and their suppliers carrying on their normal lawful business. Legitimate sales of category 1 and 2 chemicals and apparatus to school teachers, university lecturers and managers of laboratories are excluded from the Act.
>
> Victoria Police Major Investigation Division has convened a Drugs Legislation Working Party with internal and external key stakeholders including the Victorian Forensic Services Centre, Plastics and Chemical Industries Association, Scientific Industry Australia and Department of Human Services where all options and related issues will be reviewed. After these issues are further examined advice can be provided by the Working Party on the most appropriate legislative amendments.[618]

To ameliorate some of the problems associated with the control of wholesale precursors and their potential to be used for the illicit manufacture of amphetamines, the Committee makes the following recommendations:

Recommendations

26. The Committee recommends that the current industry Code of Conduct with regard to the sale and diversion of chemical precursors be established in legislation.

27. The Committee recommends that the proposed mandatory Code of Conduct incorporate the sale of pill presses, to ensure a consistent approach by all manufacturers.

Clearly there are problems associated with the wholesaling of precursor chemicals, and initiatives to deal with their criminal diversion still need to be 'ironed out'. Nonetheless, many of the problems associated with the illegitimate production of amphetamines seem to arise not so much from the diversion of wholesale chemicals as from the synthesis and extraction of amphetamine from household pharmaceuticals easily available at the local chemist. The role of retail pharmacies in preventing these criminal practices is the subject of the next section.

---

618 Submission of Victoria Police to the Drugs and Crime Prevention Committee, Inquiry into Amphetamine and 'Party Drug' Use in Victoria, November 2003.

Domestic controls – Pharmacies and precursor control in Victoria

Pharmacies and retail chemists play a vital role in containing the spread of illicit amphetamine manufacture. The Committee has heard from a number of pharmacy-related organisations with regard to the way pharmacies can curtail the diversion of pseudoephedrine and other precursors from being used in the manufacture of illicit drugs. Such organisations have included:

- The Pharmacy Board of Victoria
- The Pharmacy Guild of Australia (Victoria)
- The Pharmaceutical Society of Australia (Victoria).

Although each of these bodies made separate formal submissions to the Inquiry, and in the case of the Pharmacy Board also gave evidence at a Public Hearing, on most issues each body was in agreement.

There had been a perceived need for changes to the way in which pseudoephedrine products were sold and displayed in pharmacies. The background to the changes that ensued is outlined in the following submission from the Pharmacy Board of Victoria.

> Around mid-1998 the Board started to receive anecdotal reports from pharmacists and other authorities of frequent and sometimes multiple requests for sale of single ingredient pseudoephedrine products. By early 1999 reports of increased sales of large packs (packets of 90 tablets) of single ingredient pseudoephedrine products were being received and a meeting was held between representatives of the then Victoria Police Drug Squad, Department of Human Services, Pharmacy Board of Victoria (PBV) and the largest manufacturer of these products.
>
> The Board also became aware of reports of a number of large sales of large packs of single ingredient pseudoephedrine products by pharmacists interstate and that there was to be consideration of a change in scheduling for large pack sizes at the September meeting of the National Drugs and Poisons Scheduling Committee (NDPSC).
>
> The Board supported the proposed change and issued a statement to pharmacists on 18 August 1999[619]... The Board reproduced the statement in its Special Circular No.44 issued to all pharmacists in December 1999.[620]
>
> In September 2001 the scheduling of pseudoephedrine was changed to restrict over-the-counter (OTC) sales of single ingredient pseudoephedrine products to packs of 30 tablets or less, larger pack sizes being restricted to supply on prescription only.
>
> In February 2002 following discussion between the Victoria Police Major Drug Investigation Division (MDID), DPU and the Board it was agreed that it would assist pharmacists if more information could be provided and through the

619 Attached as Appendix 18.

620 Attached as Appendix 19.

> Pharmaceutical Society of Australia–Victorian Branch (PSA) a presentation was given at a continuing education lecture by Det Sgt G Sayce and the concept of a poster was born.[621]
>
> The MDID, DPU and PBV invited the Pharmacy Guild of Australia–Victorian Branch (PGA) and PSA to join with them in developing the concept of two posters to assist pharmacists in their communications with consumers, which in some cases had led to angry interchanges following a refusal to supply a pseudoephedrine product by the pharmacist.
>
> A letter to all pharmacists explaining the purpose of the posters and media releases were prepared in late July 2002 in preparation for a launch.
>
> On Friday 9 August 2002 following a successful raid and seizure by the MDID with some media coverage it was decided to release a statement. On Monday 12 August the matter received widespread media coverage.[622]
>
> The previously planned releases were subsequently made and posters distributed to all Victorian pharmacies.[623]
>
> In September 2002 MDID, DPU & PBV representatives attended the 6th National Chemical Diversion Conference where it was resolved that the Victorian model, using the posters to inform the public of the problem with regard to the purchase of pseudoephedrine products, should be adopted nationally and that a national working group would be established.
>
> In December 2002 a National Working Group on the Diversion of Chemical Precursors met for the first time and in June 2003 met again where it resolved to establish four action groups including one on awareness raising...
>
> In December 2002 following discussion with the MDID and DPU the Board adopted a new policy with regard to the storage and supply of pseudoephedrine containing products which it published in Circular No.51 to pharmacists issued in January 2003.[624]

As indicated above one of the first concrete steps initiated was the reduction of the sizes of available of packets of pseudoephedrine based cold relief preparations.

The Registrar of the Pharmacy Board of Victoria, Mr Steve Marty, explained this procedure to the Committee:

> We supported a change to the standard for the uniform scheduling of drugs and poisons. That is the reference document that is used by each jurisdiction. In Victoria that is through the Poisons Code[625] for setting what can be

621 See Appendix 20.

622 See for example: 'Drug alert: Crackdown on common cold and flu tablets to thwart crime gangs', Paul Anderson, *Herald-Sun*, 12 August 2002, p.1; 'Holding back the drug tide', Steve Perkin, *Herald-Sun*, 31 August 2002, p.23.

623 See Appendices 20 and 21.

624 Submission of the Pharmacy Board of Victoria to the Drugs and Crime Prevention Committee, Inquiry into Amphetamine and 'Party Drug' Use in Victoria, October 2003.

625 See *Drugs, Poison and Controlled Substances Act 1981*.

> available with prescription and what can be available without prescription. What happened at that time was that it restricted the sale of single ingredient pseudoephedrine products to packs of 30; anything else had to be only available on prescription. That resulted in those products disappearing off the market because no-one is going to go to the doctor and get a prescription for 90 when it is not on the national health scheme and they are going to pay a large amount, and at the same time it would arouse suspicion.[626]

These measures were thought to be increasingly necessary due to the alarming rise in pharmaceutical theft from chemists (see Roddis 2000). Related crimes such as the stealing of prescriptions or prescription pads from doctors' surgeries or even in some cases the impersonation of a doctor to obtain drugs from a pharmacist over the telephone have also been noted.[627]

Of particular concern was the use of 'runners' to deplete pharmacies of their pseudoephedrine stocks.

> The immediate effect of reduction in the size was that it became very evident that runners would come in, perhaps two or three in a car, and you would get a request in a pharmacy for somebody wanting a pseudoephedrine product, and 2 minutes later another person would come in and ask for the same product, and then another person. They would be observed to perhaps go to a pharmacy down the street, and of course they have become very adept at stories to present. They will know all the symptoms of rhinorrhea et cetera. They will put cottonwool up their noise so they will sound very stuffy in the nose. They know all of the stories to present.
>
> One of the things that we were concerned about was how we got this information to pharmacists in an effective form, so in February last year Detective Sergeant Graeme Sayce from the major drugs investigation division, who was involved with the clandestine labs unit, came at our invitation and gave a presentation to pharmacists at a continuing education evening. He has since done that regionally on a number of occasions. We then got together and worked out how we could ease some of the pressure on pharmacists because they end up having arguments with legitimate consumers who want to buy an over-the-counter product.
>
> ...[w]e started to talk about how we could improve information and alert the public that pharmacists were both legally and professionally obliged to discriminate and determine whether somebody had a therapeutic need in selling things from a safety perspective. Certainly there were arguments between pharmacists and customers and between pharmacists and people

626 Mr Steve Marty, Registrar, Pharmacy Board of Victoria, evidence given to the Drugs and Crime Prevention Committee, Inquiry into Amphetamine and 'Party Drug' Use in Victoria, Public Hearings (Melbourne), 27 October 2003.

627 See for example, Pharmacy Board of Victoria, Special Circular No 50, November 2002, p.8. Although this particular case in question concerned the fraudulent obtaining of pethedine, anecdotal evidence suggests similar ruses have also been tried with regard to other drugs.

seeking these for the wrong reasons.[628]

A submission from the Department of Human Services Victoria, a key player in the control of precursor chemicals, has expanded upon some of the problems Victoria Police face in combating criminals who purchase or steal precursors for diversion.[629] These groups:

- are well organised and deliberately and systematically seek products from many pharmacies each day
- request both single and multiple ingredient pseudoephedrine products
- generally do not appear to be drug-affected and have a good story justifying therapeutic need (perhaps better than the legitimate purchaser)
- have ready access to false identification
- don't visit any single pharmacy often enough to arouse suspicion on the basis of frequency
- even recruit (and pay) local people to purchase on their behalf.

Enormous profits can be made. Police advise that one pack of 30 tablets each containing 60mg pseudoephedrine (total 1.8G pseudoephedrine) available in pharmacies for around $10 can produce more than 300 doses of methylamphetamine which retail on the streets for between $2000 and $8000.

The problem is quite different from the usual situation faced by pharmacists in respect of misuse of over-the-counter medicines. The more common situation is where the purchaser is the person who has been the misuser; for example, of cough mixtures, antihistamines or analgesics. In those cases the pharmacist is in a better position to ascertain whether there is a therapeutic need and make a more informed decision about whether it would be appropriate to supply. In the case of pseudoephedrine-containing products, the prospective purchaser is not (usually) the misuser and is likely to have a well-rehearsed story with symptoms which would justify the need for a pseudoephedrine-containing product. On occasion the pharmacist may not be able to discern a person seeking the product for abuse from a genuine purchaser.

As well, it is clear that while single-ingredient products are probably favoured by the trafficker, multi-ingredient products are also attractive, as the pseudoephedrine is still readily accessible for conversion to methylamphetamine. Police report that trends in products found at clandestine laboratories indicate that multi-ingredient products are now more commonly used than single-ingredient products.[630]

628 Mr Steve Marty, Registrar, Pharmacy Board of Victoria, evidence given to the Drugs and Crime Prevention Committee, Inquiry into Amphetamine and 'Party Drug' Use in Victoria, Public Hearings (Melbourne), 27 October 2003.

629 It is not only 'outside' criminals who seek to divert precursors. As discussed in Chapter 9 amphetamines [and other drugs] are also abused by health professionals who may have ready access to them. Pharmacists are no exception as indicated in Pharmacy Board Circulars. See for example, Special Circular No 48, November 2001, p.2.

630 Submission of Human Services Victoria, Drugs Policy and Services Branch to the Drugs and Crime Prevention Committee, Inquiry into Amphetamine and 'Party Drug' Use in Victoria, November 2003.

Jurisdictional divergence

Although scheduling of pseudoephedrine packet size was pursuant to national agreement,[631] some states are allegedly less vigilant than Victoria in 'policing' the sales of these products. This can lead to some trans-border issues whereby runners from one side of the border may go interstate and stock up on large quantities of product from chemists in that state.[632] Certainly one of the tasks of the recently formed National Working Group on the Diversion of Precursor Chemicals has been to work toward consistent penalties and offences across all state and territory jurisdictions.[633]

One important area where there is a divergence of practice between states is the issue of recording the details of purchasers of pseudoephedrine products and the production of identification before a purchase can be completed. For example, in New South Wales, South Australia and Western Australia such recording and/or identification may be required.[634] Such stringent regulation is opposed in Victoria by all the major players in this area, including Victoria Police, Human Services and all the major pharmacy/pharmaceutical organisations. Victoria Police state in this regard:

> Victoria Police is opposed to the introduction of a pseudoephedrine based substances scheduling/notification system similar to New South Wales...It has been noted that in New South Wales, a fake ID industry has developed since the introduction of the scheduling/notification system. This is an unintended negative consequence. Victoria has an opportunity to learn from this experience and avoid a similar negative consequence here.[635]

In a similar vein the Pharmacy Board comments:

> The next level of control on the availability of pseudoephedrine in solid dose forms would be to restrict it to supply on prescription only. This would possibly result in visits to medical practitioners for self-limiting conditions with an increase in Medicare costs and an increase in cost to the consumer for the products and also the possibility of the condition being over-treated...

---

631 Scheduling of Drugs and Poisons at national level is done subject to the recommendations of the National Drugs and Poisons Schedule Committee (NDPSC) established under the *Therapeutic Goods Act 1989* (Cth). NDPSC recommendations are adopted in Victoria through the Poisons Code of the *Drugs, Poisons and Controlled Substances Act 1981* and regulations made subsequent to this Act.

632 For example, according to Sergeant Feeny of the Queensland Police Service Chemical Diversion Desk, some runners specifically target Tasmania because of the relative absence of legislative controls in that state with regard to pharmaceutical controls (Sergeant Feeny, Queensland Police Service, in conversation with the Drugs and Crime Prevention Committee, Brisbane, 27 June 2003).

633 See Joint Media Release, *National working group on diversion of precursor chemicals into illicit drugs* , Senator the Hon. Christopher Ellison, Minister for Justice and Customs and The Hon. Trish Worth, Parliamentary Secretary to the Minister for Health and Ageing, 4 December 2002.

634 In Western Australia, Pharmaceutical Council guidelines require identification for the purchase of even one packet of pseudoephedrine based medication.

635 Victoria Police, Submission to the Drugs and Crime Prevention Committee, Inquiry into Amphetamine and 'Party Drug' Use in Victoria, November 2003.

> Given that these products are only suitable for two to three days treatment, a further reduction in pack size availability could be considered, however, the unit cost to the consumer is likely to increase. For example, a pack size of 10 doses....
>
> There is little point in recording the sale with the name and address of the purchaser when it is not an offence to provide false information. What identifier would be acceptable given that photographic identification might be thought appropriate? What products are to be recorded – single entity and/or combination products?
>
> If this step is to be undertaken then there is little point in recording the information if it is not going to be used. To be effective, this would require the timely collection of data from all pharmacies and suppliers, collation and interpretation and possible action as a result. This would be a very resource intensive operation and would encounter possible conflict with privacy legislation. This procedure is not undertaken in Victoria for Controlled Drugs and it is suggested that the current spirit of cooperation is producing results.
>
> Recording of pseudoephedrine sales (single entity) is required in some other jurisdictions and to date the Board is unaware of any action arising from this collection of information.
>
> Some pharmacists already require identification as part of an individual practice policy whilst acknowledging the problems discussed above. Police report and it is well known that false ID is readily available. Given the nature of the criminal groups behind diversion, production of ID is more likely to inconvenience genuine purchasers than deter runners who could easily obtain multiple false IDs.[636]

The Human Services Department, the convener of the state Precursor Control Working Group,[637] believes that beneficial change can be made through change to professional practice and training rather than further regulation:

> On the advice of the police about the nature of the problem, the working group considered that the legislative or regulatory action that would reduce availability of products for diversion, eg. making products prescription-only, would also unacceptably hamper access by genuine purchasers and be unduly burdensome to pharmacists and possibly medical practitioners, as well as possibly increasing health care costs, eg. through Medicare.
>
> The working group has been aware that some States have moved to require pharmacists to record the personal details of purchasers of single-ingredient products (sometimes referred to as Schedule 3 recordable classification), primarily as a deterrent to "runners" purchasing. The working group considers this to be lacking in logic and likely to be ineffective in addressing the overall problem and, because of this, represents an unacceptable burden on the genuine purchaser and pharmacist in that:

636 Pharmacy Board of Victoria, Submission to the Drugs and Crime Prevention Committee, Inquiry into Amphetamine and 'Party Drug' Use in Victoria, October 2003.

637 Members of which include Victoria Police, Pharmacy Board of Victoria, Pharmacy Guild and the Pharmaceutical Society of Australia.

- both single-ingredient (Schedule 3) and multi-ingredient (Schedule 2) products are sought for diversion (recording only the single-ingredient products may decrease pharmacist sensitivity to vigilance and notification about suspicious sales of multi-ingredient products),
- if asked, criminal gangs will give false names and addresses and, if proof of identity is required to be given, they have ready access to false identification,
- "runners" have a good story to justify their purchase,
- criminal gangs enlist local people to purchase on their behalf,
- pharmacy records are not networked and so consolidation of records of supply is not feasible,
- law enforcement resources are not available to peruse pharmacy records, and
- it takes longer for the transaction in the pharmacy and pharmacists generally charge a professional fee for the service.[638]

Outcomes

The outcomes of measures put in place by pharmacy agencies in collaboration with Police and the Department of Human Services have been somewhat mixed. On the one hand reports of burglaries and theft from pharmacists seem to have dramatically decreased for a number of reasons. These include:

- Appropriate scheduling of pseudoephedrine products[639]
- Reduction in packet size
- Better training of pharmacists with regard to their rights and responsibilities[640]

---

638 Submission of Human Services Victoria, Drugs Policy and Services Branch to the Drugs and Crime Prevention Committee, Inquiry into Amphetamine and 'Party Drug' Use in Victoria, November 2003.

639 Pseudoephedrine products are listed in either Schedule Two if combination products or Schedule Three (single ingredient product) of the Drugs, Poisons and Controlled Substances Regulations (DPCSR) 1995. Schedule Two products can generally be only sold from pharmacies. Schedule Three products have added restrictions to their sale. Pharmacy Board guidelines require that pharmacist supplying a Schedule Three substance must be satisfied there is a therapeutic need for the product 'having taken all reasonable steps to ensure that a therapeutic need exists' (Regulation 61, DPCSR). The Board has issued the following guidelines determining what constitutes 'reasonable steps':

'The phrase is used to provide flexibility of approach according to the circumstances. An objective test must be applied to the particular circumstances as to whether or not the steps taken were sufficient. Such a test would involve considering if the steps taken would be in accordance with those an ordinary competent person, or member of the profession, would take if put in that situation' (Pharmacy Board of Victoria Guidelines 2003, Appendix Six – Schedule Three Substances, p.85).

Moreover, under the Guidelines:

'The sale of multiple packs of pseudoephedrine, either as single ingredient or in combination formulations, may be considered as unprofessional conduct in the same manner as other non-prescription products which are subject to abuse (Pharmacy Board of Victoria, Guidelines 2003, No 705 (c)).

640 A copy of a police training module for pharmacists with regard to the illicit diversion of pseudoephedrine is attached as Appendix 22.

- Increased liaison between pharmacists and Police, particularly through the use of a dedicated phone number by which a pharmacist can report suspicious activity and the development of a pro forma document for pharmacists to fill out when they encounter suspicious requests for pseudoephedrine products [641]
- More secure storage of pseudoephedrine products[642]
- Not having pseudoephedrine on public display
- The formation of Pharmacy Watch.[643]

The Pharmaceutical Society of Australia states that the collaborative efforts between pharmacy organisations and Victoria Police have been successful in many ways:

641 While such a practice is generally commendable, it is also, according to representatives of the Queensland Chemical Diversion Desk, very resource intensive:

'[w]e actively seek information and input from the community, and particularly from the pharmaceutical groups, but that is a two-edged sword. Because if pharmacies are calling in with the information on suspicious sales then they are looking for some sort of response for that or feedback from it. That then becomes a very resource-intensive practice if you were to respond to each one of those calls, and we simply don't have those resources. That creates a few problems for us in terms of trying to satisfy the needs of the persons providing the information' (Unidentified Speaker, Queensland Police Service, in conversation with the Drugs and Crime Prevention Committee, Brisbane, 27 June 2003).

A copy of the pro forma for pharmacists to notify Victoria Police is attached as Appendix 23.

642 The Pharmacy Board of Victoria has adopted the following policy with regard to storage and display, which is binding on all Victorian Pharmacies. Pharmacy Board Circular (No 52, October 2003) directs that:

'Pharmacists not supply more than one packet of pseudoephedrine containing product per day to any customer unless there are justifiable circumstances;

That supply of more than one packet in other than justifiable circumstances may be considered as contrary to good pharmaceutical practice;

That products containing pseudoephedrine not be available for self-selection (theft of these products has been easy);

That not more than one shelf-facing per product type be displayed;

That pseudoephedrine products not be advertised or promoted by way of window displays or in-store merchandising;

That good pharmaceutical practice includes notification of suspicious requests for pseudoephedrine to the Major Drug Investigation Division; and

That proprietors have a responsibility to ensure that all staff are aware of and observe the policy on storage and sale of single ingredient and combination products'.

An attenuated and easy to understand version of these guidelines has been produced in poster form for both pharmacists and their staff/assistants and the public alike. See Appendices 20 and 21.

See also Pharmaceutical Society of Australia – *Code of Practice- Pseudoephedrine*, September 2002.

643 Pharmacy Watch is the collective agreement and guidelines produced by the Pharmacy Board of Victoria, Pharmaceutical Society, Pharmacy Guild, Victoria Police and Human Services Victoria to train pharmacists and implement measures to curtail the theft of drugs and pharmaceuticals from pharmacies. Since its inception in 1999, armed robberies of pharmacist have apparently reduced by 33% nationally (see Roddis 2000).

Mr Steve Marty, Registrar of the Pharmacy Board of Victoria, states that between the financial years 2000–2001 and 2002–2003 there has been a 75% reduction in pharmacy break-ins; 'They were running at just over 1200 in 2000–01 to just over 300 in the last financial year' (Mr Steve Marty, Registrar, Pharmacy Board of Victoria, evidence given to the Drugs and Crime Prevention Committee, Inquiry into Amphetamine and 'Party Drug' Use in Victoria, Public Hearings (Melbourne), 27 October 2003.

- Pharmacists throughout Victoria have been informing the Major Drug Investigation Division about possible false purchasers which has resulted in some arrests;
- The value of pseudoephedrine on the street has increased, a sign that pseudoephedrine-based products are becoming hard to access;
- Pseudoephedrine 'runners' are being paid more for their efforts, demonstrating that pseudoephedrine is harder to come by on the street market.[644]

On the other hand, while package reduction has been to a certain extent successful in curtailing the availability of single ingredient pseudoephedrine containing products, there does seem to have been a displacement, with runners and 'purchasers' seeking to obtain solid dose (capsule or tablet) formulations with combination products. These are usually combinations of pseudoephedrine with the addition of an analgesic or antihistamine:

> There has been a transition to the point where runners know that there are procedures in place and that suspicion is aroused if they seek a particular product. Police advise that the runners accept sale of one packet of any product whilst acknowledging that single ingredient products have a higher value for sale to clandestine laboratories than combination products.[645]

Ongoing problems

The Pharmacy Board has outlined a number of problems that are still associated with the illicit use of pharmaceuticals. These include:

- The public, judiciary and law enforcement bodies remain largely unaware of the issue of diversion of pharmaceuticals for the illicit manufacture of amphetamines. This includes the substantial risk to communities where a clandestine laboratory is located because of explosion, fire and exposure to toxic chemicals. Similarly there are risks for the community with drivers of motor vehicles who have used stimulants and their involvement in accidents.
- As measures become effective in one area then pressure is brought to bear on another – the 'squeezing the balloon effect'. As it becomes increasingly difficult to obtain pseudoephedrine through OTC purchase of cough and cold products this increases the demand for supply of amphetamine type substances (ATS) and precursors from alternative sources eg. overseas, with the resulting difficulties of detection at the border or through the mail.

644 Fact Sheet on Pseudoephedrine. Attached to Pharmaceutical Society of Australia (Victorian Branch) submission to the Drugs and Crime Prevention Committee, Inquiry into Amphetamine and 'Party Drug' Use in Victoria, October 2003.

645 Submission of the Pharmacy Board of Victoria to the Drugs and Crime Prevention Committee, Inquiry into Amphetamine and 'Party Drug' Use in Victoria, October 2003.

- The offer of pharmaceuticals through internet orders has grown rapidly and few members of the public would be aware of the dangers of sourcing drugs and medicines in this manner nor are they likely to be aware of the legal requirements for importation of drugs for their own use.[646]
- Some precursor chemicals are used in large quantities for legitimate manufacturing and the diversion of small quantities may be almost impossible to detect.[647]

Another measure that has been tried with equivocal results has been the modification or reformulation of pharmaceutical products by scientists and chemists to make illicit extraction of pseudoephedrine more difficult without changing the safety or efficacy of the product.[648] Although research into such methods continues, it would seem that it does not take long for amateur (and professional) illicit chemists to be able to circumvent such processes.[649]

Notwithstanding such continuing problems, the collaborative approach between pharmacy organisations, police and health authorities is generally to be commended. Nonetheless, the Committee still believes that it is incumbent upon customers buying two or more packets of pseudoephedrine based medications to provide identification when transacting that purchase.

Recommendation

28. The Committee recommends that appropriate legislation be enacted to require photographic identification to be produced to pharmacists or pharmacy staff for the purchase of two or more packets of non prescription pseudoephedrine based medications or products (single ingredient or combination product). In all other cases current Pharmacy Industry guidelines and Codes of Practice should be strictly observed and enforced.

646 With regard to the Internet to access [illicit] pharmaceuticals, Mr Marty states:

'I think we should be aware of the effect of the Internet these days and purchasing drugs, both over-the-counter and prescription. I get inundated with this [Internet] material every day. I have discussed this with customs, but it cannot possibly detect all of this; it is a huge problem. There is also a significant cost to the community – from the effects that some of these drugs may have on young people who perhaps suffer serious adverse events...' (Mr Steve Marty, Registrar, Pharmacy Board of Victoria, evidence given to the Drugs and Crime Prevention Committee, Inquiry into Amphetamine and 'Party Drug' Use in Victoria, Public Hearings (Melbourne), 27 October 2003.

647 Submission of the Pharmacy Board of Victoria to the Drugs and Crime Prevention Committee, Inquiry into Amphetamine and 'Party Drug' Use in Victoria, October 2003.

648 For example, Warner Lambert reformulated the Sudafed tablet to increase the difficulty of extracting pseudoephedrine (see Roddis 2000).

649 Mr Steve Marty, Registrar, Pharmacy Board of Victoria, personal communication with Committee staff, December 2003.

Conclusion

The use of precursors to 'homebake' illicit drugs such as amphetamines is clearly an issue of grave importance. The initiatives put in place by retailers, pharmacy organisations, health and law enforcement agencies have assisted in curtailing the manufacture of these drugs and these initiatives are to be commended. There is, however, no reason for complacency. Drugs such as amphetamines are still being produced in Australia and still use retail pharmaceuticals to do so. Nor do problems end with the manufacture of the drugs. Police and law enforcement agencies must also concentrate on the distribution of the drugs once they have 'rolled off the presses'. The issue of distribution of amphetamines and 'party drugs' and the distribution networks associated with these drugs is the topic of the next chapter.

16. Distribution of Amphetamines and Party Drugs

The distribution of amphetamines and 'party drugs' once they have been imported without detection or locally manufactured can be plotted according to some fairly defined networks. Distribution of these drugs can be generally defined as macro distribution or micro distribution. Macro distribution involves the delivery of the drugs from the point of entry into Australia, or the source of production if made locally, through distribution networks or lines such as organised crime syndicates down through the 'chain of command' to local dealers. Micro distribution on the other hand pertains more to local level dealing. In the case of drugs such as 'ecstasy', these dealers can often be characterised as friendship networks or what Measham, Aldridge and Parker (2001) have termed 'mutual societies', as was discussed in Chapter 10. Because this type of dealing is so often done at a very local level it is discussed in Chapter 17, which concentrates on local level policing.

This chapter examines the wider networks of drug distribution.

The 'macro' distribution of amphetamines

In the 2000–2001 summary of the Australian Illicit Drug Report a number of key points were made with regard to the law enforcement of the amphetamine and ecstasy networks. Among other issues it was stated that:

- Outlaw motor cycle gangs continue to play a role in manufacture and distribution with evidence suggesting alignments with other criminal networks.
- The production trend towards smaller scale mobile laboratories in a number of jurisdictions continues to pose risks and challenges to law enforcement.
- Tighter domestic restrictions on the sale of precursor chemicals are resulting in increasing thefts from pharmaceutical companies and chemists, as well as increased attempts at importation.
- A wider range of pseudoephedrine-based products is being used as precursors for amphetamine-type stimulant production during 2000–2001.

- While the number of border detections dropped during 2000–2001, the average weight of detections increased from 358 grams to 1.7 kilograms; the postal stream remained the most common method of importation.
- Increased availability and use of crystalline methylamphetamine hydrochloride or 'ice' has been noted in most States and Territories.
- Use of amphetamine-type stimulants has increased partially due to an Australia-wide heroin shortage; specifically in the Australian Capital Territory, Queensland, South Australia, Western Australia and some regions of New South Wales (Australian Bureau of Criminal Intelligence (ABCI) 2002, p.34).

To take the first point, there has long been an association, at least in the public mind, between amphetamine markets and distribution and outlawed motor cycle gangs. The reality is not too far from the public perception. 'Bikie' gangs are involved in amphetamine distribution markets (and as was discussed above, clandestine manufacture) and other forms of organised drug crime.[650] The following summary from the 2000–2001 Illicit Drug Report is still an accurate reflection of the current situation:

> Methods of distributing amphetamine-type stimulants across Australia remains diverse, varying between regions, States and Territories. Outlaw motor cycle gangs dominate the distribution market. They are involved particularly in the inter- and intra-state distribution of amphetamine-type stimulants, precursors, equipment and personnel. Information from a joint agency report suggests over 50 per cent of clandestine laboratories they seized in 2000–01 had involved members of outlaw motor cycle gangs or their associates.
>
> National Crime Authority Task Force information suggests the distribution role of outlaw motor cycle gangs in and across jurisdictions varies from involvement by a whole group to just individuals within a group. Outlaw motor cycle gangs involved in amphetamine-type stimulant distribution are continuing to expand their collaboration with European and South-east Asian organised-crime groups based in Australia. However, links between traditional and other larger players in the amphetamine-type stimulant market are quite fluid.
>
> Distribution and supply of amphetamine-type stimulants are characterised by a great deal of fluidity within networks, particularly at the smaller end of the market where groups may come together to produce and distribute amphetamine-type stimulants and then dissipate. Often distributors are either connected in some other way or are known to each other (ABCI 2002, p.42).

---

650 In Adelaide, bikie gangs have also been associated with ecstasy distribution. The NDARC study by Longo et al. comments with regard to the survey of ecstasy users in South Australia that:

'There was agreement that there are two main sources of ecstasy distribution in Adelaide: bikies, and people involved in the rave and clubbing scene, with the quality of the ecstasy available from the bikies markedly higher' (NDARC 2002c, p.25).

More recently, the Australian Crime Commission (ACC) comments that there has, however, been some dynamic shifts in the illicit amphetamine market due to the links between 'traditional' and emerging players on the scene:

> The role of outlaw motor cycle gangs in the distribution of amphetamine-type stimulants varied within and across the jurisdictions, ranging from involvement of the whole group to individuals within a group. Gangs and individuals involved in amphetamine-type stimulant distribution continue to expand their collaboration with ethnic-based organised crime groups in Australia. It would appear that associations are being driven increasingly by business interests rather than race-based considerations. New South Wales Police reported that while outlaw motor cycle gang nominees and new members may be involved in distribution, users, prostitutes and other gang associates are more likely to be used to distribute the drugs. This broadening of the supply network not only enables outlaw motor cycle gangs to control the market in an area but also allows members to distance themselves from the actual distribution and associated police attention (ACC 2003, p.55).[651]

The former ABCI stated that due to the highly localised nature of methamphetamine production, there are no major or significant distribution centres feeding interstate markets:

> A sizeable portion of the interstate distribution that does occur, however, is believed to be facilitated through individuals in the trucking industry. Several jurisdictions reported that some interstate truck drivers are believed to be acting as methylamphetamine couriers for various distribution networks. The predominant method of importing amphetamines into the Northern Territory is by vehicle, often through the road transport industry. Outlaw motor cycle gangs in the Northern Territory have well established, close associations with the trucking industry, including local, regional and interstate movement of freight. Likewise, Far Northern Queensland police reported amphetamines were being couriered into the region by vehicle from other parts of Queensland, including central Queensland where several established outlaw motor cycle gang chapters are located.
>
> Other modes of transport used by interstate distribution networks include the postal system, commercial aircraft, commercial coaches and rail. Inter- and intra-state distribution by air has become increasingly prevalent in New South Wales (ABCI 2002, p.43).[652]

At the 'micro level' of the spectrum, depending on the user group:

---

651 Anecdotal evidence given to the Committee suggests that some members of OMCGs associated with the amphetamine trade are moving into the security industry, using hotels and clubs as distribution points for the drug (Mr Mal Hyde, Commissioner of South Australia Police in conversation with the Drugs and Crime Prevention Committee, Adelaide, 3 October 2003).

652 The Committee has also received anecdotal evidence that trucking groups may be responsible for the distribution of amphetamines across Queensland (Mr R. Kemp, Queensland Health, in conversation with the Drugs and Crime Prevention Committee, Brisbane, 27 June 2003).

> Low-level distribution varied between the states and territories. However, hotels, bars, nightclubs and dance parties continued to feature significantly. Several jurisdictions reported dealers were using mobile phones more frequently to prearrange meeting points for the delivery of amphetamine-type stimulants. Meeting points included public places such as car parks, take-away food outlets, public phone boxes and railway stations. Supply through the residential premises of the dealer was also common – particularly in New South Wales – with some dealers delivering the product personally to regular customers. In Queensland, hotels and motels are being used increasingly as production and distribution points.
>
> Relationships at the lower level of the distribution chain are best characterised as opportunistic. Most low-level suppliers are on-selling amphetamine-type stimulants to support their quantities of less than one gram. According to New South Wales Police, while many low-level suppliers operate semi-autonomously – sourcing amphetamine-type stimulants from single or multiple mid-level suppliers – a number are also members of networks which share a common middle or upper-level supplier. Consistent with the findings of the Drug Use Monitoring in Australia program, New South Wales Police reported that most amphetamine-type stimulant purchases were paid for in cash, with some instances of product being exchanged for stolen goods (Freeman & Fitzgerald 2002). Suppliers in the Campbelltown area of Sydney often use third parties as couriers to transport drugs. Juveniles are preferred as they are perceived to be less likely to receive custodial sentences (ACC 2003, p.55).

The Committee has also received anecdotal accounts from officers of the Queensland Police testifying to how 'new' technologies are employed to facilitate the manufacture and distribution of amphetamine:

> We have found that with the increased use of mobile phones and short messaging systems, people are [easily] able to source their chemicals. The use of the Internet has become very relevant at this stage, with a number of Internet sites available – you can get diagrams, recipes; there are also private news groups now in the underground clandestine drug scene, where they are going in, and they can publish their own stuff, and unless you are a member of that private news group you can't actually see what they are talking about, so that is also becoming an issue for us.[653]

Targeting trafficking and distribution

Supply reduction strategies that take place once the drugs have reached the country are those that seek to disrupt the market by targeting distributors and their profits. Much national and state law enforcement activity in the area of drugs has this as its focus. Agencies such as the ACC and the New South Wales

653 Detective Sergeant Jason Renwick, Illicit Laboratory Investigation Team, Queensland Police Service, in conversation with the Drugs and Crime Prevention Committee, Brisbane, 27 October 2003.

and Queensland Crime Commissions spend much of their energy and funds investigating high level 'drug players' and their associated criminal activity.[654] For example, in 2001 in the Hunter Region of New South Wales one of the biggest busts ever witnessed in Australia saw $60 million worth of amphetamine seized by New South Wales police in 'Operation Sibret'. The operation focussed on outlawed motor cycle gangs' (OMCG) involvement in:

- The large scale manufacture and distribution of amphetamines;
- Firearm trafficking;
- The rebirthing of heavy duty motor vehicles and earth moving equipment (Stas 2001, p.5).

The investigation and subsequent raids were a collective effort of NSW Police, the ABCI and cross-border co-operation with the Queensland Police Service, reflecting the latter state's high level of amphetamine manufacture and trafficking:

> Police involved in Strike Force Sibret shut down seven clandestine drug laboratories and seized $60 million worth of amphetamine, as well as a large amount of firearms and explosives from OMCG members and associates on the state's north coast...
>
> Officer in charge, Det Insp Wayne Gordon...said 20 people had been charged as part of the investigation, with more expected.
>
> 'The principal offenders were charged with the manufacture and supply of large commercial quantities of amphetamine...'
>
> Investigators have frozen more than $7 million worth of assets, including Harley Davidson motorcycles, cars, trucks and earthmoving equipment.
>
> Det Insp Gordon said 'voluminous amounts' of prohibited weapons were also located by police, including machine guns, sniper rifles, other long arms with telescopic sights, automatic pistols, revolvers, explosives, detonators and detonator cords.
>
> 'It's considered to be the most successful incursion into the organised crime activities of OMCGs in the Commonwealth of Australia', he said (Stas 2001, pp.4–5).

Cross-border co-operation is clearly an important aspect of any successful targeted drug operations. This is particularly the case given that Australia has one federal and seven state/territory criminal jurisdictions. Most cross-border operations or co-operation are based on either written Memoranda of Understanding between police forces or verbal agreements. In New South Wales a more formalised arrangement has recently been put in place.[655]

---

654 The ACC was formed in January 2003 as a result of a merger between the Australian Bureau of Criminal Intelligence (ABCI), the National Crime Authority (NCA) and the Office of Strategic Crime Assessments (OSCA). The ACC has taken over the role of the former ABCI in producing the annual Australian Illicit Drug Report.

655 The *Police Powers (Drug Detection in Border Areas Trial) Act 2004* enables Police to obtain warrants to stop and search all vehicles that are crossing a jurisdictional boundary bordering NSW for illicit drugs. Information is provided by Police to support such an application for this type of warrant.

Recommendation

29. The Committee takes note that state and interstate highways and major roads act as a conduit for the distribution of illicit drugs, including amphetamine. The Committee therefore recommends the increased surveillance of trucks and other motor vehicles.

Financial transactions legislation allowing the seizure of profits from the proceeds of (drug) crime are also in place in most jurisdictions and are a beneficial adjunct to target distributors.

The Australian Transaction Reports and Analysis Centre (AUSTRAC), formerly the National Cash Transaction Reports Agency (CTRA), also enables law enforcement agents to detect, trace and investigate instances of money laundering and transactions associated with criminal income.

Such measures apply to all types of illicit drugs, however they may be less effective when it comes to combating the amphetamine and 'party drug' trades. The following comments by Wardlaw, although somewhat dated, are still relevant:

> In the case of amphetamines, high level investigations may be of less importance in Australia… Although traditionally a significant share of the market has been dominated by a number of motorcycle gangs, in recent years the production mix has become more varied, with a large number of manufacturers at various levels of sophistication and size. It is now doubtful if it is possible to identify a small group of manufacturers or distributors whose removal would have a long term disrupting effect on the market (Wardlaw 1993, p.100).

Distribution of MDMA

The major entry points for MDMA in Australia are through Sydney, Brisbane, Perth and Melbourne (ABCI 2002). Even more so than with methamphetamine, however, few discrete groups or networks have been associated with MDMA distribution:

> Distribution networks continue to be flexible and diverse, and may include involvement by individuals who may not be members of a criminal syndicate. Several groups, however, play a significant role in the importation and distribution of MDMA. Established Southeast Asian organised crime groups are involved in all aspects of the importation and distribution of MDMA in Australia. There are also links suggesting greater involvement of these crime groups in the production and distribution of domestically produced amphetamine-type stimulants, both independently as well as collaboratively with other crime groups. Western Australia and New South Wales police report the involvement of foreign students in distribution. A growing trend is distribution networks diversifying to handle a variety of illicit drugs, depending on availability and supply.

> In the Australian Capital Territory, MDMA is believed to be sourced from Sydney to supplement locally produced methylamphetamine-based product. Ethnically-based crime groups as well as members and associates of outlaw motor cycle gangs are primarily involved in distribution.
>
> While some jurisdictions link MDMA distribution to outlaw motor cycle gangs, a number of these gangs are also closely associated with the production and distribution of methylamphetamine-based tablets. Involvement of outlaw motor cycle gangs in the entertainment/nightclub industry – from both a financial and a security perspective – provides these groups with ready access to major distribution opportunities for both imported and locally produced product (ABCI 2002, pp.55–56).[656]

Street level distribution

Law enforcement that targets high level distributors, usually through state police forces, also targets street level distributors.[657] Clearly there are heated debates about the merit and appropriateness of using law enforcement strategies to target the 'small fry' dealer or distributor, particularly when that distributor is also a user and/or addict. These debates have been aired in numerous fora and are readily available (see for instance Dorn, Murji & South 1991; Bagnall 1997; Saunders 1998).[658] This Report does not seek to 'rehash' these debates in any significant way. In any case, many of these enforcement strategies are geared towards heroin and heroin use. Although the 'heroin drought' has seen some displacement to the use of street market amphetamine, and to a lesser extent ecstasy, much amphetamine is still distributed in more private and discreet networks that are far more difficult to intercept. This is certainly the case for 'middle-class' users of ecstasy and other 'party drugs':

> Furthermore, for most people, use of stimulants is not compulsive and there is no need to buy at a particular time or with any great frequency. This means that most users can be more circumspect about their drug purchasers and need to purchase less frequently than do, for example, heroin users.

---

656 Bikies have also been associated with MDMA distribution in South Australia. See NDARC 2002c and the discussion above.

657 Somewhat disturbing are reports that in the United States some of the major criminal cartels that are distributing marijuana are also responsible for the distribution of methamphetamine:

'[As] marijuana is the illicit drug that is used most frequently by high school youth in the U.S, this suggests the possibility that there might be increased access to methamphetamine by high school students through marijuana distribution networks'... (Oetting et al. 2000, p.36).

658 For example, an interesting, if somewhat unsophisticated, article by O'Neill (1996) compares the prohibition of ecstasy with the ready availability of the anti-depressant drug Prozac. He argues that the biological and pharmacological effects of both drugs are remarkably similar, yet for a range of social, historical and political reasons one is banned while the other is prescribed. He contrasts the case of rock guitarist Richard Simpson being charged with the manufacture of MDMA:

'Another drug has a similar effect. It is used by several lawyers I know and could be taken legally by judges. But its manufacturers do not face charges; at worst they get the odd complaint that they are making excessive profits. The drug which could send Simpson to jail, MDMA, is best known by the name Ecstasy. The drug which comforts lawyers and millions of others is fluoextine, marketed as Prozac' (O'Neill, 1996, p.26).

> Finally, a significant number of stimulant users do not buy drugs themselves, but rely on friends to do so for them and share with them in a social setting. All of these factors reduce the number and public nature of drug transactions and so reduce the opportunities for vigorous street-level enforcement strategies to take place and have a major impact (Wardlaw 1993, pp.101–102).

The 'micro-distribution' of MDMA and other drugs purporting to be ecstasy is fluid and diffuse.

> Micro-distribution remains similar to that of other amphetamine-type stimulants. Wholesalers sell bulk amounts of MDMA to known associates. However, further distribution to users occurs in a variety of ways, with delivery to personal residences or selling at nightclubs and dance parties continuing to be common methods. There are increasing reports of the use of pre-paid SIM cards and mobile phone Short Message Services (SMS) to arrange delivery. The most prevalent form of supply, however, is through networks of friends (ABCI 2002, p.56).

Further issues pertaining to the 'micro-distribution' of 'party drugs' are more conveniently discussed in Chapter 17 dealing with the policing of 'party drugs' at the local level, the topic of the following and final chapter in this Part.[659]

659 See discussion in Chapter 10 with regard to the profiles of ecstasy users and how they 'score' their drugs.

17. Problems in Policing Amphetamines and 'Party Drugs' at Local Level

> The media is quick to portray dealers as the enemy who prey on innocent victims, yet the reality in the case of ecstasy is that when parents demand the arrest of 'evil dealers', they are often referring to their own children (Webb 2003, p.119).

Local policing of amphetamines and 'party drugs'

The policing and prosecution of drug crimes, particularly those pertaining to trafficking and supply, have come a long way in a relatively short time. John McKoy, the recently retired head of the Victoria Police Drug Squad, stated that:

> Enforcement of the anti-drug laws during the 1960s and 1970s was a straightforward matter for police in that offenders were charged and the courts meted out the appropriate sentence. No strategic plan existed, no rational system of data collection was in place and partnerships with other interested departments did not exist. Police commanders had only to produce arrest figures that justified their respective budgets. And the majority of arrests were for 'possess and use' illicit drugs while the major drug traffickers were relatively insulated against prosecution through police ignorance and lack of resources, technical and human (McKoy 2002, pp.74–75).

In its submission to this Inquiry the Victoria Police (Drug and Alcohol Policy Coordination Unit) outlined a number of specific difficulties associated with the policing of amphetamines and 'party drugs'.[660]

The first of these is danger to personnel as a result of the state of the person on the drugs:

> When a person uses an ATS [amphetamine-type stimulant] the effects include arousal, increased temperature and blood pressure. When intoxicated by these drugs, particularly through extended use, users can experience aggression, paranoia, hallucinations and delusions (psychosis). When coming

660 For policing issues of a legal nature, including police suggestions for law reform, see Chapter 12. For police views on 'pill testing', see Chapter 19.

> down and during withdrawal, users can experience depression, suicidal tendencies, bizarre thoughts and mood swings.
>
> Advice from the Victoria Police Negotiator Coordinator indicates that police members are experiencing greater numbers of critical incidents with people with amphetamine related drug induced psychosis.
>
> These critical incidents include violent behaviour in domestic situations, sieges, threats, assaults, suicides and unintentional self-harm that may lead to death or serious injury to themselves or others. The behaviour of these people at such incidents is further complicated and exacerbated through polydrug use.
>
> For many dependent users, particularly those that inject, the immediate and long term harms can be quite significant. Dependent users experience a range of harms associated with long term heavy use. These harms not only relate to the acquisition and administration of these illicit substances, but also the intoxicated behaviour as a result of their use.
>
> Harms associated with injecting drug use not only relate to the users but also to other persons who have contact with them such as the emergency services. For example there has been an increase in the number of needlestick injuries received by Victoria Police members. These injuries expose members to the risks of blood borne viruses including Hepatitis B and C, and HIV/AIDS. Notwithstanding the potential infection, there is the psychological trauma of undergoing testing.[661]

Conversely, Anex, the peak organisation for needle and syringe exchange programmes in Australia, argues that such problems could be avoided if law enforcement officers took a less vigilant approach to the policing of amphetamine (and other forms of injecting drug use):

> Anex believes that law enforcement agencies have a role in reducing the incidence of syringe litter in the community. Anex believes that the possession of a needle or syringe ought to be insufficient grounds on its own to establish reasonable grounds to search a person. On most occasions it may be in the greater public interest for police members to use their discretion to overlook minor 'use and possession' offences and take no further action. Removing the fear of prosecution may encourage people to dispose of used

661 Excerpt from the confidential submission of Victoria Police (Drugs Policy and Services Branch) to the Drugs and Crime Prevention Committee, Inquiry into the Amphetamine and 'Party Drug' Use in Victoria, August 2002. Quoted with the kind permission of Victoria Police.

> equipment appropriately thereby reducing the potential for needlestick injuries to members of the public.[662]

There are also problems associated with policing the venues themselves, particularly with regard to 'party drugs':[663]

> As the majority of ATS dealing and trafficking at 'street level' occurs in and around nightclubs and rave parties, this can be a difficult environment to police. Plain clothes police do attend and covertly patrol various rave and dance venues, however due to the subculture and the environment the plain clothes police presence is often obvious to the patrons.

---

662 Submission of Anex to the Drugs and Crime Prevention Committee, Inquiry into Amphetamine and 'Party Drug' Use in Victoria, October 2003.

While the Victoria Police now include the principles of harm minimisation in its training syllabi, there was originally some resistance to the idea of harm reduction, according to former Victoria Police Drug Squad head, John McKoy. In particular, the idea of needle exchange programmes was not at all palatable in the first instance:

'Police were aghast. Suddenly, from a police point of view, drug offences became decriminalised to a certain extent. Police were ordered not to patrol needle exchange sites nor to make arrests in those areas for drug offences. Consequently, drug use, assaults and thefts increased around most needle exchange sites. Liaison between police and those who managed the needle exchange sites was restricted to occasional meetings between senior police and health officials. While the general police members deeply resented NSEP, burglaries on pharmacies showed a marked decline and health officials regarded the program as a success with the spread of HIV/AIDS and other blood borne diseases being brought under control. NSEP also provided much needed data that contributed to the debate on the drug problem' (McKoy 2002, p.77).

Times change! Nowadays law enforcement agencies welcome and encourage research and data collection into the drug habits of users. As Dr Louisa Degenhardt of the National Drug and Alcohol Research Centre states, police:

'[are] actually quite interested in increasing intelligence, as they call it, rather than 'busting'; trying to understand the market rather than get me in trouble because I interviewed someone who said they used party drugs...' (Dr Louisa Degenhardt, National Drug and Alcohol Research Centre in conversation with the Drugs and Crime Prevention Committee, Sydney, 26 June 2003).

663 A comprehensive survey of 'clubbers' and drug use, particularly amphetamine use, in Britain found that many patrons of nightclubs thought that law enforcement officials were overly zealous in their policing of raves and clubs:

'Where concerns strayed beyond verbal aggression, clubbers discussed their experiences of excessive searches and strip searches by both the police and security/door staff in the hunt for drugs hidden on the person. Clubbers saw this as a clear abuse of power, and the frequency of such reports highlights the need for clarity, regulation and moderation in search policies and procedures both in clubland and on the streets' (Measham, Aldridge & Parker 2001, p.179).

Such policing, it is claimed, at least in the English context:

'[i]s ad hoc and inconsistent. It is often symbolic: an enforcement gesture because in reality the clubs cannot be comprehensively policed by the local force. There are far more pressing demands, particularly at weekends. In the end the clubs are expected to self-regulate and employ their own security and door staff' (Measham, Aldridge & Parker 2001, p.185).

On the other hand such attitudes need to be compared with the praise for the 'common sense' approach to the policing of raves such as Earthcore outlined in Chapter 10.

Many clubs such as ZoS in Prahran also have managers who welcome police involvement in their clubs and on Licensees and Safety Accords. This seems to reflect the:

'pragmatic realism of many dance club managers in [their] concern to run a club free from violence and intimidation rather than attempting what [they see] as the impossible: trying to run a club free from drug distribution and drug use' (Measham, Aldridge & Parker 2001, p.151).

> Police members are also attempting to detect small tablets often stored in inoffensive containers such as breath mint containers in dark, noisy and crowded environments. This makes detection of offences problematic for police.[664]

But these problems are relatively less difficult than the enormous problems of policing the import, manufacture and supply of these drugs on a national level.

The use of drug detection dogs

Victoria Police are enthusiastic about the use of drug detection dogs as an adjunct in fighting the illicit drug trade. In particular, the use of Passive Alert Detection (PAD) dogs has had noticeable success, particularly in New South Wales, in detecting the presence of drugs such as amphetamine in containers, luggage, freight and on the person.

A submission from Victoria Police to this Inquiry states:

> The New South Wales PAD dogs have been highly successful in drug detection and subsequent seizure. Some of the drug searches initiated by the dogs have also led to the seizure of weapons. As a crime prevention initiative the PAD Dogs contributed to a reduction in general crime in the area they were deployed. As the effectiveness of the PAD dogs became known so did the deterrent value.
>
> These dog teams are utilised in street operations in New South Wales and perform foot patrols of railway stations, shopping malls, licensed premises and places of public gathering including dance music festivals. The dog team is supported by several operational members who walk behind the dog team for the purpose of searching suspects on the dog giving a positive indication of the odour of narcotics. When the dog locates a narcotic odour it sits by the suspect indicating to the handler the presence of the odour.
>
> Between 9 October 2001–30 June 2002, 2194 searches were conducted using PAD dogs, resulting in 1434 arrests. Ninety drug trafficking offences were detected and of those the majority were for the trafficking of amphetamines (54). Additionally, 66 weapons were detected during searches, including knives and firearms. Of the 2194 searches, 391 were in commercial retail and licensed premises and hotels/motels.[665]

PAD dogs are to be distinguished from dogs used under the 'retrieval system'. The differences were explained to the Committee by Acting Senior Sergeant McGovern as follows:

664 Excerpt from the confidential submission of Victoria Police (Drugs Policy and Services Branch) to the Drugs and Crime Prevention Committee, Inquiry into Amphetamine and 'Party Drug' Use in Victoria, August 2002. Quoted with the kind permission of Victoria Police.

665 Submission of Victoria Police to the Drugs and Crime Prevention Committee, Inquiry into Amphetamine and 'Party Drug' Use in Victoria, November 2003.

> Up until now the Victoria Police dog squad has always had a drug detection dog unit which is based on the retrieve reward. I will just explain how that works.
>
> The dogs are put into a room or an area whereby they search that area. They are trained to detect the smell of heroin, amphetamines, cocaine, marijuana, and ecstasy, and their response to the recognition of that odour, if they detect it, is to try to retrieve it.
>
> In about September last year I went to New South Wales. They have undergone a training program, which was taught to them by Americans, on passive alert dogs. The system there is that the dogs still identify all those odours that I just described, but their response is to sit passively next to that odour. They do exactly the same job that we do here, other than they now have the added advantage of being able to search public areas, and if people have drugs in their pockets the dog will passively sit next to them.
>
> ...They use Labradors for that purpose because they move around people a lot more comfortably. Up until recently we have always used either German Shepherds or Rottweilers, and obviously that causes a bit of a problem in public areas, just with perceptions alone.[666]

Currently in Victoria PAD dogs are mostly used within the prison and corrections services:

> Department of Justice [Corrections] Victoria advise that the use of PAD dogs provides an effective visible deterrent to the introduction of drugs into correctional facilities. Apart from the dogs' ability to detect drugs on prisoners and visitors, there are other unquantifiable benefits derived from the dogs' presence at a prison. Visitors may be dissuaded from attempting to introduce contraband through the possibility of detection. During searches, the dog may indicate on a person who has been in the proximity of drugs but not necessarily in possession of them...
>
> Useful intelligence is gained as the PAD Dogs are able to detect people who have been in contact with drugs but may not actually have drugs concealed on them. This useful intelligence can be collated in conjunction with other information for future use.[667]

Victoria Police have also used drug detection dogs pursuant to searches under warrant. If warrants have not been obtained, for example in a roadblock search situation, case law is relied upon for authorisation.[668]

---

666 Acting Senior Sergeant Steve McGovern, Dog Squad, Victoria Police, evidence given to the Drugs and Crime Prevention Committee, Inquiry into Amphetamine and 'Party Drug' Use in Victoria, Public Hearings, (Melbourne), 10 November 2003.

667 Submission of Victoria Police to the Drugs and Crime Prevention Committee, Inquiry into Amphetamine and 'Party Drug' Use in Victoria, November 2003.

668 In particular, the South Australian case of *R v Hoare*, Question of Law Reserved (No 3 of 1998) 101 A Crim R 395. This case held that dog sniffing around luggage did not constitute a search.

Victoria Police would like to see a more comprehensive use of drug detection dogs in this state, concluding its submission to the Committee by stating:

> The New South Wales Police experience highlights the versatility, deterrent effect on drug trafficking and related crimes and enhances community safety in and around railway stations, shopping malls, licensed premises and places of public gathering including dance music festivals. Significant drug crime prevention and community safety benefits could be gained if Victoria Police had similar legislation and drug detection dogs.[669]

Policing 'low level' 'party drug' distribution

As discussed in Chapters 10 and 16, most occasional users of drugs such as MDMA 'score' their tablets from friends, colleagues and acquaintances rather than through 'professional' dealers – what Measham has described as dealing through 'mutual societies'.[670]

Some commentators are critical about the policing (and consequent prosecution) of the possession and 'lower level' dealing of ecstasy. Webb, for example writes:

> [t]he greatest obstacle to police targeting ecstasy use relates to its distribution. Unlike most drugs, ecstasy is not generally supplied via the traditional 'user versus dealer' dichotomy. Numerous studies have revealed that the vast majority (consistently above 90 per cent) of ecstasy users obtain the drug from a friend. There are many advantages – financial, security, wisdom, time, socially – to such friendship distribution networks. They are also extremely effective at guarding drug transactions from police. ...Reflecting the ACT experience, South Australian police note that 'the arrest rate is very low for ecstasy users, and that police tend to focus more on sellers and dealers'. It is more accurate to say that the arrest rate is unavoidably low for ecstasy users, and consequently police are forced to focus on upper-echelon figures (Webb 2003, p.119).

Even some senior (British) police officers have been critical about spending scarce police resources on the micro distribution of MDMA/ecstasy:

> If I felt that my officers were going into nightclubs looking for people who were in possession of ecstasy then I would say to them, and I would say publicly, that they are wasting valuable police resources...there are far more important things which cause real harm to the community in the way that

669 Submission of Victoria Police to the Drugs and Crime Prevention Committee, Inquiry into Amphetamine and 'Party Drug' Use in Victoria, November 2003. Victoria Police have since communicated to the Committee that legal advice suggests a change of legislation is not required to enable the efficient use of detection dogs in Victoria.

670 See the discussion in Chapter 10, particularly with regard to dealing in clubs. For a discussion with regard to the law pertaining to MDMA dealing, see Chapter 12. In particular, note the proposals in Britain for a 'mutual societies' compromise dealing offence that may recognise the 'not for profit' nature of many club transactions.

> ecstasy does not cause real harm to the community (Brian Paddick, Commander, Metropolitan Police Service, quoted in Webb 2003, p.121).

Criticisms of policing have not just been with regard to the arrest of (young) people who take the drugs, but the way in which operations are conducted. For example, Dr Simon Lenton of the National Drug Research Institute based at Curtin University, Perth, argues that sometimes 'raids' of clubs or searches of 'clubbers' cars can be counter-productive. He argues that while it is important for police to target high level drug distribution, policing on the ground needs to be more attuned to a harm minimisation focus:

> I'd like to see it lead to better enforcement, better education, better reducing harms in the scene and better linking of people who are having problems into treatment. I don't think that more is necessarily better, I think the way that things like law enforcement are done can be more or less harmful. We found in the work that we did that some of the police practices which were a response at that time to concerns from the public, understandable concerns, and media hysteria, are actually causing more problems than they're solving. I mean, police were setting up road blocks around raves, stopping cars, searching everyone, pulling socks off to see if there were any tablets. What young people were doing was thinking that rather than risk getting busted on the way, 'let's take them before we leave home, or in the car on the way', and then the person driving the car had the 'e' coming on earlier than expected and having the problem of people on the road following instructions on a map to get to a dance event and they were starting to be 'off-their-faces'. So that kind of policing in our view might have been more vigorous but wasn't better. We had police who were trying to break raves up and there were kids who were obviously intoxicated on hallucinogens, ecstasy and speed and the police were saying 'no you can't sit here in the car park and wait till the morning, you have to go now'. Now that's more vigorous policing, but is it better policing? No I don't think it is. So I think we need to have understandings that lead to better law enforcement, better management of venues, better prevention, better linking of people who are having difficulties into treatment.[671]

Turning Point Alcohol and Drug Centre believes in strong partnerships between police, data collection agencies and research centres. However, it also believes that both the timing and nature of law enforcement interventions need to be selectively targeted. Drawing from the work of Caulkin it states:

671 Dr Simon Lenton, National Drug Research Institute, Curtin University, in conversation with the Drugs and Crime Prevention Committee, Perth, 2 October 2003.

> [A] blind rush to saturate a market with drug law enforcement tactics has been demonstrated in the US context to be problematic.[672] This suggests that drug law enforcement should vary depending on the market location, the level of violence being used to maintain control in the market place, the nature of the street competition, the types of people doing the selling, price elasticities etc. One size does *not* fit all. Some approaches can actually increase the net harm if law enforcement responses are not well matched to the nature of the market-place (Authors' emphasis).[673]

The Committee recognises that there is a fine line between over policing those who may possess illicit drugs simply for their own use and legitimately targeting those who may also traffick, manufacture and/or distribute these drugs in order to make commercial profits. The Committee also acknowledges that there is sometimes community disquiet with regard to the sentencing penalties given or not given, as the case may be, to those people associated with the illicit 'drug trade'. The Committee therefore makes the following recommendations:

Recommendations

30. The Committee recommends that with regard to 'party drugs' police continue their efforts to reduce supply of these drugs through targeting and prioritising action against trafficking.

31. The Committee recommends that the Sentencing Advisory Council undertakes a wide ranging review of the adequacy of penalties and sentences contained in the Drugs, Poisons and Controlled Substances Act 1981 and other relevant legislation.

---

672 Morgan and Beck argue that 'The history of legal actions against amphetamine suggests that unintended consequences often become dominant forces in shaping methamphetamine availability' (1997, p.156). For example the demonisation of marijuana from the 1930s to the 1970s according to the authors 'helped steer the user towards more dangerous substances, including methamphetamine' (p.157). Grinspoon and Hedblom elaborate on this point:

'While marijuana was being brought to the public's attention as a menace capable of wreaking great havoc, amphetamines were introduced and promoted as perhaps the earliest technology derived drug to provide "better living through chemistry". Amphetamines were products of modern technology; they came from the laboratories of great corporations, and in the days before the growth of consumer skepticism this lent them legitimacy; unlike the dangerous foreign weed, they seemed to have reliable, safe, known properties. And, of course, they had the backing of medical authority' (Grinspoon & Hedblom 1975, p.289).

Another salient case in point was the official eradication programmes targeting *pakalolo* (cannabis derived drug) in Hawaii in the 1980s. Joe-Laidler and Morgan argue that the removal of this drug, an entrenched aspect of local culture and local communities in the islands, led directly to its replacement with *batu*, a stimulant from the Phillipines and *ice*, resulting in disastrous social, health and cultural consequences (Joe-Laidler & Morgan 1997, pp.163 ff.).

673 Submission of the Turning Point Alcohol and Drug Centre to the Drugs and Crime Prevention Committee, Inquiry into Amphetamine and 'Party Drug' Use in Victoria, October 2003.

Conclusion

This Part has sought to demonstrate the complexities surrounding the policing and law enforcement of amphetamines and 'party drugs'. The issues are complex: when it comes to these forms of drug, supply control must address two major levels. Preventing the importation of these drugs and the patrol of the extensive Australian border is clearly crucial. Yet equally important is the investigation, detection and prosecution of 'home grown' or locally manufactured psychostimulants. Once such drugs have been imported or manufactured locally, law enforcement needs to tackle equally difficult tasks pertaining to distribution.

There are also jurisdictional issues pertaining to the control of these drugs. Responsibility for law enforcement ranges across not only a variety of federal agencies (Federal Police, Customs, the Australian Crime Commission) but also a number of state based agencies including local Crime Commissions and state police forces who play a vital role in drug control and investigation at local level.

While the Committee has no responsibility for recommending policy at a federal level, it certainly recognises the importance of both state and federal bodies working together to produce the best outcomes with regard to supply and control of amphetamines and party drugs. Further and better collaboration between state, federal and indeed international agencies is absolutely crucial in reducing the problems associated with the production, manufacture and distribution of amphetamines and 'party drugs'.

PART F: Education, Information and Harm Reduction Issues Pertaining to Amphetamines and 'Party Drugs'

In any area of drug use, comprehensive and appropriately tailored policies and strategies with regard to education and information provision are an essential aspect of a demand reduction policy. Amphetamines and 'party drugs' are no exception. The questions that need to be raised include:

- Education for whom?
- Of what type?
- At what stage should such education be delivered?
- What role does drug education have in schools?
- How can parents be best educated about the dangers such drugs may pose to their children?
- What do professionals such as medical and ambulance officers, the police community, drug and alcohol and youth workers need to know about amphetamines and 'party drugs'?
- And what place does the concept of harm reduction have in providing information about these drugs?

Chapter 18 discusses these and other issues. It commences with an examination of the debates pertaining to drug education generally, before canvassing education issues specific to amphetamines and 'party drugs'. The discussion of information provision with regard to 'party drugs' and ecstasy in particular is focussed predominantly on the needs of young people as it is this cohort that primarily use these drugs. It notes that for the most part education strategies should draw from young people's own experiences of their drug use. It also takes cognisance of the fact that 'negative' drug education campaigns rarely have success in stopping young people either taking up drugs or discontinuing use. This is particularly true of the 'party drugs' such as MDMA. The section on 'party drugs' continues with a discussion of interventions such as outreach and peer education, before examining the role of the media in disseminating and commenting upon issues pertaining to 'party drugs'. The examination of 'party drugs' concludes with a discussion of the use of new technologies such as the Internet in providing both useful and possibly dangerous information with regard to these drugs.

The second half of Chapter 18 switches its attention to amphetamines. It is noted that the problem of tailoring education strategies to amphetamine users lies in the fact that there is such a diversity of profiles of users of amphetamine-type drugs. Moreover, it would seem that often drug information or services are rarely accessed by users who are not at the heavy and/or harmful end of the spectrum of drug use. Prevention and education strategies need to acknowledge that amphetamine users, it would seem, are notoriously reluctant to access information pertaining to their use. The section notes, however, that the use of outreach services such as both fixed and mobile needle exchanges may be an excellent way of providing educational material through the use of peer educators.

The chapter concludes with an examination of specific populations that may require specially tailored strategies relevant to their status or profile. These include medical staff, youth and drug workers, police and parents and caregivers. It is also stressed that, where relevant, educational material must be produced that is culturally appropriate to the needs of specific communities. These may include women, Indigenous people, people from culturally and linguistically diverse communities, and gay men and lesbians.

While Chapter 19 draws from some of the themes of Chapter 18, it presents a specific discussion of the third arm of the harm minimisation concept – harm reduction. It commences with a conceptual discussion of the sometimes contentious policy, noting that it is often misunderstood. It also examines some of the theoretical writing about harm minimisation and the related issue of the 'normalisation' of youth drug use.

The majority of the chapter is devoted to an examination of strategies, policies, services and programmes that aim to prevent or at least minimise the harms associated with amphetamine and 'party drug' use, particularly in the context of dance clubs, parties and 'rave events'. Such programmes are articulated from a variety of sources including drug and alcohol agencies, government departments, local government authorities and community networks.

18. 'Just Say Know': Drug Education as it Pertains to Amphetamines and 'Party Drugs'

> *A message that does not resonate in the culture of those who receive it with the meanings intended by those who designed the message is a useless (and potentially harmful) message. In order to work out what might be a useful message, one has to start with an examination of the culture(s) in which one hopes to resonate* (Moore 1990, p.333).

Drug education – General

Theory and practice

The Drugs and Crime Prevention Committee of the 54th Parliament has extensively canvassed the debates with regard to drug education in its *Final Report – Inquiry into the Inhalation of Volatile Substances*. Rather than 'reinvent the wheel', this Committee has reproduced some of that information in this section as it is equally timely and applicable to the current Inquiry.

Drug education, particularly as it applies to amphetamines and 'party drugs', takes different forms depending on the drug in question and the audience being addressed. Strategies that may be suitable for school students may not be appropriate if targeted at young adults, users of these drugs, party-goers, families of users or indeed professionals working in the field such as police, drug and alcohol workers and/or medical staff. Accordingly, drug educators realise different models need to be developed to meet the needs of these discrete groups.

Moreover, despite some commonalities across substances, drug education may have to be targeted in particular ways for different types of drugs.[674] Health educator J.T. Lee poses a number of questions that should be asked in tailoring drug education strategies to particular substances:

---

674 For example, the Drugs and Crime Prevention Committee of the 54th Parliament became aware that the approach to educating young people about volatile substance abuse needed to be quite different to models tailored for illicit drugs. See Drugs and Crime Prevention Committee, *Final Report – Inquiry into the Inhalation of Volatile Substances*, 2002.

The questions are:

- How much information?
- How relevant is the information?
- When is the information best considered?
- How is it to be offered?
- Is the information to be given by imposition or is it generated through sharing the knowledge offered by the teacher? (Lee 1989, p.332).

Often, whether one is addressing school students, young adults or drug users of more mature years, a didactic approach is taken that does not draw from the valuable knowledge of the recipient. As shall be discussed later, this applies equally to the knowledge of those who use the drug:

> Too often knowledge is offered as if to fill the empty vessel, the learner. Yet with drugs, as with most other topics of concern, [young] people may possess a great deal of knowledge and experience, often more than the teacher... Education is about people, and drug education needs to consider people and their ability to cope in a drug-oriented society and not just to see drugs in terms of 'problems'. Schools [for example] offer a marvellous opportunity to consider the areas of knowledge, attitudes and skills and self esteem, for it is there that young people can learn, share, discuss, practise, refine and adapt these attributes (Lee 1989, p.332).

With regard to school-based education, researchers from the National Drug Research Institute (NDRI) based at Curtin University, Perth, also agree that schools can, at least in theory, make useful contributions to drug prevention strategies through education. This has been reflected in a number of federal and state drug education programmes.[675] Midford, McBride and Farringdon argue that school based drug education is an attractive option for governments 'because it offers the potential to stop the next generation from experiencing drug problems' (1999, p.4). Given that schools are places of learning, 'there is a certain logical appeal to using school based drug education as a means of changing behaviour' (Midford, McBride & Farringdon 1999, p.4). Moreover:

> Drinking and other drug taking usually starts during youth. Most young people go to school and are a 'captive audience'. Most schools are places of learning; ipso facto, use schools to educate young people about the pitfalls of using alcohol and other drugs and thus keep them from harm. Despite this seemingly inherent logic, drug education has not been greatly successful, which a number of researchers put down to the emphasis of abstinence as the only acceptable programme goal. If the state programme objective is non-use, then any use, no matter how little, constitutes a programme failure (Midford, McBride & Munro 1998, p.319).

675 For example, the National Drug Strategy 1993–1997; National School Drug Education Strategy; National Initiatives in Drug Education 1995–1997; Prime Minister's National Illicit Drug Strategy 1999; School Drug Education Project 1997 (W.A); and Turning the Tide (Victoria) 1996–1997.

Problems in drug education

Over-reliance on United States drug education literature

Experts in drug education, however, do see some problems in how drug education principles are applied in Australia. One area of concern has been an over-reliance on literature on drug education from the United States and a lack of critical analysis about the applicability of this to Australian settings (Midford, McBride & Munro 1998; Midford, McBride & Farringdon 1999).[676] When the Committee met with drug education expert Dr Richard Midford of the NDRI he expanded on this theme:

> The problem with drug education is so much of the literature is American based and the problem with that is that it mandates abstinence as the outcome. You really can't look at harm minimisation. The problem with mandating abstinence as the only outcome you achieve is that you then ignore a whole lot of other useful outcomes...[Looking at these is] what we want to do. If we took a harm minimisation project, could we take the model of education further and look at educating people not to necessarily stop using but to use in a way that minimises harm. In some situations, a perfect strategy is abstinence or reduced use because that would reduce harm. Abstinence isn't necessarily the goal, it can be a means to achieve less harm but it's not the goal in its own right. I think that's a good paradigm to look at in the education area.[677]

Inconsistent support and application

A second area of concern is that there is no consistency in how drug education is supported and applied at state level, notwithstanding some national frameworks in the past:

> The infrastructure for drug education, as opposed to one off funding strategies or initiatives...are extensive in some Australia states and limited in others. Commitment to ongoing funding and long-term infrastructure seems to be somewhat cyclical and is determined by departmental priorities, political ideology and community demands based on reactions to drug use incidents. Currently New South Wales has the most extensive and longstanding infrastructure which incorporates drug education support staff in each region of the state. Consequently there is a relatively high support staff to teacher ratio. Queensland, by comparison, has recently downgraded its in-house support of drug education...replaced in the main by individual schools purchasing drug education support from the community (Midford, McBride & Munro 1998, p.323).

---

676 For an interesting analysis of the difference between British and American approaches to drug education in the context of (volatile substance abuse), see Ives 1994. Ives believes that American education approaches (at least up until 1994) were more focussed on the general harm to health that (volatile substances) pose, whereas British strategies were based more on preventing deaths (Ives 1994, p.44).

677 Dr Richard Midford, NDRI, in conversation with the Drugs and Crime Prevention Committee, Perth, 2 October 2003.

Ignoring social–cultural theories

A third issue recognised by Australian educators, drawing from British research, is that too often drug education and health promotion is inadequately supported by theory and that it too often ignores the social and cultural contexts of health and well being. Those who support social–cultural bases for drug education argue that too often such approaches are eclipsed by more conventional psychological theories of drug use, such as self-esteem deficits.[678] A recent report on Drug Education by the Health Education Board of Scotland (HEBS) (2002) comments on the importance of understanding the drug user in his or her cultural, social and historical milieu:

> Yet within drug education relatively little attention is given to the consideration of cultural factors in shaping and determining individual action. This is a crucial omission in developing effective interventions... In particular, there has been almost no systematic investigation of drug use that is perceived by the user or other individuals as a taken for granted aspect of everyday life. For example, investigation might consider the socialisation of drug use and the way which it manifests itself in youth culture (HEBS 2002, p.1).

This accords with d'Abbs and MacLean's exhortation that drug interventions and strategies, including education initiatives, must take account of Zinberg's analysis of 'drug, set and setting' discussed earlier. It is pertinent to repeat their discussion of this here:

> Successful strategies involve the use of a range of concurrent interventions addressing three variables labelled by Zinberg (1979, 1984) as 'drug, set and setting'. By these Zinberg means: the pharmacological-toxicological properties of the substance (drug); the attributes of persons using the substance, such as personality and physical health (set); and aspects of the social and physical environment in which consumption occurs (setting). No intervention strategy is likely to ameliorate...[substance abuse] and the problems associated with it unless it addresses each of these factors, and the interrelated effects engendered by them (d'Abbs & MacLean 2000, p.v).

---

678 For a critique of such theories including self-esteem deficits, see Coggans et al. 1991; Health Education Board of Scotland (HEBS) 2002.

A report of the HEBS in 1991 states:

'An assumption underlying much drug eduction is that young people experiment with drugs because they are in some way lacking in self esteem or are socially inadequate. While there is some evidence that people with positive health practices have higher self esteem, positive health practices or high self esteem do not necessarily preclude use of drugs' (Coggans et al. 1991, p.11).

Eleven years later HEBS reinforced this message:

'Self esteem theories...which focus on a presumed lack of self esteem provide a less than complex explanation for drug use... A recent review of the relationship between self esteem and use identified a number of methodological and statistical problems with the body of research, including deficiencies in measurement, invalid drawing of inferences from correlational studies and misrepresentation of data. The authors concluded that the evidence relating self esteem to drug use was insufficient to justify esteem enhancement as the basis for drug prevention interventions' (HEBS 2002, p.5).

In the classroom, such an approach might involve drawing upon the student's understanding and experience of drug use as referred to previously by Lee (1989). On the dance floor or at the nightclub, outreach workers and peer educators may be able to tap into some of the knowledge that ravers and clubbers have about their own drug use and the ways they try to minimise harms associated with it. Such an approach is in part premised on the idea that drug education should 'work with rather than against popular culture' (Backett & Davidson 1992, p.55).

Too didactic an approach

A fourth area of concern, and aligned to the previous point, is that much drug education material produced in Australia tends to be of the factual information provision type. As will be discussed later in this chapter, this didactic approach may be viewed in some circumstances as counter-productive among those people who do not consider themselves 'drug users or abusers', particularly those who take MDMA/ecstasy. As important as accurate factual information is, there has been very little education material that explores 'issues involved in decision making' about drug use (Midford, McBride & Farringdon 1999, p.6).

Lack of differentiation of target groups

In addition to these areas of concern, there is also the problem with some approaches to drug education that they do not differentiate between different groups of children or adolescents:

> One of the reasons that drug education has been so ineffective may be that only a small proportion of those targeted are likely to progress beyond experimentation with drugs or low levels of recreational misuse. On the other hand, problematic drug users (those with physical, psychological or legal problems arising from their drug use) are likely to be beyond the limited potential of most drug education interventions aimed at adolescents. There appears to be a need to develop variable and targeted interventions which account for the needs of different groups. The educational needs of most young people who may or may not pass through a phase of 'normative' use will differ from the needs of those who have the potential to develop drug use problems. On a continuum of drug use from no use, through experimental and recreational use to problematic use, it is possible to view normative users as those whose experimental or recreational misuse does not result in perceived physical, psychological, economic or legal problems. It is important to note there is often a significant disparity of views between young people and adults (health/social care professionals, legal authorities and policy makers) as to what constitutes misuse. The difficulty here is to have any degree of confidence in being able to distinguish, at an early enough age for proactive interventions, between those likely to be non-users and normative users, on the one hand, and problematic users, on the other (HEBS 2002, p.10).

Suggestions for overcoming problems in drug education

These areas of concern about drug education are being recognised by many organisations working in the field of drug use and abuse. The Victorian Alcohol and Drug Association (VAADA), for example, comments that tailored interventions that recognise the diversity of drug users are an essential part of an overall education strategy:

> [y]oung people are not a homogenous group. There are a number of ways of portraying messages that are appropriate to users including through face to face contact with users, the supply of information packs at venues, through the provision of updated information on websites and email alerts.
>
> VAADA recommends that strategic and targeted information about ATS [amphetamine-type stimulants] be tailored to a range of users in different settings and contexts (eg. clubs, raves, polydrug users, occasional users etc) and that provision of a diverse range of available information that is relevant be made available to individuals through a variety of avenues including websites, email alerts, mobile telephone messages, and access through peer networks. However, in all instances, feedback from users will provide the most current and viable information available.[679]

Johnson in a study examining the age of initiation into illicit drug taking also stresses the importance of devising education programmes that distinguish between different age groups:

> Generally, education and prevention programs are designed to be applied to the whole population of young people, yet ...people do not initiate drug use at the same time in their lives. Thus, timing of education programs is a concern. If drug education occurs too early it may stimulate experimentation, but if it is introduced after people have begun using drugs then it will not be effective (Johnson 2001, p.4).[680]

Similarly, the Youth Substance Abuse Service (YSAS) based in Melbourne believes the diversity of responses to drugs and drug use by young people militates against any 'one size fits all' drug strategy:

> [w]hile some young people will never use illicit drugs and some will use them intermittently, others will use them in a problematic manner. Some of those using these substances in a problematic manner will do so despite knowing the

679 Submission of VAADA to the Drugs and Crime Prevention Committee, Inquiry into Amphetamine and 'Party Drug' Use in Victoria, October 2003.

680 This ties in with the views of Measham, Aldridge and Parker 2001 that older (party) drug users generally have a 'bank' of knowledge available to them about safe drug use which younger 'neophyte' users may not. Older drug users:

'[h]ave more information available to them regarding how to deal with the negative effects of drug use, have a wider bank of experience upon which to draw, and/or are more willing or able to implement strategies. All this strongly suggests the importance of the cumulative effects of years of drugs "education", via dance club culture, drugs agencies and the media, combined with becoming "drug wise" and learning through their own and friends' experiences. Again this finding has relevance to secondary prevention messages' (Measham, Aldridge & Parker 2001, p.131)

> potential and actual risks and harms associated with use, but will simply want to manage those risks – a 'just say no' or abstinence message will not be heard by these people. Others will use these substances without caring about the potential and actual risks and harms; in fact, these people enjoy pushing the envelope and perceive messages about risks and harms associated with drug use to be a challenge to experiment further.[681]

Dr Richard Midford of the NDRI also considers the *timing* of drug education as important as its content. For example, he argues that with the possible exception of tobacco it is best to commence drug education at secondary rather than primary school:

> [i]t's better to initiate drug education at the beginning of high school and have a good coherent program that goes right through high school that deals with the various drug issues at an appropriate developmental level in high school...you've got to do drug education at a time when it becomes relevant and if you start drug education too early, it's not relevant at that particular point in that child's life. If you get into alcohol education, three or four years before the child is thinking of initiating alcohol use, it's a waste of time, they'll just sort of say what the hell's this all about. Timing of education is really important, you've really got to look at when uptake starts and get in just before that.[682]

The Victorian Education Department holds a slightly different view. It states that:

> Current research into school drug education programs, and the specific contextual experiences of schools, suggest that grades 5 and 6, and years 7 through to 10 are appropriate for drug education focusing on illicit drugs.[683]

Nonetheless, the general consensus remains that drug education messages should at all times be tailored specifically for the audience that is to receive them.

Finally, some Australian researchers have bemoaned the lack of sophisticated evaluation studies of drug education programmes in this country, particularly those that are schools based. Midford, McBride and Farringdon state:

> Despite commitments of tens of millions of dollars for the provision of illicit drug education, there is currently no research being undertaken in Australia as to what constitutes the best approach and how that can be translated into routine practice (Midford, McBride & Farringdon 1999, p.6).

Drug education, particularly in schools, is therefore clearly a complex matter. This chapter now examines education and information provision relating to the specific context of amphetamines and 'party drugs'.

681 Submission of Youth Substance Abuse Service (YSAS) to the Drugs and Crime Prevention Committee, Inquiry into Amphetamine and 'Party Drug' Use in Victoria, October 2003.

682 Dr Richard Midford, NDRI, in conversation with the Drugs and Crime Prevention Committee, Perth, 2 October, 2003.

683 Submission of Department of Education and Training to the Drugs and Crime Prevention Committee, Inquiry into Amphetamine and 'Party Drug' Use in Victoria, February 2004.

Drug education, prevention and information provision – 'Party drugs' and amphetamines

Much of what has been stated in the previous section is generally applicable to the specific drugs that are the subject of this Inquiry. This section examines some of the issues and problems pertaining to drug education and prevention programmes as applied to amphetamines and 'party drugs'.

At the outset it should be stated that one of the concerns some groups have with regard to drug education is that there is a risk of enticing, encouraging or condoning drug use when information about drugs is provided. These concerns are particularly felt and expressed with regard to the contentious issue of harm minimisation and harm reduction, an area that will be discussed in detail in the next chapter.

Ecstasy and other 'party drugs'

A recent comprehensive international review of ecstasy and its effects included an analysis of education and prevention programmes (Gowing et al. 2001). After an extensive review of the international literature it concluded that the underlying principles supporting effective education programmes were premised on the fact that 'drug use is part of wider social problems and is a health problem with multiple antecedents'. Moreover:

> While no individual strategy has been found to be effective in the long term there is considerable consistency in the identification of the criteria for effective programmes (Gowing et al. 2001, p.37).

Some of these criteria are:

- Programmes should target specific settings and cultures;
- Strategies should be carefully tailored to clearly defined target groups;
- Include multiple components addressing individuals, families, school, media, community organisations and health providers;
- Ensure that components are well integrated and messages are consistent;
- Use an evidence based approach incorporating research at all stages of the design, implementation and evaluation of the programme;
- Involve the community and target groups in defining the problem and finding solutions;
- Target groups at higher risk require higher intensity interventions;
- Strategies applied early in life are more effective for children at higher risk;
- Longer term programmes have a longer lasting impact (Gowing et al. 2001, p.37).

How appropriate is the educational information provided?

In the specific context of ecstasy, Gowing et al. (2001) state that prevention programmes need to take into account the reasons (young) people *give* for using ecstasy and 'acknowledge the personal and social functions which ecstasy *serves* for young people' (p.37, Committee emphasis). This is as true of amphetamines and other drugs as it is of ecstasy.

The importance of function in terms of prevention strategies cannot be overestimated according to Annabel Boys and her academic colleagues at the National Addiction Centre (London). Negative messages with regard to substance use, including ecstasy and amphetamines, were found to have limited effect on the respondents to a cross-sectional survey on substance use among young people (Boys et al. 1999). Moreover:

> Statistically significant associations were observed between the reported frequency of taking substances and the perceived social/contextual and/or mood altering functions cited for their consumption... If these findings are confirmed in larger studies, educational and preventative efforts may need to acknowledge the positive personal and social functions which different substances serve for young people (Boys et al. 1999, p.1043).

The authors continue:

> A common approach in drug prevention in the UK has been to highlight the potential negative effects from use. However, we found that in our sample correlations between the life time experience of negative effects and the frequency and intensity of substance use were low. It appears for this group of young people, negative experiences arising from substance use had not been sufficient to discourage future consumption. The implications from these data are that education and prevention programmes may be strengthened by using new approaches to deter use...
>
> From the results of our regression analyses it appears that the perceived likelihood of taking a substance in the future may be understood in terms of the functions served by its use. For cannabis and alcohol, perceived mood alteration and social/contextual functions, together with the extent of peer involvement predicted intentions to use. For amphetamines and ecstasy, our analyses suggested that there may be a tendency for social/contextual but not mood altering functions to be more influential on future use.
>
> Overall, our findings support the recommendation that educators and prevention programme planners should recognise the complexity of the reasons behind substance use and then encourage young people to seek alternative ways of fulfilling them (Boys et al. 1999, pp.1048–1049).

Scare tactics or negative campaigns have been shown to be particularly counter-productive. This was highlighted in the case of the education/advertising campaign following the tragic death of Leah Betts in England, supposedly from complications following the ingestion of an MDMA tablet. The key promotion in the 'Sorted' campaign were advertisements and posters with the statement 'Sorted. It took one pill to kill Leah Betts':

> [i]t was a resounding failure because drug users knew either intuitively or through the 'grapevine' that the odds of dying from taking MDMA were about 1 in a million risk exposures. They had personal experience of going to large parties at which nobody left in an ambulance as a direct result of taking MDMA...Not only did MDMA use increase after the campaign [that used a photograph of Leah Betts] but a commemorative ecstasy pill appeared called the 'Leah' (Jansen 2001, pp.195, 230).

Jansen comments further:

> With some exceptions, wholly negative drug education campaigns have often had little success. Most drug-related statistics rise and fall for reasons that do not appear to be linked to these large and expensive campaigns (Jansen 2001, p.16).

Other international surveys cited by Gowing et al. have also shown that the positive reasons for using ecstasy 'appear to be more influential in decisions to initiate or continue use than knowledge or experience of negative effects' (Gowing et al. 2001, p.37). For example, the research surveys of Italian youth by Schifano (2000, cited in Gowing et al. 2001) found that 31 per cent of the 2107 young people sampled did not think of ecstasy as a drug of abuse and 33 per cent emphasised its positive effects.

The Gowing et al. review indicates that across the world:

> Social context, fashion and peer group norms appear to be significant influences on the initiation and maintenance of ecstasy use... Prevention programmes [therefore] targeted at influencing these factors, such as peer interventions and the promotion of alternative trends and fashions to provide group identity, may be of benefit in preventing ecstasy use (Gowing et al. 2001, p.37).

In the United States there have been concerns expressed about the apparent exclusion of education and information with regard to MDMA/ecstasy in drug education curricula at both high school and college level. Although this has changed to some degree in recent years, there is still a noticeable emphasis on heroin, marijuana and amphetamines, to the exclusion of MDMA and 'party drugs'. The following remarks by Elk are still pertinent:

> The absence of apparent immediate negative or debilitating effects of this drug coupled with the lack of information being taught to students in drug education programs where other frequently encountered drugs are discussed may encourage students not to question initial or subsequent use of MDMA. By excluding discussions of MDMA within such programs, awareness of its potential dangers may be minimised if students perceive this drug not worthy of discussion or that it is of minimal risk or danger compared to other drugs that are included in the curriculum. If anything, the lack of information about the use of MDMA should be interpreted and portrayed to students as an even greater danger in itself. Therefore, including discussion of some of the

> consistent data gathered thus far can only assist students in becoming more aware of the dangers of taking such a drug and possibly deter their initial or future use of it (Elk 1996, p.355).

This concern with regard to a lack of information about ecstasy and its effects is not restricted to America. Drug researchers and workers in Australia have also stated that there is not enough information available about ecstasy. For example:

> The Alcohol and other Drugs Council of Australia (ADCA) says there should be more education programmes for younger people on the health risks of using ecstasy. They also say that these programmes should not exaggerate the risks for people who occasionally have small doses of ecstasy, but talk more about the risks of larger and more frequent doses of the drug (Shannon 2002, p.25).

This information particularly needs to be supplied while young people are still at school. The comprehensive research done by Dr Simon Lenton and his colleagues from the NDRI is testament to this need. Lenton et al.'s study of ecstasy and 'party drug' use among young people at dance and rave parties in Perth revealed that to a large extent the use of dance drugs by young people began while they were enrolled at school. As Lenton et al. state, this 'potentially [has] implications for the content of drug education offered in school' (Lenton, Boys & Norcross 1997, p.1329).

The authors continue:

> That [drug education] which focusses exclusively on 'saying no' to drugs and resisting 'peer pressure' will not help young people like these to minimise their drug related harm once they begin using these drugs. While the study was not designed to be representative of the school population, substantial numbers were in school and smaller numbers were in other education. Although there are often hurdles, such as school policy and perceived parental or community concerns about providing information to students about strategies other than 'abstinence only' messages regarding illicit drug use, this issue is too important to avoid. Appropriate, credible harm reduction orientated drug education on a range of drugs, including cannabis and the 'dance drugs', should be provided in secondary school. This should be relevant to those who are currently using the drugs or may do so at some time in the future. Perhaps if community outrage about the death of young people associated with the use of dance drugs such as ecstasy[684] can be channelled into support for sensible and workable harm prevention strategies, school based harm reduction drug education about the use of these drugs will gain more support (Lenton, Boys & Norcross 1997, p.1335).

One of the problems about supplying credible information about ecstasy lies in the fact that there is still so much about the drug that even medical researchers and drug workers do not know. Such problems are compounded when the media might exaggerate or over-dramatise its risks and effects:

---

684 The Anna Wood case being the prime example, see Chapter 6.

> The problem Ecstasy poses for drug and alcohol workers is to provide information about the very real hazards associated with use of a drug which is much safer than many other drugs. The difficulty is to provide credible, accurate information about a drug which has killed some people and made others very ill, but which produces no discernible ill effects in the vast majority of users. The challenge is risk communication [but] communicating the risks of Ecstasy use is something that has so far not been done particularly well. Much of the information spread about Ecstasy is 'folkloric and distorted to the point of legend'... In many parts of the media, Ecstasy has been portrayed as a highly lethal drug, while many occasional users consider it completely harmless (Griffin 1996, p.9).

While the article from which the above quote is taken is somewhat dated, its message is not. As will be discussed in detail in Chapter 21, much research, medical and social, quantitative and qualitative, is still needed regarding the use of and effects of 'party drugs' and amphetamines. Moreover, education and information provision, particularly from a harm reduction focus, needs to be targeted not only at users but also at general medical practitioners, nurses, police and teachers.[685] It is still at least partly true to state that:

> [f]or a drug that seems to be so widely used, there are a surprising number of things we don't know about ecstasy. We don't know exactly what's in the ecstasy tabs sold on our streets. We are not sure how many people in Australia now take it. We don't know [for certain] what the long term effects of use are (Griffin 1996, p.10).

Engaging with the users' view of the problem

Users of ecstasy and 'party drugs' are reluctant to seek information about the drugs, their drug use and services available to assist them. Researchers suggest that this resistance is, at least in part, because of the culture of drug use and users' perceptions of these drugs. As Moore states:

> Much of the information available on [harm reduction] is cold, calculated, detailed and informative. It is 'clean' and impersonal and somehow doesn't fit the reality of the social worlds of recreational drug use. Worse still, in the long run, much information is not seen as credible but rather as scare or 'cry wolf' tactics and regarded with suspicion... Such impersonal and/or discredited information is incorporated into such networks very slowly, if at all (Moore 1992, p.86).

Dr Richard Midford argues that it is important to provide young people, particularly those still at school, with what he terms 'utility knowledge':

685 This is particularly the case, given that many users of amphetamines may not access specialist drug and alcohol treatment services but prefer to seek advice from general practitioners. Many of these may be ill-equipped to deal with the problems associated with amphetamine abuse (see Wickes 1993a; Vincent, Allsop & Shoobridge 1996; Hando, Topp & Hall 1997; Gowing et al. 2001 and the discussion in Chapter 20.

> [Y]ou give people information in terms that they find of immediate use, because that's the most relevant. There's no point telling a fifteen year old that drinking will cause them cirrhosis of the liver in their fifties. If you talk to them about drinking alcohol and driving, getting picked up and losing their license or crashing or something like that, that's more relevant, then going beyond that, it's not just telling them what the issues of concern are, its giving them the skills to better deal with those sorts of things as well. There's no point telling them look, you shouldn't be doing this, or this is bad for you, if you can't give them a way of dealing with that in a more functional manner.[686]

The harm reduction agency RaveSafe stresses the importance of giving realistic information to students, particularly senior students, as it is RaveSafe's experience that many are already using 'party drugs'. Victorian RaveSafe Peer Education Officer, Natalie Russell, states in this regard:

> To address this issue, RaveSafe offers safe partying workshops for senior students, years 10 to 12, that provide information on current party drugs and harm-reduction tips for safe using.
>
> Requests for these workshops have come direct from students after seeing RaveSafe at an event, or through word of mouth or referral from the Australian Drug Foundation. RaveSafe works with each school to ensure the appropriateness of the training and that it meets the needs of the individual school.[687]

Maintaining 'street cred'

Moore argues that at least part of the answer with regard to information provision is to be found in an understanding of ethnography: understanding the value of the drug user's networks and the culture within which drug use takes place.

> Those working in public health have recognised the implausibility of solely individually-based health promotion and have proceeded to the general community level, with messages about healthy behaviour. But they have missed an intermediate level, that of social contexts, within which all individuals interact and exist. Unlike public health and its research arm, epidemiology, ethnography provides very detailed rich material about actors within specific social contexts. To say this is not, of course, to suggest that mass promotion techniques [such as media campaigns] are necessarily redundant. Smaller scale measures are not intended to replace such initiatives but to complement them. It means mediating the monolithic messages of such broad based campaigns and translating them into messages (and media) more appropriate to the numerous and overlapping social worlds which make up modern pluralistic societies (Moore 1992, p.89).

---

686 Dr Richard Midford, NDRI, in conversation with the Drugs and Crime Prevention Committee, Perth, 2 October 2003.

687 Ms Natalie Russell, Peer Education Officer, RaveSafe, evidence given to the Drugs and Crime Prevention Committee, Inquiry into Amphetamine and 'Party Drug' Use in Victoria, Public Hearings (Melbourne), 27 October 2003.

Some of the ways in which these 'monolithic messages' can be mediated are explained by Dr Simon Lenton, researcher with the NDRI:

> I think that you need to think about what sort of information, at what places, at what times is going to be most useful. The good work that's been done on what sort of interventions ought to be done at venues like nightclubs and raves and so on. Clearly there are things about managing the venues themselves, how the venues are run, whether there's free water, appropriately trained staff, exits and all that sort of stuff. There may be sorts of places like convenience advertising, information behind toilet doors, or above urinals, that people might read for those three minutes that they're standing there. There's a company that specializes in that kind of information, Convenience Advertising Australia. At dance events, there's often places like chill out rooms where people go to cool down and rehydrate and have a bit of a break from the music and dancing and that's obviously a physical environment where there might be less noise and people might be able to get information. Importantly, outreach looks to be quite successful in those venues. Helping people deal with some of the problems that they're getting, maybe providing them with a link which they might like some information about getting help later on. *What's important is we need to ask the people who are using these drugs in these venues about what they think would be useful.* They've got the internet, [they] go to the internet to get information about drugs. There's also the venues where people go to buy their music, tickets and those sort of places are where people will pick up things, read them, that's how we recruit people for these studies, we put flyers out.[688] (Committee emphasis)

Many of the strategies that Dr Lenton mentions – peer education, the Internet and outreach work – are well worth considering and form the basis of the following sections.

Peer networks, peer education and outreach

The importance of peer education in the area of drug use has been stressed to the Committee by numerous community organisations and young people with whom the Committee has met.

Moore (1992) argues that a focus on the networks and bonds apparent in groups of young people who may use drugs can give clues to how health promotion material can best be disseminated. Personal networks and contacts have an instrumental function in addition to their expressive or emotional ties:

> [p]ersonal contact is highly valued...and information from a personal source rather than a booklet, other printed material or some other 'official' source is more likely to be understood and assimilated. For these reasons, most knowledge about using drugs is almost exclusively derived from other drug users (Moore 1992, p.87).

688 Dr Simon Lenton, NDRI, in conversation with the Drugs and Crime Prevention Committee, Perth, 2 October 2003.

How can knowledge of these cultural networks be best used to provide appropriate information with regard to drug use and its potential dangers? Moore argues that detached or outreach street work and outreach methodologies are the best ways of connecting with (young) people who may otherwise be resistant to receiving such messages.

The YSAS in Victoria puts such principles into practice. Relationships are initiated between problematic drug users and YSAS staff through their outreach teams:

> Some of our staff would be encountering young people in the places that they generally congregate. For example, in the central business district our outreach workers would go out three or four evenings of the week, and they would spend time in and around the entertainment zones. They would get to know young people cold, if you like, off the street. That is one key function of our outreach staff.[689]

The use of 'peer educators' to disseminate non-judgmental drug information has also been utilised in a number of government and non-government programmes. For example, a submission from the community agency RaveSafe testifies to the importance with which they view peer education strategies:

> As RaveSafe continues to implement Peer Education as its main strategy, we also are undertaking evaluation to reflect the importance of this work.
>
> The client satisfaction with the peer education component of the project can be demonstrated by the feedback received on the RaveSafe surveys under the section asking 'what did you think of RaveSafe's services at this event?'
>
> RaveSafe received comments like:
>
> 'You guys are great, honest, friendly and informative'
>
> 'There should be more of this...knowledge is power.'
>
> 'RaveSafe made my night unreal!! It was just what I needed – Good people.'
>
> 'I think you all are wonderful. I feel so much safer with them here. My friend isn't well and they are looking after her so well. I would hate it if no one was here to help who didn't understand and judged us.'
>
> 'Thanks for being a safe focal point; you really embody the spirit of a rave.'
>
> 'Keep up the good work...you guy's rock!'
>
> RaveSafe continues to receive emails and appreciative comments from partygoers...to demonstrate the success of the Peer Education component of RaveSafe.

---

689 Mr David Murray, Executive Officer, YSAS, evidence given to the Drugs and Crime Prevention Committee, Inquiry into Amphetamine and 'Party Drug' Use in Victoria, Public Hearings (Melbourne), 27 October 2003.

> There are limitations, however, that RaveSafe has identified in providing 'Peer Education' to party drug users. With our current target group existing of ravers/clubbers and those who attend dance events, there are many other party drug users, eg. gay men, that would benefit from receiving peer education.
>
> Whilst RaveSafe has provided peer education in several Melbourne clubs, our capacity allows us to concentrate only on the traditional 'rave' venues, while there are many more commercial clubs that would also benefit from a peer education program.[690]

Kelly Weekley of the Drug and Alcohol Services Council (DASC) of South Australia also testifies to the importance of using peer educators in the dance, rave and party scenes:

> We provide training to the staff of Fresh FM, *Onion* and RaveSafe so that they are aware of drug and alcohol issues, because the way they operate they are peers within that group. They are seen as important people by those who participate in the scene because they are DJs or people who write for their main magazine and they actually participate in the scene. Peer education is one of the strongest ways that we see of getting these messages out and these agencies have been quite good in wanting to do that.
>
> We have also been looking at the kinds of education resources we can provide to people within the scene. Whilst they want to know things about drug and alcohol areas, they also want to know about health issues. For example, when they have been partying on amphetamines for days at a time, sleep is the main issue that they need to deal with, and we need to be able to give them information about how they manage those aspects of their life. We have been working with regulatory authorities and people within the scene to get some guidelines for operating safer dance parties. We have worked with the promoters, people who are in regulated venues, as well as those that operate some of the large outdoor raves…
>
> One of the project officers [with DASC] was a DJ within the scene. He still does DJ'ing at rave parties, so he has a very good knowledge of what goes on out there and has a reputation such that people will respect drug and alcohol information coming from him within that environment.[691]

The use of peer educators would seem to be a useful and worthwhile addition to education models, although further evaluation needs to be undertaken.

Youth workers, street outreach workers and indeed ethnographers all have a part to play in providing non-judgemental, accurate and impartial advice about drug use. Importantly, such advice may be given in a setting or context where the user

690 Submission of RaveSafe to the Drugs and Crime Prevention Committee, Inquiry into Amphetamine and 'Party Drug' Use in Victoria, October 2003.

691 Ms Kelly Weekley, Manager, Harm Reduction, Drug and Alcohol Services Council of South Australia, in conversation with the Drugs and Crime Prevention Committee, Adelaide, 3 October 2003.

is comfortable – a rave party, dance club or gay sauna for example.[692] Moore compares outreach methodologies with other secondary prevention strategies such as mass media campaigns, finding the latter less effective, at least with regard to those who may already be using:

> Although mass media campaigns might reach much larger audiences, outreach networks will reach drug users *in an effective and culturally resonant way*. Outreach strategies build on a cultural emphasis that most information comes from other drug users in face to face interaction and in this way outreach does not seek to alter social and cultural processes but to make use of existing ones. Perhaps most importantly, outreach programmes may provide the kind of dialectical forum in which input from both drug expert and drug user may be combined to construct a much-needed middle ground (Moore 1992, p.88). (Author's emphasis)

Dr Simon Lenton has made similar observations to the Committee:

> One of the questions is "what's the most credible source of that kind of [drug education] information and how you best get that sort of information to people". And one of the real risks about focusing on the negative stuff coming from official sources is that, for many people, it doesn't fit with their immediate experience of using the drug. And many young people think that its being hyped up in order to scare them from using these drugs.[693] One of the dangers of that is that they dismiss any messages that are about the negative effects of the drug. [Yet many of] the people that we interview [who] are often interested in the information that they receive, they seek out information, they go to the internet to get information. They're not adverse to recognizing there are harms associated with these drugs and wanting information, but the scare tactics can often have a counter intuitive effect in terms of being dismissed. I think things like information that's designed with young people in mind, you can get to peer outreach where users getting information from people who have probably used these drugs and know the scene, know what the good things are about using as well as the harmful things, and know of the medical complications and how to reduce them. That sort of method of getting

---

692 The dissemination of material or equipment or the giving of advice at venues or places at which the recipient is comfortable avoids the problems discussed by Moore (1992) with regard to the criminal nature of the user's behaviour. For example, Moore argues that some users may be disinclined to attend needle exchanges or specialist drug agencies for fear that they may be under police surveillance. Others may be reluctant to go to such venues because they may be perceived as 'junkies', a label that does not accord with either their self-image or their sense of their own drug-taking behaviour (see Moore 1992, p.85).

693 Professor Hilary Klee is more direct about the perceived hypocrisy some young people may feel towards official exhortations against using psychostimulants:

'[T]he forces for good in some quarters appear to have feet of clay. An example in the developed world is the value attached by some governments to revenue from alcohol and nicotine consumption that undermines their credibility among more clear-sighted young critics' (Klee 2001c, p.170).

> information to people is probably going to be more credible than another government pamphlet.[694]

The use of outreach and peer educators is not only about disseminating information. Engaging with young people and users is also a way of gaining or receiving valuable information from users and their networks which can then be 'put back into the loop' of knowledge with regard to 'party drug' use. As David Murray, Executive Officer with YSAS told the Committee:

> It is important that in any strategy dealing with this issue, the people using these substances themselves need to be consulted.... we have a substantial number of people using these substances who are well educated, who are engaged in employment, and who are not marginalised. They are in the mainstream, and I think we need to be consulting them, because we are not seeing them typically in drug treatment services generally.[695]

Ms Natalie Russell has made observations about the importance of getting information from users during her work with RaveSafe:

> At the events we also collect data from party drug users by means of a survey that examines the prevalence and frequency of their party drug use... These surveys are able to inform the type of resources we should be providing to party goers and the information that would be beneficial to them.
>
> We collect information on the prevalence and influence of party drug use not only through surveying but anecdotally when conversing with party goers. One of the key benefits of peer education is the openness and honesty of the party goers towards the RaveSafe peer educators. They will inform us of their personal drug use and the issues that affect them.[696]

The role of the media

> *News media are increasingly becoming the most significant public forum for debates about social policy* (Franklin 1999, p.2).

Mr Paul Dillon, Information Officer/Media Liaison Manager with the National Drug and Alcohol Research Centre (NDARC) in Sydney and a man with many years experience in drug education argues that it is essential that education strategies start with the reasons young people may think it is fun or cool to partake of 'party drugs':

> It really comes down to we have to really look at how we talk about drugs, what information we give and why we give it. So much of the information we give about drugs is political – it's, "We can't tell them the truth, we have to tell

694 Dr Simon Lenton, NDRI, in conversation with the Drugs and Crime Prevention Committee, Perth, 2 October 2003.

695 Mr David Murray, Executive Officer, YSAS, evidence given to the Drugs and Crime Prevention Committee, Inquiry into Amphetamine and 'Party Drug' Use in Victoria, Public Hearings (Melbourne), 27 October 2003.

696 Ms Natalie Russell, Peer Education Officer, RaveSafe, evidence given to the Drugs and Crime Prevention Committee, Inquiry into Amphetamine and 'Party Drug' Use in Victoria, Public Hearings (Melbourne), 27 October 2003.

> them the worst possible case scenario" because that's what the community wants to hear.
>
> I do a lot of work with the media, and *A Current Affair* executive producer once told me, "We would love to do a story on ecstasy and tell the whole story, but our ratings would plummet if we did. We would have people ringing to complain if we showed the other side because the community wouldn't accept it". And I think that is what politicians think as well. We can't say all the truth, because if we told all the truth – and all I'm saying is we don't tell them this is the greatest drug in the world, because that's not the truth – but we tell them, "Here are the good things; this is why people are using it". Once you've actually told them that, you can challenge them with the negative consequences. But until you actually accept why young people are doing this, you have no chance at all, and that's the battle we face all the time.[697]

Paul Dillon is viewed as having a great deal of authority in the area of harm reduction information provision because of his work in youth media, particularly talking about drugs on radio station Triple J FM.

Drug and alcohol agencies have generally been positive about the use of the media, particularly youth and alternative media to get the 'message across' about healthy behaviours and harm reduction strategies:

> I think media is becoming as segmented as the population itself at the moment. In terms of media that target youth culture and which are perhaps some of the most important tools for our work, we find a great deal of support around harm minimisation and health promotion. In my mind, one of the great strengths of mainstream youth culture is how health oriented it is. Even in the dance party scene, it has enormous protective factors around drug harm, an intolerance of violence within the community and a quite sophisticated understanding of how to reduce harm in terms of their behaviour. There are enormous protective factors in that scene.[698]

Professor Jason White of the South Australian DASC states that generally their organisation has had a fairly good relationship with not only the youth media but also the more mainstream print and visual media. One of the reasons he posits for this is the nature of the party scene whereby 'It is not quite so easy to differentiate "us" and "them". "Them" could be the kids of "us"'.[699] He continues:

> We cannot tell the difference; they look exactly the same. And, hey, our kids go to nightclubs, so how do we know they are not 'them'? People have a vision, for example, that heroin users look different. Some of them do, but lots

697 Mr Paul Dillon, Information Officer/Media Liaison Manager, NDARC, in conversation with the Drugs and Crime Prevention Committee, Sydney, 26 June 2003.

698 Ms Simone Cormack, Director of Population Health Programs, Drug and Alcohol Services Council, in conversation with the Drugs and Crime Prevention Committee, Adelaide, 3 October 2003.

699 Professor Jason White, Drug and Alcohol Services Council of South Australia, in conversation with the Drugs and Crime Prevention Committee, Adelaide, 3 October 2003.

> of them do not. They do not know that, so they stereotype people as all looking the same if they are heroin users, and they look like 'them' and not 'us'. I think the party drug scene has changed things completely because people cannot tell the difference.
>
> In general terms, I think the media here have been quite reasonable. We do not, as in some places, have a battle with the media. It is not a matter of trying to change them because they have completely different views. I think they are reasonably open. I do quite a lot of the work as media spokesperson for DASC and I do not find them particularly difficult. They are generally quite cooperative and they virtually always understand and seem quite reasonable when you explain why things are done
>
> ... We would get a very sympathetic view from the media. I have one personal experience of doing it, of having a research project where we needed to recruit more people. I told the media people through the university rather than through DASC. I do not know how many radio interviews there were; I spent two days of doing nothing but media.[700]

Such a view of the media is refreshing. However, it is not necessarily typical of approaches in other states.

The media play a significant role in informing and shaping popular perceptions of news, opinion and policy-making.[701] For the majority of Australians, knowledge about criminal, quasi-criminal or social 'deviance' activity within the community does not stem from first-hand experience, nor does it come from academic research. For most people this comes as second-hand knowledge and is transmitted through sources such as the daily newspaper or nightly news broadcast. As such, the images produced and articulated through the printed media permeate popular consciousness and influence societal perceptions of social behaviour in a way that is largely beyond the scope of other sources of information on crime such as police, policy advisers or academics. As Bessant points out, 'The enormous communicative power, the reach of the media and its capacity to influence community ideas and perceptions is unprecedented' (1997, p.23).

The Committee recognises that mainstream print and visual media often do perform a valuable public service in presenting issues of social concern, including drug issues, to the public. For example the recent use of the media by the Department of Human Services to get across information about illicit drugs to young people was viewed as a success:

> The Drugs Policy and Service Branch conducted the Illicit Drug Community Education and Advertising Campaign between July 2001 and February 2002. The campaign comprised three advertisements targeting heroin, ecstasy and marijuana. The campaign was aimed at 15–18 year olds, and included a

700 Ibid.

701 For a discussion of whether the media create drug problems or merely reflect them see Klee 2001b and the references listed therein.

> website, speakers bureau, directory of services and a helpline staffed on a 24 hour 7 days a week basis. At the end of each advertisement, viewers were invited to call the Campaign helpline number for assistance. 8.3 per cent of drug-related calls to the Campaign helpline were related to ecstasy use, which is more than double the level reported in calls to Directline, the general drug and alcohol helpline, for the same period (3.9 per cent), highlighting the effective targeting of this group through the media campaign.
>
> An evaluation of the campaign undertaken by Sweeney Research found that awareness of the campaign was high with 95 per cent of the high risk target audience (16–24 years of age) and 85 per cent of the general public target audience claiming awareness of one or more or several of the campaign's three commercials.[702]

Despite such positive examples of the use of the mainstream media as a harm prevention or demand reduction aid, there *are* sometimes valid misgivings about how some elements of the media present drug issues.

Paul Dillon has been particularly scathing of the way in which the print and other media 'totally exaggerate' the negative effects of MDMA/ecstasy. He told the Committee:

> We are not about overplaying the problem, because if you actually hear us speak, we say realistically for most of these drugs the chances of death are quite extreme… It [MDMA] is very low toxic. Most of them ['party drugs'] really aren't particularly dangerous… [T]he vast majority of people [emergency staff]…see with party drug stuff – panic attacks, anxiety, they are a little bit frightened about being a little bit too hot – they come in, look after them and push them back out. Some of the coverage – particularly in the Melbourne newspapers like the *Herald-Sun* – [are] just ridiculous.
>
> … The reality is that the greatest harm when it comes to most of these drugs is that they are illegal, and if you get caught with them you may have your life ruined. That's not to say they are harmless, but let's be realistic about the harms. Unfortunately what we tend to concentrate on when we actually do anything around harm, is death, and that is so unlikely.[703]

'Party drugs' and much earlier amphetamines are of course not benign substances. Yet being targeted as the latest in a long list of substances that are regularly presented as 'number one teen killer' or words to that effect is not helpful.[704]

---

702 Submission of the Department of Human Services Victoria (Drugs Policy and Services Branch) to the Drugs and Crime Prevention Committee, Inquiry into Amphetamine and 'Party Drug' Use in Victoria, November 2003.

703 Mr Paul Dillon, Information Officer/Media Liaison Manager, NDARC, in conversation with the Drugs and Crime Prevention Committee, Sydney, 26 June 2003.

704 The phrase is taken from Jenkins (1999). His book *Synthetic Panics* chronicles how a new 'drug nightmare' or wave of 'moral panic' reporting erupts every five years or so, each time concentrating on a different drug. This has ranged from marijuana in the 1930s and 1940s to amphetamines in the 1960s and 1970s to the designer drugs of the 1980s and the new 'Ice Age' of the 1990s:

'Methamphetamine, for instance, becomes the "crack of the nineties" as critics apply the scripts previously applied to that better-known drug' (Jenkins 1999, p.4).

As stated earlier in this chapter, negative drug education campaigns often run by state agencies are sometimes of questionable utility. When they are channelled through mass media outlets they can be counter-productive, particularly when accompanied by 'scare tactics' (Gowing et al. 2001.p.43).[705]

In the United States, leading academic in the field of amphetamine-type substances research, Marcia Rosenbaum, argues that many American drug education campaigns have been unequivocally counter-productive. Campaigns with regard to ecstasy have been no exception:

> Beginning with the "fried egg" commercials ("this is your brain on drugs"), American youth have been bombarded with antidrug public service announcements (PSAs) since they were small children. The effectiveness of such messages is problematic at best, and may well be counterproductive (Fishbein et al. 2002). Understanding that adults have an abstinence-only agenda, young people often write off such messages, knowing adults will say just about anything to get them to abstain. The effect is to create a huge credibility hole; in the end, hysterical warnings only make for joke fodder, and may even result in increased drug use among teens.
>
> This new anti-Ecstasy campaign is actually nothing new. For the past two years, the government has disseminated warnings about MDMA though their websites and on flashy postcards. Still, year after year Ecstasy use rises. When I ask teenage users why they have not heeded government warnings of possible brain damage, these veterans of "just say no" express deep cynicism. "Oh yeah," said one 19-year old regarding problematic brain changes attributed to Ecstasy, "they told us about that with marijuana too. But none of us believes we have holes in our brains, so we just laugh at those messages" (Rosenbaum 2001).
>
> For over two decades adults have been telling young people to "just say no". For a variety of reasons, including living in an anything-but-drug-free America and being risk-prone youth, despite admonishments to abstain, many young people say "sometimes" or "maybe" or "yes" (Rosenbaum 2002; Volberding 2000). A fallback strategy is needed that holds safety as its number one priority. An effective Ecstasy campaign should be designed to save lives and reduce health problems, rather than merely preaching total abstinence, which might not be the choice of all individuals (Rosenbaum 2002, p.5).

Indeed one of the problems facing drug educators is that media reports exaggerating the consequences of taking drugs such as ecstasy run the risk of making users blasé about the legitimate concerns held about the drug. Australia

705 In one British survey of ecstasy users, some respondents actually welcomed sensationalist media coverage. Their reasoning was that if media pressure resulted in shutting down clubs where ecstasy was known to be used this could ironically result in an enlivening of the 'scene':
'If the media get their way, what will happen is that they'll just drive everything underground...but that'll make it a lot easier for us to get on with it! Because the scene was underground at the beginning, you know... I'd like it to get back to what it was' (quoted in Hammersley, Khan & Ditton 2002, p.91).

has had its own version of the Leah Betts tragedy referred to earlier in this chapter. In this case, the sad death of Sydney school girl Anna Wood. For example Libby Topp, researcher with NDARC, commenting on the publicity surrounding Anna's death remarks how young people get frustrated at what they perceive as 'ecstasy myths'. She states:

> "We really need to get off the idea that everyone who has ecstasy is going to die" she says (Topp quoted in Sweet 1997, p.6).

There is also the fact that some harm minimisation projects such as *project e*[706] are viewed by some members of the community as signalling a green light for drug abuse or at least condoning it. For example, in the context of *project e*, pharmacologist Greg Chesher states:

> What I found was very, very sad was Mr Wood [Tony, father of Anna] saying project e is encouraging drug use...the very sad thing is that if his daughter had this information she would very likely still be alive today (quoted in Sweet 1997, p.6).

Catharine Lumby, a prominent journalist herself, while acknowledging the possible dangers associated with 'party drugs', particularly ecstasy, calls for some perspective:

> [W]hy does the media feel obliged to treat every story about young people using recreational drugs with the kind of moral outrage normally reserved for cannibals? To put it more bluntly, why do journalists who work in an industry where plenty of people take party drugs approach the subject as if they were Julie Andrews on her first night out of the convent?... If you put illicit drug use into [this] context, you start to see why it is totally counter-productive from a harm reduction point of view to treat drugs as if they weren't a normal part of everyday life.[707] Young people today are savvier than ever before and they hate being lied or patronised to... If we want young people to take the messages about the consequences of drug abuse seriously, we've got to start by accepting that drug use is normal, not aberrant. People do these things for a good reason – they're fun.[708]

While Lumby's remarks are in many ways pertinent, they perhaps minimise the concern which is raised by some of the newer 'party drugs' such as GHB and ketamine. That there are quite serious consequences associated with the use of these drugs can be seen from recent events at Melbourne Park. Although the media should never sensationalise the use of licit or illicit drugs, it is equally true that the media serves a valuable purpose in responsibly focussing attention on the risks and the attendant consequences of substance abuse.

---

706 Project e was an early harm reduction strategy developed with regard to 'party drugs', particularly ecstasy. This project is discussed later in this Chapter.

707 This concept is sometimes known as the 'normalisation thesis', see discussion in Chapter 19.

708 Catherine Lumby, 'The truth drug', *The Bulletin*, 4 March 2003, p.29.

The Committee therefore believes that the media should be encouraged to report issues pertaining to amphetamines and 'party drugs' sensitively and responsibly as outlined in the following recommendations.

Recommendations

32. The Committee recognises the valuable role the media play in disseminating information on important issues and its contribution to social policy debates.

    However, the Committee exhorts the media to report amphetamine and 'party drug' use sensitively and responsibly. In particular the Committee urges that the media:

    - avoid publishing or presenting 'how to' primers on amphetamine and 'party drug' use;
    - avoid targeting particular ethnic groups in its coverage of amphetamine and 'party drug' use;
    - avoid stigmatising and marginalising young people who engage in drug use; and
    - do not identify particular young people or their families without their express and informed consent.

33. The Committee acknowledges that there are divisions of opinion as to the appropriate nomenclature to refer to 'party drugs' and their use. Indeed, the Committee recognises the problematic use of the term 'party drugs' in itself. Nonetheless, the Committee recommends that the media should not in any way use terms or refer to these drugs in such a way that glamorises, appears to condone or encourages their use.

34. The Committee recommends that the peak agencies in alcohol and drug service delivery and information provision develop more sophisticated and informed responses and advocacy to the media on the issue of amphetamines and 'party drugs'.

A sign of the times – The Internet and new technologies

> More than any other single factor, the exponential growth of information technology has changed the context in which individual decisions about drug use are made. The range of information available through the Internet is unprecedented and some is potentially dangerous – not only how to use the drugs but also how to make them. The authorities have little control over the information and the use of the network has quickly outstripped technical developments in surveillance (Klee 2001a, p.31).

Professor Klee's comment is a salutary observation about the use of the Internet as a useful tool in providing factual and accurate information about drugs and drug harms, as well as one which facilitates access, purchase or manufacture of illicit drugs and the dissemination of inaccurate and dangerous drug (mis)information.

The Internet is clearly viewed by many people, particularly those who take 'party drugs', as an authoritative source of accurate information. The use of the Internet to ascertain 'drug alerts' with regard to the mix of what purports to be MDMA or other 'party drugs' is quite common. Such sites usually have regularly updated news on tests being done on ecstasy pills, and warnings on what batches of pills to avoid. The more sophisticated of these websites may have detailed chemical analysis of the breakdown of these pills (see Malbon 1999, p.120).

To their supporters such websites are an excellent harm reduction tool. To their detractors they are potentially dangerous instruments that, like pill testing kits, encourage illicit drug use.[709]

Jenkins argues that one of the difficulties surrounding the use of the Internet as an education tool is that few people in authority, particularly parents, have until relatively recently grasped how it is used and '[h]ow easily information about illicit stimulants can be accumulated' (1999, p.166). Jenkins continues:

> The role of the internet has revolutionized the world of synthetic drugs ...The role of the Web in disseminating such information intensifi[ed] public fears about the chances of new [drugs] spreading rapidly ...Though the new medium was poorly understood by parents, it swiftly became familiar terrain to teenagers, who seemed to their elders to be roaming out of control in this Cyberian bandit country. When in 1997 a fifteen year old girl used the Net to synthesise CAT [methcathinone – a designer drug] in her home, a drug counselor expressed the fear of many parents when she asked: "Do you want your kid reading the diaries of drug addicts who make their weeklong highs sound like a fantasy vacation? Do you want your kids seeing 'advice pages' to help them correct a bad batch of dope? Or where to shop for the ingredients?" (Jenkins 1999, pp.121, 166).

Professor Klee may be correct to warn government and community based drug education agencies that:

> The information about drugs that is available through the web is competition to be reckoned with and needs to be taken into account when mounting official information sites (Klee 2001b, p.90).

Nonetheless, the Internet has been used in constructive ways to educate and inform not only young people and potential users about drug use and abuse, but also parents, club owners, licensees[710] and people in the entertainment industry, and teachers and educators themselves. Drug websites may range from the

709 For a discussion of pill testing and pill testing kits see Chapter 19.

710 For example, the Office of the Liquor and Gambling Commissioner in South Australia is developing an online version of their illicit drugs on licensed premises 'Licensees Information Kit' particularly for licensees in rural South Australia (Ms Simone Cormack, Director of Population Health Programmes, Drug and Alcohol Services Council of South Australia, in conversation with the Drugs and Crime Prevention Committee, Adelaide, 3 October 2003).

relatively conservative or conventional which provides factual and basic information about particular drugs (for example that of the Australian Drug Foundation) to websites that are portrayed as 'cool' yet also provide accurate and non-judgmental advice about drugs and their effects. Research suggests that increasing numbers of young people view the Internet as their preferred option for ascertaining information about drugs. For example, Ms Eleanor Costello of the Drug and Alcohol Office in Western Australia comments that:

> [t]he Internet is a very, very useful tool as a medium to access services. We have a State website, it is a 'Drug Aware' website and we have a huge number of young people coming to that site. We have over 760,000 hits a month and from that we probably get about five questions a day that we then link through to our Alcohol and Drug Information Service...
>
> From recent research that we conducted early this year, 70 per cent of young people, 14 years to 24 years of age said that they would much prefer to go through a website to ask a question, even if it is just de-mystifying treatment services: 'I'm thinking about doing this but I'm not sure what to expect'.[711]

Similarly, Ms Simone Cormack of the South Australian DASC states:

> Much of the information that this ['party drug' user] group gets about their drugs and their drug use and their wisdom – the mythology around their use – is derived online. In the service industry, those of us who are, say, over 40 need to take on the challenge of becoming more sophisticated around utilising those methods and infiltrating those methods of accessing information and ensuring that credible information is available.
>
> There are some significant web sites that you can look at. Something in the order of 80 per cent of participants in the Adelaide drug scene would have a discussion after a rave. There is all sorts of information flying around on certain web sites; some of it sophisticated, some of it less sophisticated. We certainly do not have the resources at the moment to actively participate in that, but we would see that as a challenge that we do need to come to terms with, because that is where this group is getting their information.[712]

Natalie Russell also testifies to the importance of the Internet in facilitating reliable and accurate information on 'party drugs', their effects and their interaction with other drugs.

> We have identified that a large number of party goers utilise the Internet and email facilities. We have responded by accessing this group through dance music web sites. On one particular site we have a party drug information forum where party goers can ask RaveSafe safe party questions.

711 Ms Eleanor Costello, Prevention Branch, Drug and Alcohol Office of WA, in conversation with the Drugs and Crime Prevention Committee, Perth, 1 October 2003.

712 Ms Simone Cormack, Director of Population Health Programmes, Drug and Alcohol Services Council of South Australia, in conversation with the Drugs and Crime Prevention Committee, Adelaide, 3 October 2003.

> RaveSafe also emails a monthly e-newsletter to our membership list, which is currently about 250 party goers. This provides them with regular updates of the parties RaveSafe will be present at, current drug information and safer partying information. The appropriateness of this newsletter was demonstrated by an email recently received from a RaveSafe member that states:
>
> *I have been a subscriber to the RaveSafe newsletter for some time now and must admit that a lot of the information provided has been useful and the way in which your organisation reaches its clientele is appropriate. I have also been giving a lot of advice to people with information mostly from the newsletter and the informative links you guys provide!* [713]

Ms Russell adds that the Internet and the use of newsletters and email forums such as that provided by RaveSafe play a particularly important role for young people in rural and regional areas who may go to the occasional party or rave in Melbourne or major provincial centre but not have ready access to drug agencies or drug information in more traditional forms.[714]

Ms Costello, Ms Russell and Ms Cormack, and indeed many of the alcohol and drug workers with whom the Committee met, all stressed the need for agencies to move beyond traditional health responses. DASC staff view it as important for health prevention and education staff in agencies to work with the 'runners' (ie. moderators or facilitators) of youth and drug websites:

> [t]hey are keen to look at credible information and at people providing credible responses to the sorts of discussion issues that are going around. Clearly, that is a huge opening in the area of health to start looking at ways in which we can actively engage in those chats and provide credible information.
>
> At the moment this is something we are just coming to terms with here, and through our project, and the potential this has to address some of the mythologies around drug use.... Clearly, there is a significant resource issue around those things.
>
> We cannot go through every web site and every bit of information that is around. Web sites change. What was at one stage a credible web site suddenly, in a week or so, is something else. We do not have the resources to keep up. Our main push at the moment is about getting links with Fresh FM's and *Onion*'s web sites etcetera, then linking into things we think are credible, and linking back into the DASC web site.
>
> In terms of them getting on chats straight after they have been out and comparing what happened last night – actively reporting the experiences they had associated with their drug use – usually there is a degree of code, because for legal reasons the rules of a site may be that you will not discuss or promote

713 Ms Natalie Russell, Peer Education Officer, RaveSafe (Victoria), evidence given to the Drugs and Crime Prevention Committee, Inquiry into Amphetamine and 'Party Drug' Use in Victoria, Public Hearings (Melbourne), 27 October 2003.

714 Or, particularly if they live in small towns, may feel there are problems associated with anonymity and confidentiality in going to their local library, doctor or health centre (see also discussion in Chapter 11).

> drug use per se, but there is quite sophisticated code that can be used around those issues, so they are being discussed. The opportunity to interact before mythologies are created is a different way of drug service groups working and something which I think is important with this group as a potential intervention in the mainstream end of party drug use.[715]

Sometimes drug education experts will utilise outside youth oriented media such as radio, television and websites to get across the message to be promoted. For example, the South Australian Government's 'Reducing Drug Harm in the Dance Party Scene' project[716] has used a variety of media to promote harm minimisation and harm reduction messages, not the least of which has been the use of the Internet as described in a Progress Report on the project's development:

> Progress has occurred on the development of web-based communication strategies, with appropriate alcohol and other drug information and other general health (including sleep, depression and nutrition) links being identified for use on the DASC [Drug and Alcohol Services Council], Fresh FM, and Rave Safe websites, and other relevant websites, including Onion Magazine and In the Mix [rave and dance website]. Negotiations have commenced with host agencies to have this information placed on these websites in appropriate locations. Monitoring has also commenced of dance scene on-line forums as a valuable source of information from party participants [with regard to] alcohol and other drug use and safer partying.[717]

Amphetamines

Difficulties in reaching target groups

Concerns have also been expressed about information provision, educational material and programmes targeting amphetamine use (Klee 1997a, 1997b, 199c; Griffin 1997; Wood 1998a). Professor Klee, drug expert on amphetamine use, makes the following comments in the British context:

> 'Existing [education] programs are not well targeted' Prof Klee said. 'In fact there is very little targeted at British amphetamine users at all – which itself gives out a message to them that there is little to be concerned about' (quoted in Griffin 1997, p.18).

A study of British amphetamine users conducted by Klee found:

> [t]hat while some negative aspects of amphetamine were of major concern to users, other aspects were tolerated and ignored. A key finding was that providing information on physical and health effects is ineffective as a

715 Ms Simone Cormack, Director of Population Health Programmes and Ms Kelly Weekley, Manager, Harm Reduction, Drug and Alcohol Services Council of South Australia, in conversation with the Drugs and Crime Prevention Committee, Adelaide, 3 October 2003.

716 This Project conducted by the Drug and Alcohol Services Council of South Australia will be discussed in more detail later in this chapter and in the context of harm minimisation in Chapter 19.

717 *Reducing Drug Harm in the Dance Party Scene Project: Interim Progress Report*, September 2003, Drug and Alcohol Services Council, Adelaide, South Australia, p.2.

> deterrent... Prof Klee said the study showed 'you could forget about most physical damage' as a deterrent to continued use.
>
> Information and services perceived as being for heroin users were also ignored by amphetamine users, who saw themselves as a very different group to 'smackheads', and therefore regarded services targeting heroin users as inappropriate for their needs (quoted in Griffin 1997, p.18).

One of the difficulties in targeting education and harm minimisation strategies for amphetamine users (as opposed to 'party drugs') is in fact the multiplicity of substances that can come under that rubric. As Malcolm Turnbull argues:

> [I]n talking about amphetamines we are clearly faced with a diversity of both substances and users. My main concern [is] with those stimulants known colloquially as 'speed' – consisting predominantly of either methamphetamine or dexamphetamine. These drugs are used illicitly in Australia by groups ranging from street kids to truck drivers to business executives, and are variously taken as tablets, snorted or injected. It is important to keep in mind, however, that these drugs are closely linked with a range of common stimulants such as ephedrine, on the one hand and with designer drugs such as MDMA, on the other. The similarities and the popular confusion between these drugs and amphetamines is a significant factor to be considered in the framing of any strategy. In some cases it may actually be more effective to address amphetamines as part of a broader psychostimulants strategy (Turnbull 1993, p.98).

The problem with such an approach, however, does lie in the fact that there *are* such a diversity of profiles of users of amphetamine-type drugs or psychostimulants, as was discussed in Chapter 9. For example, a harm reduction programme for truck drivers who use 'speed' to stay awake may involve something as complex as structural changes to the transport industry. This approach may be very different to harm reduction measures aimed at dance party-goers. Nonetheless, education and information provision strategies could usefully be targeted at people who use amphetamine in functional ways, particularly to enhance work performance, such as people in the transport industry.[718]

Moreover, ethnographic researcher David Moore states that, at least in the context of amphetamines and ecstasy, much useful information and services seems only to be utilised by those 'at the harmful/heavily dependent end of the drug using spectrum' (Moore 1992, p.85). Turnbull states that:

> This is of particular concern because the majority of amphetamine users are casual recreational users who may only use a few times a month and are not linked to harm reduction services established for intravenous users (Turnbull 1993, p.99).

718 The community agency Anglicare also believes education strategies could usefully be targeted at groups such as 'bikies' and members of the military. The latter they see as particularly important given the 'wrong message' that use among the armed forces gives to the community. See Submission of Anglicare Victoria to the Drugs and Crime Prevention Committee, Inquiry into Amphetamine and 'Party Drug' Use in Victoria, October 2003.

As Turnbull states, amphetamines do bridge the gap between recreational, occupational and dependent use, at least in the broadest sense of the term. Recreational users, particularly those using 'party drugs', may rarely avail themselves of such information. Moreover, as Klee indicates in the earlier quote, recreational users may differentiate between themselves and 'smackheads' or 'heavy drug' users. Moore studied recreational use of amphetamines and ecstasy among young people in Perth. He argues that it is particularly difficult to get harm reduction information across to those who use amphetamines intravenously:

> Why does such information, devised with the best of intentions, fail to penetrate the various small worlds of recreational drug use? There are a number of reasons. Loxley and Davidson (1991) identify a common fear which also troubled some of my drug-using contacts – the fear of being identified by police (or by any agency or person) as an intravenous drug user should needle exchanges be under surveillance for any reason. This fear of identification as a 'drug user' also extended to those whose route of administration did not necessarily require 'picks' (needles).
>
> Some occasional intravenous users perceived educational material as targeted at 'junkies' or at least not at themselves... (Moore 1992, p.85).

Turnbull's research makes similar findings:

> Evidence from surveys suggests that young people, in particular, tend not to regard amphetamines as dangerous and even many who inject themselves with the drug do not identify as intravenous drug users and are actually very critical of heroin users. The first challenge for a harm reduction strategy [is] clearly to get the users themselves to recognise that they are at risk and to break down speed's image as a clean drug (Turnbull 1993, p.100).

Peer educators and outreach workers

As with 'party drugs', the use of peer educators and outreach may be an excellent way of reaching amphetamine users.[719] The formation of user and ex-user associations such as VIVAIDS have proved to be excellent adjuncts to more formalised or 'official' education strategies. The Committee met recently with Paul Dessauer from the Western Australian Drug Users Association (WASUA). He explained the rationale for the formation of such groups

719 For an account of an excellent outreach project among gay and bisexual methamphetamine users in Los Angeles, see Reback and Grella 1999. This study already referred to in the context of Chapter 9 employed five gay or lesbian outreach workers to collect data and disseminate harm reduction information among street users of methamphetamine. Some of the workers were also former or recovering substance abusers. Thus they were peers in terms of both their sexuality and their drug use. A loop was created where crucial research information on drug use was collated while workers were also able to impart valuable factual and referral information to users. The authors stated that these types of outreach interventions:

'[r]epresent an effective strategy for delivering HIV risk reduction interventions to populations outside treatment settings; and who are therefore potentially at even higher risk for transmission or infection with HIV' (Reback & Grella 1999, p.157). See also similar studies and programmes in Semple, Patterson and Grant 2002.

> We were actually set up by people who use drugs or who have used drugs. And that is definitely my own background as well. I spent about 12 years using methamphetamine on a pretty regular basis...
>
> My job is to try and make contact with networks of users who don't access health services normally.
>
> And that is why I was hired. Because I have got a background using and dealing and because I spent quite a few years in Perth doing that. I already had sort of networks established of old friends. The needle exchange program that we run at WASUA, I am quite convinced that that is a useful public health initiative in and of itself. Just providing clean equipment for people reduces the rate of bloodborne virus transmission full stop.[720]

Equally important is using such services as a 'hook'. In other words, the user may feel sufficiently comfortable with the peer educator after the initial contact that he or she is willing to receive further information with regard to harm prevention, reduction or treatment:

> [i]t is also kind of like the bait for all other services and people who make contact with no other health services will be coming into the exchange to get equipment. And so we have got a health centre in the same building with a nurse there.
>
> And people who don't normally make time to go to the doctor will get their blood tests done, they will get vaccinated, they will get tested for sexually transmitted diseases, and stuff like that. Because they are there already. And it only takes another 5 minutes...
>
> It has got a twofold effect, it means I am getting into networks of people that don't normally come to health services, it means I am providing clean equipment to those networks. It also means that I am getting to educate the people who are pivotal in those networks. Most people who use illicit drugs learn everything they know about what they do and why they do it from their immediate circle of peers or from the person that they score off. So if I can target the people who are socially prominent within those networks then they are doing my job for me, they are disseminating the information.[721]

Particularly impressive is the fact that Mr Dessauer is employed as a consultant educator with many bodies outside the drug user networks. For example, he conducts on-ward training on illicit drug use for mental health workers, particularly in the area of amphetamine psychosis. He also trains the recruits at the Western Australian Police Academy on issues pertaining to illicit drug use in addition to advising the Alcohol and Drug Co-ordination unit of the Western Australian Police Service. He comments that the value of such training lies in the fact that:

---

720 Mr Paul Dessauer, Outreach Worker, Western Australian Substance Users Association (WASUA), in conversation with the Drugs and Crime Prevention Committee, Perth, 1 October 2003.

721 Ibid.

> I am getting to educate and influence the attitudes of people that my clients need to help them, but basically I can feed information both ways and I could help make services that are around more responsive and more relevant to my clients' needs because I am seeing the emerging trends as they emerge because I am there when people are using.[722]

Clearly, for injecting and heavy users of amphetamines, the use of peer educators and outreach workers employed by Needle and Syringe Programmes (NSPs) may be one way of getting across harm reduction messages. Christine Tindall from Eastern Region mobile needle exchange programme explains how their service goes well beyond the provision of clean needles:

> We are in a very unique position, where we are in contact with clients on the street. As far as education is concerned, first of all, it is about building rapport and trust. Often, particularly with younger people, they will be very apprehensive about meeting new people, about people rolling up in a car, about who we are, why we are there and who we are going to tell. A lot of it is about building that rapport and, from there, they will start saying, 'Look, I'm having a problem with this,' or, 'I don't have anywhere to live,' or, 'Can you give me some information on that?' That is certainly part of what we do as workers... Quite often the interaction is very quick, particularly if there are other people around. They do not want anyone to know what they are doing, so they have to feel that we are respectful of their needs – that is, that they need to get their equipment and go very quickly, but another night they may well have time and they may well want to spend more time with us.[723]

Nick Stafford, another worker from the programme, adds:

> When we meet someone for the first time we give them our spiel – it is very short – which is, 'We operate 365 days a year. These are our hours. We have needles for you. We can give you any information you want. If you want to know about detoxes, we have them; counsellors, we have them; blood-borne viruses; safe using; whatever you want, we've got it and if we haven't got it we'll get it for you.' It is basically that, and then they just go, 'Oh, all right, no worries. Thank you,' and then they leave. Then we know that if they want to speak to us they will.
>
> When you think of needle exchange or education, you think of safe using information. The topics we cover, though, are so broad. It is just unbelievable. It is, 'Can I get a lawyer? Can I get a counsellor? Can you just sit and talk to me, because I'm really scared tonight. I've just been threatened by that person there,' to, 'I'm having problems with my mum.' It can cover anything... We

722 Ibid.

723 Ms Christine Tindall, Whitehorse Community Health Centre, evidence given to the Drugs and Crime Prevention Committee, Inquiry into Amphetamine and 'Party Drug' Use in Victoria, Public Hearings (Knox), 11 November 2003.

> end up providing a whole range of levels of support, companionship, information and education.[724]

Anex, the peak body for NSPs in Australia, fully supports the approach of services such as those spoken of by Ms Tindall and Mr Stafford but states that despite being ideally suited to engaging with amphetamine users many such programmes are restricted in doing so because of the reality of funding and staffing constraints:

> While the network of NSPs in Victoria have established a good reputation and relationship with injecting drug users, its capacity to engage meaningfully with clients is limited. The majority of outlets are based at community health centres and hospitals with the client contact occurring, in the majority of cases, over-the-counter at a general waiting area.
>
> This restricts the level of meaningful engagement that staff may have with clients as it restricts conversations on topics of a sensitive and confidential nature. Additionally most NSP staff have other duties aside from the provision of NSP-specific services which hampers the amount of time they may spend in working with clients to achieve better health outcomes.
>
> Anex believes these are issues of priority that require consideration in the review of strategies for dealing with amphetamine use. The potential of NSP to minimise harm to current users of amphetamines and to make adequate and appropriate referrals to primary health care and drug treatment services remains untapped.[725]

It would seem essential that agencies such as NSPs have sufficient resources to undertake this broader information and support service as outlined in the above evidence.

Devising education strategies for the gay community

As has been noted throughout this Report, there is a relatively high use of amphetamine and particularly methamphetamine among some sections of the male gay community, often in unsafe circumstances, and especially within the dance scene. It seems particularly apposite that tailored strategies designed by and for members of that community be developed or extended which continue to educate gay men, particularly young gay men, about the dangers of methamphetamine use and its relationship to unsafe sexual practices. Commenting on the seeming trend for younger men to be engaging in risky sexual and drug-taking behaviours, Lewis and Ross pose the following question:

> What factors other than lack of knowledge account for this recalcitrant risky sexual behaviour?

724 Mr N. Stafford, Outreach Worker, Primary Needle and Syringe Program, Eastern Region, evidence given to the Drugs and Crime Prevention Committee, Inquiry into Amphetamine and 'Party Drug' Use in Victoria, Public Hearings (Knox), 11 November 2003.

725 Submission of Anex to the Drugs and Crime Prevention Committee, Inquiry into Amphetamine and 'Party Drug' Use in Victoria, October 2003.

They continue:

> Perhaps these educational messages (including their content, argot and symbolic language) are too general or do not address the dominant attitudes or belief systems that underpin risky sexual behaviour [and drug use] that occurs among younger gay men in specific social contexts (Lewis & Ross 1995, p.3).

It is imperative that education strategies for this population, as with any specific group, start by acknowledging the importance of the milieu in which drug use takes place and the importance attached to such use if the strategies are to be successful.

Training and information provision for families, professionals and other affected parties

There are a number of groups apart from school students, clubbers and ravers and young people generally who may require appropriately targeted information and education about 'party drugs' (and amphetamines). These include but are not restricted to:

- Teachers and educators
- Doctors, nurses, hospital emergency staff, mental health and other health workers
- Social workers, youth workers and alcohol and drug workers
- Police and ambulance officers
- Parents and caregivers
- Indigenous workers and communities
- Workers from culturally and linguistically diverse communities
- Editors, journalists and media representatives.

Issues regarding some of these groups are discussed in the following sections.

Medical staff

David Murray, Executive Officer of the YSAS has stressed the importance of providing appropriate and up-to-date training and resources for 'generalist health staff to understand more fully what they are seeing when someone is presenting with the effects of psychostimulant use'.[726] Such a need was reinforced by the evidence of Dr Chris O'Donnell, radiologist at Frankston Hospital, who gave evidence to the Committee about the increasing number of patients he is seeing with complications as a result of amphetamines. He has been instrumental in attempting to get medical staff at his hospital more aware

726 Mr David Murray, Executive Officer, YSAS, evidence given to the Drugs and Crime Prevention Committee, Inquiry into Amphetamine and 'Party Drug' Use in Victoria, Public Hearings (Melbourne), 27 October 2003.

of the issues pertaining to the ingestion of amphetamines and the side effects and medical sequelae following from this use:

> What we have done at the hospital is spoken to all the emergency physicians, so that when anyone comes in with apparent complications as a result of amphetamine use, instead of leaving them to sleep it off in the department we are actively encouraging them to get involved with our neurologist and to order MRIs so that we can detect these changes as quickly as possible. So within our hospital we have been proactive in trying to get these people into the system. I might say there has been some reluctance, not by the doctors but by the people involved; they want to go home.
>
> By my presentation at the college of radiologists meeting I am trying to make my colleagues at least aware.[727]

Professor Steve Allsop of the Western Australian Drug and Alcohol Office believes that part of the problem stems from a lack of commitment to drug education as part of medical training and a subsequent paucity of material being taught in this area:

> I think firstly we need to get addiction studies, for the want of a better term, into the under-graduate and the post-graduate curriculum. .... But we are now running a [drug] program for registrars and in fact, most of the people who attended our first program were country GPs, [it is an] accredited program that builds up their expertise and it includes a range of things including amphetamines.
>
> I think by getting it [drug education] into the curriculum, you give people the knowledge and the skills but it also says: "this is part of your job". Part of the problem was because drug studies wasn't part of university education: [the reaction was] "Oh, it's not part of my role, if I wasn't taught it and examined on at university it is not part of my job".[728]

Measham, Aldridge and Parker state that:

> Whilst Accident and Emergency staff, have, through increasing clinical experience, come to recognise the costs of alcohol and drug misadventures…it is unrealistic to expect most family doctors to spot underlying morbidity, especially if they are not told the full facts (2001, pp.190–191).

In Victoria, Professor Margaret Hamilton has made similar comments with regard to the relative lack of knowledge some general practitioners have with regard to illicit drugs. This is despite the fact that for many amphetamine users in particular general practitioners may be the only health professionals they seek assistance from:[729]

---

727 Dr Chris O'Donnell, Radiologist, Frankston Hospital, evidence given to the Drugs and Crime Prevention Committee, Inquiry into Amphetamine and 'Party Drug' Use in Victoria, Public Hearings (Melbourne), 27 October 2003.

728 Professor Steve Allsop, Drug and Alcohol Office, Western Australia, in conversation with the Drugs and Crime Prevention Committee, Perth, 1 October 2003.

729 See also discussion in Chapter 20.

> I think a lot of our treatment people need to have further information about harm reduction and what might be important. General practitioners are probably the group which is least familiar with these drugs, what to look out for and how to respond if and when they see them. Often they get caught in prescribing things, wondering what is happening and not being sure what to do about it. That is a target group that might be worth looking at in terms of reducing harm for those who are using.[730]

Welfare, youth and alcohol and drug workers

Clearly it is imperative that workers on the 'front line', those who engage with (young) drug users or potential users, need to have accurate, comprehensive and up-to-date information with respect to a variety of drugs and their effects. Yet with regard to some drugs and particularly 'party drugs' sometimes not even alcohol and drug workers may have knowledge of the latest drugs or latest trends. VAADA has reported that many drug agencies are grappling with the complexities of 'party drug' use and their apparent increasing use, particularly among younger users:

> Our sector has reported to us that they are not necessarily knowledgeable around some of the issues, particularly with newer party drugs and the combination and interactive effects of party drugs and amphetamines with other drugs. Our sectors indicated that they would like to know more about what these drugs are, what their effects are, some of the harms, and particularly effective treatment approaches to dealing with people who present at treatment agencies with this particular problem.[731]

Parents and caregivers

Education materials for parents need to be easy to understand and access, and culturally sensitive to particular groups from culturally and linguistically diverse backgrounds. Some agencies believe they may also need to incorporate harm minimisation strategies. This is particularly important given the levels of misunderstanding and ignorance about 'party drugs' in particular. Professor Margaret Hamilton comments in this regard:

> [t]here is a lot of community concern about party drugs, probably related more particularly to media coverage and the types of people who are using those drugs and the environments of their use, and people like me being unfamiliar with those environments except through my research. Something I do not know tends to be more anxiety provoking than something I do know, so many parents are very anxious about party drug use but perhaps less anxious about

730 Professor Margaret Hamilton, Director, Turning Point Alcohol and Drug Centre, evidence given to the Drugs and Crime Prevention Committee, Inquiry into Amphetamine and 'Party Drug' Use in Victoria, Public Hearings (Melbourne), 27 October 2003.

731 Ms Carol Bennett, Executive Officer, Victorian Alcohol and Drug Association (VAADA), evidence given to the Drugs and Crime Prevention Committee, Inquiry into Amphetamine and 'Party Drug' Use in Victoria, Public Hearings (Melbourne), 27 October 2003.

> their teenagers using alcohol. And yet what we know is that alcohol is probably causing far more harm than the teenagers' use of party drugs.[732]

Hammersley, Khan and Ditton argue that rarely when it comes to drugs are parents (and indeed schools) the appropriate source for the provision of the sort of drug information that is required (factual and non-moral):

> Overall, it seems that parents will need far more educative input than their children before they are in (and are believed to be in) a position to listen, let alone help (Hammersley, Khan & Ditton 2002, p.146).

This may be all the more reason to ensure parents are aware of harm minimisation and harm reduction messages. There is some evidence that there are trends towards getting parents involved in school drug education programmes outside of the classroom.[733]

Midford, McBride and Munro advise, however, that any attempt to use harm minimisation strategies with parents must be done carefully and cautiously:

> Parents generally have concerns that stem from the desire to keep their child safe and they want to believe that this can be done by stopping drug use. Discussions with parents, however, indicate that they are aware of the widespread use of drugs, particularly use of alcohol and cannabis, and that realistically 'just say no' or narrow non-use approaches are not useful ways of skilling their child to make safer decisions. A number of Australian-based studies involving work with parents suggest that if harm reduction is to be used as a basis of school drug education this requires explanation, reflection and exploration of issues and concerns to ensure a certain level of comfort with the approach (Midford, McBride & Munro 1998, p.323).

Initiatives of the Department of Education and Department of Human Services Victoria that will enable parental drug training to be accessed within and outside the school system in a variety of community settings are a positive 'first step'. These initiatives include:

- The 'Creating Conversations' which is delivered in schools and aims to encourage conversation between young people and their parents on drug issues (Department of Education).
- The ABCD parenting programme which is a statewide parenting drug education program (Department of Human Services Victoria).
- Family Drug HelpLine has been established to assist parents to deal with and manage issues of drug abuse in the family setting (Department of Human Services Victoria).

---

732 Professor Margaret Hamilton, Director, Turning Point Alcohol and Drug Centre, evidence given to the Drugs and Crime Prevention Committee, Inquiry into Amphetamine and 'Party Drug' Use in Victoria, Public Hearings (Melbourne) 27 October 2003.

733 See for example, the transcript of evidence of Ms Eleanor Costello, Drug and Alcohol Office of Western Australia, in conversation with the Drugs and Crime Prevention Committee, Perth, 1 October 2003.

Culturally and linguistically diverse communities

As acknowledged in Chapter 9 people from culturally and linguistically diverse (CLD) backgrounds face many barriers in accessing, or being referred to, appropriate drug information and services:

> These barriers include, for example, language difficulties, lack of knowledge about the availability and nature of services and lack of cultural awareness among workers and agencies. Other factors can also have an impact, including:
>
> - Parents' assessment of their children's involvement in drug use against a variety of factors that can be quite different from the reality of school/street life in Australia
> - Families comparing their current lifestyle against memories of their home country without taking into account that country's current drug situation
> - 'Traditional' families responding to drug usage with a variety of methods to cover up or deny the activity, for reasons of shame and fear of stigmatisation
> - Some families embracing a 'zero tolerance' approach, and others attempting to 'solve the problem' by sending the young person 'back home' (DrugInfo Clearinghouse 2003b, p.1).

A recent project that aims to address some of the problems outlined above is the Bilingual Information Educator course, an accredited training and education course aimed to meet the needs of culturally and linguistically diverse communities:

> The course was first developed as a part of the City of Maribyrnong's Illicit Drug Strategy, with support from the Department of Human Services and various State and national drug agencies. It has since been delivered to communities in the Cities of Yarra, Moonee Valley and Kingston.
>
> To date, fifty-three graduates, representatives of CLD community organisations from communities as diverse as Vietnamese, Horn of Africa, Chilean, Bosnian and Chinese backgrounds have qualified to work in their own communities and in their own languages. Workers from many of these community agencies have taken on the task of mentoring the bilingual graduates and, in turn, will be advised by the graduates on cultural issues (DrugInfo Clearinghouse 2003b, p.1).

The course's programme, structure and content promotes the National (Illicit) Drugs Strategy's focus on harm minimisation. It aims to:

> - equip participants with a good foundation knowledge of relevant drug-related issues
> - enhance participants' skills in presenting drug information to people of CLD backgrounds (2003, p.2).

The course includes such topics as:

- The nature of drug use and dependence
- The pharmacology of drugs and the physiology of drug use
- Effects of problematic drug use on the user and the user's family, carers and friends
- Drug use and the changing political, economic and social contexts
- Central philosophies of the alcohol and other drugs sector
- Legal and policy issues
- Risk factors
- Public and personal safety
- Treatment alternatives
- Drug prevention
- Preparing and delivering information to people of culturally and linguistically diverse backgrounds.

The Bilingual Educators Course, although focussing upon a wide range of illicit drugs, is a valuable addition to the knowledge building required in the area of amphetamine and 'party drugs'. This is particularly the case for communities who have not been well served by traditional drug education services.

Indigenous communities

The Committee is aware of the degree of powerlessness and frustration felt by many members of the Indigenous community when it comes to the issue of alcohol and substance abuse. The Committee notes with satisfaction, however, that in the area of education the Koori Drug and Alcohol Workers training courses run by Ngwala Willumbong in partnership with Swinburne TAFE includes comprehensive educational materials on drug abuse, including amphetamine abuse, as part of its syllabus. Committee research staff have been privileged to attend parts of this course during the Committee's previous Inquiry into Volatile Substance Abuse and they have found the instruction and material to be of a high quality.

Nonetheless, as in the non-Indigenous community there is still not enough good quality culturally relevant materials being produced in the area of amphetamines and 'party drugs'.[734]

Professor Dennis Gray, an expert in substance abuse issues among Indigenous people, emphasised to the Committee how drug education materials produced for a general audience can so often be inappropriate for Indigenous populations. For example, with regard to injecting use of amphetamines and heroin he stated:

> The prevalence of current injectors is twice as great as non Aboriginal population. There are a whole lot of issues around in unsafe injecting. We were

734 Although as stated in Chapter 9, these are probably less of an issue or problem in Indigenous communities than they are among non-Indigenous populations.

> concerned about the spread of Hepatitis C amongst Aboriginal people so there is a need to provide good quality information to people about injecting. The WA Substance abusers group puts out some materials and there's various other bits and pieces around but one of the things that we found was that most of it was unsuitable for Aboriginal people. The stuff we looked at, for example, you almost needed a PhD to understand what they were going on about, yet most Aboriginal people had left school by year 10 and there are many who are functionally illiterate so we need to be targetting health promotion material to that group in a way that makes the information accessible to them.[735]

Whatever education based interventions are devised for Indigenous communities they need to be culturally appropriate to the target audience. d'Abbs and MacLean outline the factors that must be taken into account in providing education and educational materials to Indigenous youth and Indigenous communities. Although the authors are writing in the particular context of petrol sniffing, their exhortations are for the most part applicable, or at least adaptable, to the needs of Victorian youth who may use amphetamines, or indeed any drugs. They state:

> Education-based interventions, in sum, appear to have a useful role to play, provided that they:
>
> - are targeted at the community, and selected groups within the community such as parents of [sniffers], rather than at [sniffers] or young people not sniffing;
> - if directed at [sniffers], focus on effects of petrol sniffing which are likely to deter rather than encourage the practice, avoiding shock tactics;
> - promote caring and coping capacities within the community, rather than spread alarm and despondency;
> - are culturally appropriate;
> - occur in conjunction with other interventions aimed at reintegrating [sniffers] with their families and the community; and
> - are evaluated, so that subsequent programs can learn from them (d'Abbs & MacLean 2000, p.42).

The Committee therefore makes the following recommendations:

735 Professor Dennis Gray, NDRI, in conversation with the Drugs and Crime Prevention Committee, Perth, 2 October 2003.

Recommendations

35. The Committee recommends that, for the most part, education training and information provision with regard to amphetamines and/or 'party drugs' are most usefully developed for groups, in addition to children and adolescents. These groups should include:

    - Teachers and school support staff;
    - Parents and parent groups including those from Indigenous and culturally and linguistically diverse communities;
    - Police, ambulance officers and other emergency personnel;
    - Youth, social and community workers (including culturally appropriate education strategies for those from Indigenous groups);
    - Workers from culturally and linguistically diverse communities and agencies;
    - Drug and alcohol service workers;
    - Residential care workers;
    - Doctors, nurses and other health workers;
    - Dance club, party venue, outdoor rave staff and promoters;
    - Crowd controllers;
    - Users and user organisations;
    - Local government staff, particularly those working in areas such as recreation, parks and gardens and amenities; and
    - Journalists and media representatives.

    In particular, these groups and individuals need to be thoroughly informed of the nature and consequences of amphetamines and 'party drugs'. They should also be trained or advised of appropriate ways of assisting a person who appears to be intoxicated through amphetamine and 'party drug' use.

36. The Committee recommends that relevant professional bodies should examine the adequacy of current training regarding amphetamine and 'party drug' use and should determine the basic level of knowledge on amphetamine and 'party drug' use appropriate to their professions.

37. The Committee recommends that in-service and multi-disciplinary training on drug issues include amphetamine and 'party drug' use. Within training and education programmes for personnel working in the field, instruction should be provided giving accurate and comprehensive knowledge of harm minimisation policy and practice.

38. The Committee recommends that sufficient and appropriate ongoing training be given to medical, nursing and ancillary staff with regard to amphetamines and 'party drugs'.

39. The Committee recommends that the curricular for medical, nursing and health workers incorporate sufficient information, education and training on alcohol and drug-related issues, in particular amphetamine and 'party drug' issues.

From this discussion of needs of various groups in the community, the next section will concentrate on some programmes and projects that are currently seeking to address how and to whom drug education information can best be delivered in the area of amphetamines and 'party drugs'.

Recent national, state and local information programmes

Notwithstanding the above criticisms, in recent years there have been a number of national, state and local programmes that have endeavoured to provide information and educational materials with regard to amphetamine and ecstasy use that target audiences such as young people, ravers, clubbers and school students. Apart from fact and information sheets compiled, written and/or distributed by various drug resource and information groups, other projects have drawn from the ethnographic methodologies referred to by researchers such as Moore. For example, not only does the Australian Drug Foundation, the peak drug information body, produce standard resources such as Information Sheets, conduct research and maintain a library and information clearing-house, but it also hosts and manages a youth website called 'Somazone'.[736]

> This website was developed *by* young people for young people. A key feature of the site is the question and answer section where young people can submit questions which are answered by people with expertise on the relevant issue. The drug related questions are answered by ADF staff members. The questions and answers are posted on the site so that the information is available to all who visit the site. Currently there are 25 questions with answers listed for amphetamines, 13 for ecstasy, and 8 for hallucinogens. However it is the type of questions which young people are asking about these drugs which is enlightening, giving some indication of the level of knowledge (and ignorance) that exists about these drugs, attitudes to their use and actual practice.[737]

An early national initiative to try and make young clubbers aware of the potential dangers of ecstasy and other 'party drugs' was *project e*. This was an education kit produced for dance party patrons funded by the Commonwealth government and developed jointly by drug and alcohol agencies in Queensland, New South Wales and South Australia. The kit had four elements:

- A booklet for venue operators that suggests initiatives which encourage the safe organisation and management of dance parties. It addresses

736 www.somazone.com.au

737 Submission of the Australian Drug Foundation to the Drugs and Crime Prevention Committee, Inquiry into Amphetamine and 'Party Drug' Use in Victoria, August 2002. (Committee emphasis)

issues such as first aid requirements, provision of chill out areas, access to water, security arrangements and liaison with emergency services;

- An educational brochure about the effects of ecstasy, explaining the drug and its effects, safety risks, water consumption and how and when to seek medical assistance;
- Four wallet sized cards summarising the effects of ecstasy and what actions are necessary if someone is suffering the effects of taking ecstasy;[738]
- Two educational A4 sized poster for display in venue toilets (reproduced in Wood 1998a, p.19).

As with many such projects, whether they are dealing with ecstasy or alcohol, much of their effectiveness depends on the willingness of venue managements to fully participate in their implementation. This is not always forthcoming. Another criticism of the *project e* material was that it did not to any extent focus on or draw attention to the very real dangers of poly-drug use in conjunction with ecstasy or it did so in very generalised ways. For example, messages such as 'It is dangerous to take ecstasy when using other drugs' are not very helpful if the types of drug interactions and their consequences are not spelt out. As Wood, quoting from leading drug educators, states in this context:

> 'If concurrent use of more than one drug is a common practice among users of dance drugs, the effectiveness of harm reduction messages advising users not to mix their drugs could be questioned'... But in fairness to drug educators, what else can they do in light of the dearth of research into drug combinations? (Wood 1998a, p.19).

School based drug education

Victorian Education Department – Individual School Drug Education Strategy

At state level, the Victorian Education Department addresses the issue of drug misuse through the implementation of Individual School Drug Education Strategies which, as the name suggests, allows individual schools to develop appropriate education strategies tailored to specific needs:

> The Department has a comprehensive drug education program that all Government and 80% of non-government schools are implementing. The Individual School Drug Education Strategy ensures that schools develop prevention programs and drug education curriculum for all students.
>
> Specifically, the Department and schools address the issue of amphetamines and "party drugs" through:

738 The cards included messages with regard to safe water consumption, the effects of over-heating and how to prevent it or address it, and other medical advice to use during an emergency (see Webb 1998).

- The implementation of Individual School Drug Education Strategies that emphasise the need for consultation and the identification of local drug-related issues (including amphetamines and "party drugs")
- Student welfare support that focusses on the early identification of students experiencing drug-related issues
- Collaborative partnerships between schools, parents and community agencies such as the police, drug and alcohol agencies and Community Health Centres
- The provision of resources such as *Get Wise* which provides comprehensive curriculum and teaching materials on illicit drugs and which includes activities that specifically focus on amphetamines and "party drugs".[739]

In a submission to this Inquiry the Department states that concerns of schools and teachers with regard to amphetamines and 'party drugs' are at this stage 'minimal'. Nonetheless, as with Local Council Action Plans it is thought the school plans are adaptable to cover all forms of drug and drug education.

The locally developed school strategies enable schools to:

- implement relevant and comprehensive drug education as an ongoing core component of the curriculum
- provide each student with appropriate drug education prevention and intervention programs
- develop and review drug-related school-based policies
- provide a supportive environment that involves parents and the wider school community in drug-related curriculum and welfare issues.

> The Individual School Drug Education Strategy model also encourages schools to consult with parents, students and the broader school community to identify strategies particular to their school situation and to implement appropriate responses to locally identified issues such as amphetamines and 'party drugs'.[740]

Victorian drug education policy is based on harm minimisation principles:

> This involves utilising a range of approaches to prevent and reduce drug-related harm including abstinence from drug use, prevention, early intervention, specialist treatment, supply control and safer drug use. The approach aims to reduce the risks associated with drug use and to promote healthy behaviours.
>
> The Individual School Drug Education Strategy model is underpinned by the implementation of the *Framework for Student Support Services in Victorian Schools* which has an emphasis on primary prevention designed to enhance

739 Submission of Department of Education and Training to the Drugs and Crime Prevention Committee, Inquiry into Amphetamine and 'Party Drug' Use in Victoria, February 2004.

740 Ibid.

> the emotional and social health of all students. Much of this primary prevention is aimed at building resilience in young people through establishing a supportive environment where a sense of belonging and wellbeing are strengthened. The presence of these elements within a young person's environment are protective factors against depression, substance misuse and suicide, and assist them to deal with their problems more effectively.[741]

While the approach taken to drug education is generic in the sense that there are no specific approaches with regard to amphetamine and 'party drug' use, schools with need for specific information or support to address particular drug issues can access the services of Senior Program Officers in Drug Education located in each education region.

The Department of Education will be conducting a review of drug education, curricula and resources throughout 2004. Such a review will 'include a review of amphetamines and "party drug" use and how well this issue is currently being addressed'.

Recognising the debates and the complexities surrounding drug education, the Committee awaits the result of the review with interest.

Programmes in schools – Responses from the community

Many of the education and information provision projects that are being run in local areas concern various harm minimisation and reduction strategies aimed at reducing, if not eliminating, the deleterious effects associated with amphetamine and ecstasy use. Several school based programmes incorporate both peer education strategies as well as information sharing with parents and parent groups with regard to drug issues, including amphetamines and ecstasy.[742] As discussed above, many Victorian schools are involved in planning drug education programmes and policies through the Individual School Drug Education Strategy.

Nonetheless, there have been criticisms that schools could be doing more and doing it differently. In a submission to this Committee, the Victorian Catholic Education Office states, 'There is a need for schools to be...responsive to new situations and to adopt new approaches that promise to be effective'.[743] It continues:

> Schools should do more to provide age appropriate drug education for students in the senior secondary years (Years 11 and 12). Because of the

741 Ibid.

742 For example, the City of Monash's Parent Drug Education Program 'seeks to educate parents of secondary aged young people regarding drug and alcohol issues, as well as providing drug and alcohol service delivery information and encouraging parents to communicate with young people about substance abuse' (Submission of the City of Monash to the Drugs and Crime Prevention Committee, Inquiry into Amphetamine and 'Party Drug' Use in Victoria, August 2002).

743 Submission of the Catholic Education Office to the Drugs and Crime Prevention Committee, Inquiry into Amphetamine and 'Party Drug' Use in Victoria, August 2002.

> pressures on students and schools to succeed academically in the VCE and other senior secondary programs, schools have difficulty in finding time in the teaching programs for such matters as drug education and drug related student welfare programs...
>
> In addressing safety issues for young people using amphetamines and 'party drugs', especially in combination with alcohol, young people need to be encouraged to act on their feelings of friendship and care that they have in their groups, to support each other and seek help when needed. Schools should continue to build supportive environments for their students, so that at all levels young people experience connectedness and support. This should foster a readiness to seek advice and to talk to those who can provide advice and help.[744]

One school based strategy that seems to have achieved some success is the Schools Nurse Program in Queensland. Throughout state schools in Queensland school nurses have been employed. The crucial point according to representatives of Queensland drug programmes is that the nurses are employed by Queensland Health and not by Education Queensland:

> And they are there in a counselling capacity as well as just speaking to kids about a whole range of topics. They also run particular programs in the schools as well. It works in terms of Mary Jane could come and say, "Look, I'm worried about Phil, I think he has a [drug] problem" and the school nurse can approach them. They have even had instances where they have gone home with Mum and Dad to tell them that Jane's pregnant, ... as well as trying to encourage kids to look at the safe behaviours in the school environment. But they are specifically Queensland Health employees; the principal or whoever does not run them in each school. That is proving to be a very, very successful program in Queensland because it is creating an environment where we can intervene at a whole number of levels.[745]

Many drug, youth and community agencies agree that interventions with regard to ecstasy and 'party drugs', and amphetamines used in the party context, need to be focussed differently compared to traditional drug education contexts. The harm reduction agency RaveSafe believes that there needs to be a standardised approach across all schools for harm reduction education with regard to drug use. Although RaveSafe gives workshops to senior students in various schools,

---

744 Submission of the Catholic Education Office to the Drugs and Crime Prevention Committee, Inquiry into Amphetamine and 'Party Drug' Use in Victoria, August 2002. This submission also makes reference to the hitherto mentioned 'Celebrating Safely – 'The Later Years Project':

'This project is designed to examine the approaches used by schools to prepare their students to make wise decisions about alcohol and drug use at key celebrations, particularly those associated with the end of Year 12. The project involves working with a small number of schools, conducting focus groups with students, surveying teachers and parents, identifying good practice and collating useful information and making it available to schools'.

The Celebrating Safety project is federally funded and applies to all Australian schools, state and private.

745 Mr Robert Kemp, Manager, Queensland Availability Support Program, in conversation with the Drugs and Crime Prevention Committee, Brisbane, 27 June 2003.

requests for these workshops are usually direct from students (after seeing RaveSafe at an event), through the Australian Drug Foundation, or by word of mouth. In a submission to this Inquiry, RaveSafe stated:

> The difficulty for RaveSafe in achieving this key performance indicator [of student drug education] is that an individual school's curriculum does not identify the need for training on these issues and it is only at the discretion of the school that party drug issues are addressed.
>
> RaveSafe believes that Year 10, 11 and 12 drug education needs to be targeted more appropriately and through the Department of Education.
>
> Regulations need to be in place to influence not only the type of drug education implemented, or issues addressed, but also the provider of this information. [X agency] is a private organisation that provides workshops to Senior Students about how to keep themselves safe when they start to go to licensed venues (nightclubs, bars, raves) and parties. With no regulation or accountability on the information they are providing it is concerning that we are unsure what, if any, harm reduction advice is being given.
>
> With few controls in place for the type of drug education that can be implemented within schools, there is opportunity for the myths and unsafe using practices to be apparent when school students enter the partying scene.[746]

Finally it should be added that whatever the strength or otherwise of school based programmes, for some adolescents most in need of information or intervention with regard to drug use they will be of little value. This may be for the simple reason that these young people may seldom attend school (truants) or do not attend school at all.[747]

Non-school projects

The Big Book on Party Drugs

A recent project which seems to typify the sometimes polarised views about providing information on drugs and their effects, particularly to young people, is a publication of the Uniting Care alcohol and drug agency Moreland Hall, based in Melbourne. They have recently produced a *Big Book on Party Drugs*, similar to their highly successful *Big Book on Drugs*. The aim is to distribute accessible and non-judgemental information on 'party drugs' to young people and students through school and youth networks across Victoria. The booklet is illustrated in cartoon form and gives information on such topics as:

- Drug classifications
- The drug, the person, the environment

746 Submission of RaveSafe to the Drugs and Crime Prevention Committee, Inquiry into Amphetamine and 'Party Drug' Use in Victoria, October 2003.

747 See for example Howard, Stubbs and Arcuri 2004, in prep.

- If things go wrong
- Talking about a rave-o-lution (A snapshot of the subculture, including music and dance styles)
- Safer partying
- Detailed and comprehensive guide to the nature and effects of major drugs, including alcohol, amphetamines, marijuana, LSD and 'party drugs' such as ecstasy, ketamine and GHB
- Legal issues, including the new laws on drug driving.[748]

The booklet has received a mixed reception. To its critics it is seen as promoting or at least condoning drug use. To its supporters, often people working in the drug and alcohol field, it is a realistic and highly useful publication that can address the harms associated with young people's drug use, particularly of 'party drugs'. These reactions typify the divide felt over the contentious issue of harm minimisation, which will be discussed in more detail in the following chapter.

The Reducing Drug Harm in the Dance Party Scene Project (South Australia)

This is a collaborative project between the DASC and the South Australian Police Department. It focusses on the dance music scene in Adelaide, South Australia, and aims to prevent the uptake of 'party drugs', reduce harm among users, and encourage users to access the primary health care system. This project is underpinned by the principles of harm minimisation and consequently will be discussed in detail in Chapter 19 dealing with this topic. At this stage, however, it is appropriate to discuss one aspect of the Project which is of relevance to the issue of drug education and information provision – the use of popular culture to disseminate harm reduction messages to young 'party drug' users. In this case, through the use of the magazine *Onion*, a free, bi-monthly dance music magazine, and the peak printed media of the dance music scene in Adelaide:

> This magazine enjoys a wide distribution (8000 copies per fortnight to over 500 outlets) throughout Adelaide, being available in a range of locations frequented by young people, including universities, bars, nightclubs, cafes, music stores, and other retail outlets. It is also estimated that each copy is read by between 3–4 individuals, giving the magazine considerable readership. Magazine content ranges from clubbing and raving information to dance music news and youth lifestyle issues. The project [Reducing Drug Harm in the Dance Party Scene Project] will collaborate with *Onion*, a key project partner, to develop appropriate AOD [alcohol and other drug] related content for publication in the magazine. The project's key strategies in working with *Onion* include:
>
> - Developing tailored AOD messages with a harm reduction focus for regular publication in *Onion*

748 See, *The Big Book on Party Drugs*, John Hartley for Uniting Care Moreland Hall, 2003 Education and Training Unit, Moreland Hall, Moreland, Victoria.

- Developing feature AOD articles for publication in *Onion*
- Developing and delivering AOD training for *Onion* staff
- Developing AOD/harm reduction related web communication strategies for the *Onion* web-site (Lymb et al. 2003, p.4).

This project is still in its infancy and the use of media such as *Onion* is merely one aspect of its overall strategy. Nonetheless, it is an example of the increasing trend for harm minimisation and harm reduction strategies to draw upon the milieux and subcultures in which drug use takes place to reinforce important information which users need to be aware of.

Streetwize – 'On the Edge'

Streetwize[749] is a series of comics targeted towards young people and the issues that concern them. Drug use is one of the key aspects of youth culture that is covered by these publications. A specific edition of the comic dealing with amphetamine and other psychostimulant use has been published titled 'On the Edge'.

Many youth workers and educationalists believe *Streetwize* and similar publications serve a valuable role in providing accurate, non-judgemental and timely harm minimisation advice to young people and those who work with them. For example, Dr John Howard of the Ted Noffs Centre in Sydney is one leading educationalist who gives a qualified endorsement to this particular type of education material:

> In prevention and harm reduction much emphasis has been placed on information conveyed at schools, or raves and dance parties. As mentioned in the risk and protection literature these prevention strategies and harm reduction initiatives need to better target 'at risk' groups (eg. homeless youth, juvenile justice youth, non school attending youth) and other settings like parties and general celebrations where young people are likely to partake of these substances. One such attempt was the development of a psychostimulant specific *Streetwize* comic entitled "On the Edge". This was distributed to youth centres, refuges, and the like. Integral to the development of this publication was qualitative research carried out via focus groups into the information needs of young psychostimulant users. The final result is a language appropriate publication, in the form of a comic, that addresses the issues of side effects (in particular drug induced psychosis), harm reduction techniques and treatment availability and accessibility. Whilst no evaluation currently seems to be available as to the effectiveness of this particular issue, other evaluation reports have consistently shown that comics are more successful than other print media in disseminating information to young people. Additionally, research on previous issues has shown that 80% of young people recalled the main message of a *Streetwize* comic up to four months after they had read it. Research has also shown that young people are more likely to

749 See www.streetwize.com.au/publications

pass *Streetwize* resources onto their friends with every *Streetwize* comic being read by an average of 8 people (Howard, Stubbs & Arcuri 2004, in prep).

The content of drug education information campaigns – The Glasgow Study

Before completing the discussion in this chapter it is salutary to draw together some of the themes that have been raised by examining the findings of a survey conducted by Hammersley, Khan and Ditton into 'party drug' use in Scotland during the late 1990s. Young users of 'party drugs' were surveyed as to what education materials and strategies they found useful among a range of options including pamphlets, videos, television campaigns and school based education. The responses were instructive. The authors found a fair lack of knowledge about possible medical consequences of ecstasy:

> There is considerable ignorance coupled to considerable apprehension about the long-term effects of Ecstasy. It is ironic that the very area that users are most concerned about is also the area that medical, or other, science is least able to help with information. There is a strong desire to be accurately and honestly informed about health risks. The level of misinformation currently held is worrying, and the desire for information is certainly matched by need. Users don't say that they want to talk to their parents, but they certainly, in the main, are not able to. Their feeling is that it is their parents who need educating, not themselves (Hammersley, Khan & Ditton 2002, p.156).

Conversely, however, there certainly seemed to be a lack of credible information options available that resonated with young people:

> The evidence collected...has uniformly and consistently pointed to the need for more information, at this stage disseminated in leaflet form. Friends and other young people are the most trusted sources of information, but this seems to be not least because existing written materials are:
>
> - the wrong size (too big),
> - the wrong type (not always in colour),
> - are in the wrong form (too much writing),
> - take the wrong tone (humourless),
> - give the least useful information (don't take drugs), and
> - are compiled by those least able to gain credibility with drug users (ie., by non drug users) (Hammersley, Khan & Ditton 2002, p.157).

In this survey, a number of 'party drug' users were asked their opinions on a variety of drug education and information materials. These ranged from large sized colour magazines with a mixture of cartoons and drug information text (similar to the Moreland Hall publication discussed above) to laminated postcards with minimal but relevant dot points on basic issues such as drinking water at dance clubs.

With regard to the first mentioned format, some respondents thought they could be ideally placed in doctors' waiting rooms:

> 'cos there's lots of pictures to keep you going along the way [and] cos you've always got to sit for a half an hour anyway, so you would read it' (Female respondent surveyed in Hammersley, Khan & Ditton 2002, p.157).

On the other hand, one respondent stated:

> '...dead, dull and boring...just looking at that big book, as if you'd sit and take time and sit and read a chunk' (Female respondent, p.157).

The laminated cards generally got a far better commendation. The following response is typical:

> 'these ones are just like one sheet...are great...like you see the picture, it attracts you, and you just turn it over, and its just got like a little paragraph...If these were out in a club, I wouldn't pick up the ones that you had to flip through, you know like 3 or 4 pages, of like, just text, but these ones like...these are really good' (Male respondent, p.162).

And from another male student an imaginative suggestion as to how club pass-outs could incorporate harm reduction information:

> 'I think the thing about those little flyers...d'you know how like some clubs give you like a little ticket pass thing to get in and out...if you're going out the door and come back in you need it, if you had, like that information on the back of their flyer, then maybe you're gonna keep it in your pocket, then you'll take it...cause you need it if you want to go out and come back in again. Next day when you empty your pockets or if you're sitting on a bus doing nothing you might look at it'... (Hammersley, Khan & Ditton 2002, p.163).

The Glasgow survey revealed definite preferences as to how harm minimisation messages are best delivered to and received by young people in the dance, rave and party scenes. Summing up their responses, Hammersley, Khan and Ditton state:

> There seems to be a role for at least three different sizes of publication: Magazine size, A5 leaflet size and small postcard size. Colour is definitely in. There is some ambivalence about whether or not they should be in standard English, and this will probably be best resolved by producing different products for different target groups. A cartoon style is almost universally preferred. As for content, straight information preferred over warning messages; humour preferred to seriousness; safe using advice is preferred to non-using advice; the choice between information from friends and officialdom is harder to make.
>
> Different products should be placed in different locations, but the number of locations should spread from the current drug agencies to also include: schools, shops, cafes, clubs and raves. There are indications that for 16–20 year olds, magazines (like the Big Blue Book) might find an interested audience in GP waiting rooms, health centres and schools. A5 size leaflets (such as Peanut

> Pete and Emma E Head) will be most acceptable in drug agencies and youth clubs. Small glossy (because of the heat) postcard "info bites" would find an appreciative audience if distributed to those leaving raves and clubs, and if slipped into mainstream magazines and CDs.
>
> Very generally, for this group of young Ecstasy users, leaflets are broadly believed to be the best form of information delivery. They agree that all leaflet type materials should be colourful, humorous, and eye-catching. They should stress harm minimisation rather than drug use prevention, should be peer developed, and they should give straightforward factual information. Pictures are more powerful than words.
>
> Different materials should be produced for different socio-economic groups. Some of our interviewees had University degrees, others could barely write their names. It is absurd to imagine that one product will find its way to both groups. We feel that there are two main groups: "casuals" and "yuppies/clubbers". Within each, there are drug using initiates and experienced drug users. Both of these, too, need different materials. A fifth group is parents. Participants felt that it was this group which was most in need of drug education (Hammersley, Khan & Ditton 2002, p.165).

That there need be a multiplicity of education strategies tailored to different groups and individuals within the community is recognised in the following recommendations of the Committee:

Recommendations

40. The Committee recommends that users, including occasional users and poly-drug users, should be provided with accurate and relevant information in relation to the effects of amphetamine and 'party drug' use and how to obtain help when needed. Such an approach provides pathways and access points to treatment services.

41. The Committee recommends that strategic and targeted information about amphetamines and 'party drugs' which is tailored to a range of users in different settings and contexts (eg. clubs, raves, schools, universities, workplaces, sports and community clubs) be made readily available, particularly to young people.

42. The Committee recommends the provision of a diverse range of relevant and available information and harm reduction messages to individuals. These should be facilitated through a variety of avenues including written guidelines, websites, email alerts and mobile telephone messages, and be accessible through peer networks.

Conclusion

Drug educators and many organisations connected to the field of drug use agree that some of the bases of drug education regarding amphetamines and 'party drugs' in Australia need to be revised or changed. These include choosing appropriate drug education literature as information sources for policies, ensuring consistency in support and application of programmes and tailoring material to specific drug user groups.

Young people who take ecstasy do not necessarily view themselves as 'taking drugs' and are therefore unlikely to appear at specialist drug services. Peer educators and outreach workers would seem to be better situated than traditional information outlets to provide them with practical information and influence their attitudes to drug-taking.

The Drug and Alcohol Services Council of South Australia makes the salutary point that those who use 'party drugs' are a population that are very hard to reach, particularly once they have left home and/or school and school/youth networks:

> As the dance club scene has developed so has the increase in availability and the consumption of recreational dance drugs such as ecstasy and amphetamines. This has led to a 'normalisation' of recreational drug use within contemporary youth culture with the consequence of a potential increase in drug related harm. One of the key issues in providing harm reduction and prevention information to ecstasy and other party drug users is accessing the target group. This target group is quite different to other licit or illicit drug users and difficult to access through traditional, mainstream media outlets. Previous studies have found that most users are in their early 20s and can not be accessed through other program areas, such as the Clean Needle Program, as most have never injected drugs.[750]

For different reasons which are outlined in Chapter 20 amphetamine users are also seldom likely to access either information or treatment services with regard to their use.

The Committee has received submissions from a variety of groups, which are often local government based, outlining many projects that provide such services. These projects and initiatives are most conveniently dealt with in the following chapter pertaining to the issue of harm minimisation.

750 Submission of the Drug and Alcohol Services Council of South Australia to the Drugs and Crime Prevention Committee, Inquiry into Amphetamine and 'Party Drug' Use in Victoria, August 2002.

19. Policy Debates, Harm Minimisation and Harm Reduction

Introduction

This chapter examines some of the more contentious issues and debates concerning drug policy, particularly as it applies to amphetamines and 'party drugs'. A key aspect of the chapter is a discussion of the third aspect of harm minimisation – the concept of harm reduction. The other two aspects of the harm minimisation model, those of supply and demand reduction, have been discussed in previous chapters.[751] Before examining harm reduction in detail, however, the chapter opens with a discussion of some of the more general and theoretical approaches to addressing the use of illicit drugs.

Old wine in new bottles: The debates continue

The history of drug use and drug control shows that the concerns expressed at any given point in time are rarely original. The drugs may change but the debates remain the same as generally do the protagonists. Drug policy, whether it concerns alcohol in the 1920s or methamphetamine or ecstasy in our own era, tends to be an issue struggled over by conservative hardliners on one side and permissive liberals on the other, with of course many shades of opinion in between. This section briefly examines some of these polarised views in the context of amphetamines and 'party drugs'.

It is in the United States that these often diametrically opposed ways of looking at drug use are most vocally played out. As will be discussed later in this chapter, America does not embrace concepts of harm minimisation or harm reduction to anywhere near the extent that is done in Britain, Australia or many European countries. It is certainly not an official platform of American health policy as it is in this country.

---

751 See Part E and Chapter 18. Aspects of harm reduction are also discussed in Chapter 20 pertaining to treatment issues.

Debates concerning MDMA/ecstasy policy

In the United States in particular there are somewhat polarised positions with regard to the directions in which drug policy should head. The debates have been most pronounced in recent years with regard to MDMA/ecstasy and it is this drug that will be used to illustrate the divide in opinion. Pentney (2001) sums up the current position:

> The dangers involved in consuming MDMA [or MDA] have been the subject of heated debate for over a decade. Some believe that one dose will cause irreversible damage, while others believe that these drugs are relatively harmless. Both sides are exceedingly vocal, and the argument will most likely continue for quite some time (Pentney 2001, pp.213–214).

Agencies such as the Drug Enforcement Administration would naturally be expected to take a 'tough on drugs', zero tolerance approach. Yet to a certain extent they are joined by groups such as 'Partnership for a Drug Free America' and the key umbrella organisation for drug and health policy in the United States – the National Institute on Drug Abuse (NIDA). In July 2001 the Director of NIDA, Dr Alan Leshner, gave testimony to the Senate Subcommittee on Governmental Affairs during its hearings on 'Ecstasy Abuse and Control'.[752] Dr Leshner's testimony unequivocally concentrated on the negatives of use, including mortality, irreparable brain dysfunction and cognitive impairment. The most controversial aspect of the testimony, however, and the one that raised the ire of drug experts who took a more permissive stance was the fact that Dr Leshner indicated he spoke on behalf of the whole research community. Certainly there are high profile MDMA experts such as George Ricaurte who have been expounding such views for many years and warning of the dangers of a harm reduction approach (Ricaurte et al. 1988; Ricaurte et al. 1990; Ricaurte & McCann 1992; Ricaurte et al. 1993; Ricaurte, Yuan & McCann 2000).

Researchers such as Koesters, Rogers and Rajasingham 2002 have deplored what they see as being the wrong messages being sent out by those who propose or expound harm reduction programmes:

> Unfortunately, perceptions that the club drugs can be safe endure. Some groups, such as the Multidisciplinary Association for Psychedelic Study, continue to lobby for the legalization of MDMA for research purposes. DanceSafe is an organization that seeks to educate the "nonaddicted" user to decrease the risks. The DanceSafe Web site offers tips on the safe use of MDMA, such as attention to hydration status and ambient temperature. It also offers free testing of tablets submitted by mail and sells home testing kits to determine the content of pills sold as "ecstasy."
>
> Although much remains unknown about the long-term consequences of MDMA and the club drugs, there are clearly enough short-term dangers to prompt more aggressive education and surveillance for its use. Scare tactics

752 See: www.drugabuse.gov/Testimony/7-30-01Testimony.html

> and exaggerations often are ignored, while Web sites fully of anecdotal or incomplete information may lead the unaware user to increased use. Organizations such as DanceSafe imply that proper education decreases addiction and that only uneducated users or addicts suffer the life-altering consequences of drug use. The fallacy in the mission of educating "nonaddicted" users is evidence. Peer-based education, with a focus on both the short-term dangers and long-term consequences, may be a more effective approach (Koesters, Rogers & Rajasingham 2002, p.22).

At the other extreme, proponents of the transcendental benefits of MDMA such as Dr Alexander Shulgin,[753] the so-called 'ecstasy guru', have attracted criticism for his seemingly uncritical lauding of a mind altering drug that *can* have negative outcomes.

However, to some American researchers who occupy the middle ground, particularly those working in state public health agencies, community organisations and the university and research communities, the type of categorical testimony given by Leshner was 'alarmist' and easily misused by irresponsible media representation.[754]

Marcia Rosenbaum, for example, one of the foremost experts on MDMA in America has called the politics of ecstasy and the policy reaction to it 'America's new "reefer madness"'. She outlined the government's response to the perceived ecstasy 'crisis' in the wake of a sensationalist media campaign conducted in late 1999 early 2000:

> By the Spring of 2000, a number of governmental agencies had jumped into the Ecstasy frenzy. In May, Senators Bob Graham of Florida and Charles Grassly of Iowa introduced the Ecstasy Anti-Proliferation Bill, which would increase penalties exponentially for distribution as well as possession.
>
> The Drug Enforcement Administration held a conference, "Ecstasy and Club Drugs: Dancing with Darkness," in July of 2000. The Chief of Operations, Richard Fianno, set the tone for the conference with his opening remarks: "Every city in the U.S. has experienced some rise in Ecstasy use over the last several years… The kids believe that Ecstasy is safe, they enjoy the rave experience, but actually what is happening is that over the next couple of days after taking Ecstasy their brain cells are actually being programmed to die".
>
> Dr David Gauvin, a DEA pharmacologist, warned: "Lately raves are just a venue for drug purchases. They are no more than analogous to a crack house in which you go, buy the drug, and go out the back door"… (Rosenbaum 2002, p.3).

---

753 Dr Shulgin is best known for his publication *PIKHAL: A Chemical Love Story* (the acronym stands for Phenethylamines I Have Known and Loved). *PIKHAL* has become a cult classic, particularly among chemistry students. For a brief account of Dr Shulgin's life and work, see Brown 2003.

754 For an account of the way the American print and electronic media picked up the ecstasy issue, see Jenkins 1999 and in particular Rosenbaum 2002.

One particular issue that has been most contentious in the United States has been the placing of MDMA in the most restrictive schedule category, whereby even therapeutic use of the drug has been disallowed. Pentney argues that the scheduling of MDMA has '[l]ed to the distribution of contaminated, or falsely represented, Ecstasy tablets, and prevented responsible research into the detrimental and therapeutic effects of these drugs' (2001, p.213). This accords with Webb's view that it is '[m]ore the case that MDMA is dangerous because it is banned than that MDMA is banned because it is dangerous' (2003, p.113).

Pentney's belief is that 'the validity of studies that portray entactogens [MDMA and similar drugs] as beneficial therapeutic tools seems to outweigh the relevancy of detrimental findings' (2001, p.214). Pentney also points out that findings with regard to MDMA's neurotoxicity are often based on flawed experiments that use amounts of the drug far in excess of the average person's use at any given point in time (2001, p.218). Moreover, Pentney believes that NIDA's 'control' over postgraduate research funding and the research agenda can result in biased research:

> The scientific community is very competitive, and proposed research topics involving illegal drugs often need to suggest that the findings will be useful in advancing an anti-drug stance if they are to be funded (Pentney 2001, p.219).

Even the *Journal of the American Medical Association* (JAMA), by no means a radical tome, has given print space to those who would advocate relatively commonplace (at least by Australian standards) harm reduction approaches:

> "Ecstasy is seen as relatively benign," said Robert Carbon, PhD, an addiction researcher at Wright State University of Medicine in Dayton, Ohio. "[Prevention] messages are not getting across, and something needs to be done."
>
> "Scepticism about government studies, perception that ecstasy is safer than other drugs (including alcohol and tobacco), and willingness to take calculated risks all factor into the ecstasy equation," said Patricia Case, ScD, director of the program in urban health at Harvard University. "A lot of [ecstasy users] make clear decisions, despite the known or unknown risks, that the benefits outweigh those risks," she said.
>
> With considerations like these, Carlson and his colleagues are emphatic that one-size-fits-all campaigns hyping the dangers of ecstasy fail to sway users. Instead, they want messages that reflect reality: the effects of ecstasy feel good, different groups use it for various reasons in a range of settings, and evidence of addiction remains scant.
>
> Claire Sterk, PhD, professor of behavioural sciences at Emory University's Rollins School of Public Health, Atlanta, GA, would drive proponents of "Just Say No"-style campaigns crazy. "We'll be better off having a campaign [poster] that says, 'Ecstasy can...make you feel really good. It increases your sensory awareness, it makes you feel music.' It's okay to acknowledge that," she said. "And then have a big comma and say, 'But there are consequences.'"

> In contrast, NIDA's prevention campaign uses scare tactics. The oft-seen image of a brain before and after ecstasy provides a prime example. Split in half, a brain scan displays a lurid orange hemisphere on the left – the "plain brain." On the "brain after ecstasy" side, muted tones and a missing chunk of cortex offer vivid testimony of the drug's propensity for destroying serotonin neurons, according to NIDA, which has distributed thousands of postcards and handouts displaying the graphic.
>
> What the materials don't say is that the "after" scan comes from someone who abused multiple drugs and took several hundred doses of ecstasy, a huge amount the average user will never approach (Vastag 2001, p.777).

Some researchers are not so much promoting the use of ecstasy as a recreational drug as asking for a rescheduling of the drug so 'responsible research into the detrimental and therapeutic effects of the drug' can be carried out (Pentney 2001, p.219).

Such exponents argue there is much hypocrisy in drug research when other arguably more dangerous drugs have been given approval by bodies such as the American Food and Drug Administration. Klee states:

> A good case study is Prozac, now appearing on the illicit market, which is prescribed for anxiety, loss of confidence and depression – symptoms for which people take amphetamine. The complex mix of vested interests, moral arguments and health warnings about drugs is confusing without competent, credible, consistent and authoritative guidance (Klee 1997c, p.314).[755]

The Committee neither endorses nor condemns any of the views presented in this discussion. The inclusion of these debates is to illustrate that, as in any area of social policy, polarisation is not conducive to good policy development. In Australia the debates have not been as divided nor choices as stark. It is hoped that this state of affairs continues, particularly with regard to the national and state sanctioned policy of harm minimisation

Harm minimisation – General strategies and initiatives

The sometimes controversial issue of harm minimisation has been thoroughly canvassed by the literature.[756] The interested reader is referred to the *Final Report* of the Drugs and Crime Prevention Committee's Inquiry into the Inhalation of

755 For further discussion on a comparison between MDMA/Ecstasy, Prozac and the scheduling of drugs, see Jenkins 1999, Concar 2002. In the context of amphetamine, Klee comments somewhat ironically that 'Starting out as a legal synthetic cure all for many common ailments [amphetamine sulphate] seems to have been espoused by the medical fraternity in the 1930s as enthusiastically as Prozac in the 1990s' (Klee 2001a, p.22).

756 There is a wealth of literature explaining the concept of harm minimisation and the related principles of risk reduction. In an Occasional Paper these principles are thoroughly outlined (Drugs and Crime Prevention Committee 1998). There are also many good secondary references on the subject that can be consulted. In particular the text by Hamilton, Kellehear & Rumbold (1998) offers an excellent overview. A recent worthwhile publication is that of Ryder, Salmon & Walker (2001). See also Erickson 1995; Hawks & Lenton 1998; Lenton & Midford 1996; Midford, McBride & Munro 1998; Single 1995; Strang & Farrell 1992.

Volatile Substances (2002) for a detailed account of the theoretical and practical debates surrounding this contentious issue. However, there are some basic concepts from that Report that bear repeating at this stage prior to examining the issues as they specifically apply to the area of amphetamines and 'party drugs'.

Harm minimisation as defined by the Commonwealth Government refers to:

> Policies and programmes designed to reduce drug-related harm. Harm minimisation aims to improve health, social and economic outcomes for both the community and the individual and encompasses a wide range of approaches, including
>
> - Supply-reduction strategies designed to disrupt the production and supply of [illicit] drugs;
> - Demand-reduction strategies designed to prevent the production and supply of [illicit] drugs;
> - A range of targeted harm-reduction strategies designed to reduce drug-related harm for individuals and communities (Commonwealth Department of Health 1999, pp.15–16).

Harm minimisation is not necessarily a consistent policy. It takes different forms depending on the drug in question and the group that is being targeted. Harm minimisation is also often used interchangeably, and sometimes confusingly, with harm reduction. For the purposes of this discussion, harm reduction will be examined as one specific form or 'subset' of harm minimisation.[757]

The broader concept of harm minimisation has an extensive literature. The rationale for harm minimisation is based on the view that:

> Neither law enforcement (prohibitionist) policies nor prevention through information and education strategies have succeeded in curbing either the supply of drugs or the demand for them, and many treatment responses have met with only modest success. This has led to the emergence over the past decade of a new way of thinking about drugs: harm minimisation. Harm minimisation tries to assess the actual harm associated with any particular drug use and asks how this harm could be minimised or reduced. This approach accepts that:
>
> - Psychoactive substances are and will continue to be part of our society;
> - Their eradication is impossible; and
> - The continuation of attempts to eradicate them may result in maximising net harms for society.
>
> The objectives of the harm minimisation model are:
>
> - The identification of the harmful consequences for individuals, those around them and the community overall; and

757 For example, as stated earlier, the Commonwealth government definition of harm minimisation would also include demand and supply reduction principles. These have been considered separately in Chapters 18 and Chapters 12-17 of this Report.

- The implementation of strategies to minimise this harm (Hamilton, King & Ritter 2004, pp.134, 135).

Conceptually, Erikson et al. (1997, quoted in Hamilton, King & Ritter 2004) identify the following elements as being part of harm minimisation strategies:

- A value-neutral view of drug use;
- A value-neutral view of users;
- A focus on problems or harmful consequences resulting from use;
- An acceptance that abstinence is irrelevant;
- A belief that the user has and should continue to have an active role in making choices and taking action about their own drug use (Erikson et al. quoted in Hamilton, King & Ritter 2004, p.136).

These conceptual elements ideally produce practical strategies that:

- Seek to maximise those strategies that lead to harm reduction;
- Support pragmatic programmes that can be eclectic and flexible;
- Incorporate any scheme that will assist in net harm reduction;
- Aim to be user-centred, including users in planning;
- Emphasise choice, taking account of the users' own interests and the responsibilities they retain in their societal context (Hamilton, King & Ritter 2004, p.136).

The concept of harm minimisations can be pictorially represented by the following figure taken from a report on the harm minimisation concept by the Drugs and Crime Prevention Committee of the 53rd Parliament of Victoria.

Figure 19.1: The concept of harm minimisation

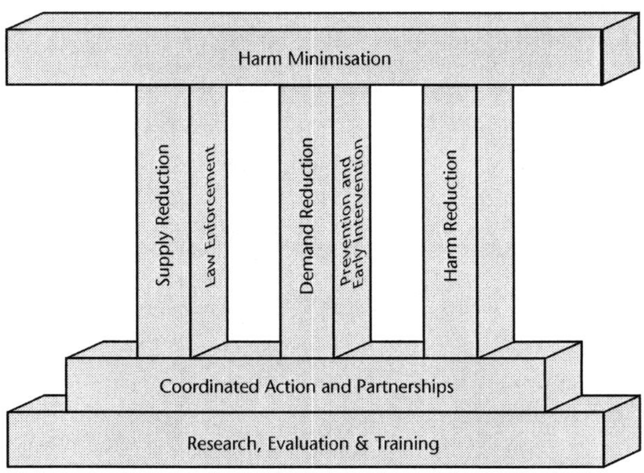

That Committee described the figure thus:

> It is useful to picture the structure of a harm-minimisation framework in terms of an archway (see Figure 19.1), where achievement of the goal of harm-

> minimisation (the roof) rests on the three strategically placed pillars of supply reduction interventions (law enforcement), demand reduction interventions (prevention and early intervention), and treatment and rehabilitation[758] interventions. Those pillars, in turn, are embedded and supported within foundations of coordinated action, and research, evaluation, and training.[759]

As useful as this figure is in giving an overview of the principle of harm minimisation, it does not fully explain the interconnecting aspects of the model. In other words, there is clear overlap between the three concepts of supply, demand and harm reduction. For example, education strategies and information provision with regard to particular forms of drug use could be viewed as both a demand or harm reduction strategy depending on the circumstances. This overlap can best be exemplified by the following Venn Diagram (Figure 19.2).

Figure 19.2: Interconnecting aspects of harm minimisation

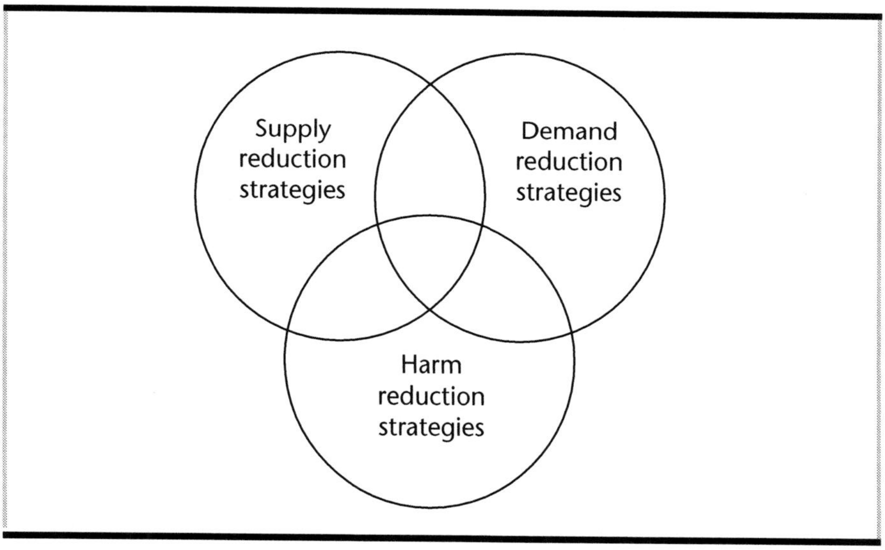

Source: Turning Point Alcohol and Drug Centre 2003, Submission, October.

While acknowledging that there are people in the community who use drugs, harm reduction policies neither condone nor encourage drug use.

In current drug policy, needle exchange programmes are a clear example of the harm reduction aspects of harm reduction to reduce the transfer of blood-borne diseases. With regard to amphetamine use, a common harm reduction approach is to attempt to persuade users not to use amphetamines intravenously or if they do to only use new and sterile needles.

758 While harm reduction may include treatment and rehabilitation initiatives, this Committee believes harm reduction encompasses much more than this. In particular, it consists of many practical community programmes and projects that aim to minimise the harms associated with substance use that fall short of 'treatment'. A typical example may be the distribution of clean syringes to prevent blood-borne diseases. See discussion later in this Chapter.

759 Drugs and Crime Prevention Committee, Parliament of Victoria 1998, p.14.

Misunderstandings about harm minimisation

Much of the misunderstanding concerning harm minimisation seems to stem from the fact that harm minimisation would appear to mean different things to different people. For example Professor Hamilton of Turning Point Alcohol and Drug Centre alerted the Committee to the confusion often found in this area, such as the distinction between use prevention and harm prevention:

> We need to think differently about preventing use and preventing harm. They are related but they are different. I think sometimes in the community's mind prevention is all about just preventing use. That is extremely hard to achieve, terribly expensive and we do not have very well, fine tuned successful interventions. We have much more knowledge and experience of preventing harm. We need both, but we need to recognise that the return on investment varies depending on where you place it.[760]

It also runs the risk of being loaded down with ideological meanings across the political spectrum that have little to do with what the term or the concept actually means.[761] A worker from the Youth Substance Abuse Service (YSAS) giving evidence at the Inquiry into the Inhalation of Volatile Substances exhorted the former Drugs and Crime Prevention Committee to be clear as to what the concept does and does not mean. It is worth reproducing this statement as it is an extremely lucid and clear exposition on the nature of harm minimisation:

> It is important to look at the philosophical underpinnings of harm minimisation. Harm minimisation is actually a goal rather than a strategy or set of policies, so it is a position a worker in the field might adopt when trying to provide care for a young person.[762] It is absolutely essential to mention that the only method to divine whether an activity is harm minimisation is by the

760 Professor Margaret Hamilton, evidence given to the Drugs and Crime Prevention Committee, Inquiry into Amphetamine and 'Party Drug' Use in Victoria, Public Hearings (Melbourne), 27 October 2003.

761 Some agencies have expressed concern to the Inquiry that there has been a shift at Commonwealth government level since the publication of the Report *'Road to Recovery'* (Commonwealth of Australia 2003).

For the agency Anglicare the concern is centred on their perception that the 'Policy is changing from harm minimisation to harm prevention. We believe that harm minimisation as a strategy is more conducive to behaviour change' (Submission of Anglicare (Victoria) to the Drugs and Crime Prevention Committee, Inquiry into Amphetamine and 'Party Drug' Use in Victoria, October 2003.

Maroondah City Council has similar reservations about the direction in which it perceives federal policy heading:

'As part of the consideration of best practice strategies to address the issue of amphetamine and party drug use Council would recommend the identification of a model which has a balanced harm minimisation and prevention approach rather than a sole prevention and treatment focus as recommended at a federal level. The juxtaposition between state and federal government policy directions need to be addressed and clarified to allow for illicit and licit drug issues and responses to be dealt with consistently within a broader community health and well-being framework' (Submission of Maroondah City Council to the Drugs and Crime Prevention Committee, Inquiry into Amphetamine and 'Party Drug' Use in Victoria, October 2003).

762 This idea of harm minimisation as a *goal* rather than a policy per se is echoed in the academic literature, in particular in the work of Midford, McBride & Munro (1998) and Midford, McBride & Farringdon (1999).

> observation of the consequences – does it reduce harm? A lot of people seek to put zero tolerance at one end of the continuum and say that harm minimisation or harm reduction is at the other end of the continuum. In fact harm minimisation is a goal that is off that continuum altogether. If you could show or demonstrate that zero tolerance was able to reduce harm, you could embrace that as a harm-minimisation strategy or approach.
>
> People often say that harm reduction or harm minimisation does not work for adolescents, which in some ways is a ludicrous thing to say because what would be the alternative – maximising harm for adolescents because it is a goal? What they are often talking about is that adolescents have a need for structuring and nurturing containment, as well as that need to take risks, bust out and find their own identity. People often react to that need for some sort of containment. Young people are often involved in very chaotic behaviour that can be very harmful, and so people will often seek a response like zero tolerance, which is an extreme response...
>
> For harm minimisation strategies to work, you need to get as much information or evidence as possible about the circumstances presenting in front of you, whether that is at a broader policy level, around how the media responds, or from a youth worker with a young person in front of them who engages or has engaged in volatile substance inhalation. Secondly, all the needs of affected individuals and groups need to be considered. It is not just looking at the actual individual but at other stakeholders and other people involved.
>
> Also, we need to deal with the unique specific circumstances that present. Given that we are looking at a goal rather than a set of strategies, one strategy that reduces harm in one circumstance may actually increase it in another, so we should not adopt strategies holus-bolus because of their effectiveness in one context.
>
> Last is the importance of monitoring and evaluation, and that is in the short and long term. To come up with an effective harm-minimisation strategy you would need to consider all those factors. I contend that is the most responsible measured approach because it focusses particularly on the needs, the health and wellbeing of the person who is involved in the act of volatile substance inhalation and not just on the drug use itself. One of the problems with a lot of policies and strategies that are implemented is that they focus on the use regardless of the consequences for the individual or the other stakeholders involved.[763]

Moreover, the development of rational drugs policy is sometimes compromised by the sending of conflicting or contradictory messages and/or misinformation, exaggeration and hyperbole. There is also the concern that the public promotion of harm reduction projects may be viewed by some members of the community as signalling a green light for drug abuse or at least condoning it. Yet behind the

763 Mr Andrew Bruin, YSAS. evidence given to the Drugs and Crime Prevention Committee, Inquiry into the Inhalation of Volatile Substances, Public Hearings, 9 April 2002.

scenes practical measures can nonetheless be tacitly approved. This is certainly the case in Britain where a harm reduction approach such as the distribution of 'safe' drug use literature may be disapproved by the Home Office at the same time as it is promoted by the Health Department.

Measham, Aldridge and Parker are particularly scathing at what they see as this hypocrisy felt towards harm reduction policies by the British government, and some sectors of the media and public:

> To officially and openly sanction harm minimisation and public health measures for clubbers is to agree that such drug use is widespread and that with some 'really useful' guidance and regulation probably no more immediately risky than many outdoor pursuits. The public health imperative is thus uniquely muffled in respect of recreational drug use. It is acceptable for problem drug users who can be medicalised or seen as a wider health threat to the public but for 'normal' people, with no excuses then the response must primarily be enforcement. Carefully considered calls to review the Misuse of Drugs Act in respect of reclassifying ecstasy and rethinking legal definitions of drug dealing – 'sorting' friends – are thus dismissed (Independent Inquiry, 2000).
>
> This is why the management of recreational drug use has not developed from the centre. It is also why government, whilst maintaining the public 'no discussion, no compromise' position, also quietly sanctions local harm minimisation initiatives and 'safer dancing' programmes (Branigan and Wellings, 1999). Because of a lack of national guidance and encouragement, however, such initiatives are currently patchy and inadequate (Measham, Aldridge & Parker 2001, p.187).

This apparent contradiction in policy-making approaches has certainly been the case in recent years with regard to ecstasy. In the United States, for example, Concar alludes to the mixed messages being sent to the community when different agencies, often within government, take opposing approaches to addressing drug use. He describes a project approved by the US Food and Drug Administration in which victims of trauma and violent crime are given ecstasy under controlled conditions as part of a trial to determine the effect of the drug as an anti-anxiety medication. Such experiments are not looked upon with favour by the US Drug Enforcement Agency:

> In other words, while bona fide doctors supported by one US government agency get ready to dole out 'E' as medicine, other agencies are doing their utmost to warn teenagers off the drug. It's all very confusing. And you will find equally mixed messages elsewhere. Take Britain, last year the government introduced a tough new law making it a crime for club owners to permit the use of ecstasy on the premises. This year it issued a booklet telling the same club owners to lay on chill out rooms, treatment areas and plentiful supplies of water (Concar 2002, p.27).

These 'mixed signals' are inimical to good policy making, particularly policies that incorporate harm reduction messages.

How relevant are harm minimisation and reduction principles in the context of amphetamines and particularly 'party drugs'? The next sections will discuss these issues in detail.

The 'normalisation thesis' and its relation to harm reduction

According to some commentators the 1990s and beyond has seen the gradual shift from those who use recreational drugs, particularly ecstasy, as 'addicts' to 'consumers' (Measham, Aldridge & Parker 2001, p.46).

In other words, the use of drugs such as ecstasy is viewed by a sizeable proportion of the adolescent and post-adolescent population as part of a package of lifestyle choices that include dance, fashion, music, travel, clubs, alcohol and illicit drugs.[764] However regrettable:

> [w]e find evidence that the drugs pathways from early adolescent drug trying into early clubbing and related recreational drug use cover only a few years. Today's young clubbers, the children of the 1990s, have tried a whole range of drugs, and in a recognizable order, several years earlier than their club elders... [Y]ounger dance drug users appear to be consuming similar drugs in similar quantities and roughly as often as their older counterparts. All this fits consistently with the normalisation of adolescent recreational drug use across the 1990s and the fall in the age of initiation across the board (Measham, Aldridge & Parker 2001, pp.102–103).[765]

Drug taking for the 'party generation' becomes an exercise in conspicuous consumption and the enjoyment of leisure time:[766]

> One key reason for this is that the *majority* of today's young adults have taken drugs and lived unscathed to tell the tale. Another is that whilst there will always be a minority in any age cohort who hold strong 'anti' views about something, be it smoking or illegal drug use, it does seem that [even] non drug users who are outgoing come to accept that those around them may take drugs. Because in the main this behaviour is benign in respect of friendships, informal parties, romantic relationships, socialising and dancing, then there is accommodation and tolerance (Measham, Aldridge & Parker 2001, p.17. (Authors' emphasis)

---

764 See for example, in the European context, Tossmann, Boldt and Tensil 2001.

765 See also the work of Measham, Newcombe and Parker 1994.

766 Williams and Parker argue that this stress on leisure and consumption is part of the trend towards *individualisation*:

'[t]he notion that today's younger citizens must navigate through a new more uncertain, rapidly changing world which requires flexibility and makes risk taking a functional necessity...with delayed settling down markers like home ownership, a permanent job, marriage and parenting being the demographic norm – a related delay in moderating drinking and drug use will also occur' (2001, p.399).

The increasing availability[767] and accessibility of drugs such as ecstasy and their *perceived* benign and risk-free nature sees them as favoured additions to a poly-drug repertoire. For some users these drugs may be seen as less dangerous and more pleasant than alcohol or nicotine. At the very least many consumers of 'party drugs' blur the distinction between licit and illicit drugs and view those who criticise the latter while condoning the former as hypocritical. Rather than being drug 'fiends', drug use has become normalised rather than pathologised (at least among the users' peers) because they are used by 'normal' people, be they students, bank clerks, doctors, 'housewives'[768] or ditch diggers. At least with regard to the 'party drug' users, the real drug 'addicts' may be those who shoot up heroin on the streets.[769]

Much of the literature on 'normalisation' is British.[770] This does not mean, however, that the same shifts in drug use and its acceptance by some young people and their peers is not being seen in Australia. As Klee states, in Western culture at least there are 'already signs of a global [ecstasy] culture among the young' (2001b, p.82). The growth and spread of such use is exacerbated by the Internet, relatively high disposable income among Western youth and a transitory youth population that is relatively well travelled. In the Australian context Dr David Moore of the National Drug Research Institute states in a submission to this Inquiry:

> The prevalence of recreational drug use (particularly of cannabis but also of psychostimulants in the context of clubbing) has risen to the point where explanations for drug use that emphasise pathology (whether individual or social) or deviance are no longer tenable... Rather than the use of drugs being 'deviant' or 'pathological' they have become part of a 'consumer lifestyle'.[771]

The Committee later met with Dr Moore who stated further:

> I'm just thinking of normalisation...there's a whole section of young people now where the use of party drugs, amphetamines, cannabis are part and parcel of a very normal existence so all kinds of notions of epidemics or infections or pathology, whether it be social or individual or family or some

---

767 British research has shown that the age of taking amphetamines and 'party drugs' such as ecstasy has become increasingly younger in the last decade. :

'We can see how in general as adolescence unfolds, illicit drugs become more and more available to young people with offer rates of amphetamines at over 40 per cent for the 15 year olds and over 50 per cent for the 17 year olds in 1998... Rates for ecstasy use are also clearly rising with age' (Measham, Aldridge & Parker 2001, p.14).

768 For a discussion of the normalisation of recreational drug use among British women, including housewives or homemakers, see Hinchcliff 2001.

769 For a discussion of the 'snobbery' of drug use, see Chapters 8 and 9.

770 A work currently being written by Dr Cameron Duff of the Australian Drug Foundation discusses whether the 'normalisation thesis is equally applicable to Australia' (Duff 2004, in press).

771 Submission of Dr David Moore to the Drugs and Crime Prevention Committee, Inquiry into Amphetamine and 'Party Drug' Use in Victoria, November 2003.

> kind of dysfunctional sort of model are really almost irrelevant. It becomes difficult to continue to use those kinds of explanations when you've got such large numbers of people…[using].[772]

Dr Moore's colleague, Dr Simon Lenton agrees:

> [t]he understanding of why people use is incomplete, it doesn't include [a focus on] culture and it just focusses on the drug …What is needed is an understanding of how [drug use] its normalized within this culture. This is part of the experience, just like the fashion, just like the music, just like the lighting, just like the venue, just like the underground nature of the drug use, it is a part of that scene. If we just think about it in terms of pathology and a disease process we [are] really only understanding one aspect of the whole thing.[773]

Indeed the popularity of drugs such as ecstasy is such that it is increasingly being taken in contexts outside the dance floor. Ms Natalie Russell of RaveSafe states in this regard:

> [w]ith the increase in popularity of ecstasy and its current status as a 'mainstream' drug, users are taking the drug not only in dance environments, but at home, parties and even the pub. At all these locations alcohol is quite common; but most importantly ecstasy is being viewed as a common substance to take on a night out, not just for attending a dance event.[774]

While the concept of the normalisation of recreational use gives rise to understandable concern, it is necessary to understand that drug use of any kind is a dynamic practice, not a fixed practice. This is illustrated by the issue of tobacco smoking:

> [Smoking] is now being challenged by changing knowledge about health risks, the attitudes and behaviours of non-smokers, ex-smokers, and often those who want to give up. Consequently smoking is becoming less socially acceptable in the wider population. Normalisation can be reversed therefore and so the day may thus come when a particular era of…youth rejects psycho-active drug use, thereby pushing back the normalisation process and redefining such drug taking as unacceptable and requiring effective sanction (Measham, Aldridge & Parker 2001, p.2).

Until such a change occurs, however, if the users of 'party drugs' and to a lesser extent amphetamines 'live in a peer world where drug taking is normal…given the problems they feel they face are understandable, and above all rational' (Hammersley, Khan & Ditton 2002, p.132), how can such users be assisted to make appropriate choices or at least less dangerous ones with regard to their drug-taking behaviour?

---

772 Dr David Moore, National Drug Research Institute, Curtin University in conversation with the Drugs and Crime Prevention Committee, Perth, 2 October 2003.

773 Dr Simon Lenton, National Drug Research Institute, Curtin University in conversation with the Drugs and Crime Prevention Committee, Perth, 2 October 2003.

774 Submission of RaveSafe to the Drugs and Crime Prevention Committee, Inquiry into Amphetamine and 'Party Drug' Use in Victoria, October 2003.

Harm reduction – Amphetamines and 'party drugs'

A variety of harm reduction measures have been established across the Australian states (and internationally) over the last ten years to minimise the dangers associated with using 'party drugs' and to a lesser extent other amphetamines. These have taken the following main forms:

- Mass media education and information campaigns;
- Safe rave or safe dance party guidelines aimed at club owners and rave promoters;
- The use of outreach workers to provide support and assistance to those who use 'party drugs' (often located at raves and venues);
- Testing stations or kits for 'party drug' pills and tablets;
- 'Self regulation' harm reduction measures of users themselves;
- Information pertaining to harm reduction and 'safe' drug use provided and shared at international and national conferences and seminars;[775] and
- Harm reduction strategies and education campaigns that are targeted at particular times of the year where it is thought ('party') drug use may be particularly prevalent.[776]

The first five of these approaches will be discussed in the remainder of this chapter. The latter two points with regard to information and education strategies have been dealt with in the previous chapter.

The use of media campaigns

The issue of the media as a provider of harm reduction messages has been canvassed in Chapter 18 and is not repeated further in this chapter, other than to state that mass media campaigns with regard to ecstasy and amphetamines have been utilised in a number of jurisdictions both within Australia and overseas. These are generally viewed as less effective, particularly if accompanied by 'scare tactics' (Gowing et al. 2001, p.43). Indeed one of the problems facing drug educators is that media reports exaggerating the consequences of taking drugs such as ecstasy run the risk of making users blasé about the legitimate concerns held about the drug. For example Libby Topp, researcher with the National Drug and Alcohol Research Centre, states:

> [t]hat many ravers call a good night out an 'Anna Wood'[777] night, as an expression of their frustration at ecstasy myths. "We really need to get off the

775 A foremost example being the *Club Health* conferences. These are international forums for debate and exchange of information on 'nightclub policy and practice', particularly with regard to health, substance abuse and harm reduction issues. The third international conference is to be held in Melbourne, Australia in April 2004. See www.clubhealth.org.uk

776 New Year's Eve, the Gay and Lesbian Mardi Gras or 'Schoolies Week' may be cases in point. See Degenhardt, Darke and Dillon 2003, p.204.

777 A 15 year old Sydney schoolgirl who tragically died as a result of complications after having taken ecstasy. For an account of the Anna Wood tragedy from the perspective of her parents and the police attached to the case, see Messenger 1998.

idea that everyone who has ecstasy is going to die" she says (Topp quoted in Sweet 1997, p.6).

A healthy settings approach

A healthy settings approach draws from the drug, set and setting concept discussed in Chapter 10 of this Report. It incorporates a harm reduction policy and is endorsed as a key health promotion strategy through the World Health Organisation:

> A healthy settings approach recognises that the effects of any particular setting on an individual's health are related to the general conditions within that setting, perhaps more than they are to provision of health or other care facilities. The nightclub setting at its most basic is a building that provides loud music, often with a repetitive beat, a dance area that usually has low background light and intermittent bright lighting effects and a licensed bar. Developing this environment as a healthy setting must recognise that large numbers of clubbers regularly consume substances such as alcohol, drugs and tobacco (often in combination) and consequently experience a variety of psychological and physiological effects. Furthermore, the criminal nature of some drug use and environmental factors such as poor ventilation mean substance consumption can directly affect staff, for example, pressure of door staff to allow drugs into clubs and passive smoking affecting bar staff, respectively (Bellis, Hughes & Lowey 2002, p.1027).

Some of the healthy setting initiatives Bellis, Hughes and Lowey (2002) suggest be put in place to reduce the harms associated with the dance club environment include:

- Training and registration of door staff
- Good lighting and ventilation
- An integrated public transport system
- Owners of club venues contributing collectively to the employment of a police officer to patrol outside their premises.

A wider range of environmental responses aimed at reducing substance related harm can be seen in the following table that summarises and synthesises some of the academic and practice writings in this area:

Table 19.1: Some wider club health issues, their relationship with substance use, and developing a setting response

Health risk	Relationship to substance use	Setting response	Groups involved
Dehydration and Hyperthermia	Ecstasy alters thermoregulation (McCann, Slate, & Ricaurte, 1996) Increased energetic dancing Alcohol consumption causes dehydration	Prevent overcrowding Well ventilation and temperature control Cool and quieter chill outs areas or ability to leave and re-enter Access to cool, free water Information on effects of taking drugs Pill testing First-aid room and staff training	Club owners/staff Drug outreach workers Health promotion groups Licensing authority Club goers Local A&E
Fire	High levels of smoking among club goers Intoxication leads to disorientation when exiting clubs Flammable clubbing clothes (eg. PVC)	Prevent overcrowding High visibility and accessible emergency exits Availability and maintenance of all fire equipment Ensure electrical equipment is safe Encourage use of non-combustible material	Club owners/staff Fire authorities Building inspectors Licensing authority Club goers
Damage to hearing	Alcohol and drugs reduce awareness of potential hearing damage Greater exposure to noise due to prolonged dancing	Set maximum levels on systems Restricted areas around speakers Make earplugs available Information on the effects of excessive noise Information on signs of hearing damage	Club owners/staff Club goers Environmental inspectors Licensing authority Health promotion Club goers
STIs and unwanted pregnancies	Alcohol and drugs reduce inhibitions (Calafat, 2001) Substances help forge safe sex message (Clarke et al, 2001)	Easy availability of condoms Information on safer sex	Health promotion Public health department Contraception services Club owners Club goers
Accident Glass Burns Falls General	Disorientation Anaesthetising effect of substances (European Monitoring Centre for Drugs and Drug Addiction, 2000) Lack of fear and increased confidence Increased risk-taking	Toughened glass or plastic bottles No drinking/smoking on dance floor Provide places to dispose of cigarettes Well-lit and clear stairwells Restricted access to potentially dangerous areas Secure fixtures and fittings are secure On-site first-aid	Club owners/staff Public health departments Health promotion groups Licensing authority Club goers
Violence	Alcohol and drugs increase aggression Drug dealing (Morris, 1998) Steroid and cocaine use by door staff (Lenehan & McVeigh, 1998) Increased risk-taking, lower inhibitions	Stagger closing times Increase public transport availability through out night Plastic/toughened glass Registration and training of door staff Complaints procedures and Policing	Club owners/staff Police Licensing authority Club goers Transport authority
Drink/drug driving	Increased confidence Lack of coordination Increased risk-taking, lower inhibitions (Crowley & Courney, 2000)	Provide cheap soft drinks Public transport taxis, buses, and trains available Information of safety issues Special club buses provided by clubs Adequate ventilation (especially behind the bar) Adequate "break areas" for staff No smoking areas Information on dangers of smoking	Club owners Outreach workers Smoking prevention groups Health promotion groups Licensing authority Club goers

Source: Bellis, Hughes & Lowey 2002, 'Healthy nightclubs and recreational substance use. From a harm minimisation to a healthy settings approach', *Addictive Behaviours*, vol. 27 pp.1028–1029.

The promotion of a healthy settings approach in clubs and at 'raves', as part of an overall harm reduction strategy diverts attention away from a focus *solely* on the drug:

> This means key individuals and organisations (including club owners, staff, promoters, and major industries) can be engaged in a harm minimisation agenda that includes drug use along with alcohol, tobacco, transport, security and other environmental issues. Furthermore, tackling a broad range of issues in the night time environment reaches groups that are difficult to reach through education or occupational settings, such as those who play truant or are unemployed (Bellis, Hughes & Lowey 2002, p.1032).

Dance/rave guidelines and outreach

Using guidelines to making 'partying' safer and employing outreach staff at such parties are attempts to use the environments in which young people congregate to make them more informed about the choices they are making. It is argued that this is a far more effective measure to get across messages with regard to the dangers of drug use than banning the activities in which the drug use is seen to flourish.[778] As Lenton, Boys and Norcross comment:

> Raves and other venues where people in the scene go (such as certain nightclubs, music and clothing stores), provide channels for distributing harm reduction information materials to this population. Banning raves, or making the regulations which apply to them so restrictive that they are unworkable, could result in events being driven more underground rather than reducing drug use. Such actions are more likely to undermine cooperative alliances between people in the scene, health workers and event promoters to institute workable harm reduction strategies (Lenton, Boys & Norcross 1997, p.1336).

It is only relatively recently that clubs and venues in Australia have introduced guidelines and safety measures, often in conjunction with government health promotion units, to minimise and reduce harms associated with amphetamines and 'party drug' use. In Britain such measures have been in use for much longer. As early as 1991 a variety of approaches were being used by club owners in consultation with drug agency workers and educators. Some of the advice given to club owners included the following:

---

778 It is interesting that in the relatively early days of MDMA, some commentators had called for the drug to be legalised as a harm minimisation measure. For example, the following comments by Fitzgerald reflect a time in which MDMA was viewed pharmacologically as a benign substance, 'relatively free of contaminants':

'The arguments to change the legal status of MDMA are: firstly, that at the current use levels, MDMA poses a low health risk to the user; secondly, users may be suffering because of the illegal status of the drug; thirdly that there may be costs to society because of its illegal status; and finally, that MDMA may have significant therapeutic value' (Fitzgerald 1991, p.1).

Since the above comments were written, many if not all of the above factors have been if not disproved at least resiled from to a significant degree.

- Safety: rave organisers need to provide more than the legal minimum, and this probably extends to crush barriers, better ventilation, chill zones and rest areas;
- Security: trained bouncers, chosen in consultation with the police;
- Silence: minimise public nuisance by staggering raves away from residential areas, supplying good maps, transport and parking;
- Supply: permitting supply of illegal drugs on the premises is illegal and neither this nor promotion of drugs should be tolerated;
- Sense: pass health information to ravers to help minimise harm...
- Site: for drug workers nothing beats working on site, where bouncers and other rave staff can be persuaded to become part of an informal paramedical team capable of dealing with all incidents (Pearson et al. 1991, p.11).

In Australia, research conducted by Hando et al. (1997 cited in Webb 1998) led, at least in part, to a series of formal and informal protocols being established to maintain a safe environment for dance clubs and venues.[779] Hando's research found that venues where ecstasy was being consumed 'were typically too crowded, noisy, smoky and hot':

> The study's authors concluded that there was an urgent need for health and safety information about venue organisation and facilities to be distributed to

---

779 Some harm minimisation projects indirectly associated with club drugs, particularly GHB, have been recently developed to combat the practice of drink spiking, usually of young women's drinks. For example, the Whitsunday Spiked Drink Awareness Program is a Queensland programme based in the Whitsunday Islands that was a result of the concerns of local police and health workers regarding the numbers of sexual assaults on young women, ostensibly as a result of disinhibiting drugs such as GHB being put in unattended drinks of young women, often tourists and backpackers. With the backing of local licensees and funding from the Queensland government the project aims to give information on the dangers of drink spiking through the placement of posters and other informative material in pubs, clubs, toilets and bars. The information in the posters included:

- 'What drink spiking is
- Harms associated with the practice, such as assault, rape, unsafe sex and robbery
- The physical effects of various drugs associated with drink spiking, particularly rohypnol and GHB
- Appropriate contacts to seek assistance or further information' (McKey 2000, p.23).

Drink Spiking Harm Reduction Programmes in Queensland are now co-ordinated and implemented by a Drink Spiking Working Party established by Queensland Health in conjunction with the Queensland Police Service, Liquor Licensing and a variety of Queensland community agencies (Personal communication to the Committee by Detective Senior Constable Fiona Hinshelwood, Queensland Police Service, 27 June 2003).

Similar projects and programmes have been established throughout Australia. See, for example, the 'Keep your eyes open' drink spiking campaign promoted by the Bendigo Safe City Forum in Bendigo, Central Victoria:

'The program is a six month pilot with an evaluative component that targets females, potential and actual perpetrators and bar staff in nightclubs. Program material consists of three A4 messages with take away information that are displayed in the toilet environments. The objectives of the program are to reinforce drink spiking as a criminal offence, recognise that nightclub staff have a duty of care, and provide behavioural practices to protect people from drink spiking' (Submission of the City of Greater Bendigo to the Drugs and Crime Prevention Committee, Inquiry into Amphetamine and 'Party Drug' Use in Victoria, July 2002). See also the discussion in Chapter 7.

venue operators and dance party promoters. The researchers recommended that such information should cover:

- Provision of adequate water;
- Toilet conditions;
- Ventilation and air conditioning;
- Crowd control;
- First aid procedures;
- "Chill out" areas which are quieter, cooler and less active; and
- Regular monitoring of patrons (Webb 1998, p.96).[780]

Many of the Hando recommendations were incorporated into the *National Protocols on Conducting Safer Dance Parties* developed by the National Drug Strategy Committee (NDSC) (1997 cited in Wood 1998a). Other suggestions that have been incorporated into such guidelines include the provision of entertainment other than dancing at venues, for example computer games etc to encourage patrons to take breaks from continuous dancing, and encouraging the wearing of loose clothing at dance parties. It has also been suggested that the provision of water at dance venues should be *free of charge* (Gowing et al. 2001),[781] a matter that has been recently taken up by the Victorian state government in collaboration with clubs and the entertainment industry (see below).

Numerous submissions have made a number of recommendations to the Committee with regard to safe guidelines for dance parties and clubbing. Doutta Galla Community Health Services, for example, makes the following suggestions:

> Harm reduction policy is the best policy response to party drug use.
>
> Safe partying guidelines should be designed and implemented. These guidelines should include:
>
> 1. All dance events should have access to free clean water
> 2. There must be a recognised first aid team available
> 3. Bar staff should have first aid training
> 4. There should be an adequate quiet location for people to withdraw from the party
> 5. All fire exits must be cleared
> 6. Safe and appropriate syringe disposal facilities must be available
> 7. Clean syringes should be available during the party or at all clubs

---

780 For other information on the use of guidelines for the conduct of dance parties, see Fromberg 1998; Kamienicki et al. 1998 and Spruit 1999.

781 Sometimes this advice may change as more information about the drug and its effects is ascertained. For example, recent harm reduction advice with regard to ecstasy/party drug use and water consumption stresses that 'water is the "antidote" to dancing, not ecstasy. That is, drink 250ml of water every hour if *not* dancing, increasing to 500ml every hour if dancing' (Kong 2000, p.420).

8. Condoms should be available during the party or at all clubs
9. Drug education should be available during the party and at all clubs
10. Cars should not be allowed to enter an event.[782]

Such an approach is endorsed by the YWCA, which recommends similar measures in its submission to this Inquiry:

> Harm minimisation and harm reduction practices can be implemented simply and effectively in relation to drug use in 'party' scenarios and in the community generally. These include:
>
> - The easy and free availability of sharps, and extensive distribution of safe sharps disposal units in acknowledgement that amphetamines are used as an intravenous drug
> - The availability of free water in licensed premises and at dance parties so that people are not discouraged from re-hydrating their bodies
> - Extensive security camera coverage in licensed premises and at dance parties to monitor activity and assess drug related emergency situations
> - The provision of 'chill-out' spaces for people who need to cool down and relax
> - The availability of drug testing kits or facilities for people to test the purity and relative safety of the drugs they have purchased
> - Compulsory training of staff to deal with drug related emergencies
> - The availability of confidential support and assistance for decreased drug dependency in various languages
> - Integrating harm reduction strategies into other areas such as primary health care and community participation
> - Confidential first-aid assistance, unless hospitalisation is necessary.[783]

In the context of MDMA and dance parties, YSAS makes the following recommendation to this Inquiry:

> Mandating the appropriate management of temperature, provision of chill-out spaces, the availability of isotonic drinks and free water, and the availability of trained first-aid staff at venues could potentially prevent adverse reactions, and would be in accordance with harm minimisation principles.[784]

---

782 Submission of Doutta Galla Community Health Service to the Drugs and Crime Prevention Committee, Inquiry into Amphetamine and 'Party Drug' Use in Victoria, August 2002.

783 Submission of the YWCA to the Drugs and Crime Prevention Committee, Inquiry into Amphetamine and 'Party Drug' Use in Victoria, August 2002.

784 Submission of the YSAS to the Drugs and Crime Prevention Committee, Inquiry into Amphetamine and 'Party Drug' Use in Victoria, August 2002.

Specifically, YSAS gives the following pointers with regard to reducing the harms associated with MDMA use, particularly in the context of dance parties:

'If in doubt, always ring an ambulance.

How much water you should drink depends on the context in which you are taking MDMA/ecstasy. While MDMA/ecstasy will tend to raise your temperature, particularly when the external ambient temperature is high, you are going to get hotter in some situations than in others.

Two of the major issues that arise from the recommendations and suggestions outlined above and which need to be addressed with a healthy settings approach in mind are those pertaining to transport and security at clubs and other venues. These are the focus of the next two sections.

Transport issues

One aspect of providing a safe environment for clubbing that has received much attention in Britain has been the need for a more comprehensive and integrated system of transport (public and private) to enable clubbers and 'ravers' to travel safely between clubs and from clubs to home:

> Transport is a key issue for the facilitation of clubbers' safety. Taxis were either unavailable or unaffordable for many clubbers and were seen as a problem, with considerable numbers of clubbers having had frustrations and bad experiences with taxis in the past. Public transport proved to be non-existent outside big cities and inconvenient or unreliable within them. This resulted in nearly half of clubbers using private cars to get home from clubs, a finding of particular concern in relation to road traffic safely. The numbers of clubbers driving on Britain's night-time roads who have consumed legal and/or illicit drugs is cause for concern, although their attempts to minimise the risks of such behaviour and the low level of reported accidents is heartening. Clubbers have strong motivation to go clubbing and hundreds of thousands of young people need safe and reasonably priced transport to and from dance venues. The issue to address, therefore is not a new peel [sic] of punitive measures to police Britain's roads but the prospect of affordable alternatives in the form of public transport and organised private-hire taxis, minibuses and coaches (Measham, Aldridge & Parker 2001, p.180).[785]

Although this quote reflects British experience there are similar concerns held with regard to Victoria. Unlike Measham, Aldridge and Parker, the Committee does not have problems per se with the recently introduced changes to road safety legislation facilitating the testing of drivers for drugs in addition to

---

If you are dancing for hours on end in a hot and sweaty club or party, then you should aim to drink about a 500ml bottle of water to which one teaspoon of salt has been added every hour. Alternatively, consume isotonic drinks which will replace the salts and minerals lost through sweating, or eat a salty snack such as crisps or peanuts. MDMA/ecstasy increases body temperature, and water should be drunk when taking it to avoid overheating and dehydration. However, it must be emphasized that *water is not an antidote to the chemical effects of ecstasy.*

Drinks should be sipped rather than gulped.

Relying on drinking water to reduce body temperature is insufficient – taking breaks from dancing, spending time in specially designated chill-out spaces are also important interventions. In some venues, volunteers spray dancers with water.

Endeavour to urinate, even if it's difficult.

Club situations are not the only concern. The need to drink enough water and not to get too hot is just as vital when taking MDMA outdoors on summer days (at music festivals, for example) or if hiking in the bush' (Submission of the YSAS to the Drugs and Crime Prevention Committee, Inquiry into Amphetamine and 'Party Drug' Use in Victoria, August 2002).

785 In Measham, Aldridge and Parker's survey of clubbers 24 per cent of the sample stated they regularly had problems getting home from clubs (2001, p.159).

alcohol.[786] Indeed, it supports the random testing of clubbers and 'ravers' outside venues and at outdoor raves. Such a measure promotes the safety of all, including clubbers and ravers. Nonetheless, it agrees that there are few integrated or affordable transport options for young people going to and from entertainment venues. However, the responsibility should not only lie with public transport authorities. There is much to be said for the suggestion that club owners and club networks contribute to a subsidisation of transport for their young patrons:

> [w]ith entry ticket reduction vouchers to hire local minibuses and coaches to take them to the popular long distance venues, whereby the drivers stay at the venue and ensure all the passengers return to the transport and get home safely, could be particularly effective...this approach of taking responsibility for clubbers' safety should be routine, every weekend, practice (Measham, Aldridge & Parker 2001, p.192).[787]

Recommendations

43. The Committee recommends that a Review of the current provision of public and private transport services, including taxi services, be undertaken with the aim of ensuring that adequate provision is made so people, especially young people, can return to their homes directly after attending nightclubs, dance venues and outdoor 'raves', particularly in high activity precincts.

44. The Committee recommends that consideration should be given to the extension of public transport hours that service such high activity precincts.

Security issues

The issue of security and crowd control at public entertainment venues has been one of great controversy in 2004. Much of the concern has arisen from the death of former test cricketer David Hookes. As regrettable as such an incident was, Mr Hookes' death simply served to highlight concerns about the security industry that were already in evidence prior to January of this year.[788]

It should be recognised that in many respects club security are placed, however misguidedly, in a dilemma, particularly in clubs which have a reputation for being 'drug clubs'. For some security personnel it may be seeking a balance between 'efficient club security and the facilitation of a good club night' (Measham, Aldridge & Parker 2001, p.167):

> It's a balance between not letting people deal and take drugs openly... And on the other [hand], to accept that people are here to have a good time,

786 See discussion in Chapter 7.

787 This is also done to a certain extent at large Australian rave events such as Earthcore where in 2003 charter buses transported 'ravers' from Adelaide and Sydney to the relevant Victorian location.

788 Mr Hookes died on 19 January 2004.

> dance and take drugs. And if they weren't here we wouldn't have a job (2001, p.167).[789]

One of the main concerns expressed by people associated with the club and 'rave' scene, particularly those who promote a harm reduction focus is that some security personnel are insufficiently experienced at or trained in first aid procedures. In particular, many are simply unable to distinguish between alcohol intoxication and that caused by the ingestion of dangerous drugs such as GHB. This can have serious consequences, as commented on by Mr Ben Horan, harm reduction/first aid officer with many years' experience working in nightclubs:

> Without naming venues and purely conveying a patron's experience, clubs face a definite issue if they have a high prevalence of illicit substances. Then their revenue options are door fees or water or spin-offs of those. I have seen clubs that run remarkably hot, uncomfortable environments with hot water in all their taps so there is no availability of cold water anywhere – that is, bar staff will not serve you a glass of iced water; it is purely buy their bottled water or faint.
>
> Coupled with a fairly common trend among clubs, which is a strict eviction policy, if someone presents as chronically affected by drugs or alcohol they are evicted from the venue. From a health perspective that is incredibly dangerous if you are dealing with someone who, for example, is overdosing on gamma hydroxy-butyrate (GHB). The symptoms of GHB are not dissimilar to alcohol, so as I said if you've got a GHB affected patron, they're not necessarily showing that much difference from someone who's intoxicated [by alcohol]...now if they're drug affected, if they're heading towards an overdose, and GHB is one of the substances that I would classify as a high overdose risk, and you take them out of the club that's overheated, you're taking them from one temperature extreme to another. Their body is already fighting desperately to sustain itself. To throw them outside where they are suddenly suffering a 15 degree temperature drop, leave them unattended and uncared for – it is my experience that a lot of venues are doing that – I think is of deep concern. That's the best way to put someone into shock. We need to take more of a harm-minimisation approach and appreciate that looking after the patrons whom venues admit is part of their duty of care.
>
> In a lot of cases, clubs appear to be trying to get them out of the venue because if the incident happens on the street out the front, "well that's not a black mark against the licensee", but if the patron collapses in the club well that comes back on them so they'll ditch the patron in public places, it's usually the back street or back alley or whatever and if they're feeling particularly generous, they'll call an ambulance... I think it's only a matter of time before you see a mortality. If the average ambulance response time is eight minutes, you've got to hope they stay breathing for eight minutes because with GHB in particular...it's not long

789 It is not helped by the fact that some security personnel may have taken illicit drugs themselves. It was certainly the view of some members of this Committee that at least one 'bouncer' was 'high' on an illicit drug while on duty during the Committee's club tour.

> before they can stop breathing. You've got something like a minute and a half, two minutes, once that happens...they're unlikely to revive successfully.[790]

Mr Horan is particularly concerned that security personnel are inadequately trained in first aid procedures and that there is no incentive (or compulsion) for ongoing or updated first aid training. Very few 'bouncers' know the 'right questions' to ask:

> It's something crowd controllers don't tend to want to do, they don't want to talk about it, try and find out what they've [drug users] had, what they've done. Most of these people [drug users] will tell you what they've had if you approach them in a non threatening way... Certainly its taken a couple of months but the atmosphere in some clubs is such that I don't get the standard response that I used to get which is "What did you have?" "Oh, nothing". Now they're a lot more open and they respond to my questions because they aren't threatened by me...[791]

Despite some current rudimentary requirements that crowd controllers have some first aid training, Mr Horan pithily remarks that in his experience:

> I've yet to meet a crowd controller who'd feel confident about putting on a band-aid.[792]

These views were echoed by National Drug and Alcohol Research Centre drug educator Paul Dillon when he met with Committee staff:

> Ninety five per cent of problems in clubs, many of the incidents I hear about, have to do with bad calls by security. Security officers really don't have the people skills, and they often make decisions, which I don't think they are capable of making. I believe security need to have basic first aid. What I try to do with clubs that I have worked at, is to say, there needs to be a liaison between security and the hotel or club staff, management, with a [designated] person in charge who is able to make those calls... You know, everyone is on radio now, every single place, no-one doesn't have radios, you know, it's a matter of getting the radio, getting the liaison down, this is a call I'm making, and it gets put in the incident book.[793]

---

790 Mr Ben Horan in conversation with staff of the Drugs and Crime Prevention Committee, 25 November 2003.

791 Ibid.

792 Ibid. Mr Horan's concerns are well founded if a recent survey of British dance party clubbers is an accurate representation. Fifty-eight per cent of a sample of 250 British clubbers had claimed to feel unwell at some time or other at a dance event. Many of these had taken one or more ecstasy tablet or other 'party drug':

'What sort of help did they get when feeling unwell? Who provided it? Not much, and mostly from friends is the short answer. In rather more detail, 65 (50%) of the 131 answering this question claimed that they received no help at all. Of the other half of the unwell group, 32 (24%) just received general sympathy, 19 (15%) were given water, 6 (5%) were guided to fresh air, 4 got medical attention, with 5 specifying some other kind of help. Most of this help received by the 66 who received it was provided by friends, according to 48 (73% of the group), with 6 (9%) getting trained medical help, 3 (5% assistance) from club staff, and 9 (14%) from strangers' (Hammersley, Khan & Ditton 2002, p.78).

793 Mr Paul Dillon, Information and Media Liaison Officer, National Drug and Alcohol Research Centre in conversation with staff of the Drugs and Crime Prevention Committee, April 16, 2004.

Mr Dillon also alludes to the fact that many clubs and venues have an incredible turnover of security staff and that in itself causes problems:

> I mean the places I work with up here, [Sydney] the security problems are enormous. And this is because many of them [security officers] actually are employed from security companies and every weekend or whatever, you never see the same people twice...So you don't develop relationships, and the security personnel don't understand the crowd, it gets very messy. [794]

Mr Dillon concludes his comments with regard to security issues by stating 'when you have a club that has good security, you don't see problems'.[795]

Rightly or wrongly crowd control in today's environment encompasses (or should encompass) more than just 'doorkeeping'. Particularly in the entertainment/dance club environment the responsibilities of crowd controllers are many and onerous. While it may not be either necessary or appropriate for every nightclub to have a dedicated harm reduction officer, at the very least crowd control personnel should nonetheless be trained to question whether a patron may be drug affected and/or seek further assistance before acting unilaterally.

Finally, while many promoters and other people involved with the dance party and 'rave' scene welcome the type of harm reduction regulation canvassed in the previous commentary and endorsed in our recommendations, they are fearful that an over emphasis on 'policing' may result in raves and dance parties being banned or closed down. Such views are not fanciful given the publicity pertaining to the recent Two Tribes function. Organisers such as Tim Harvey from the environmental rave group Transplant profiled in Chapter 10 of the Report sound a salutary warning:

> In regard to outdoor dance parties, over the last couple of years we have probably seen a fairly large increase in the number of parties that have been shut down by the police and the Environment Protection Authority. I have noticed in the last 12 months that that is pushing the parties underground.
>
> We have a very good working relationship with the police, so do most outdoor dance parties, and I have spoken to many police on many occasions. They are more than happy to just sit in their cars because they know that generally nothing is going to happen and it is usually a fairly peaceful process to go through. I have noticed that there has been monitoring of web forums so the police know prior to where the party is going to be and then they go and shut it down. The one thing I would say is that increased policing is probably going to do you more harm than good. If you build a better mouse trap, you are going to build a better mouse. These guys are not stupid. They know how to hide it and they know how to push it back underground.

---

794 Mr Paul Dillon, Information and Media Liaison Officer, National Drug and Alcohol Research Centre in conversation with staff of the Drugs and Crime Prevention Committee, April 16, 2004.

795 Ibid.

> The general acceptance in some communities of the scene has been a good thing because it has allowed it to come out from being underground and to be more in public view. What you possibly risk over the next couple of years is that if you put the hammer down you will push it straight back underground. You will lose all ability to control it, which I have got to say I do not think is particularly much at the moment. You will tend to lose that if you are not careful in the next couple of years by putting too much pressure on it. I can guarantee you it has been going on for so many years that it is not going to stop. You can just displace it; it is going to go somewhere else.[796]

The Committee believes that at this stage the 'banning' of dance parties and outdoor raves would be a precipitate and unwarranted step. The Committee does believe, however, that a mandatory regulatory framework for club venues and outdoor raves needs to be implemented. Such a conclusion is drawn not only from the Committee's own observations but also after having ascertained the views of many experts in the field. For example the views of drug educator Paul Dillon of the National Drug and Alcohol Research Centre are timely and apposite.

> I think without some teeth, guidelines are pretty useless and they tend to get forgotten. It is about time someone actually took the bull by the horns and said "OK well, we need to make some rules, and give someone the power to enforce them". Though I don't think they should be, you know, pages and pages long, if you make 4 simple rules, something about – cold flowing water, chill out spaces, certain types of security guard regulations or, and give them to you know the local command of police to look after, at least you send the message that you are serious about it.

Mr Dillon believes that such a simple regulatory code is best enforced through an audit system conducted by local area police commanders, in a manner similar to the policing of liquor accords and liquor licensing:

> Well, you have to make it simple, it's got to be very simple. It's got to be a team of two, walking in, you know, whatever time, they have a checklist. It's as simple as three ticks, signed off, yes, you passed, you got those three things, it gets filed. I don't think you can do any more than that… But I also believe the only way to do it is through local area [police] commanders, because, you know, most probably, they've got a relationship with them [clubs] anyway, because of the [liquor] accords, you know, there are things in place already. We shouldn't be reinventing a new system, but going to a system that already exists.[797]

The Committee therefore considers that if sensible harm reduction recommendations and regulations are adopted and enforced, and groups such

796 Mr Tim Harvey in conversation with the Drugs and Crime Prevention Committee, Melbourne, 10 November 2003.

797 Mr Paul Dillon, Information and Media Liaison Officer, National Drug and Alcohol Research Centre in conversation with staff of the Drugs and Crime Prevention Committee, April 16, 2004.

as RaveSafe have an active presence at such venues and events, many of the problems such as those that occurred at Two Tribes would not occur.

As such the Committee makes the following recommendations:

Recommendations

45. The Committee recommends a wide-ranging and comprehensive review of security issues and security personnel including but not restricted to security personnel and crowd controllers located at nightclubs, dance clubs, venues and 'rave' events. Such a review would concentrate not solely on issues involving security and violence but also those pertaining to health, training and other concerns relating to the industry.

46. The Committee recommends that, subject to the findings of such a review, more stringent requirements be placed on the initial issue and ongoing renewal of a Security/Crowd Controller licence to include the following requirements:

    a) Training modules developed to give a better understanding of illicit substances, their signs and potential hazards.

    b) Training modules developed to give a better understanding of drink spiking, the strategies that can reduce occurrences, and the consequences of non-intervention.

    c) Level 2 First Aid qualification must be maintained as current in order to hold licence (renewed every 3 years).

    d) CPR Refresher must be maintained as current in order to hold licence (recommended renewal every 1 year).

    e) Mandatory reporting of violent incidents involving Crowd Controllers for review of their licence holding.

    f) Training in the detection of drug trafficking or distribution at clubs and associated venues.

47. The Committee recommends that random drug testing of security personnel should be undertaken by Police on a regular basis.

48. The Committee recommends that a regulatory framework for dance and club venues and indoor and outdoor 'raves' be established that mandates the appropriate management of these facilities and locations. This should include but not be restricted to:

    Mandatory licensing conditions to be developed to govern patron health and safety at venues and events, including:

    a) Adequate ventilation and sensible climate controls (generous airflow, and ambient temperature around dance areas to be of a comfortable level for high exertion).

    b) Well ventilated seated areas ('chill-out' space) sufficient for the expected patronage.

c) The ready availability of free potable cold tap water, and where appropriate isotonic drinks.

d) For venues or events that cater for less than 500 patrons, a Level 2 First Aid qualified staff person should be in attendance. The requisite standard of first aid equipment should be provided.

e) For venues or events of more than 500 patrons, a Level 2 First Aid (or higher) trained staff member should be assigned the specific duty of patron care (monitoring for concerning signs of drug influences, intoxication or overdose and providing appropriate care).

f) Venue managers and promoters should take responsibility for the care of drug affected patrons where health risk is imminent until such patrons are delivered into the care of ambulance officers, emergency services workers or other suitably qualified staff. In particular, venue or event staff should not evict patrons who appear to be drug affected or at risk until the first aid staff person has been consulted.

g) It is recommended that a comprehensive manual of patron care be developed to govern the detailed management and treatment of patrons who may be affected by amphetamine, 'party drug' and/or poly-drug use.

49. The Committee recommends that appropriate licensing agents regularly inspect clubs and associated venues for compliance with the regulations as established in Recommendation 48.

The next major section profiles a number of current strategies and initiatives that concern harm reduction with regard to the use of 'party drugs' and to a lesser extent amphetamines.

Many of the projects canvassed could be classified as incorporating a 'healthy settings' perspective as previously discussed.

Specific Australian projects

South Australian projects

South Australia has been one of the most proactive states in addressing amphetamines and 'party drugs' from a harm reduction perspective. Many of the harm reduction strategies developed in South Australia have been a result of the comprehensive Drugs Summit hosted by the South Australian government in June 2002. The initial government response to the Summit and its recommendations specifically recognised that consumption of recreational dance drugs including amphetamines and MDMA was part of the 'normalisation' of drug use within youth dance party culture.[798] In a submission to this Inquiry the Drug and Alcohol Services Council (DASC) of South Australia

798 *South Australian Drugs Summit: Tackling Drugs: Initial Government Response and Initiatives for Immediate Action,* December 2002, Government of South Australia, Adelaide.

outlines the following strategies designed to 'address the prevention of uptake of 'party drugs' as well as reducing the harms associated with 'party drug' use'.[799]

Illicit Drugs and Licensed Premises Project

The DASC is currently working in partnership with the Office of the Liquor and Gambling Commissioner, Australian Hotels Association (SA Branch), Clubs SA, Royal Adelaide Hospital and SA Police to develop a health promotion strategy addressing psychostimulant use by young people within South Australia.

The aim of the project is to decrease the harms associated with illicit drug use in and around licensed premises. This aim will be met by improving the capability of licensees to address illicit drug use issues through:

- developing and implementing education strategies for licensees; and,
- broadly disseminating clear, credible and accurate harm reduction and prevention information to patrons of licensed premises relating to illicit drug use.

Specific resources developed by the project will include social marketing tools, including posters and stickers, together with a licensee education kit which will be integrated within current licensee education and training sessions. The project was piloted within three licensed premises in August 2002, with the project resources on offer to approximately 200 licensed premises by December 2002.[800]

The following update is an account of the success of the licensing kit currently in circulation:[801]

> - The IDLP kit was piloted in three licensed entertainment venues attracting young people: one country, one metropolitan, and one CBD. Feedback from the pilot suggests that licensees find the information within the kit easy to read, clear and credible, realistic and, for the most part, useful. Most respondents indicated that the kit had increased their confidence in addressing illicit drug issues within their licensed premise. The kit encouraged the development and, in part, the reiteration of strategies between licensees and their staff. In particular, the development of operating procedures and training activities for staff, on how to respond to illicit drug use, were implemented in pilot venues. This feedback determined the content of the final kit and the full implementation of the project.

799 Submission of the Drug and Alcohol Services Council (DASC) (South Australia) to the Drugs and Crime Prevention Committee, Inquiry into Amphetamine and 'Party Drug' Use in Victoria, August 2002.

800 Since the submission was received the Committee has been informed that this project has commenced with the relevant information kits being sent out to targeted licensed premises in December 2002 (Personal communication between DASC and Committee staff member, 14 May 2003).

801 Some examples of the resources included in the kit are attached as Appendix 24.

- The IDLP kit was distributed to 1000 licensees in December 2003 through direct mail by the Office of the Liquor and Gambling Commissioner. Licensees were selected on the basis of providing late night entertainment and a perception of a high numbers of young people frequenting the premises. Additional patron information was made available for licensees through the Alcohol and Drug Information Service. This option was not taken up by many licensees.
- The IDLP was officially launched by Health Minister Lea Stevens on December 18th, 2002. Media coverage for the event was extensive including television coverage on channels 2, 7, 9, 10 in addition to coverage in The Australian newspaper and across all major radio stations in Adelaide on the launch day. Local licensee newsletters also highlighted the availability of the kit.[802]

Due to the popularity of the resource an extra 500 copies had been reproduced by September 2003. Other positive results from the initial launch and distribution have included:

- Specific training and information sessions have been delivered in partnership with Local Drug Action Teams, at police request.
- The Office of the Liquor and Gambling Commissioner are now investigating amendments to the Liquor Licensing Act's Code of Practice in order to incorporate some of the strategies contained in the kit as part of required licensee practice.
- A PowerPoint training session has been developed and distributed in partnership with licensee training providers within this state. All Liquor Licensing and Responsible Service of Alcohol training providers within the state have agreed to incorporate the training information within the delivery of their sessions.[803]

The Committee has been most impressed with the kit and its contents and commends the DASC and its partners for its excellent work in the area of harm reduction. It is a model that could usefully be emulated in Victoria.[804]

---

802 Illicit Drugs and Licensed Premises Kit, Update report, September 2003, Drug and Alcohol Services Council, Adelaide.

803 Ibid.

804 In particular it has been impressed with the variety of posters and information sheets produced as part of the kit. These include easy to read drug information sheets on most drugs found on licensed premises (a copy of the poster on GHB is attached as Appendix 25); a concise ready reckoner on the drugs, reactions to them, adverse health effects and indicators to them being on the premises (see Appendix 26) a general information sheet including the benefits to licensees in managing illicit drug issues on their premises (see Appendix 27), and a guidelines for licensees poster, given in useful question and answer form (see Appendix 24).

Another excellent innovation has been a series of role-plays developed to instruct licensees or managers what they should be doing if a staff member, including security staff, came to them with news of a drug-related emergency (see Appendix 28).

The Reducing Drug Harm in the Dance Party Scene Project

The Reducing Drug Harm in the Dance Party Scene Project, a collaborative project between the DASC and the South Australian Police Department (SAPOL), focusses on the dance music scene in Adelaide, South Australia, and aims to prevent the uptake of 'party drugs', reduce harm among users, and encourage users to access the primary health care system.

Lymb, Weekley and Creaser from the Harm Reduction unit of the DASC describe the project as follows:

> Strategies promoting abstinence from drug use are a key part of the harm reduction philosophy; however, this approach also aims to reduce harms among individuals who continue to use drugs. A harm reduction approach is therefore considered to be the most realistic and achievable platform for the successful delivery of the project objectives, as this approach can also effectively address continued drug use among the target population by reducing the harms associated with this use.
>
> There is a need for the dance party industry to develop their capacity to address drug related harm within the dance music scene, and for accurate, culturally relevant information be available within this scene. The project will be engaging with the dance party industry to develop guidelines for the operation of dance parties, which will provide methods of best practice for the industry. The project will collaborate with the dance music industry, including dance event organisers, venue operators and staff, DJ's and dance scene media, to build the capacity of the dance music industry to develop and implement strategies to reduce drug use and the harm associated with this use.
>
> It is planned that the project will achieve the following outcomes:
>
> - Reduced use of party drugs amongst young people in the dance scene
> - Increased referral into treatment
> - Reduced harm arising from party drug use in the dance scene
> - Sustainable partnerships between the health, law, non-government, youth and commercial sectors that address prevention and harm reduction
> - Establishment of dance event environments which prevent and reduce the potential for drug related harm
> - Development and distribution of dance event guidelines for safer dance parties in Adelaide (Lymb, Weekley & Creaser 2003, pp.2–3).

The project utilises the assistance of three key and influential agencies involved in the party scene in Adelaide, namely RaveSafe (South Australia), *Onion* Magazine, and youth radio station Fresh FM.[805]

Other aspects of the project are:

- Developing, testing, distributing and maintaining up to date education resources targeting ecstasy and other 'party drugs', including information to be inserted on tickets to raves, information to be utilised by specific CD retailers focusing on dance music, information for licensed premises (eg. coasters, signage in toilet areas), and posters for licensed venues, CD retailers and health services.
- Developing web-based communication strategies, providing appropriate alcohol and other drug information and links for use on the DASC, Fresh FM, Rave Safe and other relevant web-sites.[806]

---

805 *Onion* Magazine and Fresh FM have already been discussed in the context of education strategies in Chapter 18. To reiterate the roles and functions of these information providers:

Fresh FM, a key partner in the project, is an Adelaide based dance music radio station popular among young people. This station attracts a range of volunteers, Adelaide DJs and professionals, and boasts a membership of 5000 subscribers who support the station. Fresh FM is vital to the success of the project as it has a large, expanding audience base, currently estimated at approximately 100,000 listeners, the majority of whom are young people between the ages of 18 to 24. The project's key strategies in working with Fresh FM include:

- Collaborating with Fresh FM staff in the development of tailored, appropriate AOD community service announcements (CSAs) with a harm reduction focus for regular broadcast by Fresh FM and the distribution of these CSAs to regional community radio stations for broadcast.
- Providing AOD training for Fresh FM staff.
- Facilitating a range of AOD-related guest speakers for regular interview style segments broadcast on Fresh FM (such as 'Morning Fresh' and 'Fresh Forum').
- Developing AOD/harm reduction related web communication strategies for the Fresh FM web-site.

Onion, a free, bi-monthly dance music magazine, is the peak printed media of the dance music scene in Adelaide, and provides the opportunity for significant access to the target group. This magazine enjoys a wide distribution (8000 copies per fortnight to over 500 outlets) throughout Adelaide, being available in a range of locations frequented by young people, including universities, bars, nightclubs, cafes, music stores, and other retail outlets. It is also estimated that each copy is read by between 3-4 individuals, giving the magazine considerable readership. Magazine content ranges from clubbing and raving information to dance music news and youth lifestyle issues. The project will collaborate with *Onion*, a key project partner, to develop appropriate AOD related content for publication in the magazine. The project's key strategies in working with *Onion* include:

– Developing tailored AOD messages with a harm reduction focus for regular publication in *Onion*.

– Developing feature AOD articles for publication in *Onion*.

– Developing and delivering AOD training for *Onio*n Staff.

– Developing AOD/harm reduction related web communication strategies for the *Onion* web site (Information taken from Lymb, Weekley & Creaser 2003, pp.4–5).

806 Submission of DASC to the Drugs and Crime Prevention Committee, Inquiry into Amphetamine and 'Party Drug' Use in Victoria, August 2002.

Victorian projects

Victoria has also been developing a variety of strategies and programmes relating to amphetamine and 'party drug' use. These include:

RaveSafe

RaveSafe is a peer education initiative, targeting high-risk illicit drug users who frequent rave parties. RaveSafe, which has been funded by the Drug Policy Unit since 1996/1997, is auspiced by Victorian Drug User Group (VIVAIDS). Consisting of a team of trained peer educators, RaveSafe has been extremely successful in educating thousands of people who frequent the rave scene about safe drug use practices in a way relevant and acceptable to the culture. In 2000, 30 volunteers also received training and assisted RaveSafe at rave parties.

RaveSafe provides both verbal and written information and resources to reduce the risks of illicit drugs (generally in relation to 'party drugs'.) A team of five peer educators were recruited through a comprehensive recruitment process, to provide peer education and support to partygoers to reduce the misinformation and dispel some of the myths and unsafe using practices within the scene.

RaveSafe undertakes other strategies including workshops for 'party drug' users and workshops for promoters and event organisers to encourage them to provide a safe environment. The strategies and implementation of RaveSafe is overseen by a Reference group whose membership includes St Johns Ambulance, Ambulance Victoria, Dept of Education and Training, Victorian Police, Enlighten, VIVAIDS, Australian Drug Foundation, Turning Point Alcohol and Drug Centre, Department of Human Services, Pt'chang Non-violent Community Safety Group, RaveSafe Peer Educators, and promoters, security and DJs.

PARTY SAFE WORKSHOPS

RaveSafe has also conducted Peer Education Workshops aimed at young people who are involved in or likely to be involved in the rave scene. The messages in the workshops included planning for a safe night, look after your mates, seeking assistance and first aid, harm reduction and 'party drugs', 'party drugs' and their effects. Workshops were held at RMIT Health Services, Southern School of Natural Therapies, NMIT Collingwood and Preston Campuses, Monash University and at VIVAIDS.

RaveSafe has identified some of the key strategies for dealing with 'party drug use' as:

- Peer Education
- Working with and upskilling event organisers and promoters
- Developing appropriate resources
- Developing and maintaining partnerships between appropriate agencies
- Influencing of legislation (eg. free cold water in clubs, introduction of pill-testing)

- Upskilling of AOD workers.[807]

In conjunction with the Victorian Department of Human Services and the Australian Drug Foundation, RaveSafe has developed a draft document entitled 'Guidelines for Running Safer Dance Parties', for distribution to organisers within the dance party industry. This document has yet to be finalised but was used to form the basis of the audit tool developed by RaveSafe and a draft RaveSafe booklet for promoters entitled 'Recommendations for providing a safe dance environment'.[808]

PRESENCE AT CLUBS AND RAVES

A key role of RaveSafe is its presence at dance clubs and major dance and music festivals and outdoor 'raves' such as Earthcore. Ms Natalie Russell, RaveSafe Peer Education Officer, explained this aspect of the organisation's work to the Committee at a Public Hearing:

> As a team of six well-trained and well-equipped peer educators, we attend a mixture of dance events – from 200 people in size up to 8000 or 10 000, from indoor events at Melbourne Park to outdoor bush events near Bendigo.
>
> We set up a marquee with blankets and beanbags, which acts as a safe chill-out space where party goers can sit and chat with us about party drugs, safer partying and other health issues. We also distribute safer partying packs, which contain safe partying tips, information on chlamydia, a condom, lube and lolly. We hand out fruit and earplugs, are licensed to provide sterile injecting equipment discreetly upon request, and we also comfort and reassure party goers who may be anxious, unwell or freaked out.
>
> We collaborate with first-aid services at events to ensure that any unwell party goers or overdoses are passed from us to them. In turn, the first-aid services communicate with us as to effects of particular drugs on individuals who they are not familiar with and refer party goers onto us.[809]

WORKING WITH EVENT ORGANISERS AND PROMOTERS

The promotion of collaborative approaches and working partnerships is a key aspect of a harm reduction strategy. RaveSafe endorses and incorporates a partnership approach into all aspects of its harm reduction work, particularly with regard to working with promoters and club owners:

> RaveSafe's experience has been very positive when dealing with promoters and event organisers as they have embraced the project and overwhelmed RaveSafe with response for service. RaveSafe believes this is in part due to our

807 Submission of RaveSafe to the Drugs and Crime Prevention Committee, Inquiry into Amphetamine and 'Party Drug' Use in Victoria, October 2003.

808 For further details see Submission of Department of Human Services to the Drugs and Crime Prevention Committee, Inquiry into Amphetamine and 'Party Drug' Use in Victoria, October 2003. For a copy of the RaveSafe Audit see Appendix 29.

809 Ms Natalie Russell, RaveSafe Peer Education Officer, evidence given to the Drugs and Crime Prevention Committee, Inquiry into Amphetamine and 'Party Drug' Use in Victoria, Public Hearings (Melbourne), 27 October 2003.

> negotiations and liaison with promoters from the peer education perspective and not imposing our principles or strategies upon them. RaveSafe Peer Educators have been promoters themselves which creates a sense of understanding and familiarity with other event organisers/promoters.[810]

Unfortunately, such co-operation was not apparent at the recent Two Tribes rave and dance party held at Melbourne Park from which 11 people were taken by ambulance to hospitals with signs of apparent GHB intoxication.[811] Ms Natalie Russell has confirmed that the promoters of this 'mega rave' had been approached by RaveSafe with the aim of providing six trained advisers to assist with harm reduction support:

> Ms Russell said it was unusual for the offer to be rejected, particularly as RaveSafe was a free service funded by the Department of Human Services.[812]

Despite such an incident RaveSafe has had an excellent track record in working with promoters and venue owners:

> Rather than employing strict guidelines for each promoter, such as 'RaveSafe will only provide services if they allow Needle Syringe Exchange at parties', we work with what the promoters will allow and build up our relationship from there. This approach develops trust and understanding between RaveSafe and event organisers, which provides benefits for RaveSafe, promoters and partygoers.
>
> By having promoters/event organisers on the RaveSafe reference group they have influence on the strategies of RaveSafe and can advise on how best to work with promoters/club owners.[813]

RaveSafe audits

The RaveSafe audit identifies issues for consideration that may impact on the safety of a dance environment and reports them to the promoter/event organiser.

At the time of submitting to the Committee, RaveSafe had completed ten audits of clubs and venues in Melbourne. It has identified that most venues are of acceptable standard with only one not providing free cold water. An example of a RaveSafe audit checklist and questionnaire is attached as Appendix 29.

RaveSafe workers and volunteers also ascertain important information about drug using and harm reduction practices in less formal ways:

> We collect information on the prevalence and influence of party drug use not only through surveying but anecdotally when conversing with party goers. One of the key benefits of peer education is the openness and honesty of the

---

810 Submission of RaveSafe to the Drugs and Crime Prevention Committee, Inquiry into Amphetamine and 'Party Drug' Use in Victoria, 27 October 2003. Members of the Committee's staff have attended a promoter and peer educator training session held by RaveSafe. They found this session professional and most informative.

811 Held on 7 March 2003.

812 Quoted in 'Police to monitor dance scene after rave overdoses', Bridie Smith and Jamie Berry, The *Age*, 10 March 2004, p.7.

813 Submission of RaveSafe to the Drugs and Crime Prevention Committee, Inquiry into Amphetamine and 'Party Drug' Use in Victoria, 27 October 2003.

> party goers towards the RaveSafe peer educators. They will inform us of their personal drug use and the issues that affect them.[814]

RaveSafe communicates their findings to the Department of Human Services through partnership on a reference group and continues to work with them on ways in which to promote harm reduction strategies in venues, clubs and at 'raves'.

THE RAVESAFE NEWSLETTER

Rave Safe's 'e-news' is as the name suggests an electronic newsletter designed to inform and educate people with an array of information pertaining to clubbing and 'raves', emphasising a harm reduction perspective to any drugs they may take while clubbing. A typical newsletter may include the following:

- Information profiles on particular drugs
- Safety issues and harm reduction tips
- Competitions (rave tickets often being a prize)
- Surveys and Questionnaires[815]
- Community Service Announcements (for example, calls to become participants in research projects)
- An on-line chat forum
- Drug and pill warnings and alerts
- Calendar of Events
- Music news and reviews.

RaveSafe has been given glowing endorsement and support by a number of local government and community agencies.[816] Not everyone, however, is as enthusiastic about groups such as RaveSafe or indeed the concept of harm reduction in itself. The Committee acknowledges the views of people like Josh Brooker, a young man with whom the Chairperson and staff of the Committee met in November 2003. His views are encapsulated in the following quote:

> For the last five and a half years, I've raised issues in the media with my concerns regarding drug use at rave parties. In particular, young kids accessing the rave environment. With my experience, when I started up my campaign, I was sixteen at the time, a lot of my friends were going to rave parties as nightclubs and pubs were near impossible to get into unless you had proper, half legible ID. The rave industry, any aged child can frequent them and they do, as is now happening with my younger sisters, they don't go but their

814 Ms Natalie Russell, RaveSafe, evidence given to the Drugs and Crime Prevention Committee, Inquiry into Amphetamine and 'Party Drug' Use in Victoria, Public Hearings (Melbourne), 27 October 2003.

815 A copy of a newsletter is attached as Appendix 30.

816 For example, see testimonies contained in submissions from City of Yarra, City of Melbourne, Turning Point Alcohol and Drug Centre, YSAS, to the Drugs and Crime Prevention Committee, Inquiry into Amphetamine and 'Party Drug' Use in Victoria.

> friends at school are asking them to go. It's just not an environment for young kids to be around... You've got thirty five year old dirty men there, you've got chill out rooms, they set up mini hospitals in raves, why? The government's breaking the law, how is that harm minimisation really? Having a paramedic there. If I was going to drop my first pill, I'd love a paramedic to be there, I'd feel more inclined to take the drug, knowing that there's first aid on hand ready to pump you back to life or try to anyway. I'm just astounded that I'm so sick of reading in the newspapers that young kids do illicit drug use and I've been saying this for five years, every year, whether it be on radio, whether its to a paper, etc, etc.[817]

The Committee appreciates being privy to Mr Brooker's sincere and earnestly held beliefs. Nonetheless, the Committee generally supports the broad principles of harm reduction and the specific work of agencies such as RaveSafe. The Committee wishes to add its own commendation of the work RaveSafe undertakes and the professional manner in which it is performed. As such it makes the following recommendation:

Recommendation

50. The Committee acknowledges the valuable contribution of peer network organisations such as RaveSafe in providing information, training and practical assistance at events, clubs and other venues. The Committee recommends that these services be expanded and adequately funded to meet the current needs.

Department of Human Services initiatives

ILLICIT DRUG HARM PREVENTION PROJECT FOR INJECTING DRUG USERS

The Drug Policy and Services Branch are currently working with VIVAIDS targeting injecting drug users at high risk of drug overdose through peer education and information workshops. The project was initially aimed at the prevention of heroin overdose but re-designed in order to provide a response to current trends in drug use including the misuse of psychostimulants.

THE DIVERSION OF PSEUDOEPHEDRINE STRATEGY

> The Drug Policy and Services Branch of the Victoria Police, Pharmacy Board of Victoria, the Pharmacy Guild of Australia, and the Pharmaceutical Society of Australia have worked together to develop strategies to address the diversion of pseudoephedrine products (used as a precursor in the illicit manufacture of amphetamine in clandestine laboratories) from pharmacies. Strategies include:
>
> - a letter to all pharmacists advising of the problem;

817 Mr Josh Brooker, evidence given to the Drugs and Crime Prevention Committee, Inquiry into Amphetamine and 'Party Drug' Use in Victoria, Public Hearings (Melbourne), 18 November 2003.

- a poster for pharmacists and staff providing strategies to assist in limiting the diversion of pseudoephedrine products; and
- a poster advising customers of the prevention strategy.

Future strategies of the Department based on harm reduction principles include the distribution of *Guidelines for Running Safer Dance Parties* aimed at promoters and the dance party industry; a *Party Survival Guide* aimed at party goers 'with harm minimization tips, before, during and after rave parties'; a wallet card for party goers warning of the risks associated with amphetamines and 'party drugs'; and an education and information kit to be developed for general practitioners regarding the effects and misuse of psychostimulants.[818]

Voluntary Water Guidelines

As a result of the concerns expressed by a number of agencies and individuals (including many of those profiled in the Committee's *Discussion Paper* and this Report) on 22 June 2003 the Victorian Government announced that Voluntary Guidelines to provide free or low-cost drinking water on licensed premises would be developed. This measure was considered necessary following recent concerns that the lack of available free or low-cost water on some licensed premises has been impacting on the health and welfare of patrons in Victoria.

The Guidelines were launched by the Minister for Health the Hon. Bronwyn Pike on 20 January 2004. The rationale for their development was outlined in greater detail in a circular:

> It is essential that drinking water is readily available in order to prevent dehydration, which is often associated with the consumption of alcohol and some illicit drugs. The drinking of water can also slow down alcohol consumption and minimise the potential for intoxication. While the government does not in any way condone illicit drug use on licensed premises, all possible actions should be taken to minimise any health risks associated with licit or illicit drug use.
>
> While many operators and owners of licensed premises are currently offering appropriate drinking water facilities, it is proposed that these Voluntary Guidelines will provide a standard framework for the provision of drinking water at all licensed premises.
>
> The Guidelines have been developed by Government and industry stakeholders following a consultation process that included: the Department of Human Services, Liquor Licensing Victoria, the Victoria Police, and representatives from the industry including the Australian Hotels Association and the Nightclub Owners Association and Restaurant and Catering Victoria.[819]

818 Submission of Human Services Victoria (Drugs Policy and Services Branch) to the Drugs and Crime Prevention Committee, Inquiry into the Use of Amphetamines and 'Party Drugs', August 2002. See also discussion in Chapter 15.

819 Circular, *Voluntary guidelines to provide free or low cost drinking water on licensed premises*, Department of Human Services, 20 January 2003.

The guidelines were developed and endorsed by the Minister for Health, the Nightclub Owners Association, the Australian Hotels Association and Restaurant and Catering Victoria. For those operators and owners of licensed premises who adopt the guidelines it will be a requirement that:

- Free or reasonably priced drinking water will be available to patrons at all times on any premises where liquor is sold or supplied.
- Water should be sold or supplied at or near liquor service points, or by the same method that liquor is sold or supplied.
- When free drinking water is not feasible, a reasonable charge for drinking water will apply and must be less than the lowest price at which any alcoholic or non-alcoholic drink is sold on the premises.
- To comply with the Guidelines operators and owners of licensed premises can also choose from various options for providing drinking water including:
  - Water by the glass/carafe from the bar or by waiter service (to a dining table);
  - Bottled water; or
  - Using a water cooler.

For health and hygiene reasons, cold unadulterated water should be available in all bathrooms and toilets, however directing patrons to a venue's bathroom to obtain drinking water does not comply with these Guidelines.[820]

The Committee believes these guidelines are a valuable 'first step' but the provision of water should be a mandatory rather than voluntary requirement. Water supply needs to be seen, however, in conjunction with a whole range of harm reduction guidelines and practices that should regulate the operations of night clubs and similar venues. Available water is a necessary but not of itself sufficient step to ensure a safe 'clubbing' environment as indicated in the Recommendations enumerated previously in this Chapter.

The Committee also makes the following recommendations in relation to harm reduction strategies for clubs, dance parties and raves:

820 Ibid.

Recommendations

51. The Committee recommends that appropriate educational material in a variety of forms, including signage, leaflets and posters, be clearly displayed and available at clubs and associated venues, including 'raves'. Such material and signage should include warnings and alerts as to the risks associated with amphetamine and 'party drug' use.

52. The Committee recommends that a manual be developed for events managers and promoters which details all appropriate legal, regulatory and harm reduction strategies required in organising events such as raves and dance parties.

53. The Committee recommends that consideration be given to the Transport Accident Commission providing voluntary testing of people for both alcohol and amphetamine at 'raves' and outdoor dance parties.

The role of local government and harm reduction: Strategies and initiatives

The Committee acknowledges the importance of local government as a main player in matters affecting local communities. It has been therefore particularly keen to ascertain the views of local government authorities as to the extent and nature of amphetamine and 'party drug' use in their shires[821] and municipalities and any (harm reduction) strategies developed by local authorities to address drug use in their communities. Harm reduction strategies have been promoted and endorsed at a local government and community level, as evidenced in many submissions to this Inquiry.[822]

Some local government initiatives and suggestions with regard to guidelines for 'safe partying' have already been discussed in a previous section.

The role of local governments with regard to drug issues has recently been espoused in a paper produced by the Victorian Local Government Association (VLGA):

> Local governments have played a variety of roles in responding to drug issues affecting their communities. Since 1999, local governments have either coordinated or facilitated the development of specific local drug strategies and

821 The role of local government in rural shires may be particularly important with regard to drug policy and services. For example rural local government agencies may be the only possible entity that is in a position to administer programmes such as clean syringe exchange or disposal. Unfortunately, the Committee has received very little information on the role of local government in rural Victoria with regard to drug misuse. See also the discussion on rural and regional issues in Chapter 11.

822 See for example the submissions of: City of Greater Bendigo; City of Melbourne; City of Monash; Uniting Care, Moreland Hall; Youth Substance Abuse Service (YSAS); Doutta Galla Community Health Service; St Kilda Community Legal Service; YWCA Victoria to the Drugs and Crime Prevention Committee, Inquiry into Amphetamine and 'Party Drug' Use in Victoria, (all the above submissions dated August 2002).

> action plans in over 30 municipalities across Victoria. Some councils have adopted drug policy statements stating their commitment to tackle drug issues in partnership with their community. Other initiatives developed by local governments include: prevention and early intervention programs; provision of information on local drug and alcohol agencies and support services; and public space management.
>
> A range of networks have been established by local governments on drug issues. The Local Government Drug Issues Forum (LGDIF), a statewide network of local government officers responsible for responding to drug-related issues in their municipalities, meet regularly to share information about effective programs and strategies. The Victorian Local Governance Association (VLGA) also convenes a Drug Issues Working Group, involving councillors, council officers and representatives from drug sector agencies. Local governments in developing and implementing local drug strategies have formed steering committees and working groups to ensure key stakeholder input and community ownership.
>
> With the support of the State Government, local governments have played an active role in coordinating strategic responses to drug issues affecting their communities. However, as much as the situation is suggestive of a strengthened role for local government in drug policy development, there are concerns about how sustainable that role is into the future.[823]

Each of the 78 local government authorities in Victoria was sent a copy of this Committee's *Discussion Paper* accompanied by a series of questions designed to gauge how big a problem amphetamines and 'party drugs' are in their respective communities. Ten councils responded with submissions.

Local government views

The local government submissions indicate that there are themes that are common and particular to local governance:

- Very few councils see amphetamines and 'party drugs' as being a problem in their shire or municipality. This is the same for both rural and metropolitan areas:[824]

---

823 *Local Government roles in responding to drug issues: A Discussion Paper.* Produced by the VLGA and the Local Government Drug Issues Forum, Melbourne, 2002, p.2.

824 Most Councils relied on feedback from agencies, particularly schools, drug or youth agencies, within their shires or municipalities to ascertain this information. Sometimes this information is contradictory. The response from the City of Monash is indicative of many:

'The extent of amphetamine or 'party drug' use in Monash varies, but it is apparent that no community stakeholder considers this type of drug use to be a critical or vast issue.

Monash secondary schools have consistently indicated that the nature and extent of 'party drug' use and amphetamine use amounts to either an extremely small percentage, or nil...

Police have reported that in the twelve months to the end of 2002, only four offences were listed in relation to amphetamine use, one of which was driving under the influence of a drug. Whilst this is considered to be a small number relative to other areas, "a lot" of offenders have admitted to using amphetamines, but are seldom charged solely on their own admissions.

The service provision sector within the City of Monash has reported that anywhere up to sixty

- Some councils now have Drug Strategy Plans (DSPs) or the equivalent. However, few of these specifically include amphetamines and 'party drugs' being more generalist in nature. Many councils say, however, that their DSPs are flexible to include amphetamines and 'party drugs' strategies should the need arise;
- Most Councils who responded to the Discussion Paper were concerned about access to sufficiently comprehensive data on general drug use and specifically on amphetamines and 'party drugs'. A submission from the City of Monash based in Melbourne's southern suburbs is instructive in this regard:

> [a] lack of statistical data relating to amphetamine use remains an issue for the development of localised strategies. Information that points to the regularity and impact, both social and health impact, of party drug use remains a challenge for all stakeholders in producing effective programme responses to amphetamine use. Localised data such as ambulance and hospital admissions, Police arrest and offence data, as well as clinical research studies with a particular focus on the local area would assist in the development of evidence based targeted program delivery. Further detailed information relating to the profile of a typical amphetamine user would also assist in this process.[825]

The City of Moreland based in the northern suburbs of Melbourne has stated that it is not only the lack of data that is frustrating for local government authorities, it is also the way in which the data is collected that gives rise to difficulty. It has made a recommendation to the Committee with regard to this issue:

> Ambulance attendance data and emergency hospital presentation and admissions data currently bundle incidences of drug overdose into the catchall 'other drug' category unless they are primarily heroin-related or alcohol-related. This aggregation masks rather than illuminates the drug issues associated with amphetamines, 'party drugs', pharmaceuticals and some other substances.

---

percent of clients have tried amphetamines or 'party drugs' in the twelve months to the end of 2002. There was no suggestion that any of these clients were experiencing problematic use issues with amphetamines, or any ill health effects as a result of using the drug. Each service has indicated that amphetamines are becoming more readily available, and that a trend of increased use of amphetamines in emerging...

A conflicting view of amphetamine use within schools relates to the age group of users. Whilst some schools are of the opinion that amphetamines are used by older adolescents, a small number thought it more common among younger adolescents.

Police and service providers have so far been unable to identify any typical demographic profile of an amphetamine or 'party drug' user in Monash' (Submission of the City of Monash to the Drugs and Crime Prevention Committee, Inquiry into Amphetamine and 'Party Drug' Use in Victoria, October 2003.

825 Submission of the City of Monash, to the Drugs and Crime Prevention Committee, Inquiry into Amphetamines and Party Drugs, October 2003.

> Research data based on full drug screens and at local government level should be resourced to enable appropriate analysis, planning and strategy development.[826]

- Some councils are concerned that drug use generally is a 'cross-border issue'. Strategies should therefore be best devised and implemented in co-operation with and co-ordinated by neighbouring authorities to minimise displacement. Ironically, some councils are concerned that the risks of displacement are greatest when neighbouring councils have implemented intensive, well funded and effective drug strategies in their areas;
- A common response from local government authorities is that it is difficult to implement a comprehensive policy with regard to issues such as amphetamines and 'party drugs' and indeed health prevention generally without appropriate levels of funding.[827] For example, in responding to the Committee's previous Inquiry into the Inhalation of Volatile Substances the City of Casey has stated that one of the main functions of local government is to advocate for increases in funding and its equitable distribution from state and federal government in order to provide appropriate programmes.[828]

  Certainly many councils argue that they are witnessing an increase in the number and type of responsibilities being undertaken by local authorities but without a commensurate allocation of funding. Such a trend was remarked upon in the recent Report commissioned for the Australian National Council on Drugs (ANCD):

  > [T]here has been a trend in western societies to reduce spending on infrastructure, and towards devolution of responsibility to the local community level. Devolution can be a good thing, given the importance of community influences on drug use and variants between communities in such influences. However, there has not been a transfer of funds to the local level along with the transfer of responsibility. Spending on developmental health needs to be seen as a social investment in societal adaptability and economic prosperity, rather than simply as a benefit to individuals (ANCD 2001, p.23).

---

826 Submission of Moreland City Council to the Drugs and Crime Prevention Committee, Inquiry into Amphetamine and 'Party Drug' Use in Victoria, October 2003.

827 Funding for local government drug initiatives is generally through the state government's Municipal Drug Strategy (MDS) funding. This is particularly concentrated on the five 'drug hotspot areas', that is local government areas that are thought to have particularly high concentrations of (illicit) drug use within their boundaries:

'Over the next three years [as from 2004] each of the five hotspot municipalities will receive annual funding of $720,000 for their primary health care services. All other MDS funding (approximately $1.5 million in the current year) will be collapsed into a centrally determined $800,000 per year/over three years funding pool' (Victorian Alcohol and Drug Association 2003, p.2).

828 Submission of the City of Casey to the Drugs and Crime Prevention Committee, Inquiry into the Inhalation of Volatile Substances, February 2002, p.7.

Funding is seen as particularly crucial with regard to collecting reliable data on the extent of the problem.

- Local councils acknowledge that their staff need to be better educated with regard to drug use generally. This is particularly true of youth services staff, recreation staff and parks, gardens and maintenance staff.

With regard to this area of need, Ms Kym Neville, Community Development Officer with the Shire of Yarra Ranges states:

> Another problem is a lack of knowledge and understanding about what the impacts really are around amphetamine and party drug use. At a number of meetings that I go to we all talk about it and we all have an understanding as adults, but we are not at the parties and we do not really know what goes on. Maybe that is a good thing sometimes. Another issue for local government is probably their role as advocate in ensuring that the right services are available for people. There has been evidence – and, again, this will be backed up by speakers after me – that service providers, particularly in detox, have issues around the behaviour that clientele are now exhibiting, particularly people who are using methamphetamine Ice. They become quite violent and aggressive, and staff have real issues and difficulties in working with these people. They are used to working with heroin users, who are more docile and are not likely to act up or harass other people who are also accessing that service. An issue for local government is how do they advocate to ensure that service providers have funds to give their staff appropriate training on how to deal with these differences in behaviour?[829]

Most councils are not direct providers of drug and alcohol information, treatment or counselling services. Most local government authorities act as brokers, tendering such services out to community agencies. Nonetheless, many councils do view themselves as having a limited role in addressing amphetamines and 'party drugs' within their communities.

Ms Neville states in this regard:

> [Local government's] unique position at the interface means that it has quite a bit of local knowledge, as long as they have the right partnerships. It is this knowledge that enables local government to address their local issues, with their own local solutions. I believe that local government should develop an alcohol and drug action plan of some sort. That demonstrates leadership to the community, and to other levels of government, and also demonstrates that they are aware that these issues exist and that the community is finding it quite difficult to deal with things.[830]

829 Ms Kym Neville, Shire of Yarra Ranges, evidence given to the Drugs and Crime Prevention Committee, Inquiry into Amphetamine and 'Party Drug' Use in Victoria, Public Hearings (City of Knox), 11 November 2003.

830 Ibid.

The need to facilitate community partnerships

Many of the common concerns outlined in the previous section were raised in a forum/public hearing convened by the Committee in one local government area of Melbourne – the City of Knox, based in the eastern suburbs. This forum brought together representatives of the Knox Council and other proximate local government authorities, local police, and community agencies to discuss problems relating to the issues of amphetamine and 'party drug' abuse within this municipality.

One of the key participants was Ms Kim Neville, Community Development Officer with the Shire of Yarra Ranges.[831] She stated broadly the role local government and its agencies play (or should play) with regard to the issue of drugs in their communities:

> In relation to the role of local government in addressing amphetamine and party drug use, I think that local government's unique position at the interface between the community and other government agencies means that it can monitor local amphetamine and party drug use, develop strategies to address local issues and ensure that state government bodies and agencies are aware of changing patterns of use and the demographics of users. It is this unique position at the interface between other tiers of government and the community that enhances local government's capacity to address local issues at the local level, taking into account things like the geographic location and size of the LGA, the population and the dispersion across the LGA, the demographics of alcohol and drug users, transport, service availability, access to services and the different drug scenes, such as the type of drug that is most commonly used, where it is most commonly used, how it is purchased and how it is used.
>
> Local government is, therefore, in a prime position to develop programs targeting local solutions to local issues and, importantly, involving the community in the development and implementation of the programs.[832]

Without doubt most councils see their role in this area as being facilitative. In other words, councils are best placed to bring together and in some cases fund meetings of concerned stakeholders in their communities with regard to amphetamines and 'party drugs'. This may take the form of convening steering committees or holding community forums. Community partnerships between local, state, and federal governments, private enterprise and industry and community agencies and individuals are seen as essential. The City of Moreland, for example, seems to have taken a partnership approach that 'is working to

---

831 Although the forum was hosted by and located in the City of Knox, the only representative *directly* employed as a local government officer was Ms Neville who came from the neighbouring Shire of Yarra Ranges, one of the biggest interface local government areas (LGAs) in Victoria. An interface LGA is one that straddles both rural or semi-rural and outer suburban areas.

832 Ms Kym Neville, Shire of Yarra Ranges, evidence given to the Drugs and Crime Prevention Committee, Inquiry into Amphetamine and 'Party Drug' Use in Victoria, Public Hearing (City of Knox), 11 November 2003.

create the social, physical and economic environments that can best minimise the effects of these drugs in the community'.[833] The Council's submission continues that its Drug and Alcohol Plan:

> [enables] people to have access to a broad range of leisure activities, community information and community support to reduce the misuse of such drugs. Through facilitating partnerships with such groups as schools, police, liquor licensees, community health services and community organisations Council can assist collaborative strategies to be developed to address drug and alcohol misuse issues.
>
> Moreland City Council has [also] established a 'Moreland Health, Safety and Wellbeing Leadership Group' which brings together senior people from a range of government agencies and local services including VicPolice, Department of Education, VicRoads, community health services and hospitals. This group provides advice on emerging issues in the community and initiates partnership action to address them. The Leadership Group has provided input to the development of our Municipal Public Health Plan and the associated Community Safety Plan. Such forums facilitated by Local Government can provide a powerful mechanism for collaborative action at a local level. The extent of specific action on amphetamine and 'party' drugs would depend on having a good understanding of the local issues, the extend to which 'general drug strategies' can pick up on the more specific drug use issues and resources made available.[834]

Addressing amphetamines and 'party drugs' – Local initiatives

With regard to the specific issue of amphetamines and 'party drugs' a very few number of Councils have initiated programmes that, while largely generalist in nature, do try and address some of the specific issues surrounding these drugs, particularly from a harm reduction focus. The following are some examples.

City of Maribyrnong

The City of Maribyrnong based in the western suburbs of Melbourne has stated to the Committee:

> Access to local information on broader 'drug' use is either very limited, or unavailable. Council is currently undertaking a substance misuse needs assessment which will broaden the focus to licit drugs such as the prevalence of overuse of prescription drugs. Through this research we will attempt to collect evidence based data on drug use, and develop a better understanding of the local 'drug' use issues within our municipality. The local needle and syringe program, Western Region AIDS and Hepatitis C Prevention Program (WRAP) will be contributing to this research by conducting a survey of their clients on the types of drugs currently being used. This will help inform the

---

833 Submission of the City of Moreland to the Drugs and Crime Prevention Committee, Inquiry into Amphetamine and 'Party Drug' Use in Victoria, October 2003.

834 Ibid.

> extent of amphetamine and "party" drug use within this client group. Anecdotal evidence suggests that "party" drugs are not the drugs of choice by WRAP clients, but rather heroin, amphetamines and methamphetamines are commonly used. The injection of prescription drugs such as morphine tablets and benzodiazepines (for example temazepam is also practiced).[835]

They have also produced a Drug Information Kit:

> To date internal reviews of the drug strategy and anecdotal evidence has shown that Council and its strategy partners have conducted effective community education and information dissemination programs. These have included the development and distribution of a Council drug information kit which includes an information booklet "Understanding Drugs", a pamphlet on safer handling of syringes and postcards explaining Council's syringe collection hotline. This has been translated into 12 different languages. Community education sessions on drug awareness, safer handling and blood borne virus management have been delivered to schools, community groups, traders, child care centre and Council staff by Council and local drug and alcohol service providers. WRAP has implemented education sessions aimed at injecting drug users accessing their service.[836]

As stated in Chapter 18 in areas such as Maribyrnong with high levels of people who speak languages other than English, it is crucial that such materials are not only linguistically accessible but also culturally appropriate.

City of Stonnington Accord and the Nightclub Precinct

As has been discussed previously some local government authorities have devised accords between the Council, police and emergency services and local nightclub and licensed venues. Many of these accords, however, are specifically tailored to issues pertaining to alcohol and alcohol-related problems. This is understandable given that alcohol is a much more widely used and in many ways problematic drug than the illicit drugs. Nonetheless, in many areas, particularly those in which there is a high proportion of dance party and nightclub venues, 'party drugs' are increasingly posing problems for local authorities.

The City of Stonnington, which includes the nightclub strips in Chapel Street and Commercial and Toorak Roads, Prahran, has attempted to deal with the problems associated with illicit drugs by developing a collaborative accord with police and local venues. Although titled a 'Liquor Accord' it does include policies by which participants in the Accord can address illicit drug use and have their premises audited for compliance with the voluntary code and guidelines.[837]

---

835 Submission of the City of Maribyrnong to the Drugs and Crime Prevention Committee, Inquiry into Amphetamine and 'Party Drug' Use in Victoria, October 2003.

836 Ibid.

837 See City of Stonnington, Safe Venues Liquor Accord, 2003, City of Stonnington.

The Accord promotes a harm reduction approach to drug use, for example through participating premises making cold water readily available, having well trained 'first aiders' on site and each venue having a drink spiking deterrence policy.[838] At the same time the Accord emphatically states that drug dealing and drug usage are not to be tolerated on venue premises. Such an approach according to Professor Steve Allsop of the Western Australian Drug and Alcohol Office (DAO) is not contradictory:

> I think it [such strategies] can be seen as inconsistent but I don't think it necessarily is so. It is illegal to 'speed' but we also have strategies to try and reduce and discourage this. It is illegal for people to allow drugs on their premises, I think it is still legitimate to say, "we don't accept that we will have drugs on our premises, we will also have strategies to prevent people doing themselves harm from drug use".
>
> In fact, a large amount of harm from drug use doesn't occur from drugs that are used on the premises... A lot of people will actually use the drugs before they go to the venue so that they are less likely to get charged with possession. So in fact I think we can have both messages. I think we can have a message that it is not appropriate to allow drug use on your premises and also to have strategies to prevent people doing themselves harm if they choose to ignore the law.[839]

Ms Eleanor Costello, also with the DAO, states that increasingly both local government and venue operators will view such accords and collaborative approaches as in their best interests:

> They [venue owners] have started acknowledging even amongst security staff and amongst their own venues, issues with just not being able to control the situation and recognising that there is something else needed. And they are recognising that they need to do something about it ...[840]

This has certainly been recognised by Matthew Deveson, part owner of the ZoS Night Club in Chapel Street, Prahran, one of Melbourne's biggest dance venues. When he met with the Committee he extolled the virtues of collaborative ventures such as the Stonnington Accord:

> We have spent a lot of energy and time developing a Safe Venues Accord with the police and other licensees in Stonnington... I work very closely with the district [police] inspector on developing our policies, and the policy we have is a two-tiered approach. Firstly, drug dealing is prohibited and what we do is evict dealers and give the information to the police. We have about 35 cameras throughout the venue, and that footage is kept for about six weeks... We also do feel that our duty of care does extend beyond our walls... We try to work

838 For a copy of the Illicit drug section of the Accord, see Appendix 31.

839 Professor Steve Allsop, DAO, in conversation with the Drugs and Crime Prevention Committee, 1 October 2003.

840 Ms Eleanor Costello, DAO, in conversation with the Drugs and Crime Prevention Committee, Perth, 1 October 2003.

> with the resources of the community available to us. We have installed a camera on our roof that overlooks a particular nasty corner, and that has dial-up capability to the police station, so the police can dial up and look at that camera 24-hours a day and see the images, as well as check on what happened there three or four weeks ago. Also we provide security guards that escort people to the car park as well, but it is a community problem and we try to get involved through the accord, which is a fantastic initiative for tackling the problems. If everybody is working together, including the community resident groups, the licensees, the police, even Vicroads, we have a much better chance of solving the community problems on the outside as well.[841]

ZoS Nightclub has also employed Mr Ben Horan as a dedicated harm reduction/first aid officer to oversee and monitor the club during the busier nights of the week. Mr Horan explains his role in promoting harm reduction strategies as follows:

> I have been lucky in joining ZoS as, particularly this year, they have taken a number of initiatives that are rare in other venues, but I hope they become more commonplace.
>
> To deal with your amphetamine side of issues, you are typically worried about dehydration, hyperthermia and similar things. ZoS has installed a chilled water cooler in the nightclub area that is available free to all patrons, so if patrons need to refill their water bottles or get a cool drink, that is available to them without any hassles. ZoS also has installed a number of additional coolers and exhaust fans around the main dance area, so unlike a lot of clubs where you walk in and feel like you are melting – it becomes a very hot, clammy environment – we have taken that issue of overheating almost away by keeping the whole club at a generally much more comfortable level. There are numerous seated areas and relaxation areas available. At present there is a female powder room as well. So there are numerous places where patrons can relax, cool down, just have a rest and revive.
>
> ZoS employs me on their main nights basically to patrol in a first aid and harm-reduction role. My job is to detect anything from possible symptoms of drink-spiking victims right through to GHB and depressant overdoses or chronic effects and to take a non-judgemental intervention into that just to ensure that patrons leave ZoS happy and healthy wherever possible.[842]

The club's sense of being a good 'corporate citizen' has even extended to them commissioning Dr Cameron Duff of the Australian Drug Foundation to do research at the club 'to help us develop our strategies for going forward'.[843]

---

841 Mr Matthew Deveson, ZoS Nightclub, in conversation with the Drugs and Crime Prevention Committee, 10 November 2003.

842 Mr Ben Horan, ZoS Nightclub, in evidence to the Drugs and Crime Prevention Committee, 10 November 2003.

843 Mr Matthew Deveson, ZoS Nightclub, in evidence to the Drugs and Crime Prevention Committee, 10 November 2003.

The City of Stonnington and the venues such as ZoS with which it is associated in this collaborative process are to be commended for their attempts to reduce the use and abuse of illicit drugs in the local community.

City of Melbourne –Licensed Venue Workshops

The City of Melbourne in conjunction with VIVAIDS is developing information sessions targeting 'party drug' use for licensed venues owners in the Melbourne municipality. In a submission to the Committee the Council states:

> A series of workshops will be facilitated by Council to raise awareness and provide information on the effects of party drugs in venues. The workshop will provide up to date information on practices to encourage safe club environments for clients under the influence of 'party' drugs and to anticipate and address possible problematic situations or behaviours associated with drug affected clients.
>
> It is anticipated that these pilot workshops will be run on a needs basis with venue staff and management and developed to incorporate the needs of staff in venues likely to attract 'party' drug users.[844]

Family and Community Strengthening Programmes[845]

Many Councils have testified to the importance of family and community strengthening programmes as one way of helping to prevent the uptake of illicit (and licit) drugs. Moreland City Council, for example, has stated that 'The availability of early intervention and family support programs are key strategies for addressing misuse of drugs'.[846] As such they have developed the Moonah Community Strengthening Project, facilitating it in a public housing estate in Brunswick. The programmes that are part of the project are aimed at preventing and/or addressing 'poor social, economic and environmental behaviours and conditions, including drug misuse'.[847] Similarly the Shire of Yarra Ranges has implemented the 'Best Start' Project in lower socio-economic areas of the Shire:

> This project aims to improve the social, emotional and physical well-being of children aged between birth and 8 years, improve the capacity and

844 Submission of City of Melbourne to the Drugs and Crime Prevention Committee, Inquiry into Amphetamine and 'Party Drug' Use in Victoria, October 2003.

845 Similar programmes have been instigated in the school system, often under the auspices of the Health Promoting Schools Framework. Such programmes, as with local government family strengthening projects :

'[a]round resilience, values, bullying and personal skills ensure that young people are connected to the school, by feeling safe, by developing positive self regard, and by having an adult and a peer group to whom they can relate. Crucial times such as transition from primary to secondary school where young people are vulnerable to risk-taking behaviours, including experimenting with drug use, are times when teachers especially deliver drug education programs which concentrate on the positive aspects of decision making and life-long skills' (Submission of the Catholic Education Office to the Drugs and Crime Prevention Committee, Inquiry into Amphetamine and 'Party Drug' Use in Victoria, October 2003).

846 Submission of the City of Moreland to the Drugs and Crime Prevention Committee, Inquiry into Amphetamine and 'Party Drug' Use in Victoria, October 2003.

847 Ibid.

> competency of parents and carers, and assist communities to become more child friendly.[848]

Community participation and information provision

Some councils have produced Drug and Alcohol Projects that are based on community development models in which the main aim is the reduction of alcohol and drug-related harms through the encouragement of community participation. An example of one received by the Committee by way of submission is that produced by the City of Monash. Similarly some councils have been instrumental in developing Alcohol and Drug 'Expos', particularly aimed at parents, teachers and young people. Ms Kym Neville from the Shire of Yarra Ranges spoke to the Committee about the Expo held by the Shire:

> At [the] expos we also talked a lot about amphetamine and party drug use and drink spiking... We want to roll that out into a number of schools. That expo targeted parents. However, at our expo we did have a number of young people. Parents brought their kids along, which was good. We are hoping that we can do a similar thing in a number of schools and target both young people and their parents, but perhaps the parents after hours and the young people for maybe a half-a-day activity, and get key speakers in. But we want to make it fun, not preach to these kids. We want to talk to them about what the real issues are, but make it a bit of fun, and give them some responsibility and input into the day.[849]

Community workers recognise that in this particular area of drug education, dissemination and promotion of harm reduction and prevention material can be difficult. For example, Doutta Galla Community Health Services based in the inner north of Melbourne argues that one of the difficulties in getting drug education messages across to 'party drug' users is the fact that these people rarely associate themselves with 'drug users':

> This creates a challenge when packaging educational resources. The resource must be presented in a format that is conducive to the users' way of thinking – ie. does not identify them as 'illicit drug users' – and it is recommended that it is presented by peers from the dance party scene.
>
> This also highlights the limited services available to party users when drug use becomes an issue; they would be unlikely to consult drug and alcohol services and be more likely to go to their local General Practitioner (GP). Identifying the drug use may be difficult for the GP as the symptoms of lack of appetite, sleep deprivation may be diagnosed as depression. There is limited study into the

---

848 Submission of the Shire of Yarra Ranges to the Drugs and Crime Prevention Committee, Inquiry into Amphetamine and 'Party Drug' Use in Victoria, October 2003.

849 Ms Kym Neville, Shire of Yarra Ranges, evidence given to the Drugs and Crime Prevention Committee, Inquiry into Amphetamine and 'Party Drug' Use in Victoria, Public Hearings (City of Knox), 11 November 2003.

effects when anti depressants and ecstasy are combined. Some evidence suggests that it can have an adverse reaction.[850]

Given the important role local authorities play with regard to these issues pertaining to licit and illicit drugs in their jurisdiction, including amphetamine and 'party drugs', the Committee makes the following recommendations:

Recommendations

54. The Committee recognises that the problems amphetamine and 'party drug' users experience are caused by a range of social and economic variables as well as the use of the drug itself. The Committee therefore recommends that a key focus of Government policy should be the development of programmes which engage vulnerable groups in recreation, leisure, family strengthening and support, and community projects to support health, safety and economic well-being generally. Such programmes should be targeted at a local level.

    Such programmes should be supported along the continuum of prevention, early intervention and treatment services for groups and individuals that are vulnerable to substance misuse.

55. The Committee recommends that commensurate with their powers and responsibilities, local councils should ensure raves, dance parties and clubs and other venues fulfil the appropriate regulatory requirements applicable to the conduct of such activities. These include but are not restricted to issues such as the availability of medical advice and support, ventilation and appropriate use of space, availability of free drinking water, food, toilets, chill-out spaces, transport and general amenity considerations (such as parking and noise).

56. The Committee recommends that those local government authorities, licensees and club owners who have not produced or are not currently a member of a Licensee and Safety Accord or equivalent should endeavour to formulate or become part of such an accord.

57. The Committee recommends that all accords should also include reference to and strategies for managing illicit drugs, particularly amphetamines and 'party drugs'. To date, most Licensee Accords concentrate solely on alcohol.

850 Submission of Doutta Galla Community Health Services to the Drugs and Crime Prevention Committee, Inquiry into Amphetamine and 'Party Drug' Use in Victoria, August 2002.

Work Hard Play Safe – A harm reduction initiative from Hong Kong

The Committee includes one example of a harm reduction initiative from overseas because of its unique nature. The Work Hard Play Safe Team are a group of outreach workers employed by the Caritas Youth and Community Service in Hong Kong. Rave culture and associated 'party drug use' is very popular in Hong Kong with as many as crowds of 4000 to 5000 clubbers packing dance party venues to capacity on Friday and Saturday nights (Chan Wai Leung 2003, p.1).

Most ravers and clubbers in Hong Kong use ecstasy and ketamine; other drugs, including GHB are apparently rare (Chan Wai Leung 2003, p.4). Of interest is the fact that, according to recent surveys of Hong Kong clubbers, an overwhelming majority would only ever use 'party drugs' at raves or clubs and 'despise those who use ecstasy or ketamine in other places and at other times. They consider these people to be the real drug users' (Chan Wai Leung 2003, p.6).

The unique nature of the Work Hard Play Safe project lies in its extensive outreach initiatives. A team of three full-time and one part-time social workers and nurses are present at venues on Friday and Saturday nights. They set up mobile stations outside the venues and have workers and volunteers present inside the clubs:

> Young drug users will never say they need help or go out to seek it. Therefore meeting them in their gathering place is one of the most effective ways to understand, locate and connect with them.
>
> Each working night our workers would be stationed in or outside the venue. We would wear a uniform so that the young people could identify us. In order to facilitate the initial person-to-person contact, we would give the young people some trendy and useful souvenir as a personal gift, like wet tissues (useful in the hot and humid dance venue, or after snorting ketamine) and a neck pocket (for them to use to store their belongings inside the venue). This outreach approach established an appropriate culture context for the worker and young people to build relations and communicate (Chan Wai Leung 2003, p.9).

Such an outreach approach is not very different from that taken by groups such as RaveSafe. The novel aspect of this project is the use of the 'mobile centre'. This seven-seater car serves as a recreational leisure centre (videos and games provided), a 'library' with useful drug and harm reduction information supplied, a counselling service, an escort service in case of emergencies and most importantly an on-site health check service (see Gosling 2003). Partygoers can take advantage of the latter service for a free check up, which may include having their pulse, body temperature, blood oxygen levels, hand/eye co-ordination measured and blood pressure taken. Participants received a copy of their health record which they could bring back the following weekend to monitor their health status. Many people who had had check-ups took the initiative to later obtain a full medical check-up.

Gosling claims that initially 'Western' approaches to harm reduction that focussed solely on drug use were evaluated as culturally inappropriate to Hong Kong's young clubbers. Most users resisted talking about their drug use or claimed they did not use any:

> In contrast, the concept of health promotion is a familiar concept in Chinese society. People use a variety of ways to keep healthy on a day to day basis, such as drinking health soup or using Chinese herbs. So the Caritas program highlighted ways to reduce the harmful effects of Party Drugs, such as drinking iced lemon tea or using Chinese herbs to detoxify.
>
> Leveraging the health approach made it possible for the Caritas team to create a more acceptable and less threatening atmosphere for young drug users to talk about their drug use.
>
> The health checks provided a framework, a direct and undeniable demonstration of the physical effects the drugs were having on the young people attending clubs and taking these drugs.
>
> This stark realisation of the state of their health would sometimes represent a turning point for young drug users and make them reconsider their drug habit (Gosling 2003, pp.14–15).

The Committee does not necessarily believe that a programme such as Work Hard Play Safe can be simplistically extrapolated to a different cultural milieu such as Victoria. Nonetheless, there are certainly elements of the programme such as the use of the 'mobile centre' that it would seem could be usefully incorporated into the work of agencies such as RaveSafe.

Pill testing

Sometimes harm reduction advice is clearly not going to be palatable to some members of the community, least of all the popular media.[851] Any distaste may be as much for the way the advice is expressed and the language used as for the content of the message.

An aspect of harm reduction that is bound to be viewed as controversial is that of the testing of psychostimulants such as ecstasy, a form of 'quality control' for which there are both committed supporters and trenchant detractors.

851 A submission from the Eastern Drug and Alcohol Service argues: 'that the scare mongering that occurs in the media inhibits the development of appropriate harm minimisation strategies that would foster a pragmatic approach to reducing the harms associated with use. For instance environmental changes in clubs and dance venues' (Submission of the Eastern Drug and Alcohol Service to the Drugs and Crime Prevention Committee, Inquiry into Amphetamine and 'Party Drug' Use in Victoria, August 2002).

The testing of psychostimulant drugs, either through self 'testing kits' used by the consumer[852] or at testing stations conducted at dance venues is clearly problematic:

> You want a good night out, the people running the rave or nightclub don't want you swallowing anything really nasty. So here's the deal. You provide a crumb or two of your ecstasy pills for the checkers to inspect and test. They tell you what they think the pills contain and what the risks of swallowing them might be.
>
> Depending on who you talk to, it's either a pragmatic way to curb the harm ecstasy tablets can do or a dubious step toward quality control for illicit drugs that can only create more users (Ainsworth 2002, p.32).

Pill testing in overseas jurisdictions

In some countries (Spain, Holland, Austria, France and Germany) drug screening at raves, clubs and venues, if not approved by the state, is at least unofficially sanctioned in the interests of preventing fatalities and casualties caused through the use of adulterated tablets.[853] Even in the United States the private sector organisation 'Dance Safe' has worked in collaboration with law enforcement authorities to ensure clubbers who produce pills for testing are not arrested for possession. Dance Safe is fairly typical of testing organisations. It is based in Berkeley, California and present in at least eight major American cities:

> *Dance Safe* sets up tables at raves, where users can get information about drugs and also have ecstasy pills tested... A Dance Safe worker shaves off a sliver of the tablet and drops a solution on to it; if it doesn't turn black quickly, it's not MDMA.

---

852 Such testing kits have been available in Australia for some time, often sold in music and record or clothing stores for approximately $25.00. For example, a test called 'E – a Quick and Simple Test' was developed in 2001 by a consortium of Melbourne chemists called Chemical Generation (see *User News* 2001, p.3). Other testing kits including those produced by Dance Safe are purchasable from the United States and Holland via the Internet (Shannon 2002, p.24).

A Sydney based group called 'Enlighten' also provides free substance testing at dance events and sells test kits:

'Enlighten is a volunteer organisation dedicated to raising safety awareness in the dance community. It is an organisation founded and run by "people like you" [users/clubbers]... [This] grassroots organisation provides data sheets on ecstasy, GHB, LSD and substance test kits. Knowledge about responsible substance testing is absolutely key information...' (Thomas 2003, p.10).

Other testing kits available on the market in Australia or via the Internet include E1 (Marquis reagent), E2 (2nd Defence) produced by Chemical Generation (Australia), EZ Test (UK and Europe), Green Party (UK) Test Kit and DanceSafe Kits (USA).

For an account of these various tests, see Submission of Victoria Police to the Drugs and Crime Prevention Committee, Inquiry into Amphetamine and 'Part Drug' Use in Victoria, October 2003.

853 In 2001 the Drugs and Crime Prevention Committee of the 54th Parliament visited the Vienna Social Projects Association. Since 1997 the Association has operated an innovative project 'Check it!' In addition to testing drug substances in an on-site laboratory during 'raves', the project has a strong prevention component. Street workers offer information and counselling to the ravers on ecstasy and other drugs. In the tent where samples are handed in, information and counselling is provided, as well as seats, drinking water and a 'relaxation zone'.

> The organisation has found that as much as 20% of the so-called ecstasy sold at raves contains something other than MDMA. Dance Safe also tests pills for anonymous users who send in samples from around the nation; it has found that 40% of those pills are fake. Late last year, Dance Safe workers attended a 'massive'...rave in Oakland, Calif. Nine people were taken from the rave in ambulances, but Dance Safe confirmed that eight of the nine had taken pills that weren't MDMA (Cloud 2000, p.52).

Not all commentators are as enthused by either the testing kits or drug screening conducted at dance parties. Claims are made that these tests can be imprecise and create a dangerous and false sense of security among users:

> The commonest method, called the 'Marquis test', involves scraping some of the pill into a colourless reagent containing sulphuric acid and formaldehyde. MDMA turns the reagent violet/purple and then slowly blue/black. The problem is that some ingredients in fake ecstasy pills trigger the same colour changes. Others, such as PMA, cause no colour change at all. So tablets made of these will pass the test provided they contain a trace of MDMA (Ainsworth 2000, p.32).

To circumvent these uncertainties, the Netherlands has utilised more sophisticated testing methods:[854]

> While stopping ad hoc chemical testing in nightclubs, it runs an official pill testing service at 23 drug prevention and treatment centres. Dutch ecstasy users can take their pills to any of these centres, where trained employees note down the pills' colour, dimensions and logo, and run a Marquis test. They then log on to a database that holds details of all the pills tested more rigorously by an independent lab service in the previous six weeks. If the pill doesn't match any of the known profiles, it can be sent off for rigorous testing and added to the database. Any evidence about potentially dangerous pills is available to clubbers within days (Ainsworth 2000, p.32).

Pill testing in Australia – support and opposition

'Pill testing' in Australia, particularly through the use of self-testing kits, is also

---

854 Since 1992, the Netherlands government has funded the Drug Information and Monitoring System (DIMS) As an official part of Dutch drug policy, one of DIMS' tasks is to chemically analyse ecstasy pills:

'Users anonymously submit tablets at one of 23 offices, where trained employees note down the pills' colour, dimensions and logo. They then log on to an Internet database that holds details of all the pills tested in the previous six weeks. If the pill does not match any known profile, it is sent off for laboratory testing and added to the dataset. The contents of a pill are available to clubbers within days' (Webb 2003, p.126).

Winstock, Wolff and Ramsey 2001 describe the technicalities of the Dutch system as follows:

'Preliminary analysis is by thin layer chromatography (TLC) followed by gas chromatography (GC) with nitrogen phsoporus detection for quantification and GC-mass spectrometry for identification of any unknown compounds. Any worrying findings (unusually high dose pills or the presence of unusual compounds) are made the subject of warning notices which are distributed to the relevant venues' (Winstock, Wolff & Ramsey 2001, pp. 1143–1144. See also van de Wijngaart et al. 1999; van Laar & Spruit 1997).

In some cases DIMS has launched public news campaigns 'directed at producers...in order to persuade them to withhold their pills from being marketed and to adjust the doses' (van Laar & Spruit 1997, p.264).

contentious. Agencies such as Bluelight advertise testing kits on their web site, publish test 'alerts' advising of potentially dangerous batches of drugs in circulation and hosts Internet forums whereby users and forum participants can seek advice or swap information with regard to the pills they are using.[855]

Opinions with regard to pill testing tend to be (fairly predictably, but not exclusively) divided between those working in the area of health and harm reduction (RaveSafe type organisations, user groups, some health agencies) who give qualified support and those in law enforcement and state agencies who would generally oppose such measures. Yet ambivalence is found among even those who have harm reduction uppermost as part of their brief. For example, Ms Simone Cormack of the DASC in South Australia expresses a disquiet that is fairly typical of those working in the field:

> This issue has come up quite recently in our steering committee for our party drugs project. I would suggest that there are benefits to looking at trials in this area to see the impact but it needs to go ahead within a more sophisticated environment of understanding the risks and problems associated with it. This needs to be more fully discussed with groups like police and all the concerns need to be sorted out before such a trial might proceed. We would see it potentially as something you would use to engage in brief intervention, taking that opportunity to interact with users. It is a carrot, if you like, for doing that. There are enormous risks that have to be considered around it as well, from my point of view, in terms of these projects.
>
> We are preparing a discussion paper at the moment on the matter, to raise the level of debate about this, certainly in government but in all the stakeholder groups. What I have found, when some of the concerns about pill testing come up with participants in rave scenes, is that it is an 'Aha!' experience. They have not thought through the problems it might cause. Certainly the commercial pill testing kits are anything but definitive and potentially quite dangerous if there is any confusion about what they are telling you. They might tell you about the presence of a drug but not all the other drugs that may be in it. What we have found, in talking about a discussion paper raising the issues and canvassing the issues, is that the user groups themselves are also second-thinking about whether they want it.
>
> I think there are a number of issues. What we would like to do is raise the level of debate, have perhaps a more informed discussion with people in the community as well as groups like the police, and consider whether or not we could put together a trial. It is important that it would be rigorously evaluated in terms of unintended consequences before we go ahead with it. Certainly I am not dismissive of them. I think there is potential. It is just not the time.[856]

---

855 See www. bluelight. nu, www.pillreports.com, www.enlighten.com. For an example of a web forum with regard to pill testing, see Appendix 32.

856 Ms Simone Cormack, DASC in conversation with the Drugs and Crime Prevention Committee, Adelaide, 3 October 2003.

Although recognising some of the uncertainties associated with pill testing, Mr David Murray, Executive Officer with the Victorian YSAS, gives some qualified support to the idea as a way of giving users valuable knowledge about which drugs *not* to take:

> The notion of providing people with information about what they can expect is important, particularly around the likely adverse results of use of amphetamines. One of the key issues here in relation to all illicit substance use is that people are taking substances of which they do not know the contents, either in terms of the purity or the actual content.
>
> This leads to the point around pill testing. You have undoubtedly heard the toing and froing of arguments around pill testing. There needs to be some consideration given to the availability of pill testing, given what I previously said about a demography of users who are using in the knowledge of the risks and harms, but often using substances, the contents of which they have absolutely no idea about. Much of what is marketed as ecstasy we know is speed, not ecstasy at all, and there are other even more dangerous substances that are mixed within these pills and marketed as ecstasy.
>
> Therefore we understand there is a paradox that is contained within harm reduction. On the one hand you do not want people to use these substances because they are dangerous; but on the other hand there is a need to have some type of process by which they can do so more safely. We understand the paradox, but we think, just the same, that there is evidence from overseas – from the Netherlands in particular – to suggest that this is an effective strategy for dealing with the harms associated with the use of these types of drugs.[857]

Tony Palmer, also from YSAS, acknowledges that the accuracy of pill testing can be low but believes there are:

> [s]ome examples of where drug testing would have been useful. The paramethoxyamphetamine deaths that were occurring in the United States would undoubtedly have been picked up by the test because it would have informed you that you were not actually taking MDMA.
>
> So although the test is not specific enough to give you actual information about the substance you are using, what it does do is tell the tester that it is not what you purchased; it is not what it was advertised as.
>
> We are saying that in combination with groups like RaveSafe and other things that were already happening, like Internet alerts, you would eventually come up with a system that would warn people that there are substances out there, that this is the description of pills, we have seen them before, and they contain toxic substances like paramethamphetamine (PMA), for example.
>
> There was a large batch [of PMA] in the United States that was being marketed as ecstasy, even down to being stamped with the Mitsubishi sign, which was

857 Mr David Murray, YSAS, evidence given to the Drugs and Crime Prevention Committee, Inquiry into Amphetamine and 'Party Drug' Use in Victoria, Public Hearings (Melbourne), 27 October 2003.

> a common and popular sign on the ecstasy pill at that time. And PMA has this unfortunate profile in that when you take a standard recreational dose you get what appears to be a very weak ecstasy effect.
>
> What we have therefore assumed is then happening is that people have taken a pill, have had that weak effect, have assumed it is really weak ecstasy, and so have then gone back and brought a couple more pills. The real problem with PMA is that the difference between a recreational dose and a toxic dose is very small, so people would then overdose and be in a critical condition. I think there were 10 deaths in the United States in one year from PMA being marketed as ecstasy.
>
> Those tests would be able to inform testers of that fact, and if we started a system of alerts between, say, police forensics, between the testers and using the Internet you would actually have quite a sophisticated alert system.
>
> ... I am not suggesting that we test for PMA, I am saying that you have purchased a pill you believed was ecstasy; the test can tell you whether it is or is not. If it is not, then you have a second tier where you look at your Internet alerts and the information that is coming out of forensics; and when you start to combine these, you get a convergence of data that then gives you a risk profile around a particular pill.[858]

The formal written submission of YSAS to this Inquiry puts their support of pill testing into recommendation form as follows:

> Consistent with a harm minimisation approach, users in Victoria should be able to quickly test and verify any substances being sold as MDMA/ecstasy in order to reduce the risks associated with 'party drug' use. One of the hazards associated with MDMA/ecstasy use is the unknown content of the pills. On-site testing facilities at venues in Holland enable the provision of accurate information to users and medical support staff in relation to the contents of pills submitted for testing, and potentially prevent adverse reactions through a system of 'alerts'. The provision of testing facilities has also been found to reduce the incidence of substance use (van de Wijngaart et al.).[859]

Legal writer, Timothy Webb, states that government analytical laboratories in Australia only analyse 'party drug' pills for police prosecution or forensic reasons. He argues that such laboratories should be using their technology to test pills for harm reduction purposes as in Holland:

> [Australian laboratories] could analyse a far greater number of ecstasy pills and publicly disseminate the results via an Internet database. There are several ways the drug could be acquired: users could discard pills into 'amnesty bins' placed in clubs;[860] users could anonymously mail pills to the laboratory; or legislative

858 Mr Tony Palmer, YSAS, evidence given to the Drugs and Crime Prevention Committee, Inquiry into Amphetamine and 'Party Drug' Use in Victoria, Public Hearings (Melbourne), 27 October 2003.

859 Submission of YSAS to the Drugs and Crime Prevention Committee, Inquiry into Amphetamine and 'Party Drug' Use in Victoria, October 2003.

860 For a discussion of the use of such dance party 'amnesty bins' for the purposes of toxicological research in London, see Ramsey et al. 2001.

> amendment could allow licensed individuals to collect street samples from dealers.
>
> Such a proposal has numerous advantages. First, it would alert users to the range of dangerous adulterants present in ecstasy. The information would also allow users to adopt suitable harm reduction practices for pills that do contain MDMA. Second, the data would be invaluable to emergency departments. Ecstasy users that present to hospital can require vastly differing treatment depending on the substance ingested. Third, and most persuasively, the proposal would assist drug law enforcement. The Australian Bureau of Criminal Intelligence admits that drug testing provides much useful information: seizures can be linked by comparative analysis to assist prosecutions; the grouping of otherwise unconnected samples can indicate a common source; insight can be gained on the extent of local production compared with importation; and drug purity can be an indicator of the economic behaviour of the market. With the ultimate success of law enforcement operations 'arguably more dependent upon the availability of good intelligence than on any other single factor', laboratory data on ecstasy could become an essential police resource.
>
> A concern may be that the availability of purity data may encourage the use of ecstasy. Dutch studies have shown, however, that ecstasy use was not higher, and was sometimes even lower, in those places where testing facilities were available. Even in the absence of such reassurance, the proposal is still worthwhile. Legislators must ask: would they prefer to see a 5 per cent reduction in use if this meant a 5 per cent increase in harm, or a 5 per cent reduction in harm if this meant 5 per cent increase in use? With harm reduction a central plank of Australia' national drug policy since 1985, the latter option must be preferable. Furthermore, by helping users to minimise neurotoxicity and mortality, laboratory pill testing addresses the fundamental justifications for prohibiting MDMA in the first place (Webb 2003, pp.126–128).

One of the arguments that is used in support of pill testing is the multiplicity of logos that adorn ecstasy tablets. It is argued that users:

> [p]erceive labels or brands as symbols that distinguish between 'good and 'bad' tablets and help the user to identify the specific types of effects…that one should expect from a particular brand (McElrath & McEvoy 2002, p.205).

Testing, it is argued, can assist users to not be lulled into such a false and misguided sense of 'quality control'. Ironically, it is the fact that some users may believe some pills safer than others that can contribute to some critics thinking pill testing is superfluous or of dubious value (Winstock, Wolff & Ramsey 2001). Certainly testing or at least checking testing web sites and alerts is one of the ways in which clubbers may prepare during the 'planning phase' discussed in Chapter 10.

> 'When we started taking them [ecstasy] we looked up on the internet every bit of information on Es to find out what roughly, the effects were. We tried to work out what a safe dose was, we tried to work out what we were taking, 'cos

> there's so many different sorts. We tried to get as clued up as we could' (Female 'clubber', quoted in Malbon 1999, p.120).[861]

Carol Bennett, Executive Officer of the Victorian Alcohol and Drug Association (VAADA) also acknowledges that there is a degree of division among agencies within the alcohol and drug sector over pill testing:

> That was very much highlighted through our party drugs symposium, where you had very divided opinions about whether drug testing per se was a good thing or not.
>
> We thought about this for quite some time and decided that the issue is really about the kind of information that drug users receive. If you are putting people in a situation where they believe they are getting a certain type of information that may indicate the level of harm they might experience related to their drug use, then they need to have the information that will enable them to make that decision. That is why we came down in favour of information being available to drug users. Clearly the current testing system is inadequate in terms of the range of information it can provide, so it is important that users have information about the limitations of that – what it does not actually tell you.
>
> It is not that we do not support drug testing. We know that lots of young people do use that drug testing and that is the reality. I guess it is around quality control and if there was a quality mechanism for undertaking that testing where full information was provided to the users of those drugs then we would probably support that.[862]

---

861 One of the most comprehensive surveys of clubbers and their drug use (n = 760) was undertaken in Britain recently (Deehan & Saville 2003). Most of those interviewed were aware of the risks associated with 'party drugs', had actively sought out information about physical and mental health consequences and had taken measures which they believed would minimise those risks:

'Interviewees did recognise the potential health risks attached to drug taking. Most had sought out information to verify that their drug use was not physically or psychologically harmful and many felt they had developed risk reduction techniques to minimise the impact of their drug taking. However, whilst some of these were sensible and based on actual harm reduction strategies (eg. keeping hydrated), others were based on urban myths and not proven to be of any benefit (eg. taking vitamins)' (Deehan & Saville 2003, p.3).

862 Ms Carol Bennett, VAADA, evidence given to the Drugs and Crime Prevention Committee, Inquiry into Amphetamine and 'Party Drug' Use in Victoria, Public Hearings (Melbourne), 27 October 2003.

In VAADA's written submission to the Committee they gave some qualified support to the idea of testing as indicated in Ms Bennett's testimony quoted above. The submission states:

'VAADA has grappled with the vexed issue of pill testing. The work of non police based pill testing experts at parties is occurring and does enable users to test 'first hand' what is actually contained in pills. VAADA acknowledges, however, that this is an illegal activity. Pill testing experts argue that not only do they identify the most current data and statistics in relation to the content of ATS, but they can also inform law enforcement agencies and governments about what is currently available on the ATS market.

In addition, non police based pill testing experts are often one of the first to be made aware of the re-branding of different drugs under the one logo and can often portray this message to the authorities and also to users who would have otherwise believed they were buying a drug from the same 'batch' as previously bought due to the logo.

VAADA is of the view that pill testing is an area that should be addressed in terms of ensuring that users are aware of the strengths and limitations of the results' (Submission of VAADA to the Drugs and Crime Prevention Committee, Inquiry into Amphetamine and 'Party Drug' Use in Victoria, October 2003.

Victoria Police, however, leave no doubt as to their misgivings with regard to either official testing stations or self-test kits:

> Where persons establish drug testing stations at venues to test the purity of drugs before others use them, a number of issues are raised. The process of testing tablets may be perceived as giving a seal of approval to certain drugs, based on test results. As there is an element of potential harm in all drugs, this type of testing could send out the message that those drugs are safe to use, particularly when a so-called positive result is obtained.
>
> Irrespective of assertions that testing kits are a bona fide harm minimisation response, there may well be duty of care issues to be considered. If a person suffered serious harm or died after taking a substance that had been tested using a drug testing kit, the substance tester may face litigation for negligence.
>
> From a criminal law perspective,[863] the possession or trafficking in illicit drugs is an offence. Persons facilitating the testing of illicit drugs could arguably be viewed as aiding and abetting the commission of the offence, even if the user, who is already liable, actually conducts the test. Where a third person tests an illicit drug on behalf of a potential user, at the very least they commit an offence of possession of an illicit drug.[864]

A summary of Victoria Police's attitude towards testing kits in particular is presented in a written submission to this Inquiry:

- Producers and distributors of the ecstasy testing kit in Australia and overseas promote the kits as a harm minimisation approach claiming the harm associated with using ecstasy is reduced if users are able to determine if tablets/powder they intend to use is shown to contain ecstasy like substances such as MDMA, MDEA and MDA.
- It is important to note that adverse reactions, including death, have occurred when MDMA appears to have been the only drug used. Knowledge that MDMA is contained in the drug consumed is not enough to protect the user from adverse effects.

---

863 In Britain the legal position of pill testing is similar. Winstock, Wolff and Ramsey state:

'Since MDMA and many of the other drugs found within pills sold as ecstasy are controlled under the Misuse of Drugs Act in Class A, possession and supply are serious criminal offences carrying the risk of custodial sentence. It is difficult to see how onsite testing could be carried out without infringing the law. Merely handling a tablet to a third party for analysis could constitute supply, the law not recognizing a lower limit on how many drugs are required before an offence is committed. Laboratories carrying out this work in the United Kingdom are thus required to have licenses issued by the Home Office and these are unlikely to be granted for consumer-oriented testing. Those supporting testing suggest that law enforcement agencies could benefit from the information obtained by the regular analysis of new pills as they appear on the market; that is, as a means of profiling (fingerprinting) the chemical composition of a pill in a similar fashion to the forensic work of amphetamine profiling in the 1980s (Jonson & Stromberg, 1993; Rashed, Anderson & King, 2000). Such information is clearly useful, but we feel that it could be equally attainable by a more rigorous routine analysis of confiscated pills or those deposited in an amnesty bin' (Winstock, Wolff & Ramsey 2001, p.1146).

864 Superintendent Paul Ditchburn, Victoria Police, evidence given to the Drugs and Crime Prevention Committee, Inquiry into Amphetamine and 'Party Drug' Use in Victoria, Public Hearings (Melbourne), 10 November 2003.

- Based on available scientific evidence, drug testing kits currently on the market:
  - are not able to provide clear identification of a particular drug;
  - at best and when used under optimum conditions they provide an indication of a compound/drug class, which may be present;
  - no information is provided on the non drug components which may be present in a sample;
  - where drug mixtures are concerned (a common occurrence in street drugs) the results become misleading;
  - drug levels and toxicity are not addressed at all by this testing method – drug level (purity) and toxicity are critical issues in drug use and harm minimisation;
  - interpretation of the results is extremely subjective, and the variation inherent in this testing regime is a significant limitation;
  - a false sense of security is bestowed upon the user which may in fact increase the risk of drug taking; and
  - the kits themselves contain hazardous chemicals (concentrated acids) that would cause irritation, injury and damage upon contact with person (skin) or other surfaces.
- Given that the various testing kits available on the market match different colours to the chemical reaction which takes place when the reagent is applied to the substance, there is even more potential for the user to misinterpret the result. The user may rely on familiarity with a particular test, not realising that colour readings differ between the various kits and thus mis-interpret the results if using a new kit for the first time.[865]

Academic opinion

It is not just community representatives who are polarised over the issue of pill testing. Academics and medical professionals also seem divided over the utility and accuracy of testing, particularly self-testing kits. The medical and other academic journals, including their letters pages, air the opposing sides of the debates. For example, a relatively recent article by Winstock, Wolff and Ramsey (*Ecstasy pill testing: harm minimization gone too far?*) clearly shows misgivings about even some of the more sophisticated methods of testing ecstasy and other 'party drug' pills such as the state sponsored Check It programme in Vienna:

> A more recent innovation in Austria has been the use of high performance liquid chromatography (HPLC) equipment with diode array detection. This has been transported on site to large rave parties where accurate and rapid testing

865 Submission of Victoria Police (Drug and Alcohol Strategy Unit) to the Drugs and Crime Prevention Committee, Inquiry into Amphetamine and 'Party Drug' Use in Victoria, November 2003.

An opinion on the technical aspect of pill testing and pill testing kits prepared by Dr Cate Quinn, Manager Chemistry Unit, Victoria Forensic Services Centre is attached as Appendix 33.

> (15–30 minutes) has been performed with the aid of extensive technical support. The machines probably cost in the order of 35,000 [pounds sterling] each and require experienced laboratory personnel to operate them and interpret the results. The results are posted anonymously on a board and the individual consumer is able to identify his/her pill by means of a code. Although providing extensive information, this is a costly and time-consuming process that would be impractical to operate in a widespread manner (Winstock, Wolff & Ramsey 2001, p.1144).

It is not only the prohibitive costs that give the authors concern. The usefulness of the testing procedures, particularly those that are less sophisticated than those used in Austria and Holland, are open to question:

> Although the introduction of pill testing was seen initially as a means of monitoring pill composition and encouraging information exchange, for the user the primary concern was presumably to confirm the presence of MDMA in pills. It is possible that many users see such affirmation to imply quality and even 'purity'.
>
> There are three issues that need clarification for the user. First, colour-testing methods give no indication that many harmful substances may be present in the pill. Secondly, the user, even with the knowledge that a pill contains MDMA, is unable to gauge until after consumption what the true psychoactive effect of the tablet will be. Confirming that MDMA is present in a pill will not reduce the risk of idiosyncratic adverse effects (responsible for many of the MDMA associated fatalities, eg. from liver failure). Thirdly, colour tests gives no information regarding the strength of a pill and cannot differentiate between optical isomers and unless chiral chromatography is available, neither can HPLC or GC-MS. Precise isomeric composition of pills reflects the availability of the precursors and remains largely unknown.
>
> Furthermore, factors such as variations in metabolism caused by genetic differences cannot be identified through pill testing and such variation may contribute to individual vulnerability to adverse events (Tucker *et al.,* 1994; Kreth *et al.,* 2000). False reassurance through misinterpretation of the information that MDMA has been identified in a pill meaning it is a 'safe' pill is a particular worry.
>
> The belief that pill testing may be viewed as a harm reduction approach is based upon the assumption that the knowledge made available to users from testing will in some way influence their drug-taking and lead to behavioural change. However, evidence for this is not substantiated. In a recent study of over 1000 UK clubbers, subjects were asked how the quality of ecstasy pills would influence the amount of drug they consumed. Subjects indicated that if the quality of pills was considered to have become worse over 20% would take more, just over a third would take less, with 40% reporting no impact upon their ecstasy use. Conversely, and perhaps more worrying, if pills were thought to improve, 40% reported they would take more, just over 10% would take less, with nearly half reporting that it would make no difference to their use

> (Winstock, Griffiths & Stewart, 2000). Wijngaart *et al.* (1997) found the presence of testing facilities to be unrelated to participants' drug use and the consumption of ecstasy. In terms of harm reduction this finding could be interpreted as a failing of pill testing, since it suggests that the results have little impact upon reducing subsequent use.
>
> Viewed in the broader context of harm reduction, a pill testing service may be regarded as a pragmatic attempt at minimizing or avoiding consumption of potentially more harmful substances than MDMA. However, specific knowledge of this kind can only be achieved a priori with sophisticated laboratory techniques (HPLC or GC-MS) and not colour tests. There is paradox in prevention in that the potential for harm associated with use of dance drugs is mediated through the pattern and context of their use. Accepting this, the most significant harm reduction impact upon dance drug users could be achieved through detailed information on minimizing harm associated with use (Winstock, Wolff & Ramsey 2001, pp.1145–1146).

The concerns expressed in the Winstock article, although not necessarily refuted, were addressed by those who thought that any attempts to lessen the dangers associated with taking 'party drugs' are better than none at all. For example, a letter to the journal in which the Winstock article was placed (*Addiction*) responded soon after:

> On-site tablet testing allows harm reduction organizations to provide warnings about specific tablets circulating in the venue on that night rather than posting the findings on websites weeks or even months later. This could, potentially, prevent adverse reactions.
>
> The Marquis test is of extremely limited value in determining the precise contents of tablets but one must assume that it has more value than the assurances of a friend and/or drug dealer. The authors demonstrate that the Marquis test was able to identify correctly all tablets containing MDMA. No evidence is presented that the Marquis test would have given a false positive if it was used only to identify MDMA. This does not support their assertion that the Marquis test will identify MDMA incorrectly. Further work is required to determine if the Marquis test will identify false positives.
>
> Ecstasy users want to use MDMA and because of the wide publicity given to its adverse effects it is unlikely that they are unaware of the risks involved. The authors make a large number of assumptions about the beliefs and behaviour of ecstasy users that are not substantiated. A properly controlled trial is needed to determine if the presence of sophisticated tablet testing facilities (eg. HPLC) changes the incidence of adverse reactions to the use of ecstasy. The jury should remain out until these data are available (Cole 2002, p.231).

The jury may still be out, but the jury is also obviously divided. Drug testing, particularly that which is given the imprimatur of the state, is clearly contentious. Its advocates cite the number of lives saved through alerting users to adulterated drugs, particularly those containing PMA. It is viewed by some as a particularly useful service to users at festivals such as Earthcore where many attendees, who will in any case use 'party drugs', can have *some* level of assurance that their pills may not be adulterated According to Gowing et al., a further benefit is that such programmes have 'the opportunity to monitor trends in supply and rapidly respond to changes in the market' (2001, p.38). Its detractors view such schemes as simply a back-door method of decriminalising such drugs. Those critics who are not so concerned with the use of the drugs per se, may nonetheless have deep concerns about the accuracy or otherwise of the test results. Notwithstanding these somewhat polarised views, it would seem that testing can never of itself be seen as an adequate harm minimisation strategy. Gowing et al. state that if testing is used it should always '[b]e accompanied by secondary preventive education' (2001, p.38).

On balance the Committee believes that although there are some valid and sincerely held beliefs with regard to the efficacy of pill testing stations or sophisticated pill testing laboratories they would be prohibitively expensive to establish and maintain. They also risk sending the 'wrong message' to users and potential users that taking 'party drugs' can be 'risk free'. As for self-testing kits, the evidence indicates that such instruments are inaccurate and possibly dangerous. At this stage the Committee can not support either of these measures. Instead the Committee makes the following recommendations:

Recommendations

58. The Committee recommends that the provision of accurate information in relation to the contents of pills submitted for testing be available to medical support staff, through a system of 'alerts' provided by Victoria Police Forensic Science Laboratories.

59. The Committee recommends that pill testing kits should not be available to the public as they are potentially a dangerous and inaccurate tool to measure the content of particular pills.

Harm reduction for (injecting) amphetamine users

Much of the above discussion with regard to harm reduction strategies and 'party drugs' will also be applicable to the amphetamine aspects of the Inquiry. This section will therefore concentrate on primarily injecting users of amphetamine and methamphetamine.

Harm reduction programmes, particularly with regard to injecting use of amphetamines should clearly have input from ex and even current users of such drugs in their planning, design and implementation, wherever possible. Often this may be best facilitated through the use of needle and syringe exchanges or drug user organisations and associations.[866]

866 In the United States some cable television stations have given time slots to drug user organisations to produce their own harm reduction oriented programmes. See Anderson and Flynn 1997, p.194.

Some of the first harm reduction strategies and initiatives were devised in response to the risk of blood-borne viruses such as HIV and Hepatitis C through the use of injecting drugs such as heroin and amphetamines. Those workers who engage with the 'hard end' of drug using clients argue that, however unpalatable, sometimes harm reduction includes acknowledging and accepting that users will continue to 'score' no matter how risky such behaviour may be. Ms Siobhan Foley of the Yirra Youth Service in Perth states that for the person who is determined to keep injecting amphetamines or other drugs, advice may be given as to proper vein care, 'swabbing', not mixing drugs into a 'cocktail', "Trying a bit before injecting the whole lot into yourself".[867] Her colleague, Carmen Acosta of the Youth Withdrawal Service, adds that in order to prevent more ongoing serious complications sometimes distasteful choices may need to be made:

> Going to the same dealer could be [one practical piece of advice]. As horrid as that is, at least if you are using the same dealer on a regular basis, it is someone that is going to have an invested interest in your return and is not going to be doing something that they shouldn't in terms of giving you something that they shouldn'[t be giving you. So, things like that. It can be as basic as that.[868]

Many of the harm reduction programmes or projects with regard to injecting drug use are run through needle and syringe exchanges. They may provide practical help such as the distribution of syringes, filters and filtered water, or education and information pertaining to 'safe' injecting and reducing drug-related harm.[869] In some of the larger centres, advice may be given or referrals made with regard to general medical, legal and financial assistance.[870] Some needle and syringe programmes (NSPs) may use outreach mobile teams to deliver such services. Anex, the peak body for NSPs, drawing from the work of Dixon and Maurice 2002, argues that NSP workers have a key role in promoting harm reduction measures among their clients. Some of the practical strategies that can be provided by NSPs and their staff include:

- Organising a safe and quiet environment for clients under the influence of psychostimulants to have a rest;
- Identify and organise support for a client;
- Providing information and tips to improve sleep;
- Providing information on overdose prevention, including minimising levels of drug use;

867 Ms Siobhan Foley, Yirra Youth Services in conversation with the Drugs and Crime Prevention Committee Perth, 1 October 2003.

868 Ms Carmen Acosta in conversation with the Drugs and Crime Prevention Committee, Perth, 1 October 2003.

869 See for example, the excellent publication 'Vein Care', a joint project between Queensland Health and the Victorian Department of Human Services. *Vein Care: Maintain Your Veins*, Paul Hardacre, Andrew Preston and Jon Derricott on behalf of Queensland Health/Victorian Department of Human Services, Exchange Campaigns 2003, Brisbane/Melbourne.

870 See for example, submission of Anex to the Drugs and Crime Prevention Committee, Inquiry into Amphetamine and 'Party Drug' Use in Victoria, October 2003.

- Contacting mental health services or escorting the client to Hospital emergency Departments where required, especially if the client is experiencing psychosis; and
- Identifying high risk situations with the client and strategies to reduce risk.[871]

Anex also believes that needle and syringe exchanges should be more widely accessible across the state, particularly in rural and regional centres of Victoria. The location of exchanges in stand-alone facilities should also be given consideration:

> The majority of outlets are based at community health centres and hospitals with the client contact occurring, in the majority of cases, over-the-counter at a general waiting area. This restricts the level of meaningful engagement that staff may have with clients as it restricts conversations on topics of a sensitive and confidential nature. Additionally most NSP staff have other duties aside from the provision of NSP-specific services which hampers the amount of time they may spend in working with clients to achieve better health outcomes.[872]

It also believes that needles and other safe injecting equipment could be available through automatic dispensing machines at hospitals, health clinics and other localities throughout the state. While the Committee believes that there should certainly be a greater coverage of NSP outlets and better after-hours service and more flexible hours of operation, particularly in rural and regional areas, it can not at this stage countenance the provision of needles and other paraphernalia in public vending machines. It does, however, make the following recommendations:

871 Dixon and Maurice quoted in submission of Anex to the Drugs and Crime Prevention Committee, Inquiry into Amphetamine and 'Party Drug' Use in Victoria, October 2003.

872 Submission of Anex to the Drugs and Crime Prevention Committee, Inquiry into Amphetamine and 'Party Drug' Use in Victoria, October 2003.

Recommendations

60. The Committee strongly recommends that the Government initiates the introduction of retractable single dose syringes.

61. The Committee believes that increasing access to blood-borne virus prevention equipment is of priority and recommends a number of strategies to be implemented including:
    a) Establishment of new Needle and Syringe Program outlets including pharmacy-based outlets;
    b) Further and ongoing funding for after-hours Needle and Syringe Program services;
    c) Attaching Needle and Syringe Program services to other after-hours services.

62. The Committee recommends that as a hepatitis C prevention measure, Human Services Victoria supplies Needle and Syringe Program outlets with a range of sterile injecting equipment including sterile water and filters for distribution to clients.

Self-regulation

In previous chapters the Committee examined the ethnographic work of David Moore and his study of 'party drug' users in Perth. Moore argues that his set of recreational drug users employed a number of social controls to 'minimise the legal, financial, social and health costs associated with their illicit drug use and to maximise the benefits' (1992a, p.69). Users self-regulate their use or utilise their own harm reduction measures, often drawing from the advice of friends and fellow users or the 'folkloric knowledge' of the scene. Moore states that some of these controls can be readily articulated but most 'remain part of their "taken for granted" reality' (p.69).

Some of the controls – of which several almost achieve the status of rules – observed in Moore's fascinating study include:

- Drug purchases should be conducted through a known dealer or dealers [As was observed in Chapter 10 at least in the case of ecstasy, users most often bought their tablets from friends or known acquaintances];
- Do not use drugs during the week;
- Do not use drugs with strangers (unless perhaps introduced by, or accompanying , a trusted friend);
- Seek advice from experienced drug users when in doubt;
- Do not carry drugs in public in case of arrest (although this sanction was obviously waived by those involved in drug-dealing);
- Consume drugs...in a comfortable, safe and hygienic place;

- Do not use drugs above a certain frequency (although rules concerning frequency are particularly fuzzy and vary considerably even within small drug using sets) (Moore 1992a, pp.70–71).

Moore states that while these controls/rules are sometimes broken:

> [t]hey serve to set general limits on what is, and is not, broadly acceptable. When an individual does not follow them, he or she must usually offer some justification as to why this should be so (Moore 1992a, p.71).

In the specific context of ecstasy there are similar rules or extensions thereof. For example, on the advice of more experienced users, novice users of the drug may use only half the regular dose of an ecstasy tablet compared to regular users. The advice of more experienced, often older, drug 'mentors' is viewed as invaluable for the neophyte.[873]

> [O]lder dance drug users experience fewer problems in relation to their drug use. The most likely explanation for this finding is that older dance drug users may have learned more effective ways of avoiding negative effects, and the data in fact support this hypothesis. There was a significant positive correlation between age and number of strategies employed...such that older dance users tended to employ more strategies than younger ones to deal with the negative effects of dance drug use. This suggests that older dance drug users may have information available to them regarding how to deal with the negative effects of drug use, have a wider bank of experience upon which to draw, and/or are more willing or able to implement strategies. All this strongly suggests the importance of the cumulative effects of years of drugs 'education', via dance club culture, drugs agencies and the media, combined with becoming 'drug wise' and learning through their own and friends' experiences (Parker et al., 1998). Again, this finding has relevance to secondary prevention messages (Measham, Aldridge & Parker 2001, p.131).[874]

Other sources of information from which the novice user may draw can include isolated news reports, dance/music magazines and the Internet (see Webb 1998 and the discussion and references in Chapter 10).

Shewan's ethnographic study of ecstasy use in Scotland also showed that ecstasy users consciously made efforts to minimise the harms associated with the adverse consequences of ecstasy use. Of paramount importance to this group was the preparation and planning of the 'big night out' discussed in Chapter 10 of this Report. Members of this group adhered to a number of precepts about drug taking that seemed to be well known within the group. For example, not taking ecstasy when experiencing psychological difficulties such as depression, or ensuring that the drug was taken in the presence of supportive friends in case any of the batches were adulterated. Although the users would not rationalise it in such terms, their

873 This also seems to be true of amphetamines where advice is sought from within the peer group networks, see for example, Vincent et al. 1999 and the discussion Chapters 9 and 10.

874 See also for example Forsyth 1995; Shewan, Dalgarno & Reith 2000; McElrath & McEvoy 2001; 2002.

behaviour very much incorporates testing for the factors of drug, set and setting discussed in Chapter 10.

> It is the case that these ecstasy users paid heed to existing guidelines in most UK harm reduction drug information (eg. Lifeline, 1992; Scottish Drugs Forum, 1996). Becker (1953, 1963, 1967) has described how drug knowledge, including learning the appropriate way to use a drug, is communicated among groups of drug users and this type of 'social learning' may be a feature of the patterns of drug use described here. The principles of drug, set, and setting drawn from Zinberg's work have been used in this study to analyse drug using and related risk behaviour among ecstasy users (Zinberg, 1984). McDermott et al. (1993) have described using Zinberg's principle of controlled drug use as the starting point for a health promotion initiative. It may be that the principles of drug, set and setting could be successfully implemented in future initiatives.
>
> Almost by definition, taking a drug involves an element of risk: after this decision has been made a continuum of risk becomes apparent. The users described here, on the whole, seemed to feel that observing a number of basic harm reduction principles provided them with what they felt were acceptable safeguards. For this group, this is an element of safer drug use, which they did not see as impinging on the more hedonistic aspects of their ecstasy use.
>
> The ecstasy-related risks which were, subjectively, most salient to this group, and which appear to have most influence on their behaviour are largely short-term negative experiences while taking ecstasy. In this context, the preparations which the group reported add an element of rational planning to the drug-taking episode. In terms of risk discourse (Douglas, 1986; Giddens, 1991; Beck 1992; Douglas, 1992; Furedi, 1997; Reith, 1999), this could be described as 'conservative' behaviour, rather than 'true risk taking' behaviour. In the short-term, surprisingly little is left to chance by this group when taking ecstasy, to the extent that events are under participants' control. For example, when buying ecstasy tablets there is always an element of doubt as to the actual content of the pill: that said, participants did seem to try and find out about the type of experience associated with particular designs (see Forsyth, 1995). An element of impulsive behaviour is reported verbally by some of the group, but typically this is contradicted by descriptions of actual behaviour.
>
> Furedi (1997) has argued that the greater one's perception of risk, the more conservative one's behaviour will be. This would appear to be confirmed in relation to the perceived short-term risk of the sample described here, in terms of planning, preparation and monitoring of the ecstasy experience. Indeed this pattern could be described as archetypal harm reduction drug using behaviour, both in terms of the safer drug use messages given in harm reduction leaflets, and in terms of the provision of adequate safety facilities within clubs (Shewan, Dalgarno & Reith 2000, pp.450, 451).

Similar findings were noticeable in a more recent qualitative survey of ecstasy users conducted in Perth, Western Australia, by Hansen, Maycock and Lower (2001). This study found that participants applied a 'cost benefit analysis' to their use of ecstasy. As long as the positive effects of using the drug outweighed any negative benefits (experienced or perceived) then they would continue to use:

> A number of strategies were adopted to minimise the potential for negative or adverse outcomes. These included controlling for the factors of drug, set and setting...the participants used the notion of 'acceptable safeguards'...or steps that provide an acceptable level of protection. For example, using only when with friends; using only after someone else has tried it; using a regular supplier; controlling the amount consumed; controlling the amount of other drugs consumed; monitoring others (for physical and psychological harm); guiding initiates; limiting one's supply and use; and using only when in a positive mood (Hansen, Maycock & Lower 2001, pp.191–192).

The authors also state that:

> The participants attempted to exert control over set (expectation, risk perception, mood) and setting (physical surroundings), and although it was impossible to control for the drug, they adopted measures such as using a regular supplier and having pre-taste tests as methods of semi-control. New users were initiated into the ecstasy-using experience by more experienced users who helped the new initiates to interpret the symptoms they experienced during the drug use. The data revealed evidence of user folklore and myths that served to define and influence the overall drug experience. Users came to accept certain 'norms' about the effects, benefits and harms associated with their use of ecstasy. Using this knowledge they become more expert at manipulating drug, set and setting to maximise the experience and reduce the potential risks. Thus, despite the evidence of occasions of unplanned and spontaneous use, the participants revealed highly ritualised and largely controlled behaviour in relation to their ecstasy use (Hansen, Maycock & Lower 2001, p.197).

The degree and type of harm reduction 'strategies' employed by users will also depend on the perception of risk the user has about the drug. Several surveys have included questions or discussions gauging risk perception with regard to 'party drugs' (see Hansen, Maycock & Lower 2001; Hando, Topp & Dillon 1998; NDARC 1998). For example, subjects in the Hando, Topp and Dillon survey on average tended to place ecstasy as a drug 'mid way' (5) on a risk scale (where cannabis was placed at 0, no or low risk, and heroin at 10, high risk). Such subjects tended to have reasonable knowledge about the physical effects of ecstasy; the risks posed by impurities in the drug and the unknown long-term effects of use. Accordingly, they took 'precautions', such as 'scoring' the drug from known acquaintances or monitoring their water/fluid intake, particularly after dancing (Hando, Topp & Dillon 1998, pp.36ff.).[875] Moreover, in a British survey comparing amphetamine, cocaine and ecstasy use, it was found that given knowledge (or experience) of adverse

875 Notwithstanding such perceptions of risk, in this survey:

'[M]ost subjects perceived their own use of ecstasy to be moderately (31%), quite (39%) or very safe (24%), with only 5% believing that ecstasy use was quite likely to very risky' (Hando, Topp & Dillon 1998, p.36).

effects and consequences associated with their drug use, some users may modify their drug-taking behaviour in light of those effects. In this survey (Williamson et al. 1997) more than half of the sample modified the way they used their drugs, with half of that number reducing the amount taken, in response to experiencing or becoming aware of adverse effects associated with use. As the authors conclude:

> If stimulant users in the community are able to modify their drug taking behaviour in the light of experience, then this should encourage the development of health education strategies aimed at non treatment populations (Williamson et al. 1997, p.94).

More worrying, however, are indications that over time, and as users became more 'experienced', some of these safeguards may have been followed less stringently. Sometimes the behaviour of participants revealed 'a disparity between what they claimed to do and what they recognised as safe and what they were actually doing' (Hansen, Maycock & Lower 2001, p.192). The study conducted by Hansen, Maycock and Lower revealed that:

> Though users identified a wide range of harm reduction strategies, the application of these strategies was inconsistent, with a large number of the sample indulging in occasional binges, spontaneous purchases, polydrug use and purchasing from unknown individuals in clubs/pubs. As users become more experienced, their perception of the risks associated with use tended to diminish and they exhibited greater risk taking behaviour. The majority of participants indicated an intention for prolonged future use; however, they recognised that changes to life circumstances could serve to alter their use patterns. This suggests that the cost-benefit analysis conducted by the users is a constant process and one that is periodically reviewed. It may be that interventions could be developed that alter the cost-benefit analysis so as to increase the costs while decreasing the benefits.
>
> Although aware of some of the potential long-term adverse health effects, the participants did not perceive these risks as particularly salient. These data imply that the evidence linking use to long-term negative outcomes has had little impact upon levels of use. This suggests that greater emphasis on the negative short-term effects of use is required if changes to use patterns are to be achieved. Future interventions could adopt strategies similar to recent Western Australian programs directed towards the reduction of smoking and consumption of alcohol, which focused upon adverse short-term effects (Hansen, Maycock & Lower 2001, p.197).

Despite such 'lapses', the authors state that the participants did make conscious efforts to control any harms associated with their ecstasy use. Nonetheless, further research is crucial, particularly with regard to why some harm reduction techniques or measures may be utilised and others not:

> The study points to other aspects associated with ecstasy use that need further research and careful consideration with regard to intervention programs. The socialization associated with use has potential to be used as an intervention route; however, it would be necessary for individuals to be able to distinguish between

> signs of ecstasy consumption and consumption of a product that could cause even more harm. The inconsistent application of the identified harm reduction strategies would require further research to investigate the efficacy of peer-led harm reduction interventions. The disparity between expressed harm reduction strategies and the observed action of the users reinforces the need for multiple data collection methods and the need for constant comparison between data sets.
>
> Further research is required to identify optimum intervention methods. For example, this study found evidence that as users became more experienced they appeared to be willing to engage in behaviour that they had previously identified as being risky. This has implications for the salience of intervention methods (Hansen, Maycock & Lower 2001, p.198).

Clearly, such research is important and needs to be undertaken as a matter of priority.[876] Notwithstanding much useful information coming from valuable qualitative and ethnographic research projects such as that undertaken by Moore (1992a) and by Hansen, Maycock and Lower (2001) in Australia and Forsyth (1995), Shewan, Dalgarno and Reith (2000) and McElrath and McEvoy (2001) in Europe, there is still much to be done. Moore acknowledges that there is still a great deal of knowledge to be gained about psychostimulant use in non-captive settings:

> There is [also] little known about the degree of penetration of harm reduction messages...into non clinical populations of drug users, the perceived relevance and extent of adoption of such messages, and whether there are alternative sources of information. How do drug users gain information about unsafe behaviour? Whom do they trust for such information? Which source or type of information do they act on? (Moore 1992, p.9).

It is equally important that research projects, particularly those exploring issues of risk perception and self-harm reduction measures, draw from the folklore and knowledge of users themselves The need for such research is the subject of Chapter 21.

Conclusion

Harm reduction approaches are not based on a 'one size fits all' strategy. Clearly, what works in some contexts and for some drugs may not necessarily be appropriate for others. Naturally information needs to be provided for users but should this be through (sometimes didactic) pamphlets and information sheets or via the use of

---

876 One such research project that might yield some valuable information is currently being proposed between the Melbourne Parks Trust (MPT) and the Centre for Youth Drug Studies. The MPT manages large sports venues such as the Rod Laver arena that host large-scale dance parties six to eight times per year. The MPT has approached the Australian Drug Foundation for assistance in identifying issues of importance in conducting these parties and disseminating appropriate education messages with regard to party drug use:

'The Centre for Youth Drug Studies is currently working with the Trust to develop a research project to identify the key issues and messages which will have relevance with this target group. This project will provide valuable access to this particular target group (18–25 year olds who attend large dance parties) and the findings should greatly expand our knowledge of the drug knowledge, attitudes and practices among this group of young people' (Quoted in the submission of the Australian Drug Foundation to the Drugs and Crime Prevention Committee, Inquiry into Amphetamine and 'Party Drug' Use in Victoria, August 2002).

outreach and peer networks. In addition to providing appropriate material for users, it is equally important that venue owners, bouncers, support staff, medical officers, including general practitioners, and police receive appropriate training and information. Dance party guidelines and practical measures such as the provision of water at venues (and information as to correct water consumption) are essential. The efficacy of tablet testing to ascertain their content and 'safety' has yet to be determined. Such a measure is highly contentious. It would certainly seem, however, that such a practice should never be implemented as a stand alone measure. Further research on all manner of aspects pertaining to the use of amphetamines and 'party drug' use is crucial, as will be discussed in Chapter 21. Mass media campaigns might only be effective if complemented by grassroots community based initiatives.

Harm reduction measures such as those discussed in this chapter are not always universally popular. There is a tension apparent between trying to minimise the harms associated with drug use while not giving the message that such behaviour is approved of or even condoned. Youth and outreach workers tread a fine line between promoting measures that will hopefully minimise adverse outcomes associated with taking the drug and promoting the drug itself.[877]

There are also, as many commentators have pointed out, tensions to be reconciled between strict law enforcement of illicit drug use and health promotion that incorporates harm reduction techniques and strategies. Webb argues that:

> The concept of harm minimisation need not be incompatible with modern policing practices if law enforcement officers are given appropriate training... Law enforcement personnel need to be trained about the health risks and consequences of amphetamine type stimulants and other drug use, so that their work does not conflict with that of health workers using harm minimisation approaches... Effective liaison between the Police and primary care workers is especially important when dealing with first time drug offenders (Webb 1998, p.97).

While such comments generally fit in with the approach taken in most Australian jurisdictions with regard to the issue of harm minimisation, the Committee nonetheless encourages further discussion, debate and input to this somewhat vexed and controversial area, particularly in the context of amphetamines and 'party drugs'. It believes its recommendations in this area are a useful contribution to the field.

---

877 For an account of four previously implemented preventive and harm reduction campaigns pertaining to psychostimulant use, see Kamienicki et al. 1998, pp.19–24. The authors discuss the development, execution and evaluation of the following programmes:

- Speed Wise Speed Safe (Amphetamines – Australian)
- Rave Safe Project ('Party Drugs' – New South Wales)
- Chill Out ('Party Drugs' – Liverpool, England)
- Factline '91 ('Party Drugs' – Brighton, England).

PART G: Treatment and Research Issues Pertaining to Amphetamine and 'Party Drug' Use

The following Part examines two discrete but interrelated areas pertaining to amphetamine and 'party drug' use. It commences with an exploration of some of the treatment issues surrounding amphetamines and 'party drugs'. It notes that there are very few specific treatment interventions for amphetamine users, compared to the number available to heroin or problematic alcohol users. Moreover, amphetamine users are in any case reluctant to present to specialist alcohol and drug agencies. The most common 'port of call' for amphetamine users experiencing problems with their drug use may be a general practitioner. This may be in part because there *are* few discrete specialist, particularly pharmacological, interventions available. Again this is different from the situation pertaining to heroin where substitution therapies such as methadone and buprenorphine may be viewed with favour by some users. The issue of substitution therapies for amphetamines such as oral use of dexamphetamine is contentious. The arguments for and against such therapies are canvassed in detail in this chapter.

When it comes to MDMA/ecstasy and other 'party drugs', treatment per se is of less relevance. Most users of 'party drugs' who experience difficulty with regard to their drug taking will have had either minor incidents that a first aider could address or, far less frequently, a major and possibly life threatening episode that would be dealt with by emergency or casualty departments. In any case, current knowledge suggests that there is little need for long-term treatment interventions for MDMA or other party drug users, although this may change as more evidence from longitudinal studies becomes available.

Chapter 21 in this Part concerns the need for comprehensive and targeted research into amphetamine and 'party drugs'. This issue is related to the treatment issues discussed in Chapter 20 in as much as it is crucial that further research into treatment options for amphetamine users continue, particularly in the area of pharmacological interventions. But the focus of Chapter 21 goes well beyond treatment research. It argues that a wide range of research projects and methodologies of both a quantitative and qualitative nature need to be undertaken. The chapter argues that while there is certainly a huge amount of research literature on amphetamines and 'party drugs', there is still an enormous gap in our knowledge of the effect of these drugs and the patterns of their use.

20. Treatment and Service Provision Issues

This chapter raises ongoing points for discussion and probably asks more questions than it solves. It discusses the area of treatment of amphetamine and 'party drug' associated problems and conditions. It also examines the provision of treatment services (or lack thereof) for such conditions. In particular, it examines whether there are specific treatment regimes for amphetamine-related conditions and if there are not, should there be. A key aspect of the discussion will concern the apparent lack of treatment services specifically catering to the users of amphetamines and 'party drugs'.[878]

A constant refrain throughout the academic literature and the submissions received by the Committee has been that users of amphetamines rarely use these drugs exclusively. The last section of the chapter looks at how poly-drug use compounds the issue of treatment as it pertains to amphetamines and 'party drugs'.

Clients seeking treatment for amphetamine use in Victoria

It would seem that just as there has been an exponential growth in the number of people who are using amphetamines (and 'party drugs'), so too there has been a concomitant increase in the number of people who are seeking treatment for such use from Victorian agencies. This growth can be observed in figures supplied by the Department of Human Services Victoria. Figure 20.1 below shows the numbers of clients accessing DHS-funded drug treatment services whose primary drugs are amphetamines, for the period July 2000 to June 2003.

878 A national Drug Strategy monograph on treatment intervention for amphetamine users (*Models of Intervention and Care of Psychostimulant Users*) has recently been prepared to update the publication by Kamienicki et al. 1998 cited extensively throughout this Chapter. At the time of writing, this Monograph was not yet available for public perusal.

Figure 20.1: Clients accessing drug treatment services with primary drug amphetamines

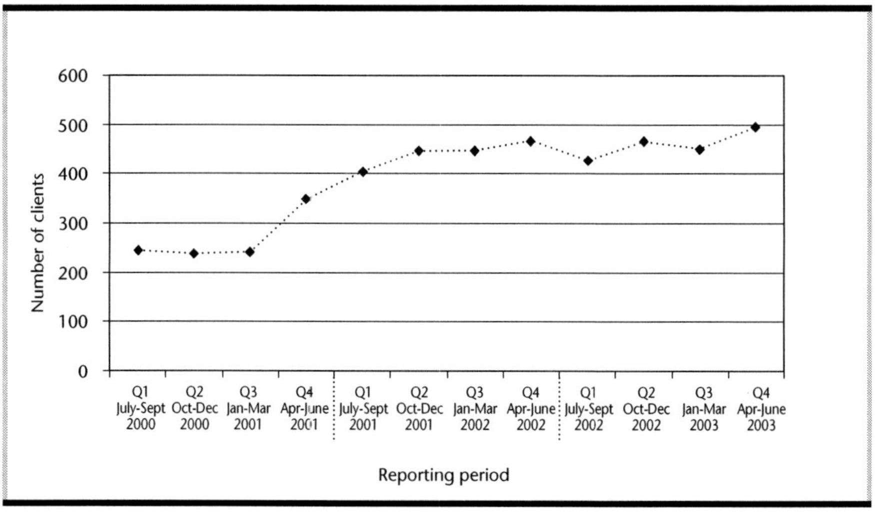

Source: Alcohol and Drug Information System 2003.[879]

The Department of Human Services Victoria comments in relation to these treatment services:

> In 2002–2003, of the clients whose primary drug of concern was amphetamines, the most commonly accessed service type was counselling, consultancy and continuing care (901 clients). These Services provide a range of services and supports appropriate to the needs of clients, including assessment, treatment and consultancy, referral and ongoing case management. The next most commonly accessed service types were residential withdrawal (233 clients), outreach (166 clients) and outpatient withdrawal (111 clients).[880]

Similar data is not available for ecstasy use because it is extremely unusual for ecstasy users to access drug treatment services. Most presentations by ecstasy users to medical services (and these are few) would be to the emergency room due to toxic complications with the drug or what is thought to be MDMA.[881]

Overview of treatment issues regarding psychostimulants

Research into treatment options for drug use is predominantly geared towards opioids such as heroin. There are few, if any, specialist drug and alcohol services in Australia catering exclusively for problematic, dependent or heavy users of amphetamines (South Australian Drugs Summit Communique 2002a; Mundy

879 Submission of the Department of Human Services Victoria to the Drugs and Crime Prevention Committee, Inquiry into Amphetamine and 'Party Drug' Use in Victoria, November 2003.

880 Ibid.

881 This applies only to people for whom ecstasy is the only or primary drug of choice. Poly-drug users may appear in treatment data for other drug categories.

2001). Moreover, research that is undertaken into treatment for psychostimulant-related conditions tends to be focussed on cocaine, despite the fact that amphetamine use is far more prevalent in Australia than cocaine use (South Australian Drugs Summit 2002b, p.15).

One of the few comprehensive studies and literature reviews of treatment options (or lack thereof) for psychostimulant users conducted in Australia comments:

> Much of the intervention literature for psychostimulant users has come from the United States and has primarily involved cocaine users. The hundreds of treatment studies for cocaine users comprise an estimated 90% or more of the total psychostimulant intervention literature. Despite the great deal of effort that has been expended in devising effective treatments for cocaine users, there is no consensus regarding effective treatment. The same is true of amphetamine users (Kamienicki et al. 1998, p.vii).[882]

Of further concern is the fact that many of the treatment interventions that are being used for illicit drug management are extrapolated from opioid and alcohol programmes. It has been suggested that many users of psychostimulants may not be willing to avail themselves of such measures because of the stigma associated with heroin use. Moreover:

> The lack of [specific] pharmacotherapies for amphetamine users is probably one reason underlying the low number of users (compared to heroin users) who seek treatment from drug and alcohol services (South Australian Drugs Summit 2002b, p.15).

Whether or not there should be separate treatment regimes for psychostimulant abuse, particularly amphetamines and methamphetamines, is a debated issue and one that will be canvassed later in this chapter. The next section will examine some of the general issues associated with treating amphetamine-related problems. It will be followed by a section outlining the difficulties in accessing specific treatments for amphetamine use.

Treatment issues regarding amphetamines and methamphetamines

The harms associated with amphetamine use, particularly chronic use, are well documented.[883] Despite this, an Australian study of amphetamine users in Newcastle, conducted as recently as 2001, comments that:

> Despite the popularity of amphetamine and its associated problems, there is a paucity of information concerning the characteristics of regular users of the drug and their readiness for treatment (Baker, Boggs & Lewin 2001, p.50).

---

882 This report comments further:

'Hundreds of empirical intervention studies have been conducted with cocaine users; the number of published and unpublished empirical intervention studies with amphetamine users is approximately 20' (Kamienicki et al. 1998, p.16).

883 See Kamieniecki et al. 1998 for a convenient summary, the discussion in Chapter 6 of this Report, and the references listed therein.

There is also still concern among medical practitioners, scientists and researchers about the lack of tailored treatment models for (meth)amphetamine users:

> The number of people presenting to drug and alcohol services with primary amphetamine problems is increasing (Darke et al 1996; Torres et al 1996) but there are no specific services for amphetamine users. All current available treatments are abstinence based. This approach unfortunately appears unattractive to a considerable number of problematic users. There are currently no recognised pharmacotherapies for amphetamine users in Australia or overseas. Amphetamine users can attend general hospital emergency, general practitioners, psychiatric services, drug counselling services, detoxification and rehabilitation services, therapeutic communities and self-help groups such as Narcotics Anonymous. Amphetamine users rarely contact these treatment services, which they perceive to be targeted at people with alcohol and opiate problems. ...This low level of engagement with treatment services is reflected in several studies which have reported between 7 and 12% of long term amphetamine users in treatment other than methadone maintenance (Hando et al 1997; Darke et al 1998; Ross et al 1994) (cited in National Drug and Alcohol Research Centre (NDARC) 1999, p.3).

There are a number of other issues associated with treating amphetamine and methamphetamine dependence that are still problematic, largely because they have been so under-researched. Some of the general areas that need to be examined in greater detail, include:

- Toxic complications from amphetamine use;[884]
- Withdrawal management for amphetamine use;[885]
- Appropriate pharmacological interventions for psychostimulant treatment, including drugs to decrease discomfort, blocking drugs, aversive agents, and substitution therapies (see Kamienicki et al. 1998);[886]
- The treatment of amphetamine use in conjunction with other forms of drug use (poly-drug use);

884 Psychostimulant intoxication is usually dealt with in hospital emergency departments (see Kamienicki et al. 1998, p.16).

885 For a discussion of treating withdrawal symptoms from amphetamine addiction and general withdrawal management, see Cantwell and McBride 1998.

886 Dr Nick Lintzeris, formerly of Turning Point Alcohol and Drug Centre in Melbourne, has commented that an effective medication to deal with amphetamine withdrawal and use is sorely needed to complement other methods:

'We're going to get many, many more people presenting for treatment and if we can give them a medication that actually works...because lots of these people will think "why bother going to treatment if all you're going to get is a bit of a talking to?", particularly when the talking to isn't even very good, and not amphetamine oriented. It will be good when we have an effective medication to link with psychotherapeutic approaches' (quoted in Wood 1998a, p.22).

For a discussion of the use of the drug *imipramine* to treat methamphetamine addiction and disorders, see Galloway et al. 1996. See also Rawson et al. 2002. For a discussion of the use of the experimental drug *ibogaine*, as an adjunct for treating methamphetamine addiction, see Wray 2000.

- The treatment of amphetamine use in conjunction with co-morbid psychiatric disorders;[887]
- Inpatient versus outpatient treatment;[888]
- Brief versus intensive treatment (Kamienicki et al. 1998; Wickes 1993a, 1993b);
- Non-pharmacological treatment interventions[889] (including behavioural, psychosocial,[890] cognitive, family oriented and supportive therapies);[891]
- The suitability of natural therapies;

---

887 In a comparison of cocaine and methamphetamine patients in treatment services, Copeland and Sorensen found that: 'Methamphetamine patients are predicted to be at especially high risk for relapse, because of the lingering depressive and psychotic symptoms that methamphetamine can produce' (2001, p.95).

888 As early as 1993 these options were being canvassed by Wickes. Ten years later there is still uncertainty as to the appropriateness of one as opposed to the other. Wickes stated in 1993:

'The value of outpatient treatment programs is supported by studies of cocaine users in the United States where 30–90% of those who remained in outpatient treatment of various modalities ceased use. Outpatient programs are also more cost effective than inpatient programs and the problem of generalisation from the inpatient to the outpatient environment does not exist.

Inpatient treatment is, however, thought to be warranted in the following instances:

- Polydrug dependence;
- Where severe withdrawal is anticipated;
- Medical complications requiring close observation or treatment;
- Psychiatric complications...;
- Absence of social supports;
- Undesirable living conditions;
- Failed outpatient treatment' (Wickes 1993b, p.11).

Anglin et al. have more reservations about outpatient treatment for methamphetamine users, at least in the American context:

'For MA abusers being treated as outpatients, the easy availability of the drug and the allure of its long action often lead to resumption of MA early in treatment. The consequence is usually patient dropout from all forms of treatment before the onset of any effects of therapeutic medication or psychotherapy' (Anglin et al. 2000, p.140).

Turning Point Alcohol and Drug Centre generally believe outpatient treatment is best practice, unless circumstances otherwise demand inpatient stays, particularly as it is difficult to retain patients in inpatient services (Submission of Turning Point Alcohol and Drug Centre to the Drugs and Crime Prevention Committee, Inquiry into Amphetamine and 'Party Drug' Use in Victoria, October 2003).

889 Kamienicki et al. define 'non-pharmacological interventions' as '[t]he treatment of psychostimulant users utilising non drug procedures with a view to decreasing/eliminating drug consumption or reducing the harms associated with continued use' (1998, p.16).

For example, Ms Carmen Acosta of the Youth Withdrawal and Respite Service in Perth emphasised the importance of alternative therapies, such as reiki and meditation as an adjunct to traditional withdrawal from amphetamines and other drugs (Carmen Acosta, Youth Withdrawal and Respite Service, in conversation with the Drugs and Crime Prevention Committee, Perth, 1 October 2003).

890 For a recent account of the use of psychosocial interventions as an intervention for problematic amphetamine use see Baker & Lee 2003.

891 For a discussion of the effectiveness of brief cognitive-behavioural interventions among regular users of amphetamines, see Rawson, Gonzales and Brethen 2002; Baker, Boggs and Lewin 2001. This study of Newcastle [Australia] amphetamine users found that:

'[B]rief cognitive behavioural therapy appears to be feasible and moderately effective among regular users of amphetamine. The results of this study suggest that a larger randomised controlled trial of the effectiveness of cognitive-behavioural therapy should be conducted' (Baker, Boggs & Lewin 2001, p.1286).

- The value of self-help groups and therapeutic communities; and
- Harm reduction measures.

This Report does not seek to discuss each of the above factors in any great detail, although the Committee has endeavoured to seek the views of experts within the field about such issues.[892] However, it is important to canvass some general issues pertaining to amphetamine treatment. One of the important questions to ask is: What interventions do users themselves seek for their (problematic) amphetamine use?

Accessing treatment[893]

> One really important piece of research that has not been done in Australia is looking at the engagement of users into treatment. What we do know is that they do not attend treatment easily, they do not find our treatment services particularly suited to their needs. Part of that is probably because there are no specific treatments for them, and treatment service staff are not very confident in dealing with amphetamine users. We certainly do not know how to attract them into treatment, how to keep them there, and what to do with them when we get them in there.[894]

As the above quote indicates there has been very little research undertaken as to why amphetamine users in particular do or do not access treatment. One study that has been conducted in this area is that of Hando, Topp and Hall (1997) who surveyed 200 regular and problematic amphetamine users in Sydney. The survey sought to determine the treatment issues and preferences of the sample. In the study the authors reviewed the international literature on the increasing number of people presenting to drug treatment services with a *primary* amphetamine problem. Most of these Australian, American and British studies showed that primary treatment programmes were either non-existent or perceived as inappropriate by users. Such views were also expressed by the sample in the Sydney study. Moreover, if 'treatment' *was* sought it was more often for the behavioural effects of the amphetamine use rather than any physiological or pharmacological problems (see, for example, the British study of Klee & Morris 1994, discussed in Hando, Topp & Hall 1997, p.106).

---

892 The Committee has found the views of Professor Margaret Hamilton and Dr Nicole Lee of Turning Point Alcohol and Drug Centre particularly useful.

893 Much of the research done in this area is British, particularly that of Professor Hilary Klee and her colleagues. The primary point to come out of such research is that for a variety of reasons amphetamine users find it very difficult to access treatment services for their addiction or drug use and if they do, find it even more difficult to stay in treatment. For a minority view, also from Britain, that disputes this finding, see Gossop, Marsden and Stewart 2000.

894 Professor Margaret Hamilton, Director, Turning Point Alcohol and Drug Centre, evidence given to the Drugs and Crime Prevention Committee, Public Hearings (Melbourne), 27 October 2003.

A submission by Turning Point Alcohol and Drug Centre adds that further qualitative research studies into the natural history of amphetamine users are required. 'What brings them into treatment? Who are they and how do they use? In other words, surveys that ask users about their experiences and the factors that may prevent them from accessing treatment services are needed' (Submission of Turning Point Alcohol and Drug Centre, to the Drugs and Crime Prevention Committee, Inquiry into Amphetamine and 'Party Drug' Use in Victoria, October 2003).

British research indicates that a frustrating loop is created whereby amphetamine users who often regard themselves as a distinct sub-group:

> [are] reluctant to attend a service where they will be in contact with opiate users. The result [in turn] is that many drug workers have relatively little experience of working with primary amphetamine users...
>
> ...Amphetamine users may therefore feel that their most pressing problems cannot be dealt with by drug agencies. In addition to this was the belief that drug workers have little experience of working with amphetamine users, and may not be able to offer appropriate help (Wright, Klee & Reid 1999, p.72).

Such views are reflected in the comments of some of the amphetamine users surveyed in Wright, Klee and Reid's research:

> 'They're just geared up for smack-heads, so they'd love it if I was a smack-head 'cos then they could help me...but sorry I'm not like that' (female amphetamine user, age 24).
>
> 'Call yourself a drug team?... why don't you call yourself a heroin team' (male amphetamine user, age 26 years)[895] (Wright, Klee & Reid 1999, pp.77, 79).

A separate study by Wright and Klee profiled a number of amphetamine users who never returned to drug treatment services after an initial presentation. Many of the original attendees viewed the attitude of drug service staff as one of the factors that militated against return visits. These attitudes were recognised and acknowledged by staff themselves:

> The majority of drug workers interviewed...acknowledged that they had little experience of working with amphetamine users. The agencies reporting greater contact with amphetamine users found them to be more time consuming because they had more problems – 'with the amphetamine user, everything is a problem' [drug worker]. They could be more difficult to manage because of agitation and aggression – 'All the A's – agitation, aggression and amphetamine' [consultant psychiatrist].
>
> Frustration was often felt by the drug workers who did not feel they were helping:
>
> '[l]ike with heroin users you feel that you've done something because you can give them methadone and that's what they need, whereas with amphetamine users sometimes I kind of flounder a bit and try to think how to make them feel better initially. That's probably more a problem for us than it is for them perhaps.'
>
> This evidence suggests that there are personal characteristics of amphetamine users which make them hard to attract to treatment, and that it is relatively easy to deter potential clients inadvertently from seeking prolonged treatment (Wright & Klee 1999, p.237).

---

895 Such quotes are also a testimony to the 'snobbery' of drug use discussed in Chapters 6 and 8.

There are strategies, however, that can be utilised to increase the attraction of treatment for primary amphetamine users, particularly around the training of drug workers and other professionals:

> It is recognized that the training needs of professionals in drug services need to be identified, and that resources should be made available to them to improve their credibility (Boys *et al.*, 1997). Services need to be designed to meet the specific needs of amphetamine users, with staff who have experience of working with stimulant users. Consequent upon such improvement, amphetamine clients would need to be made aware that services are not solely for the use of opiate users, and that appropriate help will be made available to them. Problems of access to a drug service may arise from any drug user, particularly those who work or have pre-school children. However, for amphetamine users who may only present to drug services when they have a severe crisis, and who may then be referred to a specialist service miles away, access can be a major problem. Many amphetamine users feel a strong sense of stigma associated with receiving treatment and fear the possibility of exposure to others as a drug user. These factors combine to give amphetamine users a low expectation of possible care from a treatment service, and despite overcoming the barriers to make an initial visit to services, any further hurdle may deter them from returning for continuing help (Wright & Klee 1999, p.240).

In a more recent British study also conducted by Professor Klee, preliminary findings indicated that amphetamine users presenting for treatment 'tend to do so because of a feeling that their lives are out of control and because of social isolation and psychological symptoms' (noted in Griffin 1997, p.19). Moreover, because seeking intervention may be predicated on the occurrence of a crisis:

> The motivation for treatment provided by a crisis is frequently short-lived; most users of illicit drugs are ambivalent about entering treatment and particularly about ceasing their drug use. Hence, unless a treatment response is provided quickly, the impact of the motivating factor is likely to decline, resulting in the risk of dropout from treatment (South Australian Drugs Summit Issues Paper 2002b, p.12).

A later study by Klee, Wright and Morris (1999) found that physical and psychological complications were one of the main reasons amphetamine users may seek treatment at first instance. Vascular problems were particularly indicated. Of interest, however, is the fact that while some men were concerned at the loss of weight due to their amphetamine use, women for the most part did not view this as a problem.

The need for a quick treatment response for those who *do* seek treatment is essential:

> The time between the initial approach and the first interview was recognised as a point at which clients could disappear, and often did... In some cases there

are waiting periods of several weeks before the first assessment and an amphetamine user might well fail to appear:

'If you give them an appointment for 2 weeks time, I think it's very off-putting... I'm sure it is for heroin users as well but its within the context of a 10 year heroin habit...But for a young amphet user it's a problem' [Drug Service Provider] (Wright, Klee & Reid 1999, p.80).

An Australian study of amphetamine users also found that:

> The best independent predictors of feeling the need for treatment were greater time spent unemployed, poor general health and the development of aggression since using amphetamine... Since psychological symptoms associated with amphetamine use have been found to be far more disturbing to users than physical health problems, psychological morbidity – and in particular the development of aggression – may be an important factor in precipitating treatment seeking in amphetamine users (Vincent et al. 1999, p.71).[896]

Clearly, the links between pre-existing psychological morbidity, co-morbidity and amphetamine use are ones that need to be examined in much greater detail.[897] A more detailed discussion of this issue is beyond the scope of this Report, but it must be stated that this is a much neglected area of research:

> The treatment of psychostimulant users with co-morbid psychiatric disorders has largely been neglected in the literature. Only a handful of pharmacotherapeutic intervention studies have been conducted on psychostimulant users with co-morbid psychiatric disorders. Moreover, all of these studies have included very small sample sizes and most have been uncontrolled. The results from these studies need to be replicated in larger, controlled studies (Kamienicki et al. 1998, p.viii).[898]

Of particular concern to some clinicians is the fact that there appear to have been some efforts by amphetamine users to self-treat any medical problems associated with the drug. One Australian study reported that amphetamine users were using benzodiazepines to assist with amphetamine-related problems and even using heroin as a form of 'self-medication' (NDARC 1997).

Clients surveyed by Hando, Topp and Hall in the 1997 NDARC study considered the following measures of dealing with this issue to be the most appropriate:

---

896 For a comprehensive review of the literature as to the reason why amphetamine users may (or may not) seek treatment or intervention, see Kamienicki et al. 1998, p.7.

897 See in particular Kamienicki et al. 1998; Baker, Boggs and Lewin 2000.

898 This paucity of treatment research studies is despite the fact that:

'Several studies have attested to the fact that very large numbers of amphetamine and cocaine users experience at least some psychiatric symptomatology (Gawin & Ellinwood 1988; Hall & Hando 1994; Hall et al. 1996; Hando 1996; Harrison 1994; Vincent et al. 1997). Not only do many users have some psychiatric symptomatology, many also have full blown psychiatric disorders (Gawin & Ellinwood 1988; Regier et al. 1990). This has been found to be especially true of those presenting to treatment services' (Kamienicki et al. 1998, p.18). See also section below on 'Different populations'.

> Twelve per cent of the sample (n = 24) were interested in receiving drug counselling, especially counselling which was amphetamine specific, non-judgemental and allowed a variety of goals, including abstinence and controlled use. Of the sample, 12% (n = 24) were interested in receiving natural therapies, such as acupuncture, herbal remedies and massage. A total of ten subjects were interested in participating in a detoxification program, especially home detoxification programs and programs which were amphetamine specific. Those interested in NA [Narcotics Anonymous] and TCs [Therapeutic Communities] also wanted programs that focused on amphetamine use. Six subjects wanted assistance from a GP, four subjects wanted assistance from a psychiatrist and eight subjects desired greater support from family and friends (NDARC 1997, p.110).

Natural therapies and self-help and social support were viewed as valuable adjuncts by users. However, by far the most popular treatment option from the client or subject perspective was 'amphetamine substitution'.[899] This topic is discussed further in a later section of this chapter.

The NDARC study by Hando, Topp and Hall concluded from their respondents' replies that:

> The results of the present study confirm a growing need for treatment among regular amphetamine users. However, there are few treatment alternatives available specifically for amphetamine-related problems and none have been rigorously evaluated… In Australia, amphetamine users can attend general hospital accident and emergency departments, drug counselling, consultation with a GP, psychiatric services, detoxification services, therapeutic communities and self-help groups. Traditionally these services have most often dealt with primary alcohol and opiate problems; it is still being relatively uncommon for primary amphetamine users to present for treatment (Torres et al 1996). Preliminary results from a UK study found that help-seeking amphetamine users tended to avoid drug clinics as they were seen as oriented towards heroin users. [Conversely] Drug workers considered amphetamine clients 'hard work' and believed that there were fewer incentives (such as prescribed drugs) for amphetamine users to attend (Institute for Drug Dependence 1996; Myles 1997). Most users interested in receiving treatment in the present study also recommended that it focus on amphetamine-specific issues and be relevant to them (NDARC 1997, p.110).

A lack of services

It has been six years since the Hando, Topp and Hall study was undertaken. Nonetheless, there still seem to be few specific amphetamine treatment modalities. As recently as September 2002 Dr Nicole Lee, senior research fellow at Victoria's Turning Point Alcohol and Drug Centre, stated that:

---

899 This treatment option was requested by 18% of the subjects (see Hando, Topp & Hall 1997, p.110).

> [t]here are very few treatments specifically for speed users and little research is conducted in Australia.
>
> 'There is an acknowledgement within alcohol and drug services that current treatment is not meeting client needs, staff need more training, and services need to become more amphetamine-user friendly' Nicole says (Turning Point Alcohol and Drug Centre 2002, p.1).

The submission from the Turning Point Alcohol and Drug Centre to this Inquiry was equally concerned about the ability of Victorian services to cater for this population:

> Turning Point has experienced a significant increase in amphetamine use among our existing clients and also an increase in the number of clients presenting for treatment. However, [there are] very few interventions and services oriented towards recruiting and retaining amphetamine users in treatment...
>
> Clinically, amphetamine users have different needs to other drug users. This is partly due to the pattern and context of use. Amphetamine is generally used as part of a social context and usually in a 'binge' pattern, intensely over short periods of time. Our traditional notions of what constitutes use, abuse and dependence do not always apply to this group. Typically, treatment seeking users present for short periods of time and are often in need of acute intervention. In general, they do not access traditional treatment centres, partly because of the focus on opiates and/or alcohol. Therefore treatment services require a reorientation and culture shift to increase 'user-friendliness' for this group.
>
> In short, our treatment services are not well equipped to deal with this ever increasing group – in either staff expertise or specific treatments that staff could be trained in. This process of reorienting services will involve developing and trialing new interventions specifically designed for this group and to provide training and support for staff to implement these interventions.[900] Supporting staff by providing tested best practice interventions will increase their confidence in addressing amphetamine use and assist in creating a culture shift to engage these clients more assertively.
>
> In addition, amphetamine use tends to be accompanied by more severe mental health and other sequelae than other drug use (Nutting, Lee, Jenner & Saunders 2002). Co-morbidity creates a significant challenge for treatment providers. It has been widely recommended that treatments for co-morbid substance use and mental health problems should address both disorders at the treatment agency to which they present (Jenner et al., 1998; Pennebaker et al., 2001). Yet, there are few programs specifically designed for amphetamine users within alcohol and drug or mental health services. Much of the recent research in co-morbidity has been undertaken within mental health services, for people with severe mental illness, such as schizophrenia and

900 Of interest is the fact that in Sweden there are few treatment services for discrete groups of drugs. In other words, for the most part, abusers of different drugs including alcohol, heroin and the amphetamines are treated together (see Kall 1997).

> bipolar affective disorder. However, research suggests that depression, anxiety and anger/irritability/paranoia are more commonly associated with amphetamine use – problems that are often subclinical and are excluded from public mental health services.[901]

Clearly there are problems with regard to treatment and service delivery, but most of the problems testified to in the previous quote tend to be couched for the most part in terms of metropolitan services. As has been discussed in Chapter 11, such problems are equally, if not more, prevalent and serious in rural and regional centres. This is particularly true of attracting and training staff in appropriate treatment methods and in access to detoxification and rehabilitation services.[902]

This lack of services has been felt even more since the rise of amphetamine use due to the 'heroin drought' (see Chapter 4). Miller, Fry and Dietze comment that it is natural to expect that as the heroin supply decreased more demand for amphetamine and subsequent amphetamine-related problems would result in an increased need for treatment interventions:

> This study provided evidence of increased amphetamine use as a result of the 'drought'. However, unlike benzodiazepines that frequently cause acute drug-related harms (eg. ambulance attendances), amphetamines only rarely appear involved in current monitoring systems for drug related harm. Nevertheless, stimulants such as amphetamines do present long-term harms for which treatment may be required. In this regard only a small proportion of clients of specialist drug agencies present with stimulants as their primary drug problem...and it is reasonable to expect an increase in demand for stimulant-related treatment if problems with heroin supply continue in the longer term. Typically, persons with stimulant-related problems have been characterised as difficult to manage (Lintzeris, Holgate and Dunlop 1996). Therefore the public health hazard presented by increases in amphetamine usage (as reported amongst the current sample) requires a response directed toward developing the capacity of treatment service providers (including General Practitioners) to respond to issues around amphetamine dependence. Moreover, this capacity development needs to go further than treatment service providers to include others who may come into contact with stimulant dependent persons (eg. agents of law enforcement agencies) to ensure humane management of these people... Finally, it is important to sustain current monitoring efforts around amphetamine-related harms in order to document any rise in amphetamine-related harm that may emerge as a result of the heroin drought (Turning Point Alcohol and Drug Centre 2001, pp.28–29).

Moreover:

901 Excerpt from the confidential submission of Turning Point Alcohol and Drug Centre to the Drugs and Crime Prevention Committee, Inquiry into Amphetamine and 'Party Drug' Use in Victoria, August 2002. Quoted with the kind permission and approval of Turning Point.

902 See discussion in Chapter 11 for further discussion of problems with regard to service delivery in rural communities.

> [m]any agencies were unprepared for the increased numbers and behaviour of amphetamine users who sought treatment when heroin became scarce (Turning Point Alcohol and Drug Centre 2002, p.1).

The comprehensive literature review of treatment interventions for psychostimulant users written by Kamienicki et al. raises pertinent issues pertaining to service provision for these groups of drug users:

> The majority of existing drug treatment services in Australia have been designed to manage alcohol intoxication or withdrawal from opiates and alcohol. Staff within treatment services, both in Australia and overseas, have reported feeling frustrated by their inability to adequately manage withdrawal from amphetamines. This has resulted from their lack of knowledge about the amphetamine withdrawal syndrome and appropriate management strategies, and because the lack of resources within services places strain on agencies since amphetamine users appear to require more time and effort than opioid users in withdrawal (Klee et al. 1995; Vincent et al. 1997).
>
> Many amphetamine users have reported that they have found it extremely difficult to enter traditional drug treatment services because of the perceived stigma attached to being associated with opioid users... In addition, many services have long waiting lists, which may 'penalise the amphetamine user disproportionately as their connection with the agency ...[may be]...more fragile and they would prefer to opt out if they could' (Klee et al. 1995 cited in Kamienicki et al. 1998, p.60).

This problem of managing withdrawal from (heavy or prolonged) amphetamine use has been commented upon by workers in the field with whom the Committee has met:

For example, Professor Steve Allsop of the Western Australian Drug and Alcohol Office states that withdrawal from amphetamines is not necessarily something that many drug and alcohol workers may be used to, particularly in comparison to heroin:

> [t]he services dealt poorly with [amphetamine users] people when they arrived. They were used to people whose withdrawal would peak after 2 or 3 days, which is common with alcohol and opiates, and here were these people whose withdrawals started to peak on the 6th or 7th day or 8th day and it was being misinterpreted as drug-seeking behaviour, not...and they were being discharged on the very days that their withdrawal was peaking.[903]
>
> They were turning up in emergency medicine and in the police services, much more aggression, much more behavioural problems and, again, coupled often

903 Not only are amphetamine users possibly being discharged prematurely in cases of amphetamine induced psychosis, but also Professor White of the Drugs and Alcohol Services Council of South Australia states that often such clients may not receive appropriate follow up because they 'were being dealt with in mental health facilities, not drug and alcohol facilities' (Professor Jason White, Director, Treatment and Rehabilitation Services, Drugs and Alcohol Services Council, in conversation with the Drugs and Crime Prevention Committee, 3 October 2003).

> with, well, psychotic sometimes and behaviours, a lot more depression, malnutrition, so, all the common problems that you see associated. And I think the services were ill-equipped to respond to them. I think there was also an age issue in there. In general, amphetamine users were a younger – without wishing to stereotype – but tended to be a younger age group and so you had services that were unfamiliar with dealing with young people and unfamiliar with dealing with people on stimulants. So, it was a challenge in both respects.[904]

In the United States, pharmacological treatments until very recently have borrowed:

> [f]rom treatment with cocaine dependence. Unfortunately, this approach has not met with much success since no single agent has proven efficacious in controlled clinical studies. Antidepressant medications [however] are helpful in combating the depressive symptoms frequently seen in methamphetamine users who recently have become abstinent.
>
> There are [also] some established protocols that emergency room physicians use to treat individuals who have had a methamphetamine overdose. Because hyperthermia and convulsions are common and often fatal complications of such overdoses, emergency room treatment focusses on the immediate physical symptoms. Overdose patients are cooled off in ice baths, and anti-convulsant drugs may be administered also (National Institute on Drug Abuse 1998, p.7).

But as indicated above, such measures are more geared towards dealing with the ancillary symptoms or 'by-products' of amphetamine use, not the dependence itself.[905] If, as seems to be the case from the discussion in Chapter 6 of this Report, a discrete amphetamine dependence syndrome exists, then tailored interventions may indeed be necessary to treat the physical and psychological consequences of this condition.[906]

Amphetamine substitution

As indicated above, the most popular treatment intervention sought by amphetamine users who responded to the survey of Hando, Topp and Hall (1997) was substitution therapy. The substitution therapy most often noted for treatment of problematic or dependent amphetamine users has been the controlled administration under clinical conditions of (oral) dexamphetamine

---

904 Professor Steve Allsop, Executive Director, Drug and Alcohol Office of Western Australia in conversation with the Drugs and Crime Prevention Committee, Perth, 1 October 2003.

905 In the United States, the extensive use of methamphetamine results in the users frequently accessing ambulance, emergency room and other hospital services and the resources associated with these services. However, the presentations largely concern trauma and violence associated with the use of the drug, such as stabbings, shootings, assaults and motor accidents. See Richards et al. 1999 and Chapter 7 of this Paper for further discussion of this issue.

906 This much was recognised by Huber and her colleagues in a 1997 study of possible research approaches needed for methamphetamine abuse. This study suggested that the development and application of novel pharmacotherapies for such abuse presupposed that medical science understood the clinical syndrome resulting from chronic methamphetamine abuse. This, at least in 1997, was not necessarily the case and much further research was (and is) required (see Huber et al. 1997).

substituting for street amphetamine. Substitution therapy has been available for a number of years in the United Kingdom[907] (see Strang et al. 1994; Klee 1997a, 1997b, 1997c) but has only been relatively recently considered as a method of treating amphetamine use and amphetamine dependence in Australia.

Much of the interest in substitution therapy arises out of a concern with the increasing number of people using amphetamines intravenously during the 1980s and 1990s:

> The rationale for the provision of amphetamine substitution is similar to that for heroin substitution programs. The potential benefits of such programs embody major public health goals including: prevention of transmission of blood borne viruses such as HIV and hepatitis B and hepatitis C by means of sharing of injecting equipment; improvements in the health and social functioning of drug users; reduced illicit drug use; and reductions in the associated criminal behaviour undertaken to fund drug use (Ward et al. 1998; Fleming 1998, cited in NDARC 1999, p.3).

One of the main objections to substitution schemes has been the risk that the use of dexamphetamine or other substitutes may in itself lead to dependence and/or providing dexamphetamine substitution therapy may result in the development of psychotic symptoms or episodes in the users. However, a study conducted by Shearer et al. at a primary health care centre in Kings Cross, Sydney, found that the risk of either of these complications arising was low (NDARC 1999). This study also reviewed the extensive British literature and studies on dexamphetamine substitution therapy which also found the benefits outweighed the low risk of any negative outcomes:[908]

> It has been argued that public health benefits may outweigh risks associated with the prescribing of substitution drugs (Fleming and Roberts 1994; Pates et al 1996; Charnaud and Griffiths 1998). Oral dexamphetamine substitution may allow stabilisation of some patients on a dose which causes neither withdrawal or craving and which may thereafter allow gradual reduction and eventual cessation (Bradbeer et al 1998; Sherman 1990). In a discussion of the role of substitution therapy for amphetamine users, Mattick and Darke (1995) identified four criteria of appropriateness of a maintenance treatment program. These were: i) regular frequent use (usually daily); ii) clear evidence of dependence; iii) continued use representing severe adverse complications for

907 For a comprehensive discussion of British studies on amphetamine substitution treatment, going as far back as the 1960s, see Kamienicki et al. 1998, pp.34ff. This includes a review of the *Cornwall Community Study*, an amphetamine substitution study with the largest treatment cohort in the world (as of 1998). In particular, the Cornwall study found that 'only those who had a history of psychotic episodes prior to the study experienced psychotic symptomatology during treatment' (Kamienicki et al. 1998, p.38).

908 Shearer et al. in a study for NDARC note that a survey of 149 medical drug and alcohol specialists in England and Wales:

'[f]ound that 46% of respondents were currently prescribing amphetamine and 60% saw a role for this therapy (Bradbeer et al 1998). [However] [A]lthough the practice of amphetamine prescription was found to be widespread, little scientific evidence was available to evaluate the efficacy or safety of the approach' (NDARC 1999, p.5).

> the user; and iv) the harms associated with illicit use exceed the risks associated with the use of legal substitute drug (NDARC 1999, p.4).

In a literature review of treatment options for amphetamine users, Kamienicki et al. summarise the arguments of the proponents of substitution therapy as follows:

These proponents argue that:

1. as current treatment programs are irrelevant to the needs of amphetamine users (ie. they are primarily orientated toward opioid users or rely on abrupt withdrawal) there is a need for appropriate interventions for amphetamine users;
2. amphetamine prescribing attracts users to treatment services;
3. having amphetamine users attending treatment services gives health practitioners the opportunity to distribute accurate harm minimisation and safer sex information;
4. amphetamine prescribing leads to a reduction in injecting activity;
5. the prescription of amphetamine will eliminate criminal activity associated with obtaining the drug;
6. the provision of dexamphetamine may stabilise patients on a dose which does not cause withdrawal or craving, and may subsequently lead to a reduction in dosage and eventual cessation of the drug; and
7. the high risk of contracting blood borne diseases as a result of needle sharing among intravenous amphetamine users outweighs the risks associated with prescribing amphetamines (Kamienicki et al. 1998, pp.35–36, reviewing the available literature).

Of particular importance, according to Shearer et al. (NDARC 1999), are the studies that suggest users who attend substitution programmes may also benefit from ancillary services often provided at the same clinic or treatment centre. These may include general information and advice, counselling and harm reduction measures such as needle exchange (see also Fleming & Roberts 1994; White 2000).

One of the major British studies done in this area (McBride et al. 1997) posed three questions for evaluating the use of dexamphetamine substitution therapy for a group of injecting amphetamine (sulphate) users in Wales.[909] These were:

1. Does [the therapy] attract drug users?
2. Does it retain drug users in contact with the service?; and
3. Does it change behaviour? (McBride et al 1997, p.98).

In the context of this study the authors found:

909 As mentioned earlier in this Report, amphetamine sulphate is still the most predominant form of amphetamine used in the United Kingdom, unlike methamphetamine in Australia or the United States.

> Amphetamine users attending the service described constitute a high risk group of drug users. The availability of dexamphetamine prescribing as one option in the treatment of amphetamine users increased the number and proportion of amphetamine users attending the service. The prescription of dexamphetamine significantly increased the duration of service contact. The prescription of dexamphetamine to this selected group of high risk amphetamine users substantially reduced the self reported quantity and frequency of illicit amphetamine use. There was a substantial reduction in injecting behaviour and in the sharing of needles. The incidence of all side-effects was low. The incidence of psychosis and hypertension appeared to be related to factors other than the prescribed dexamphetamine.
>
> The Study supports the developing consensus that dexamphetamine prescribing reduces high-risk behaviour in selected amphetamine users. Properly designed double blind controlled trials are now required to test the validity of these observations, but the difficulty of conducting such studies should not be underestimated (McBride et al. 1997, pp.110–111).

One barrier to treatment participation, however, noted at the recent South Australian Drugs Summit, was the cost of substitute medication. Although this was discussed particularly in the context of heroin and alcohol abuse (the cost of medications such as methadone, buprenorphine and naltrexone), the same point would apply to any existing or subsequently developed medications to treat amphetamine dependence.

The Treatment Working Group at the Summit stated:

> The cost of [such] medications...should not expose the individual to financial hardship arising from their participation in treatment. This has been identified as a significant barrier to retention in treatment. The benefits associated with continued treatment are such that measures to overcome this barrier is considered by the working group to be highly desirable (South Australian Drugs Summit Communiqué 2002a, p.11).

As a result the Working Group recommended the introduction of a co-payment system for clients where 'the fee burden is shared between the individual and the state' (p.11).

Problems with substitution therapy?

Not all commentators have supported amphetamine substitution treatment or indeed separate treatment regimes for amphetamine users. The Treatment Working Party of the South Australian Summit sounded a cautionary note about relying too heavily on new pharmacotherapies to address problematic amphetamine use:

> The inordinate amount of research effort that has been directed at pharmacological interventions for cocaine [and amphetamine] users has been to the detriment of psychosocial interventions which have good potential. Commentators in the field have recommended that further research on

> pharmacotherapies for cocaine and amphetamines factor in complementary psychological therapies, and be directed to determining whether specific pharmacotherapies add to overall treatment effectiveness. Because the safety of stimulant use is unpredictable and rates of retention in treatment tend to be poor, caution should be exercised when investigating new medications because of the possibility of additive negative effects of the trial drug and the stimulant. Indeed, it is desirable that selection of pharmacotherapies be undertaken on the basis of neurophysiological theory – the impression gained by reviewing research on pharmacotherapies for cocaine dependence is that of a scattergun approach in the hope that something interesting will emerge. Increased understanding of mechanisms of action of cocaine and amphetamines, and selection of appropriately targeted pharmacotherapies, would seem to be a more efficient approach (South Australian Drugs Summit Issues Paper 2002b, pp.15–16).

There have also been concerns expressed about the quality of the research conducted with regard to amphetamine substitution, including some of the older British studies that have been relied upon.

Mattick and Darke, for example, have sounded a note of caution, arguing that many of the analyses and studies upon which support of amphetamine substitution rely lack methodological rigour. The true efficacy of amphetamine prescribing can only be known when sufficient random and case-controlled trials are conducted (Mattick & Darke 1995). Wodak, although acknowledging that some of the studies (for example, Charnaud and Griffiths 1998) seem to hold promise, states that 'the rigour of these studies has not yet reached the standards usually required for categorical conclusions' (Wodak 2001). White, echoing Mattick and Darke, argues that without controlled trials 'there is no way of knowing whether clients who cease injecting would not have done so anyway without a prescription' (White 1996, cited in Kamienicki et al. 1998, pp.38–39).[910] In a more recent study White summarises the evidence and the findings from dexamphetamine substitution therapies as follows:

> Substitute prescribing has been regarded with suspicion by many (cf Mattick & Darke, 1995). Apart from the apparent failure of previous attempts at prescribing (Hawkes et al., 1969), and fears regarding the potential toxicity of amphetamines (Sato, 1986), there have also been concerns regarding diversion, the difficulty of monitoring illicit use and difficulty in defining an identifiable dependence syndrome (Parmeshwar, 1995, Topp & Mattick, 1997).
>
> Most agencies, however, are united in recognizing a pressing need to find effective interventions for amphetamine users, particularly injectors. Klee (1992a, 1992b) compared opiate and amphetamine users and found that, of the two, amphetamine users are at a greater risk of contracting transmissible

910 Lintzeris, Holgate and Dunlop have established comprehensive guidelines for the establishment of an Amphetamine Prescription Program and a controlled amphetamine prescription study. These bear paying attention to. See Lintzeris, Holgate and Dunlop (1996).

> illnesses. Their habit, with its potential for inducting greater arousal and sociability, makes it likely that they will be involved in a greater *range* of risk behaviours.
>
> Amphetamine substitution as a possible solution has, in recent years, been largely limited to the UK, where there is no legal impediment to prescribing amphetamines for this purpose. A survey in 1995 estimated that there were 900–1000 people in England and Wales in receipt of a prescription of amphetamines for the treatment of addiction (Strang & Sheridan, 1997). Another, more recently, reported that 46% of drug misuse medical specialists in England and Wales regularly prescribe amphetamines (Bradbeer et al., 1998).
>
> However, the practice seems to have evolved without empirical support for its efficacy. The attempts that have been made to evaluate the treatment (eg. Ford, 1993, Fleming & Roberts, 1994; Pates, Coombes & Ford, 1996; McBride et al., 1997), have yielded some promising results but, with the exception of McBride's study, they were performed with small samples and under artificial treatment conditions (eg. with very stringent entry criteria and with dexamphetamine doses fixed at a modest level) and, crucially, without a control group. Despite continued widespread prescribing, there is therefore still only very limited evidence that the treatment is effectives, and as yet no evidence to suggest when prescribing is appropriate, or at what dose and for how long (White 2000, pp.229–230). (Author's emphasis)

Even in Britain where substitution therapy has been most utilised, concerns have been expressed. Myles states:

> In the guidelines on the Clinical Management of Drug Dependence (HMSO, 1991), it is advised that the most appropriate treatment for amphetamine users is abrupt cessation of amphetamines without substitute prescribing. It has also been the consistent view, held by many statutory drugs agencies in the UK, that developing interventions that involve substitute prescribing for amphetamine users is only prolonging and expanding the extent of amphetamine use generally. It has been further the view that to prescribe a stimulant drug is dangerous in terms of the anticipated behavioural consequences and may induce more cases of amphetamine psychosis[911] (Myles 1997, p.75).

However, even commentators such as Myles quoted above recognise that there are benefits to substitution programmes:

> The balance of risks associated with prescribing dexamphetamine when compared with the alternatives – irresponsible injecting behaviour, lack of retention of stimulant users in drug services, unplanned sexual activity, and recurrent episodes of psychosis – suggests that a well controlled prescribing intervention could be reasonably recommended (Myles 1997, p.78).

---

911 It was thought particularly unsuitable that amphetamines be prescribed to patients who were also suffering from schizophrenic conditions (Myles 1997, p.78).

Medication or substitute pharmacotherapies are also seen as being a possible valuable adjunct in early days of withdrawal. In a study of effective treatments for methamphetamine addiction, Rawson, Gonzales and Brethen state:

> [I]t would be tremendously helpful to have medications that could help methamphetamine users recover more quickly from the effects of chronic use. Medication(s) that could reduce symptoms in the early days and weeks of recovery could be extremely valuable in promoting engagement and retention in behavioural and psychosocial treatments (Rawson, Gonzales & Brethen 2002, p.147).

On balance, substitution programmes do seem to have benefit,[912] although there have not been sufficient evaluative studies undertaken to make this claim with complete confidence.[913] Clearly such objective evidence is required. Professor Jason White of the Drug and Alcohol Services Council in South Australia stated to the Committee that some promising research is being conducted internationally that may yield some promising results for pharmacotherapies for amphetamine use:

> We are currently looking at practical issues such as the best available drugs and which ones we can get the pharmaceutical companies to cooperate with. It is at an interesting stage of development. I was recently at a meeting in Amsterdam at which people from the National Institute on Drug Abuse in the US presented their program of research around stimulants. They have a very structured research plan about what they want to do. There are a number of drugs that they are looking at testing. As opposed to what has happened perhaps in the last 20 years, where they have had almost a total lack of success, there are probably some drugs now that look more positive in terms of outcomes. I think we will see an increase in the range of drugs that are used for the treatment of stimulant dependence over the next five years. It may not be confined solely to the issue of substitution. There may be other alternatives. We are looking at some issues of substitution at the moment but it may be that what we do changes.[914]

Certainly DASC in South Australia will be examining the feasibility of possible dexamphetamine substitution therapies and other pharmacological interventions.

---

912 See Table G in Appendix 34 for a summary of the positive outcomes associated with amphetamine substitution therapies.

913 Myles drawing from the evidence both formal and informal of presenters at a variety of United Kingdom conferences and other academic fora claims that:

'[such] presentations clearly demonstrated certain outcomes of [substitution] treatment, most notably that drug users engaged in services when they became aware that a substitute prescribing intervention might be available and that those patients, taken on for treatment, showed a high rate of retention in treatment. Additionally they demonstrated a marked decrease in injecting practice, increased social stability and a marked reduction in criminal activity' (Myles 1997, p.77).

914 Professor Jason White, DASC in conversation with the Drugs and Crime Prevention Committee, Adelaide, 3 October 2003.

It should be noted that the Department of Human Services Victoria is also currently considering conducting a trial with regard to the prescription of oral amphetamine (dexamphetamine) as a substitute treatment for dependent injecting amphetamine users:

> This trial is expected to evaluate the safety and efficacy of prescribed oral dexamphetamine for amphetamine dependence. It will measure whether street amphetamine use decreases and if treatment retention, HIV/HCV risk behaviour, psychological and social adjustment, criminal behaviour and general health improve under this trial. It is expected that the trial will be completed by the end of 2003.[915]

As of the time of writing (March 2004), the proposed trials have not yet commenced. A feasibility study has been called for and it is envisaged that dependent upon the results of this study the trials will commence in the later part of the year.[916]

Turning Point Alcohol and Drug Centre has also given some guarded approval to the idea of running a clinical dexamphetamine trial. For example Professor Margaret Hamilton told the Committee in this regard:

> We are suggesting that there is a need to continue to look at new treatments – for example, the trial of dexamphetamine. I know a lot of people find it difficult to think that giving a drug user drugs is a way to treat them, but it is one way of dramatically decreasing harm. Getting people into treatment can often be facilitated by having medications available. That is what we have learnt with heroin users, with methadone, with buprenorphine and so on. Having a medication makes a difference as to whether they will come to treatment in the first instance. We have nothing at the moment to offer. Dexamphetamine is promising and would provide us, if we could do some research on that, with an opportunity to use that as a part of the menu of options for people with these dependencies on amphetamines.[917]

Whatever the efficacy of substitution treatments, it would seem to be essential that any form of pharmacotherapy needs 'to be supported by access to psychiatric, psychological, and medical services' (Kaye & Darke 2000, p.194). For example, one recent study undertaken in New South Wales has indicated that amphetamine substitution in combination with counselling or cognitive behavioural interventions may produce some positive results (Allen & Tressider 2003).

---

915 Submission of the Department of Human Services Victoria (Drugs Policy and Services Branch) to the Drugs and Crime Prevention Committee, Inquiry into Amphetamine and 'Party Drug' Use in Victoria, August 2002.

916 Personal communication from the Drugs and Policy Services Branch, Department of Human Services Victoria to the Drugs and Crime Prevention Committee, 4 March 2004.

917 Professor Margaret Hamilton, Director, Turning Point Alcohol and Drug Centre, evidence given to the Drugs and Crime Prevention Committee, Inquiry into Amphetamine and 'Party Drug' Use in Victoria, Melbourne, 27 October 2003.

The fact that substitution measures seem to be popular among users themselves also needs to be taken into consideration.[918] Evaluation of these and other treatment measures are an important overall part of research involving amphetamines and 'party drugs'.[919] This general issue will be discussed in the following chapter.

Different populations

Many commentators have drawn attention to the fact that while some of the basic attributes of drug treatment programmes may be comparatively similar, for example the use of particular medications, other aspects of the programme may need to be modelled specifically for different drug using populations (Kamienicki et al. 1998; Wright, Klee & Reid 1999; Anglin et al. 2000; Rawson, Gonzales & Brethen 2002). This is particularly true of an area such as amphetamines and 'party drugs' where the profiles of users are so diverse, as discussed in Chapter 9.

Young people

The needs of young people who are receiving treatment for amphetamine abuse may not be the same as their adult counterparts (Klee & Morris 1994). Treatment programmes may include components, or at least access to ancillary programmes, on literacy skills or sexuality to name a few. A safe environment where they can take 'time out' may in itself be a valuable preliminary form of 'treatment', or at least a first point in which they may start to seriously think about, if not necessarily act upon, treatment options.[920]

---

918 As stated previously, Hando, Topp and Hall's survey found that substitution therapy was the most popular of the treatment options with 18% of the subjects requesting it.

However, it should be noted, if somewhat cynically, that not all users of amphetamines who have requested substitution therapies may have done so with treatment or 'recovery' uppermost in mind.

The difference in motivation between opiate and amphetamine users with regard to accessing (or not accessing) treatment services is summed up in this quote from a drug service worker:

'Somebody who's an opiate user will be prepared to come back because they know they're going to get something...they know they're going to get methadone. Whereas an amphet [sic] user is going to get counselling or something like that' (Wright, Klee & Morris 1999, p.80).

919 One of the recommendations of the Youth Substance Abuse Service (YSAS) to this Committee has been to fund greater research into the development of alternative pharmacotherapies for the treatment of amphetamine-related disorders. See Submission of YSAS to the Drugs and Crime Prevention Committee, Inquiry into Amphetamine and 'Party Drug' Use in Victoria, October 2003.

920 For example, Professor Steve Allsop of the Western Australian Drug and Alcohol Office states that for many young people with drug-related problems, particularly amphetamine-related problems, there is a crucial need for a place where they can feel safe. At that stage in their drug using they may not want anything longer term:

'We had therapeutic communities saying [to a young person] : "oh well, would you like to go away for 6 months to a therapeutic community?"; which to a 16-year-old amphetamine user might not be particularly attractive. So, I think that the services were unattractive to the users and the services themselves were a bit unsure about how to manage them' (Professor Steve Allsop in conversation with the Drugs and Crime Prevention Committee, Perth, 1 October 2003).

The Youth Substance Abuse Service has had an increasing number of young people admitted to both their residential and non-residential services with amphetamine-related problems. They state:

> YSAS has responded to the increasing number of young people using amphetamines by ensuring that appropriate treatment services are provided for them. For example, this meant the reorientating of residential and home-based withdrawal services to address the particular needs of amphetamine withdrawal responses such as sleep disturbances and depression, whilst continuing to provide services to those requiring opiate withdrawal.[921]

However, there are particular problems associated with inpatient or residential treatment programmes for young people who use amphetamines. As Howard et al. explain:

> Howard and Arcuri (2003a) found that those clients presenting with primary psychostimulant use had the lowest rates of retention in residential treatment, with close to 60% leaving in the first thirty days of ninety day inpatient treatment. This initial finding may bring into question the effectiveness of such treatment for this group of users. However, of those clients who completed a substantial component of the program (as measured by attendance of at least 6 weeks) at three months post treatment the psychostimulant users did as well as other users on the whole; showing statistically less drug use from pre-treatment measures (self reported). The fact that the outcomes for this group were no different to the other groups of young people presenting to treatment is quite significant when one considers the more problematic pre-treatment presentation of psychostimulant clients in this study (ie. they were more likely to have self reported greater mental and physical health problems, greater money problems, more likely to have overdosed, committed person and property crimes in the last three months and were more likely to have had more sexual partners three months prior to treatment).
>
> It should be noted that residential treatment is an expensive and potentially invasive option for young people. As such, it should be viewed as the last option where external supports (eg. family, school/work, accommodation, income, etc) have broken down, are openly hostile or are non existent, or where there are significant mental health and other behavioural concerns present. Whilst residential treatment will remove a young person from their environment and thus halt or break dysfunctional behaviour patterns and associations, it also does likewise with those things that are working in the young person's life. By entering a residential treatment facility the young person is given a peer group with which to associate, all of whom have significant AOD issues themselves. The potential for "streetwise" young people with more entrenched behaviours influencing less experienced less problematic users is a real risk (Howard, Stubbs & Arcuri 2004, in prep).

---

921 Submission of YSAS to the Drugs and Crime Prevention Committee, Inquiry into Amphetamine and 'Party Drug' Use in Victoria, October 2003.

Howard et al. also state that while young people who use psychostimulants may require specialised care at particular times (such as during withdrawal or suffering from a significant dependency), generally:

> [h]owever, they require the same assistance as other young people. Research shows that early interventions have the greatest impact and multiple interventions are more effective than one-dimensional approaches. Effectiveness of programs is further enhanced by the involvement of caregivers and families. Families and the wider community need to "provide young people with opportunities to develop increasingly complex intellectual skills to express their emotions appropriately, to develop supportive friends, and to assume new responsibilities" (WHO, 2002b). In this way, young people may gain the confidence and skills to assist them to live independently and contribute to their families and communities. It needs to be noted, that while a holistic approach is implied, the suggestion is not that young people who use substances or those who develop substance-use related difficulties are deficient. Rather, treatment interventions, whilst addressing any deficits, must acknowledge and build on strengths inherent in the young person.
>
> In considering prevention and treatment options for young people efforts to date have brought varied results, and, there is a need for more comprehensive programs and more sophisticated research. Further, there is a need for increased participation by young people in all aspects of interventions for substance use-related difficulties; including prevention, treatment, assessing need, planning, delivery of interventions, monitoring and evaluation (Kirsch, 1995: WHO, 1993 & 1995). As for future research, it is recommended that secondary analyses of existing adult data sets be undertaken to explore for any effects of age and gender differences, and, in any future research, include these two variables (Howard, Stubbs & Arcuri 2004, in prep).

Women

Turning Point Alcohol and Drug Centre have expressed to the Committee the importance of further research into the discrete treatment needs of women. This is particularly true of pregnant women who may be amphetamine users. Rawson, Gonzales and Brethen comment:

> Pregnant women and women with small children frequently require increased levels of care. While it may be possible to treat pregnant women in intensive outpatient treatment, attention must be given to monitoring and promoting proper prenatal care with these women while in treatment. In addition, it is important that clinical staff be capable of working with pregnant women who relapse in treatment. Frequently, there is an extreme lack of empathy exhibited by staff and other patients toward women who relapse during their pregnancy. Clinical staff who can properly address these treatment situations and effectively move these patients to more intensive levels of care when necessary is essential. Women with small children frequently require an increased level of support either via a women's and children's residential setting or an intensive

> day treatment setting with sober housing for women and children. The combined burdens of work, home care, childcare, and other family responsibilities, plus attending treatment frequently can induce such a level of exhaustion and fatigue that MA use may appear to be the only way to acquire sufficient energy to accomplish all of the responsibilities. Clearly under these circumstances, special treatment considerations are needed (2002, p.149).

Dr Nicole Lee of Turning Point Alcohol and Drug Centre has also indicated to the Committee the need to ensure discrete populations such as women and children have their specific needs taken into consideration when examining treatment options:

> [s]ome special populations that have been identified [with regard to treatment research]: young people and their use of amphetamines and other psychostimulants – there is very little research into that area; and women, especially pregnant women...[922]

As indicated in Chapter 9 there is very little known about the natural history of women who use amphetamines (and other drugs) in general and even less about the effects of such drugs on the unborn child. Women amphetamine users are known to be even less likely to access treatment services than males. Wright, Klee and Reid posit that:

> Reluctance to be identified as a drug user is particularly strong for women who fear that social services may be informed, to check on the welfare of their children (Wright, Klee & Reid 1999, p.78 and the references listed therein).

The specific needs of female (and male) sex and street workers must also be taken into consideration when considering treatment interventions for amphetamine users in particular.

Indigenous Victorians

When the Committee asked Indigenous drug and alcohol workers how drug use of any kind among Indigenous people should be addressed the workers were unanimous in believing that socioeconomic deprivation and structural deficits, particularly in the areas of employment, education and housing, were primary reasons Aboriginal people turned to drugs and this must be taken into consideration in any areas of policy development or analysis. As Mr Rick Henderson, Acting Executive Officer of the Central Gippsland Aboriginal Co-operative stated to the Committee:

> It incorporates all those social justice issues around education, employment, health, homelessness. I put it this way: to have a home you need a house; to have a house you need a job; to have a job you need education; to have

922 Dr Nicole Lee, Turning Point Alcohol and Drug Centre, evidence given to the Drugs and Crime Prevention Committee, Inquiry into Amphetamine and 'Party Drug' Use in Victoria, Public Hearings (Melbourne), 27 October 2003.

> education you need to have a place where you feel safe, and where is that? That is a home. It goes in a circle.[923]

Mr Jurgen Hemmerling of the Open Family (Hume Region), although not referring specifically to the Indigenous community, also believed secure housing was a crucial protective factor in reducing drug consumption or initiating it in the first place. This was particularly the case for those living in rural and regional Victoria:

> [i]t is really hard to deal with someone's alcohol and drug issues if they have nowhere to live or if they have not eaten for three days. So there are some priority issues that obviously take place. The research will indicate that if people do not have safe and secure housing they will not do well regardless of what interventions you have. So that could be the priority issue and that might be the first thing we do: organise stable housing, get them a food voucher or take them out and get them a feed or whatever, and then look at the other stuff.[924]

Such comments apply equally, if not more so, to members of the Indigenous community, particularly those in rural Victoria.

Indigenous Victorians in rural and regional parts of the state are also concerned about the lack of facilities and services for drug prevention, education and treatment for their communities:

> If you think about all the factors that come into play within the Koori community, we live in a crisis from day to day, because the programs are reactive instead of proactive. It might be that your day is not planned. We work 24 hours a day, seven days a week, no matter what you do. You do not knock off at five. Laurie is on call. He is the only worker for the whole region. He is on call every day of the year, 24 hours a day. So in terms of the reactive programs versus the proactive, we would like to see money allocated to proactive programs. If I need to go to Bendin House, which is the alcohol and drug program at the co-op, to get help, the situation has gone too far already. I should not need to go there. I would see that funding should be allocated for an awareness and education program in the community.[925]

Services such as a de-tox centre in an area such as the Latrobe Valley is sorely needed. As discussed in the chapter on rural and regional issues, workers in the country are appalled that they need to transport clients to Melbourne to seek treatment. For Indigenous people this may be particularly problematic if it

923 Mr Rick Henderson, Acting Executive Officer of the Central Gippsland Aboriginal Co-operative, evidence given to the Drugs and Crime Prevention Committee, Inquiry into Amphetamine and 'Party Drug' Use in Victoria, Public Hearings (Moe), 23 October 2003.

924 Mr Jurgen Hemmerling, Outreach Worker, Open Family, Hume Region, evidence given to the Drugs and Crime Prevention Committee, Inquiry into Amphetamine and 'Party Drug' Use in Victoria, Public Hearings (Benalla), 22 October 2003. For further discussion of amphetamine and 'party drug' use in rural and regional Victoria, see Chapter 11.

925 Rick Henderson, Acting Executive Officer of the Central Gippsland Aboriginal Co-operative, evidence given to the Drugs and Crime Prevention Committee, Inquiry into Amphetamine and 'Party Drug' Use in Victoria, Public Hearings (Moe), 23 October 2003.

results in a person being isolated from family, friends and peers in an alien and in some cases culturally insensitive environment:

> Once you get sent to Melbourne, there is a sense of being forgotten by people, by your family. You are doing it on your own and are not supported. If there was something here in the country, I think it would make inroads into some of the issues that we have.[926]

Not all workers from Gippsland with whom the Committee met believed it was necessary to provide Koori-specific treatment centres. They did, however, state it was crucial that such facilities employ a sufficient number of Koori workers there.[927]

Recommending initiatives and strategies with regard to amphetamine use among Indigenous communities is difficult, especially given that there is so little hard data on the subject. Further research both quantitative and qualitative in this area needs to be undertaken, preferably by Indigenous researchers or, at the very least, with the guidance and co-operation of the Indigenous community. Nonetheless, the Committee acknowledges the concerns of organisations such as ATSIS and concerned individuals within the communities. It accepts that there are many strategies pertaining to general licit and illicit drug use which may be adaptable or relevant to specific issues around amphetamine use. ATSIS has suggested the following interventions as ways of addressing drug abuse within Indigenous communities:

- Improve school retention rates through more appropriate curriculum and more support services for Aboriginal students
- Improve and expand support services for Aboriginal families (eg. financial resources to be able to support kids to get involved in positive activities; eg. parenting skills to be able to provide better support to their kids)
- Implementation of Indigenous mentors/role models program
- Resources for Aboriginal communities to run constructive social activities, to build community and individual confidence and pride

---

926 Mr Gordon Hood, Program Co-ordinator, Bendin House, Central Gippsland Aboriginal Co-operative, evidence given to the Drugs and Crime Prevention Committee, Inquiry into Amphetamine and 'Party Drug' Use in Victoria, Public Hearings (Moe), 23 October 2003.

927 This issue of Indigenous specific versus generalist facilities was raised by members of the South Australian Drugs and Alcohol Service Council (DASC) when the Committee met with them in October 2003.

Ms Kelly Weekley, Manager of the Harm Reduction Unit of the DASC said in this regard:

'One of the significant pushes at the moment is in terms of Indigenous populations. Do they go to mainstream services or do they go to Aboriginal-specific services? The only answer we have to that is that some want to go where they are not known and some would prefer a service that meets their cultural needs. The only way we as an organisation can address it is to have more services so that they have more choices' (Ms Kelly Weekley in conversation with the Drugs and Crime Prevention Committee, Adelaide, 3 October 2003).

The issue was also discussed at length in the Drugs and Crime Prevention Committee's *Final Report into Public Drunkenness* and its *Final Report into the Inhalation of Volatile Substances*. On balance it would seem that a majority of Indigenous community representatives would like to see separate Indigenous health and welfare facilities, particularly in the area of drug services. For an in depth discussion of these issues, particularly in the context of Koori holistic healing centres, see the Reports mentioned above.

- Resources for Aboriginal communities to run programs to help build individual and community capacity, to make sure people have the skills and opportunities to make positive life choices
- Private and public sector commitment to ensuring economic and employment opportunities are accessible to Indigenous Victorians.[928]

Such initiatives should be seriously considered.

Gay men

This Report has commented previously about the disproportionately high health risks faced by gay men, particularly those who use methamphetamine as a dance or 'party drug'. Given that this drug is relatively prevalent in one aspect of gay subculture, and often in combination with alcohol and other drugs, this has implications for treatment services. As American commentators who have worked with gay dance patrons and/or male sex workers who have sex with other men state:

> The needs of gay male MA users may require special treatment programming (Frosch et al., 1996). The use of MA by gay and bisexual men frequently becomes inextricably intertwined with their sexual and social behaviors. The unique and powerful nature of this conditioned pathology presents a clinical syndrome that often cannot be effectively discussed in mixed patient groups with heterosexuals. The importance of this issue and the difficulty of discussing it in mixed patient groups frequently results in very poor treatment engagement and early treatment dropout. The importance of successful treatment with this group is of particular importance as the sexual behavior of this group is a tremendously critical vector in the spread of HIV (Reback 1997) (Rawson, Gonzales & Brethen 2002, p.149).

Psychiatric co-morbidity

As has been discussed previously, amphetamines are drugs associated with psychiatric co-morbidity. This may be associated with either the effects of the drugs themselves (amphetamine psychosis), an underlying psychiatric condition in the person who takes the drug, or a combination of both. Whatever the reason, experts in the area have stressed the importance of having treatment services that can deal with the issues of psychiatric co-morbidity. Sometimes underlying psychotic symptoms may be resolved fairly speedily. In other cases more intensive treatments may be needed. Rawson, Gonzales and Brethen comment in the context of methamphetamine:

> Those individuals who enter treatment with such severe psychiatric impairment that they are unable to safely function on an outpatient basis require admission and stabilization in a medically supervised treatment setting where short term use of antipsychotic and tranquilizer mediations can be

928 Submission of State Office (Victoria) Aboriginal and Torres Strait Islander Services to the Drugs and Crime Prevention Committee, Inquiry into Amphetamine and 'Party Drug' Use in Victoria, November 2003.

> administered to reduce paranoia, psychosis, and agitation. The duration of treatment in this setting is variable. Many individuals require only 48–72 hours to resolve these debilitating psychiatric symptoms. Once these symptoms are resolved to allow the patient to be safely treated on an outpatient basis, transfer to this setting is appropriate.
>
> However, there are individuals whose psychiatric symptomatology is not quickly resolved. These patients require longer stays under medical/psychiatric supervision and may need ongoing treatment with antipsychotic medications (Rawson, Gonzales & Brethen 2002, p.149).

Moreover, Turning Point Alcohol and Drug Centre states that mental health services in this state tend to treat primarily psychotic conditions and conversely alcohol and drug workers rarely have formal mental health backgrounds. They argue that non-specialist drug and alcohol workers need to be up-skilled not just to manage non-psychotic co-morbidity issues but to develop interventions and appropriate treatment plans (see also Nutting, Lee, Jenner & Davies, in prep).[929] Professor Margaret Hamilton, Director of Turning Point Alcohol and Drug Centre, stated in this regard:

> We need to recognise that the mental health problems they [amphetamine users] experience are particularly in the arena that mental health services do not attend to, depression and anxiety; and also the need for drug treatment services to be more active in being able to recognise, diagnose and treat those particular conditions.[930]

The problems of co-morbidity and service delivery are also alluded to by Professor Steve Allsop, Executive Director of the Western Australian Drug and Alcohol Office:

> [m]ental health and drug problems have always been an issue – but I think amphetamines have really sharpened that issue for many of the services. I think many of the services found themselves initially at odds with how to respond to this group...
>
> A large proportion of people are being admitted to mental health services with amphetamine problems, and the two systems don't work well together, the mental health system and the drug system. The best description of that was a colleague, Steven Jerdis, in New South Wales, who said the duality is in the system, not in the individual; that the system isn't geared up well to work together to manage, so people with mental health problems seen by the drug services would be pushed off to the mental health services because it's a

929 Submission of Turning Point Alcohol and Drug Centre to the Drugs and Crime Prevention Committee, Inquiry into Amphetamine and 'Party Drug' Use in Victoria, October 2003.

930 Professor Margaret Hamilton, Director, Turning Point Alcohol and Drug Centre, evidence given to the Drugs and Crime Prevention Committee, Inquiry into Amphetamine and 'Party Drug' Use in Victoria, Public Hearings (Melbourne), 27 October 2003.

> mental health problem and, of course, the people in the mental health services would see a drug problem and push back.[931]

Mr Richard Bostwick, Perth clinician and Director of the Joint Services Unit of the Western Australian Health Department, states that there is definitely 'a disparity in the levels of clinical knowledge within both [drug and alcohol and mental health] sectors'.[932]

In Western Australia there is a specific dual diagnosis service that addresses the problems associated with co-existent amphetamine and other drug-related problems in persons with psychiatric or mental health related conditions. Mr Bostwick pointed out to the Committee that:

> around 60 to 80 per cent of people presenting with a mental health problem have got a co-morbid substance problem and about 50 per cent of people with a drug and alcohol problem have got a co-morbid mental health problem.[933]

The correlation between psychiatric illness and amphetamine use is particularly high, although as indicated the precise nature of the relationship between the drug use and the psychiatric symptoms is difficult to ascertain. Mr Bostwick outlines the problems in treatment service delivery that this relationship gives rise to:

> I guess the issue with co-morbidity or dual diagnosis, people who have got a mental health problem and a substance misuse problem is that the very nature of the problem usually isn't entrenched within the individual. It is actually – it is a problem with the system and how the system deals with these individuals. Stephen Jerdis, a psychiatrist from New South Wales, made this salient comment probably about 4 or 5 years ago now, that the duality is with the system, not with the individual. And basically there he was talking about, there is a heck of a lot of duplication and redundancy within services.
>
> It is expensive both for governments and for health service providers but it is also messy and complex for people who are trying to navigate the system. So if you can imagine somebody with a mental health problem and an overlay of a substance misuse problem or vice versa, perhaps some cognitive deficits and having to negotiate the system, which is quite complex for people that actually work in the system. So with those deficits in mind, it is probably very difficult for them to work out where is the best point to access and which is the best and most effective treatment option for them.[934]

931 Professor Steve Allsop, Executive Director, Drug and Alcohol Office of Western Australia, in conversation with the Drugs and Crime Prevention Committee, Perth, 1 October 2003.

932 Richard Bostwick, Director of Clinical Services, Joint Services Development Unit, Western Australian Health Department, in conversation with the Drugs and Crime Prevention Committee, 1 October 2003.

933 Ibid.

934 Ibid.

In Victoria, the Turning Point Alcohol and Drug Centre has testified to the inadequacies of the mental health system as it pertains to drug treatment issues:

> More service research is required because mental health services generally won't accept people with non psychotic mental health conditions... So Alcohol and Drug Workers (who usually have no formal mental health background) need to be skilled in not just management but intervention.
>
> Much more research is needed into non psychotic co-morbid conditions.[935]

A positive step in Victoria, however, is the development of the Dual Diagnosis Initiative, an undertaking of the Victorian Department of Human Services. The initiative is described as follows:

> Given the prevalence of clients attending services experiencing co morbid substance abuse and mental health disorders; Victoria has developed a Statewide initiative aimed at building the capacity of existing Mental Health and Alcohol and Other Drug Services.
>
> The key activities of the initiative are the development of local networks; training consultation to cover the State. The Dual Diagnosis Lead Agencies are auspiced by St. Vincent's Health Service, Southern Health, Eastern Health and Melbourne Health.
>
> The four Dual Diagnosis teams currently sit across the 2 service systems with a total of 27 Dual Diagnosis workers employed by the 4 lead agencies. These workers are located both in metropolitan and rural areas.[936]

The role of specialist dual diagnosis workers is to provide a link between services for those people who suffer from both mental health and substance abuse problems. In particular:

> Each specialist dual diagnosis worker should be allocated a catchment for which they will be responsible for:
>
> The development of cooperative working relationships between mental health and drug treatment services within the relevant area service catchment. This should particularly address issues of access, assessment and the development of effective treatment planning.
>
> The provision of training and consultation to all mental health (including PDSS) and drug treatment services within the service catchment with a strong focus on building capacity within the services to respond more effectively to people with a Dual Diagnosis.
>
> The provision of a direct service to clients with a serious mental illness and substance use problems with a focus on developing and modelling good

935 Submission of Turning Point Alcohol and Drug Centre to the Drugs and Crime Prevention Committee, Inquiry into Amphetamine and 'Party Drug' Use in Victoria, October 2003.

936 Correspondence from Alysha Batty, Policy Officer Drug Treatment and Health Promotion, Drugs Policy and Services Branch, Department of Human Services (Victoria) to the Drugs and Crime Prevention Committee, 25 February 2004.

> practice. This may be through providing a limited direct service and intensive support/consultation to case managers on specific cases.[937]

There are also specialist positions being developed for youth dual diagnosis services. These positions recognise that co-morbidity can be as much an issue for young people as it is for adults. Funding has been provided for new clinical and support positions targeted at youth residential rehabilitation services to support young people with a dual diagnosis. Four positions have been located in youth residential rehabilitation services and four in mobile support and treatment teams (MST).

These youth positions are attached to and build on the experience and infrastructure of the existing Dual Diagnosis teams:

> Many of the features of existing dual diagnosis teams will be built into this strategy. However a number of key differences are also required to take into account the broader range of conditions and developmental issues, which are managed by adolescent and youth focused services and the different service context.[938]

The aims of the Youth Dual Diagnosis Strategy are:

> 1. Promote greater collaboration between Child and Adolescent Mental Health Services (CAMHS) and youth alcohol and drug treatment services.
> 2. Enhance the confidence and skills of workers in CAMHS and youth drug and alcohol treatment services in assisting young people with a DD.
> 3. Provide direct treatment and support to a small number of young people who have a complex presentation of both mental illness and problematic alcohol and drug use.
>
> The target group is young people aged between 16–25 years old with a diagnosed mental illness who have serious substance abuse issues.[939]

In addition to developments in Victoria, there has also been recognition at Commonwealth level of the importance of integrating mental health and substance abuse services where relevant. For example the announcement in the 2003–2004 Federal Budget by the Commonwealth Government of funding for a National Co-morbidity Initiative ($4.4 million over two years), the aims of which are to improve treatment co-ordination and outcomes for co-morbid clients, is certainly a step in the right direction.

It is not only specialists who need to be apprised of the needs of amphetamine users. Non-specialist medical and non-medical personnel also have an important role to play.

937 Ibid.
938 Ibid.
939 Ibid.

The importance of non-specialists

One of the constant themes coming from the literature is the place of non-specialist medical officers in addressing issues pertaining to (meth)amphetamine and to a lesser extent ecstasy use. Dr Nick Lintzeris, formerly medical officer with the Turning Point Alcohol and Drug Centre, stated that doctors and nurses *outside* the drug and alcohol field see more amphetamine users than do drug and alcohol counsellors:

> Certain GPs in certain areas see a lot of amphetamine use. For example, in one or two community health centres in Melbourne the doctors who work there are saying 'I've thought about becoming a methadone prescriber but there's no point – I'd see one heroin user for every 20 amphetamine users' (quoted in Wood 1998a, pp.20–21).

Many studies, both in Australia and overseas, have stressed the importance of having *well trained* general practitioners as a front line source of information and assistance for amphetamine users.[940]

Vincent et al. state it may therefore be:

> ...important to ensure that these professionals are equipped to respond appropriately to their needs. However, it has been noted that most health practitioners are largely unfamiliar with the management of amphetamine-related problems, and so require education and training on the issues. Another option may be the development of a system of 'shared care' between treatment services and general practitioners in the community. Such a system has been implemented in Britain, and although under resourced has been highly successful in many instances, particularly where services have been more pro-active in forging links with GPs (Vincent et al. 1999, pp.71–72).

In Western Australia there have been concerted efforts made to enable general practitioners to deal with problems associated with amphetamine and other drug use, or at least recognise the issues surrounding the use and abuse of such drugs. This is partly attributable to the huge land area of that state and the few specialists that may be found outside metropolitan Perth. The Director of the Western Australian Drug and Alcohol Office explained the importance of using general practitioners to the Committee:

> The international evidence and the local evidence is consistent. One of the first ports of call for amphetamine users are GPs. It's a consistent message from research in South Australia, New South Wales and the UK, one of the first places they will go is a GP, not for drug problems but for malnourishment, sleeping disorders and mood disorders. A lovely little study [was] done in South Australia with a couple of post-graduate medical students. They interviewed 11 users and nine out of 11 of them said they would go to a GP if they had a problem with their amphetamine use. And they interviewed 11 GPs and nine

940 See Klee and Morris 1994; Klee et al. 1995; Hando, Topp and Hall 1997; Kamienicki et al. 1998; Vincent et al. 1999; Baker, Boggs and Lewin 2000.

> out of 11 GPs said they would send them somewhere else. And I think that is an issue. They are using general medical practices and one of the things we have to do is look at ways in which we can provide a better link between the general medical services and the drug specialist services.
>
> We've done a little bit of work on that in this State. One of the things we've done is provided some funding to the non-Government sector and the community drug service teams, to employ medical expertise into their services, particularly in the remote areas. So a GP might be reluctant to see someone in their practice for all sorts of reasons. They may not be reliable at turning up for appointments and that can cause havoc as well as cost money. The GP may be reluctant to see them because they don't have the support services around them. Whereas a GP may be willing to see someone in a community drug service team setting and build up a collegiate network.
>
> So we've funded a number of the community drug service teams out in the rural areas to actually have access to that. Similar to other jurisdictions, we have a GP program where we invest quite considerable effort in recruiting medical staff or "seducing" medical staff, if you like, to engage in working in the drug arena, provide training and authorisation where that is required... Then providing a clinical consultancy and support service both to the GP and to other services around the GPs.[941]

Of particular concern is the need for emergency personnel to be aware of issues pertaining to amphetamine use. As Kamienicki et al. state:

> The emergency services are often the first point of contact psychostimulant users have with the health system. This occurs when medical or psychiatric complications result from psychostimulant use. Individuals may not have had previous contact with a drug and alcohol service as they may not have believed their drug use to be problematic or may not have perceived such services as attractive and/or accessible. Accident and emergency staff are ill equipped to respond to the needs of psychostimulant users. They generally lack knowledge about psychostimulant use, have limited skills in identifying psychostimulant related harm, and limited skills in responding to and managing intoxicated behaviour. It is also important that referral pathways and processes are identified for accident and emergency staff (Kamienicki et al. 1998, pp.66–67).

Dr Kevin Lambkin of Queensland Health also stressed the importance of having knowledgeable and well trained 'frontline' workers' to assist amphetamine users who often are volatile or 'hard to manage':

> One of the main findings of the recent national working group on amphetamine issues was probably that the treatment capability most needed was the ability to deal with a person at street level, I suppose, with that sort of behaviour – not so much specialist treatment personnel but for generalist

941 Professor Steve Allsop, Drug and Alcohol Office, in conversation with the Drugs and Crime Prevention Committee, Perth, 1 October 2003.

> providers like police, social workers or welfare workers who encounter these people – and what's the best way to deal with that.[942]

Needle and syringe exchanges may also be another good source of information and referral on treatment options. A submission from Anex, the umbrella agency for needle and syringe services, drawing from the research of Dixon and Maurice (2002) outlines the benefits of needle and syringe programmes for psychostimulant clients in terms of primary health care and longer term referrals. They include:

- Wound care clinics and providing material aid such as food or food vouchers are some examples of primary health interventions that may be offered. Providing a quiet space for amphetamine injectors to "chill out" is another practical response.
- Given that some amphetamine injectors may present with a number of physical symptoms such as muscle cramps, nausea and hypertension, while others may be experiencing psychosis, adequate procedures to facilitate access to appropriate crisis intervention services are important. These may include crisis assessment teams and hospital emergency departments.
- As amphetamine withdrawal may involve physical and emotional exhaustion resulting in fatigue and depression, developing clients' capacity to cope with withdrawal symptoms may be a useful primary health care strategy.[943]

Despite the benefits of access to such programmes there are also some obstacles that may mitigate against clients using them:[944]

> While the network of NSPs in Victoria have established a good reputation and relationship with injecting drug users, its capacity to engage meaningfully with clients is limited. The majority of outlets are based at community health centres and hospitals with the client contact occurring, in the majority of cases, over-the-counter at a general waiting area. This restricts the level of meaningful engagement that staff may have with clients as it restricts conversations on topics of a sensitive and confidential nature. Additionally most NSP staff have other duties aside from the provision of NSP-specific services which hampers the amount of time they may spend in working with clients to achieve better health outcomes.[945]

---

942 Dr Kevin Lambkin, Acting Manager, Alcohol, Tobacco and Other Drugs Unit, Queensland Health in conversation with the Drugs and Crime Prevention Committee, Brisbane, 27 June 2003.

943 Submission of Anex to the Drugs and Crime Prevention Committee, Inquiry into Amphetamine and 'Party Drug' Use in Victoria, October 2003.

944 Young people in particular may be reluctant or embarrassed to access the services of NSPs or pharmacies for reasons of confidentiality or to protect anonymity. This may particularly be the case in small towns or rural regions. See discussion in Chapter 11.

945 Submission of Anex to the Drugs and Crime Prevention Committee, Inquiry into Amphetamine and 'Party Drug' Use in Victoria, October 2003.

Nonetheless, as stated, it is to general health services that amphetamine users, at least at first instance, may go for assistance with any direct or indirect complications associated with the use of the drug. Yet as Kamienicki et al. also comment:

> Psychostimulant users may be reluctant to access mainstream health services due to uncertainty about the reaction of staff to their use of illicit drugs. Thus, the response they may receive initially may have an impact on compliance with treatment and future utilisation of health services. More informed service providers/clinicians are likely to be more confident in managing psychostimulant users. This may result in more positive experiences for these clients through more effective management of their problem, which, in turn, results in more effective reduction of harm.
>
> Staff in general health services should be trained to consult with clients to link them in with drug and alcohol services for assessment and on-going management beyond the acute problems, if this is required (Kamienicki et al. 1998, p.67).

Thus it is crucial to have generalist services integrated with specialist facilities and vice versa.

Many of the clinical and ancillary workers with whom the Committee has met have stressed the importance of providing a whole range of services, both medical and non-medical to people who have problems associated with their amphetamine, 'party drug' and/or poly-drug use.[946] This is particularly crucial given that many amphetamine users, as discussed, do not necessarily view themselves as either addicts or 'problem users' and thus may not access specialist drug treatment centres.

For example, Professor White of the Drugs and Alcohol Services Council of South Australia states that one of the key outcomes of the South Australian Drugs Summit was to provide better integrated treatment and service options for amphetamine users. Their project:

> [i]s looking at enhancing the ability of both specialist treatment services and primary health care to respond to amphetamine or stimulant related problems, with an emphasis on young people, since it was seen that a number of the people who used amphetamines were in younger age groups.
>
> ...What we are doing in that project is developing models of care, best practice in terms of care, putting those into practice and evaluating those to gain the evidence about their effectiveness. We then look at implementing those in primary health care, either as stand-alone in primary health care or as a shared care model with specialist treatment services. We are looking across

946 For example, the Ted Noffs Foundation in New South Wales provides a number of facilities for young people with drug-related and other problems. Although these are not treatment services per se, the residential units and day programmes attempt to integrate a number of clinical and non-clinical, leisure and educational services aimed at promoting better physical, social and mental health of the young people. These may range from school and learning services to a legal clinic staffed by private volunteer solicitors from some of Sydney's biggest legal firms.

> a range of interventions. We want to improve our ability to provide withdrawal treatment, for example, for people who come into an inpatient unit; potentially outpatient withdrawal as well but the emphasis at the moment is on inpatient withdrawal.[947]

Wright, Klee and Morris outline some of the integrated interventions that could be adopted to attract amphetamine users into treatment:

> There are several measures that could be adopted to attract more amphetamine users into services. Information about the services available to amphetamine users, and agency policies on confidentiality, should be made known and on public display. The education and training needs of health professionals should be identified, and resources made available to improve their credibility (Boys *et al.,* 1997). Specialist services that are designed to meet the wide variety of health and social needs of amphetamine users, and which offer a treatment package assembled for each individual could be considered (Lintzeris *et al.,* 1996). Drop-in centres that allow drug users to seek advice and support as soon as they identify a problem might lower the barriers to attending treatment services, as would partnerships between non-specialist services (ie. GPs and criminal justice workers) and drug agencies (1999, p.84).

The need for well informed general practitioners and ancillary health personnel is similarly crucial when addressing health interventions and assistance with regard to MDMA/ecstasy, the subject of the next section of this chapter.

Treatment issues regarding MDMA/ecstasy and other 'party drugs'[948]

If there is little information with regard to the treatment of (meth)amphetamine use and dependence, this is even more the case for the use of MDMA (ecstasy). This is of course partly attributable to the very real doubts as to whether an 'Ecstasy Withdrawal Syndrome' exists (see discussion in Chapter 6 of this Report).

It is also even more the case that MDMA users, even those who take it on a regular basis, do not present for treatment, although the Department of Human Services Victoria has notified the Committee that their Alcohol and Drug Information System (ADIS) data has recently:

> ...identifie[d] a dramatic increase in clients in treatment services with problems primarily related to ecstasy. Although the numbers presenting are small they more than doubled between July 2000 and December 2001.[949]

---

947 Professor Jason White, Drugs and Alcohol Services Council in conversation with the Drugs and Crime Prevention Committee, Adelaide, 3 October 2003.

948 While the discussion in this section will focus predominantly on ecstasy, many of the issues and concerns will apply equally to substances such as GHB or ketamine.

949 Submission of the Department of Human Services Victoria (Drugs Policy and Services Branch) to the Drugs and Crime Prevention Committee, Inquiry into Amphetamine and 'Party Drug' Use in Victoria, August 2002.

Current figures supplied to the Committee show that in the period between July 2002 and June 2003 there was a similar increase in presentations to treatment services for ecstasy-related complications. Despite a slight decrease at the end of 2002 the number began climbing again to a high of 40 presentations in approximately May of 2003. Such an increase is a cause for concern.

Figure 20.2 below shows the numbers of clients accessing DHS-funded drug treatment services whose primary drug is ecstasy, for the period July 2000 to June 2003.

Figure 20.2: Clients accessing drug treatment services with primary drug ecstasy

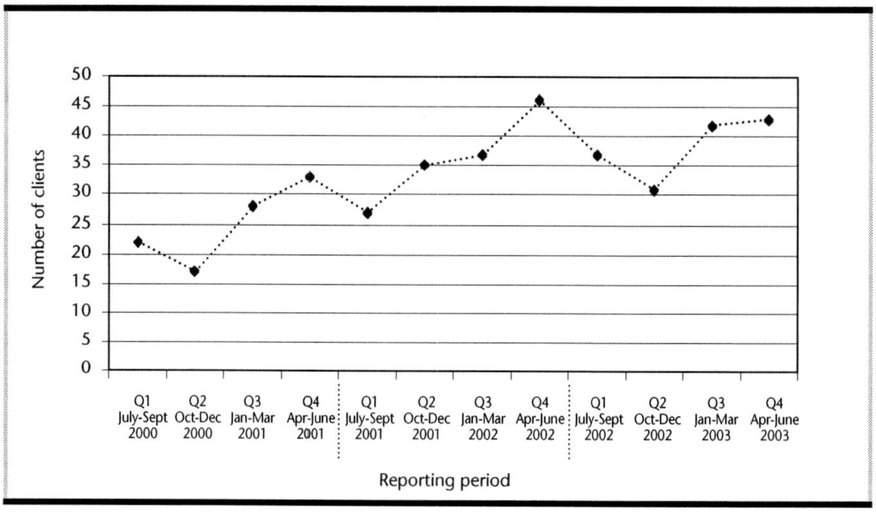

Source: Alcohol and Drug Information System 2003.[950]

It would seem, however, to be generally true that, as Longo et al. remark:

> By their very nature, ecstasy users are highly functioning members of society who are likely to be employed or engaged in studies. They are less likely to present for treatment, to have major legal problems, or to die from drug related complications. In general, they are a much less 'visible' population of illicit drug users... (NDARC 2001a, p.40).

Exceptions to this general rule of not presenting for treatment are usually medical emergencies, such as hyperthermia,[951] or when there have been medical complications as a result of taking other drugs or alcohol in association with the drug (see Gowing et al. 2001). Most interventions for the users of 'party drugs'

950 This Figure reproduced and included in the submission of the Department of Human Services Victoria to the Drugs and Crime Prevention Committee, Inquiry into Amphetamine and 'Party Drug' Use in Victoria, November 2003.

951 There is some inconclusive evidence that a drug called 'dantrolene' may be of benefit in the treatment of hyperthermia induced by MDMA consumption. See White, Irvine and Bochner 1996; Denborough and Hopkinson 1996; Kamienicki et al. 1998.

have been preventive in nature and often of the harm reduction type (see discussion in Chapter 19 of this Report):

> Moreover, there have been very few preventive interventions specifically targeted at users of MDMA; most have been aimed at users of 'party drugs' [in addition to MDMA]. Only one preventive intervention for the users of 'party drugs' has been evaluated (Kamienicki et al. 1998, p.17).

Most interventions for problematic or acute ecstasy or 'party drug' use (including 'fake' ecstasy) have been similar to those applicable to other forms of psychostimulant.[952]

> Wickes has provided guidelines for the management of acute amphetamine and cocaine intoxication. The medical management of acute MDMA intoxication is the same...with treatment of the symptom complexes as they emerge. The recommendations provided by Wickes are based on extensive clinical experience and have not been tested empirically to date (Kamienicki et al. 1998, p.28).

Similarly, the same types of intervention that are applicable to intravenous amphetamine (and heroin) users to minimise the spread of blood-borne diseases will be applicable to those (few) groups of users who inject ecstasy.

However, treatment modules for other psychostimulant users cannot be extrapolated to 'party drug' use exclusively and without qualification. As Gowing et al. state:

> While cocaine and amphetamines are related to MDMA, it should be noted that there are substantial differences in the context and patterns of use, as well as pharmacology. Furthermore, it is now generally accepted that cocaine and amphetamine use can progress to a dependence syndrome, while the existence of ecstasy dependence remains questionable (Gowing et al. 2001, p.39).

There is also doubt as to whether pharmacotherapeutic measures have any relevance to the 'treatment' of ecstasy and other 'party drug' use:

> Considerable research effort has been directed towards the identification of effective pharmacotherapies for cocaine users. To date these efforts have been largely unsuccessful and even if an effective pharmacotherapy were found, any transfer to the treatment of ecstasy is questionable because of the differing pharmacology of the drugs... Hence pharmacotherapies for ecstasy users should be innovative and specific to the action of MDMA (Gowing et al. 2001, p.39).

Given the fact that users of 'party drugs' may not consider themselves to be taking 'drugs' per se, it is even more important that general practitioners and ancillary health personnel are aware of the nature of the drugs and the dangers associated with use (Wodak 1996; Gowing et al. 2001). It is equally necessary

952 See generally, Wickes 1993a, 1993b; Kamienicki et al. 1998; Gowing et al. 2001.

that emergency personnel, including ambulance officers, have the knowledge to effectively respond to acute episodes of ecstasy, 'fake ecstasy' and other 'party drug' use.

Brief interventions

The concept of 'brief intervention' may be particularly appropriate for ecstasy users prior to the development of any problematic use. As Gowing et al. argue:

> Brief interventions aim to investigate a potential problem and motivate an individual to begin to do something about their substance use. The basic goal of a brief intervention is to reduce the risk of harm that could result from continued substance use. Brief interventions on their own can promote behaviour change, or they can act as the first stage of more intense treatment. Furthermore, brief interventions are applicable to individuals from a wide range of cultures and backgrounds, and they can be used in a variety of settings, both opportunistic or within specialised substance abuse treatment.
>
> Potential settings for opportunistic use of brief interventions to address ecstasy use include emergency departments of hospitals, subsequent to attendance for acute adverse effects; support services at major events such as dance parties; primary health care (doctors or dentists may detect ecstasy use in the context of other consultations); law enforcement settings (subsequent to being found in possession of an illicit drug); and computer based applications (the target group is likely to be high level internet users).
>
> These strengths identify the potential value of brief interventions in addressing ecstasy use, but brief interventions need to be structured and much of the evidence of their effectiveness relates to alcohol abuse. It is desirable for there to be development and evaluation, through structured research, of brief interventions appropriate to ecstasy users and the various contexts for the delivery of the interventions (Gowing et al. 2001, p.40).[953]

Baker, Boggs and Lewin also extol the benefits of tailored brief interventions:

> [t]he data show that regular amphetamine users are a diverse group of people for whom interventions need to be specifically targeted. Brief interventions should be provided for people at early stages of change within primary care settings and needle and syringe exchange schemes. Interventions for amphetamine use should be provided within methadone maintenance treatment programmes and in community settings. Services should offer assistance with amphetamine-related problems. Clearly, services need to adopt a harm reduction approach as few users wish to reduce or abstain from all drug classes. Treatment in regional areas needs to address lifestyle issues in the likelihood of long term employment. Women may need to be targeted for early intervention with the aim of preventing transition to regular

953 See also Baker, Kay-Lambkin, Lee, Claire and Jenner (2003) for a recent discussion and evaluation of brief cognitive behavioural interventions for amphetamine users.

> amphetamine use. Among people with a longer duration of amphetamine use, tranquilliser use and risk taking behaviour need to be specifically addressed (Baker, Boggs & Lewin 2001, p.55).

The Drugs and Alcohol Council of South Australia (DASC) subsequent to the South Australian Drugs Summit have incorporated brief interventions into their array of treatment options for drug abuse, particularly amphetamine abuse. Professor Jason White of DASC explains the motivations as follows:

> We want to look at brief interventions. Particularly in the primary health care setting, brief interventions may be useful, especially as a number of people who use amphetamines do not necessarily have severe dependence problems. Probably the vast majority of people that use amphetamines have relatively low-level problems. Larger scale specialist interventions may not be appropriate for them. We are looking at briefer interventions that may be able to be implemented in the primary health care setting and at long-term treatment options, both drug treatments and psychosocial therapies. Our goal is to provide that evidence on effectiveness and the models of how it is to be done in the first three years and in the last two years look at implementation in the primary health care setting, including an evaluation component of that as well. That is a major effort we are directing at the moment.[954]

Some critics have argued that while brief interventions have their place in the short term, particularly in attracting users to treatment services, they must be complemented eventually by programmes of longer duration. For example, Rawson, Gonzales and Brethen in the American context of methamphetamine treatment comment:

> Treatment funding policies that promote short duration or non-intensive outpatient services are inappropriate for providing adequate treatment for methamphetamine (MA) users. One specific practice is a managed care practice of providing a maximum benefit of 20 outpatient sessions for the treatment of individuals with MA use disorders. ...MA use disorders involve profound changes in multiple areas of human brain chemistry and brain functioning. Brief superficial treatment benefits frequently promoted by managed substance abuse benefit policies are in direct opposition to what is known about the treatment needs of MA users. In areas where MA use is a significant presence, financing policies for the treatment of these patients should be made consistent with evidence about their treatment needs (Washton & Rawson 1998) (Rawson, Gonzales & Brethen 2002, p.148.)

There has also been criticism that brief interventions may not provide any long-term structured assistance for people to 'kick their habits'. But as Ms Carmen Acosta of the Youth Withdrawal and Respite Service states, while many clients may relapse:

954 Professor Jason White, DASC in conversation with the Drugs and Crime Prevention Committee, Adelaide, 3 October 2003.

> [n]o-one ever returns to the same place they started when they walked through our doors. You can't. Because a process of change has somehow happened. You know? Some sort of contact with our staff, some sort of seed has been planted, something has happened along the way. Just even the groups that we run and that in both of our services, a lot of harm reduction groups, something has started to happen. So, they can never go back to that square 1. They can continue to use, but it will be a different type of use.[955]

For some people, particularly young people, a brief intervention may simply be about some 'time out':

> [y]oung people, the ones that are self referring, are at a time...where they're wanting that time out. And if there is one thing that we do know about young people, it is that while they may not be ready for a long term process of a 3-month program, 12-month program, they are much easier, much [more] ready to tackle a 2-week program which just means: 'I just have to think about this, I don't necessarily need to take anything on'...they're good at indicating when they really do need time out from their drug using lifestyle.[956]

It may also be finding a 'safe haven' where they can work out or at least start thinking about their drug-related problems:

> [w]here people can be kept safe in a low authoritarian nurturing environment while acute symptoms that mimic mental health problems are managed. Some people are vulnerable to psychosis that result from amphetamine use, some people it is dose related. Some people, some of the symptoms aren't psychotic but are interpreted as such...
>
> Now for a large proportion of people that symptomatology disappears relatively quickly. I mean, if any of us stayed out for three days and didn't eat anything we would behave a bit oddly. So for some people it is an acute phase and short-term management is required. For a small but significant proportion of people those symptoms last longer than two weeks and will require more specialist intervention. But we certainly need that sort of respite service, simply for a safe place to put people when the other services and families are unclear about what to do.[957]

Whatever the problems or deficits that apply to the treatment of those who use amphetamines or 'party drugs', it is often the case, particularly with (meth)amphetamine users, that these will not be the only drugs they are taking. The issue of treatment and intervention is complicated by poly-drug use, which is the topic of the following section.

---

955 Ms Carmen Acosta, Youth Withdrawal and Respite Service in conversation with the Drugs and Crime Prevention Committee, Perth, 1 October 2003.

956 Ibid.

957 Professor Steve Allsop, Drug and Alcohol Office of Western Australia, in conversation with the Drugs and Crime Prevention Committee, Perth, 1 October 2003.

Complicating treatment: Amphetamines, 'party drugs' and poly-drug use

Poly-drug use clearly has significant implications for treatment, both in terms of dealing with an emergency or acute episode (what drugs have been consumed) and with regard to long-term rehabilitation (in what context should the interventions focus upon; the treatment interventions for a problematic alcohol user may be very different to those dependent on methamphetamine). As Dr Nicole Lee from Turning Point Alcohol and Drug Centre stated to the Committee:

> Most polydrug-use people use alcohol, tobacco and all sorts of other illicit drugs, along with their psychostimulants. The implications for treatment come when they are dependent on more than one drug. That certainly increases the complexity of their presentations.[958]

The problems are even more intractable when the amphetamine user may also have psychiatric co-morbidity or when heroin is used in association with amphetamines. With regard to this last issue, Baker, Boggs and Lewin state:

> It is apparent that many people who inject drugs use amphetamine and heroin, often in combination with other drugs. Clearly interventions for amphetamine use are indicated among people who use amphetamine and heroin. In particular methadone maintenance treatment units could offer amphetamine focused interventions to users enrolled in MMT [methadone maintenance treatment] programmes. Interventions for amphetamine users not enrolled in MMT also need to be available... Interventions for people who are ready to reduce their use of amphetamine need to be accepting of polydrug use, as it is evident from the present study that polydrug use is common and readiness to change may vary between drug categories (Baker, Boggs & Lewin 2001, p.55).

It would therefore seem that interventions need to be developed that cater specifically for particular forms and combinations of poly-drug abuse and that flexibility should be the key word. As Hando, Topp and Hall state:

> The issue of polydrug use must [also] be considered. Given that most amphetamine users are polydrug users...is there a need for amphetamine specific treatment? Characteristics of the present [survey] sample clearly highlight an amphetamine dependence syndrome and a group of users who request treatment specifically for these problems... However, there is a need to assess polydrug dependence and to address it in the treatment plan (Hando, Topp & Hall 1997, pp.111–112).

Clearly further research, both medical and sociological or ethnographic, is needed on specific and general drug interactions. What Solowij, Hall and Lee stated in one of the earliest Australian studies on ecstasy is equally true today:

958 Dr Nicole Lee, Turning Point Alcohol and Drug Centre, evidence given to the Drugs and Crime Prevention Committee, Inquiry into Amphetamine and 'Party Drug' Use in Victoria, Public Hearing (Melbourne), 27 October 2003.

> It is...clear that recreational drug users are likely to experiment with various 'cocktails' or mixtures of substances, whether it be premeditated or opportunistic experimentation. Further research is needed to explore the various drug interactions, licit and illicit, before the consequences of these can be fully understood (Solowij, Hall & Lee 1992, p.1168).

Conclusion

Treatment for problematic users of amphetamines and to a lesser extent 'party drugs' clearly poses difficult problems for clinicians, drug and alcohol workers and medical researchers. The issue of pharmacological interventions, particularly substitution drugs, as an adjunct to amphetamine treatment is particularly contentious.

Although the situation is markedly improving, there also seems to be very little understanding of what may or may not 'work' for this type of drug user, compared to more 'established' or at least better understood drugs such as heroin. The problem is compounded by the fact that so many users of amphetamine may also be using other drugs, including alcohol, as part of their drug taking 'repertoire'. The need for an integrated treatment service delivery system that recognises the different types of amphetamine user is reflected in the following recommendations:

Recommendations

63. The Committee recommends that the government develop and implement a new strategic integrated framework for the delivery of drug treatment services that should be circulated to all relevant state and local government departments, service agencies and user groups working in alcohol and drug services.

    The framework will:

    a) be co-ordinated in the Department of Human Services;

    b) be supported by sustained and realistic funding;

    c) have the capacity to respond to changing circumstances such as the trend of increasing use of amphetamine-type stimulants and 'party drugs';

    d) be developed in partnership with service providers and people most affected;

    e) incorporate mechanisms to ensure improved co-ordination of services support to individuals;

    f) incorporate a research base and evaluation and monitoring processes; as outlined in Recommendation 66, p.629; and

    g) incorporate the capacity to map and describe the changing base of services provided in the state.

In developing the framework consideration must be given to current system deficits, particularly:

- crisis response, including quick access to detoxification;
- services appropriate to people with dual diagnoses (see also Recommendation 64, p.611);
- youth-specific services;
- services targeting poly-drug use, especially involving use of amphetamine-type stimulants;
- services appropriate to people from culturally and linguistically diverse communities;
- services relevant to Indigenous people including holistic healing centres (see Recommendation 7, p.224); and
- equitable access to services in rural and regional areas.

64. The Committee recognises that there is a high proportion of people who use amphetamine who also have a condition affecting their mental health. Some such people fall too easily 'between the cracks' of government and community agencies dealing specifically with alcohol and drug or specifically with mental health issues. The Committee therefore recommends as part of the Treatment Strategy outlined in Recommendation 63, p.610:

    a) That a central body be established within the Department of Human Services to co-ordinate the integration and smooth delivery of services pertaining to people with dual diagnoses of mental health and drug use.

    b) That in establishing this body reference should be made to the Western Australian Joint Services Development Unit as outlined in Chapter 20 of this Report.

    c) That the proposed body facilitate the training of workers in both the mental health and drug service fields to recognise the issues pertaining to dual diagnoses.

65. The Committee acknowledges that there is an ongoing debate as to whether treatment for amphetamine use and addiction requires specialised services. The Committee therefore recommends that a pilot service be established to trial the use of separate facilities and treatment strategies for amphetamine users.

The need for further and better resourced research and policy development appears to be as crucial in the treatment field as in so many other aspects of amphetamine and 'party drug' use. The area of well targeted and directed research will be the topic of the next Chapter.

21. The Need for Further Research

> *To understand the behaviour of someone who is a member of a group it is necessary to understand that way of life* (Becker 1983 in Malbon 1999, p.12).

A common theme that has arisen throughout the Inquiry is the paucity of appropriately targeted research being undertaken into the areas of amphetamines and 'party drugs'.[959]

This lack of focussed research applies not only to medical research pertaining to treatment but also more general quantitative and epidemiological studies, qualitative and ethnographic research projects. Such a lack of inquiry and consequent policy development is felt not only in Australia but also at an international level (Yacoubian 2001). A need for a greater research effort with regard to these drugs is the topic of this chapter.

In 1993, at a symposium on psychostimulant use in Australia, drug researchers Julie Hando and Wayne Hall identified three areas of research priority:

> First, we need much better information about what forms of amphetamines are being used. What are the major modes of administration? What are the typical doses used? What impurities do illicitly manufactured amphetamines contain?
>
> Second, we need to be better informed about existing patterns of amphetamine use to make better educated guesses about the likelihood that amphetamine use will spread. What are the major routes of administration and why do different users choose them?
>
> Third, we need to look more systematically at the potential health and social problems associated with amphetamine use by each of the major routes of administration. What are the adverse effects of acute oral and injected amphetamine use? What are the health hazards of chronic use? (Hall & Hando 1993, p.65).

Notwithstanding a range of state, federal and university funded projects over the ten years since these exhortations were made, it could still be argued that Hall and Hando's comments are as applicable today. This is as true of the

---

959 As indicated in Chapter 6, while there is now a reasonable number of medical research studies in the area of amphetamines and to a lesser extent 'party drugs', relatively few of these seem to have produced definite 'answers' to some of the more pressing issues troubling medical researchers, analysts and policymakers.

international situation as it is in Australia. In an excellent literature review pertaining to global ecstasy use, Yacoubian makes the following pertinent comment:

> Despite its history, and the major physiological and psychological problems associated with its ingestion, ecstasy has received relatively little attention in periodicals devoted to the social sciences... [O]nly 35 empirical studies have been published on ecstasy in peer reviewed periodicals devoted to the social sciences. Of these 28 (80 per cent) were conducted outside of the United States (Yacoubian 2001, p.128).

Medical and clinical research

In the area of clinical research there are still many gaps in what we know about psychostimulants and particularly MDMA/ecstasy. Much of what has been learned about (meth)amphetamine use and ecstasy has been extrapolated, not always appropriately, from research into cocaine. This has been partly attributed to an expected jump in cocaine use in Australia during the 1980s that never actually eventuated (Baker in Wood 1998a, p.19).

With ecstasy use in particular there is still a range of unanswered questions that need to be explored. In the medical/clinical area one of the key debates still focusses on the (relative) safety (or otherwise) of 'pure' MDMA:

> In scientific as well as in popular texts there is a great controversy if ecstasy is a relatively benign (and even psychotherapeutically effective) substance (Szukaj 1994) or a dangerous neurotoxin (McCann et al. 1998).
>
> There is also a lack of knowledge concerning the incidence and prevalence of ecstasy use and use disorders in the general population. Research deficits are mainly due to the fact that ecstasy studies mostly have highly selected samples...usually do not have prospective longitudinal designs, do not use specified diagnostic criteria for clinically relevant abuse or dependence patterns and focus on the initiation of ecstasy use, not on its reduction or cessation (Von Sydow et al. 2002, p.147).

Dr James Fetherston, for example, argues that it is difficult to make any pronouncements with certainty as to the long-term effects of ecstasy given that insufficient time has elapsed to do major longitudinal studies and evaluations of its use:

> You need to have a longitudinal look at the long term effects of ecstasy, and there's not been much done on that. Some of the major papers that were saying that ecstasy was particularly dangerous have recently been withdrawn as they were fundamentally flawed. The drug hasn't really been around that long so what it could actually do to people in the longer term is still very much up to question, so that has to be looked at.[960]

960 Dr James Fetherston, National Drug Research Institute, Curtin University, in conversation with the Drugs and Crime Prevention Committee, Perth, 2 October 2003.

Such clinical issues tend to be mixed up with (or alternatively are part and parcel of) political ones, often generated by the media.[961] Grob's article particularly concerns the controversy over the neurotoxicity or otherwise of ecstasy. Political agendas aside, this is an issue which has vexed clinicians for many years. In their global review of the MDMA literature, Gowing et al. make the following salient points:

> This report identifies the absence of controlled epidemiological studies and the consequent difficulties in quantifying risks of ecstasy. It is recommended that such studies be designed and initiated to establish prevalence of harms associated with ecstasy use, and particularly to assess long term functional consequences of ecstasy use.
>
> Another area where our knowledge is currently limited relates to the capacity of ecstasy to produce dependence. Furthermore, if ecstasy dependence does exist what are the central features, how should it be assessed, and does it have any diagnostic significance. That is, does it predict risk of adverse effects or appropriate treatment responses?
>
> Although animal and cellular studies have contributed much to our understanding of the effects of amphetamine derivatives, there is still much to do. Due to the unpredictability of adverse effects of these drugs and the very large number of possible chemical manipulations that can be made by illicit chemists, we are still not capable of predicting the outcome of administration in individuals... Further cellular and animal studies are essential if we are to gain sufficient knowledge of the mechanisms of action of these drugs to predict the likely adverse effects in a given situation. This indicates the importance of continued basic research in the area.
>
> Our general understanding of the pharmacology of MDMA and related amphetamine derivatives should continue to be developed... Data reviewed also indicates that a wide range of drugs are [sic] commonly used in conjunction with ecstasy. Improved understanding of the potential for interaction between these drugs may help to avert or respond to other possible interactions. Further analysis of toxicological data in fatal and non fatal cases of adverse effects would also help to determine relative toxicity of various amphetamine derivatives (Gowing et al. 2001, p.44).

There are a variety of other clinical research needs outlined in a research symposium on amphetamine use in Australia that still have relevance and still are worthy of attention today (see Burrows, Flaherty & MacAvoy 1993). For

961 For an account of the 'politicisation' of the research agenda as it applies to amphetamines, ecstasy and drugs research more generally, see Burrows, Flaherty & MacAvoy 1993, at pp.105–106; Saunders 1998; Pentney 2001; Grob 2000; Concar 2002; Rosenbaum 2002 and the discussion in Chapters 18 and 19.

Concar's article is particularly interesting for its account of the debates surrounding the views of Professor George Ricaurte of Johns Hopkins University in Baltimore. Ricaurte has been long advocating the view that ecstasy use, particularly if used regularly and over a long period of time, can have serious and damaging effects on brain function, a view to which not all in the research or medical communities subscribe (Concar 2002).

example, Wickes' (1993a) call for research into the effects of psychostimulants on pregnancy is still timely. Chesher's (1993) advocacy of research into the transition from oral use of amphetamines to injecting them may be equally applicable to the slight but nonetheless noticeable use of ecstasy intravenously. More generally, better research into the epidemiology of psychostimulant use, particularly with regard to ecstasy use, is clearly required. A specific area needing such research is the use of so-called 'party drugs' outside of the party or dance environment.

One novel idea put forward to get a better understanding of the effect of (club) drugs on users is linking the world of the researcher to that of the clinician or treatment provider:[962]

> The unique social and cultural factors that support the use of these drugs in a given population must be taken into consideration in designing intervention and treatment strategies. Research is needed to determine which elements are effective for which populations. Treatment providers who are working with club drug users have a unique perspective in understanding the role that these drugs play in social networks. Pairing clinicians with researchers may help to ensure that interventions are empirically validated and that effective treatments are disseminated as quickly as possible (Freese, Miotto & Reback 2002, p.155).

One other important issue to bear in mind in considering research agendas is the relationship between psychostimulant use, of whatever type, with other conditions. This, as has been observed in Chapter 20, is particularly important with regard to co-morbid mental illness. The Youth Substance Abuse Service (YSAS) based in Melbourne, which sees many young clients who present with co-morbid mental illness, makes the following points regarding research into psychostimulants:

> [m]uch of the current research relates cause and effect conclusions that are not justified by the data presented. Some of the confounding variables include:
>
> - Amphetamine or MDMA use is associated with the symptoms rather than being the cause of the symptoms.
> - The probability of a chance association. Of the large group of drug users within the general population, a proportion will have mental health issues regardless of any drug use. Depression and anxiety are common conditions in the general population. According to the Australian National Survey of Mental Health and Wellbeing 2000, depression and anxiety affect up to one in five Australian adolescents – three times higher than 10 years ago (reported in 'Sad statistics: the scourge that's scarring our young' *The Age* 7th July 2002). It is a statistical certainty that many users of amphetamines or MDMA will develop depression regardless of their drug use.

962 Equally if not more important is the linking of the *user* and his or her world to the clinician, researcher or service provider. See the discussion later in this chapter.

- Poor pre-morbid adjustment (a poor adjustment to life circumstances) is associated with an increased likelihood of any drug use. As such, a person's drug use in the form of self-medication of distress may be a symptom of impending or actual mental illness, or an indication of impaired judgement. Pre-existing mental illness and a family history of mental illness is common in people who develop psychiatric illness in apparent association with drug use.
- Some people with schizophrenia or bi-polar disorder may also use amphetamines or MDMA. The peak age of onset of schizophrenia is 20–30, an age group in which experimentation with drugs is relatively common. It is unknown whether amphetamines or MDMA can specifically induce a relapse of pre-existing schizophrenia or bi-polar disorder, beyond the increased risk of relapse attached to any emotional stressor.
- Demanding subjects abstain from all drugs before tests of function are undertaken can result in a mild withdrawal syndrome that could confound tests conducted during this withdrawal period. For example, ceasing regular coffee intake can result in headaches, fatigue and impaired function.
- Adequate control group monitoring. It is particularly important to carefully match for the use of *all* other drugs in order to avoid the possibility of bias for the control group to have used fewer drugs and to be higher functioning than the subjects are.[963]

Finally, as has been noted in great detail in the last chapter, there is a great deficit in treatment options and treatment research for psychostimulant users. This lack applies to both pharmacological and behavioural interventions. Recent Australian reviews (Gowing, Proudfoot, Henry-Edwards & Teeson 2001; Baker & Lee, in prep):

> [c]learly highlight the lack of well conducted research with psychostimulant users and the need to undertake research that suits the Australian treatment context. There is a great deal more research required into best practice treatment options for this group.[964]

Research is also required as to why users may or may not, as the case may be, access treatment services. Professor Margaret Hamilton of Turning Point Alcohol and Drug Centre states in this regard:

> One really important piece of research that has not been done in Australia is looking at the engagement of users into treatment. What we do know is that they do not attend treatment easily, they do not find our treatment services

---

963 Submission of Youth Substance Abuse Service (YSAS) to the Drugs and Crime Prevention Committee, Inquiry into Amphetamine and 'Party Drug' Use in Victoria, August 2002. (Emphasis in the original)

964 Excerpt from the confidential submission of Turning Point Alcohol and Drug Centre to the Drugs and Crime Prevention Committee, Inquiry into Amphetamine and 'Party Drug' Use in Victoria, August 2002. Quoted with the kind permission and approval of Turning Point.

> particularly suited to their needs. Part of that is probably because there are no specific treatments for them, and treatment service staff are not very confident in dealing with amphetamine users. We certainly do not know how to attract them into treatment, how to keep them there, and what to do with them when we get them in there.[965]

A lack of quantitative data

Notwithstanding some excellent data collection such as the Illicit Drug Reporting System (IDRS), a constant refrain that the Committee has heard during the course of this Inquiry is the lack of co-ordinated data with regard to amphetamine and particularly 'party drug' usage, especially at the state and local level. Much of this criticism has come from local government departments, particularly in the social and health service sectors. Many workers from local government units found themselves struggling to answer the questions in the Committee's Discussion Paper pertaining to drug usage in their communities because they either did not have localised data or no means of accessing it. The City of Monash's submission is typical of many in this regard:

> A lack of specific data and accurate information regarding the extent, nature and scope of amphetamine use is a key issue facing all stakeholders who seek to address amphetamine and 'party' drug use issues.
>
> Many in the community are becoming more aware of the effects of amphetamines but misinformation through some media outlets, and other sources has meant that a lot of wrong or misleading information remains an obstacle for the development of a sound harm minimisation and prevention program in the community.
>
> Furthermore, a lack of statistical data relating to amphetamine use remains an issue for the development of localised strategies. Information that points to the regularity and impact, both social and health impact, of party drug use remains a challenge for all stakeholders in producing effective programme responses to amphetamine use. Localised data such as ambulance and hospital admissions, Police arrest and offence data, as well as clinical research studies with a particular focus on the local area would assist in the development of evidence based targeted program delivery.[966]

Another concern voiced, particularly by local government and community groups, is that even when (limited) data is available it is not sufficiently disaggregated into discrete drug categories. In other words, much health data is classified into broad categories such as 'amphetamine' which give very little indication as to what actual drug has been taken under that broad rubric:

---

965 Professor Margaret Hamilton, Turning Point Alcohol and Drug Centre, evidence given to the Drugs and Crime Prevention Committee, Inquiry into Amphetamine and 'Party Drug' Use in Victoria, Public Hearings (Melbourne), 27 October 2003.

966 Submission of the City of Monash to the Drugs and Crime Prevention Committee, Inquiry into Amphetamine and 'Party Drug' Use in Victoria, October 2003.

> Comment on the true extent of some drug problems, including amphetamine and 'party' drugs, is difficult.
>
> The aggregation of overdoses attributable to a range of various substances into the 'other drugs' category, the lack of universal methodologies in data collection and the current shortcomings on comprehensive local drug data create limitations for analysis, planning and strategy development.
>
> Ambulance attendance data and emergency hospital presentation and admissions data currently bundle incidences of drug overdose into the catchall 'other drug' category unless they are primarily heroin-related or alcohol-related. This aggregation masks rather than illuminates the drug issues associated with amphetamines, 'party drugs', pharmaceuticals and some other substances.
>
> Research data based on full drug screens and at local government level should be resourced to enable appropriate analysis, planning and strategy development.[967]

The problems associated with this lack of categorical specificity were testified to by Dr Louisa Degenhardt of the National Drug and Alcohol Research Centre when the Committee met with her in Sydney:

> [w]hat we have noticed [from our own research] has been an increase in the use of certain types of drugs that you really wouldn't capture from the use of just data from hospital admissions or even from key informants because it is so new. A couple of the drug types that we have seen emerging have been the use of ketamine and the use of GHB. In terms of if you wanted to get a handle on the use of those drugs from hospital admissions, for example, you are never going to capture it because of coding systems. ... You will not even get ecstasy from emergency department admissions, from hospitals or anything like that, because they use what is known as the international classification of diseases that was developed by the WHO, and we cannot in any data source of users work out whether or not the stimulant that was used was ecstasy. So we are really trying to be quite inventive in getting different sorts of information for these newer drug types.[968]

The City of Yarra based in inner city Melbourne makes a similar point:

> There are several difficulties that local government experience regarding access to relevant data sets and drug trends information which include:
>
> - Restrictions placed upon data collection agencies on their capacity to provide responsive and timely access to research, data and analyses. There needs to be a commitment from state and federal governments to ensure that this information is provided to local government in a timely

967 Submission of Moreland City Council to the Drugs and Crime Prevention Committee, Inquiry into Amphetamine and 'Party Drug' Use in Victoria, October 2003.

968 Dr Louisa Degenhardt, National Drug and Alcohol Research Centre, in conversation with the Drugs and Crime Prevention Committee, Sydney, 26 June 2003.

> manner so that local government can plan services and work with local community agencies, services and citizens.
>
> - Difficulties with negotiating and accessing data from a multitude of government agencies and services. Often the processes in place to access the various relevant data sets are cumbersome, time consuming, fragmented, inconsistently reported (which makes synthesising and integrating the data much more resource intensive and difficult) and not made available unless by request.
> - Other than anecdotal data and ad hoc local research projects in some municipalities – local governments don't tend to be the "keepers" of drug and alcohol data. In the main, secondary data sets are accessed from state government services or government funded agencies such as Turning Point Drug and Alcohol Centre [sic].
>
> The State Government should play a stronger role in coordinating the collection and dissemination of data from its various agencies and funded agencies.[969]

Yarra Council makes the following recommendations to redress these problems:

> - There is a need for data that is centralised, co-ordinated, and timely and made available and accessible to local government (and also analyses data at local level). This is essential for any ongoing capacity by local governments to address drug and alcohol issues including those posed by psycho-stimulant drugs such as MDMA and amphetamines.
> - Quarterly provision and or analyses of these secondary data sets would assist with local governments planning and facilitation role regarding local drug and alcohol issues such as those identified in the *Drugs and Crime Prevention Committee Paper.*
> - Further research into the impacts, behaviours, needs and effects of psycho-stimulants and polydrug use.[970]

Anex, the umbrella group for needle exchange programmes in Victoria, while viewing systems such as the IDRS as valuable also argues for the need to collect and disseminate more localised data:

> Anex believes that in order to respond quickly and effectively to changing drug trends, especially at the front line, it is important that relevant information be collected and disseminated. While annual surveillance studies such as the IDRS and the Australian NSP survey are valuable in providing a snapshot of drug using patterns, Anex believes that they are unable to capture more localised changes. These localised patterns may be captured by the network of NSP outlets that has the highest number and frequencies of contact with current drug users.[971]

---

969 Submission of the City of Yarra to the Drugs and Crime Prevention Committee, Inquiry into Amphetamine and 'Party Drug' Use in Victoria, October 2003.

970 Ibid.

971 Submission of Anex to the Drugs and Crime Prevention Committee, Inquiry into Amphetamine and 'Party Drug' Use in Victoria, October 2003.

Some agencies have commented that current data collection methods are ill equipped to pick up on some 'hidden populations'. For example, the community agency Anglicare stated in a submission to the Inquiry:

> Data collection surveys from Drug and Alcohol Services do not...capture middle class drug users, as they are not accessing these services. Household and school population surveys also fail to capture young people using drugs in residential units. Those with decreased literacy are not likely to fill out large surveys. Data collection methods, therefore, need to be extended to ensure that these young people are not overlooked. In addition, many people of Asian background are not using detoxification services and therefore are also not included in any surveys.[972]

Gowing et al. also note that better systems of drug monitoring need to be implemented to give data on current drug patterns and usage.[973] This should be done particularly in emergency room situations where patients are brought suffering the effects of overdoses and other adverse effects associated with the drug and/or drug interactions.[974] The Turning Point Alcohol and Drug Centre also has called for more clear data on psychostimulant use in Victoria. In its submission to this Inquiry it states:

> Given the significant demonstrated potential for health and other harms associated with psychostimulant abuse, there is an imperative for broadening existing drug trend monitoring systems to facilitate a more sensitive mechanism for detecting trends in this area. This may be achieved by extending current monitoring methods to new sentinel groups including gay and lesbian, dance/rave attendees and others (and also through the development of new methodologies). The value of such monitoring is that it may serve as a more sensitive early warning mechanism for emergent psychostimulant trends, and thereby highlight possible areas of focus for future public health response (policy, program and research).[975]

---

972 Submission of Anglicare to the Drugs and Crime Prevention Committee, Inquiry into Amphetamine and 'Party Drug' Use in Victoria, October 2003.

973 One project that seems to be of merit is a Sentinel Monitoring System that has been recently established in Adelaide. Comprehensive information will be collected from clients presenting with drug-related toxicity at Royal Adelaide Hospital and Lyell McEwin Hospital:

'This information will enhance the evidence available to guide health and law enforcement activities in reducing harm arising from amphetamine and other psychostimulant use. In particular, this initiative will enable the development and implementation of timely prevention and intervention strategies in line with the changing picture of substance misuse and the potentially fatal consequences' (South Australian Drugs Summit 2003, p.7).

974 Gowing et al. view the United States Drug Abuse Warning Network (DAWN) as a useful model:

'An added advantage of this sort of system is that it also has the capacity to identify emerging patterns of drug use and related problems. For example, data from DAWN indicates the significance of mixing drugs, and recent increases in GHB-related problems in parallel with MDMA. Data [also] shows the young age of users experiencing adverse effects' (Gowing et al. 2001, p.43).

975 Excerpt from the confidential submission of Turning Point Alcohol and Drug Centre to the Drugs and Crime Prevention Committee, Inquiry into Amphetamine and 'Party Drug' Use in Victoria, August 2002. Quoted with the kind permission and approval of Turning Point.

One encouraging development is the Psychostimulant Monitoring Project which aims to monitor psychostimulant market trends in Melbourne. In 2003, researchers at Turning Point Alcohol and Drug Centre commenced a study designed to identify and monitor emerging trends in psychostimulant (including 'party drugs') use and harms in Melbourne. The Party Drugs and Psychostimulant Monitoring Project is an example of integrated drug trend monitoring. The research is gathering primary data from current users and secondary data from available indicator sources and interviews with key informant experts across Victoria. Turning Point Alcohol and Drug Centre's research on this issue extends the drug trend monitoring model it has applied annually since 1997 in the conduct of the Melbourne arm of the national IDRS study. The challenge in developing an ongoing monitoring capacity for psychostimulant trends is to access new sentinel groups via novel research methods. To meet this challenge the Party Drugs and Psychostimulant Monitoring Project is exploring the feasibility of Internet recruitment and surveys and computer assisted telephone interviews (CATI).

The methodology design includes a specific focus on cocaine, methamphetamines, ecstasy and other designer drugs, and will target people other than needle exchange programme clients (eg. dance/rave scene participants, gay/lesbian groups). Data sources will be triangulated against each other in order to minimise the weaknesses inherent in each one and to ensure that only reliable and valid emerging trends are documented.

In its 2002 submission to this Inquiry, Turning Point Alcohol and Drug Centre outlined the aims and methods of the project as follows:

1. To improve monitoring of the patterns and characteristics of psychostimulant use in Melbourne, including an increased focus upon target groups other than injecting drug users (eg. rave/dance scene, gay/lesbian target groups).
2. To commence strategic early warning around psychostimulant trends across Melbourne, and serve as a mechanism for supporting drug trend monitoring over time.
3. To consider the implications of emerging psychostimulant trends for health and law enforcement sector responses.[976]

Despite the clear need for greater research into epidemiological and clinical aspects of psychostimulant use, it would seem that it is equally important to continue and expand qualitative research into this area of drug studies. Such research should include social and ethnographic models.

976 Ibid.

Qualitative and social research

> Without cultural analysis all policy science is vain (Sansom 1988 in Moore 1990, p.333).

In Australia there is a dearth of research into the 'social worlds' of psychostimulant users.[977] This is particularly the case for those who use ecstasy. Conventional approaches in psychological, behavioural and psychosocial research clearly have an important role to play in the qualitative research programme (South Australian Drugs Summit Communique 2002a).

For example, most researchers, including qualitative researchers, recognise the valuable role played by monitoring systems such as IDRS. However:

> [w]hile these systems are valuable in tracking the use of these drugs, they are limited in understanding the contexts, functions and risks associated with this drug use in specific populations of users. Such an understanding is crucial if we are to develop better interventions to reduce the use and harms associated with the use of these drugs.[978]

Or, as Moore states, epidemiology is a valuable but incomplete way of looking at drug problems:

> Existing research processes can identify broad sections of the drug-using population but they cannot inform us about the cultural practices and social organisation of particular types of use, nor can they identify the material conditions that set the parameters for the creation of drug using scenes and subcultures.[979]

One of the key areas of qualitative research that has been utilised in Europe, but to some extent ignored in Australia, is ethnography. Why is ethnography important in the area of drug studies? Australian ethnographer David Moore argues that:

> [e]thnography has the ability to provide research insights, fill important gaps in our knowledge, and complement more quantitative methods. One of the main strengths of the method is the ability to get 'inside' a group and therefore to gain a fuller understanding of the social processes involved in drug use. This process in turn may generate hypotheses which might be later tested using more quantitative methods. With respect to drugs such as Ecstasy (and amphetamines), where our baseline information is poor, data collected via ethnography allow the planning of appropriate health promotion and harm reduction programmes by gaining an understanding of the origins of drug use,

977 Moore argues that this is, at least in part, because of an unwillingness of both state and private/university funding bodies to finance such research. For a discussion of the 'politics' of drug research and its funding, see Moore 2002b.

978 Submission of Dr Simon Lenton on behalf of the National Drug Research Institute, Curtin University, to the Drugs and Crime Prevention Committee, Inquiry into Amphetamine and 'Party Drug' Use in Victoria, October 2003.

979 Submission of Dr David Moore, National Drug Research Institute, Curtin University, to the Drugs and Crime Prevention Committee, Inquiry into Amphetamine and 'Party Drug' Use in Victoria, October 2003.

> the maintenance of particular drug using patterns and the social meanings of such patterns.
>
> ...Ethnographers claim to paint a picture of drug use which accords more closely with the various social contexts in which drug use occurs. The multitude of social worlds in modern pluralistic society means that simplistic messages which might be relevant to one set of people may hold little relevance for others. The challenge for health promotion and policy is to devise strategies which take into account these cultural and social differences (Moore 1992, pp.13, 83).

The value of ethnography lies in the importance it attaches to:

> [t]he ways in which drug users categorise *their* worlds, the ways in which *they* ascribe meaning to their actions and the ways in which broader structural processes shape *their* lives (Moore 2002, p.278).[980] (Committee emphasis)

For example, in Chapters 6 and 9 of this Report attention was paid to the relatively high levels of methamphetamine and other drug use among some groups of Australian gay men. Research by Murnane et al. (2000) cited in Chapter 9 provides an excellent quantitative and epidemiological snapshot about drug use in this community but it cannot answer some of the questions as to why such use occurs. Nor can it paint a picture about the life worlds of such users.[981] Moreover, much drug research concentrates on the drug only:

> The difficulty with most research projects that investigate the use of illegal drugs is that far too many questions are asked about their drug use, and far too few about all the other things they do (Hammersley, Khan & Ditton 2002, pp.94–95).

Many ethnographical studies on drug use draw either explicitly or implicitly from Zinberg's analysis of 'drug, set and setting' referred to earlier. In other words,

---

980 Moore argues that more formalised structures need to be put in place to encourage the conduct of ethnographic studies in Australia including:

'[a]n ethnographic drug research program, a dedicated 5-year, potentially renewable, funding stream housed either in an established research centre or a multicentre collaborative program involving established ethnographers with appropriate qualifications and track records. In addition to its empirical and theoretical contribution to researching the place of drugs in Australian society, and to mapping the "conditions that place people at risk of harm and those that build resilience", a further benefit would lie in training and securing the next generation of ethnographers' (Moore 2002b, p.282).

981 For example, such data cannot answer the questions posed in the forward to *A Certain Body*, Lewis and Ross' book on drugs in the gay dance party culture:

'The fact that men who frequent the dance clubs are accomplished at juggling [these] risks – indeed undertake them as a recreational activity – raises some interesting questions. Do they, in fact, perceive these risks to be dangerous? If so, do they regard them as avoidable dangers or yet another of the risks that accompany being a gay man in a big city? How is gay male drug use different from heterosexual patterns, and is drunken/drugged comportment different across gay and straight cultures? Is sex regarded by the dance club patrons as an expected part of the drug-using experience? To what extent is drug or alcohol use an expected part of sex? How are gay men socialized so that they are able to purchase drugs, use drugs, navigate urban settings while drugged and/or have sex under the influence so that they experience only a minimum of social problems/ Or is the assumption that gay men have 'only a minimum of social problems' associated with drug use, in fact, incorrect?' (Lewis & Ross 1995, p.vi).

qualitative or social research into drug use should not concentrate only on the pharmacology of the drug (drug) or the individual psychology of the use (set) but should also examine the social context within which these two variables are located and the values, beliefs and sanctions that are brought to drug use by various individuals and social groups (the setting). It is the interaction between the drug taken, the individual psychology of the user and the cultural or social milieu in which it is taken that is crucial in attempting to understand drug use and thus formulate appropriate interventions. Much ethnographic research, particularly that which is based on participant observation, also takes place in the natural settings of the user, the dance club or the rave, rather than a clinic or institution. Such a method would not concentrate exclusively on the negatives, problems or harm of drug use. This is not to condone, encourage or lionise drug use. It is simply to acknowledge that researchers, educators and policymakers need to understand the social world of the drug user in formulating effective interventions to reduce the harms that *are* associated with the drug. As Moore states:

> Researchers spend many hours devising ways of measuring drug-related harm but there is a noticeable absence of ways of quantifying the benefits of drug use. If the majority of drug users experience little in the way of negative effects, this aspect must be incorporated into our approach however difficult we might feel this to be (Moore 1992, p.83).

In short, ethnography promotes the 'insider' view of drug use as understood by the users themselves. Moore states that:

> Various types of drug experts, policymakers and law enforcement personnel all contribute to the formation of policy and practice but drug users, who are presumably entitled to some say in policy which effects them, do not. Their view is labelled 'anecdotal' and given little intellectual, political or social weight (Moore 1992, pp.82–83).

Rowe similarly argues that in the area of drug policy particularly, research must be informed by the views and experiences of those most at risk – the users themselves:[982]

> Street-based drug users remain an under-researched population, particularly in respect of qualitative and ethnographic studies. This submission urges the Committee to recommend the funding of qualitative 'bottom-up' research with those who are best placed to provide policy advice for harm prevention strategies aimed at those most at risk – marginalised, homeless and street-based injecting drug users.[983]

One way of ensuring the voices of those who use illicit drugs are heard is to encourage outreach workers to tap (with their informed consent) into their knowledge and then feed that knowledge back into policy design. Something

982 Such approaches are not without their problems. For example, Measham, Aldridge and Parker testify to the ethical and practical difficulties of doing research among clubbers in noisy environments among participants who may be drug affected. For example, how does one obtain informed consent from someone 'high' on ecstasy? See Measham, Aldridge and Parker 2001, pp.75ff.

983 Submission of Dr James Rowe, RMIT University, to the Drugs and Crime Prevention Committee, Inquiry into Amphetamine and 'Party Drug' Use in Victoria, October 2003.

similar to this is done by the workers at the YSAS in Melbourne:

> It is very hard to create one particular mechanism which, if you like, mines the terrain of young people's knowledge of the circumstances around drug use. Certainly our outreach workers would be well in touch with young people and we would be talking to them about what they are seeing. Particularly in the day program the framework is very largely around engaging young people in developing some responsibility for what goes on in the program. So it is not about us doing things to them; it is us engaging in dialogue about their circumstances and how we can work with that. So there is a continual feedback loop going on there.
>
> We are also developing a research agenda broadly within YSAS. We are encouraging and seeking researchers to come in and work with us and young people within YSAS. We are particularly interested in projects which work in a qualitative way, not at the expense of quantitative research, but in a sense respecting and honouring the stories of young people. Where we can we will support and assist people interested in research to have a dialogue with young people as part of their overall research project, so that the product ultimately is informed by the views of young people. They are the types of things we are doing. It is not an easy area; it is not straightforward.[984]

The recent comprehensive review into psychostimulant treatment and interventions by Kamienicki and his colleagues endorsed such an approach. It also recognised that:

> [c]onsumer input into research, service development, provision and evaluation, should be recognised as vitally important. User groups, established in all states and territories, and which are tasked and assisted to access psychostimulant users from a range of subcultures, would be in a key position to provide such informed input based on local needs.
>
> Psychostimulant users have useful information on their experience of, and beliefs about, drug treatment, which may facilitate treatment services attracting clients, making treatment more effective, and assist in defining measurable and achievable treatment goals which may have not been considered by service providers but which are of value to the client group. For example, while it may not result in abstinence, the interruption to an escalating binge cycle provided by a short term stay in an in-patient withdrawal service may provide important 'time out' from drug-using peers and environment and may facilitate re-establishing control over use. Thus, users of psychostimulants have a great deal to offer service providers in determining how existing services could be modified. They can also provide input into how new services, and other interventions, could be designed to better meet the needs of this group.
>
> Within the heterogenous group of psychostimulant users, there appear to be distinct sub-cultures with different social norms and drug using practices (Berg

984 Mr David Murray, Executive Officer, YSAS, evidence given to the Drugs and Crime Prevention Committee, Inquiry into Amphetamine and 'Party Drug' Use in Victoria, Public Hearings (Melbourne), 27 October 2003.

> 1994, Hando & Hall 1993, National Task Force on Psychostimulants 1995, Vincent et al. 1997). Examples include transport industry and shift workers, users of 'party drugs' in the rave and dance music scene, and regular amphetamine injectors who may also inject opioids. Treatment services which target acute and chronic amphetamine associated harm are more likely to be attractive and acceptable to potential clients if they consult with representatives of a variety of identifiable client sub-groups (Kamienicki et al. 2002, p.63).

Moreover, according to many professional researchers, users of drugs, particularly 'middle-class' drugs such as MDMA/ecstasy, are often more than prepared to assist with research programmes.[985] Dr Degenhardt of the National Drug and Alcohol Research Centre told the Committee that such users:

> are often interested in doing it because they are keen to help, they are keen to generate a body of knowledge about the use of these different drugs; and they often want to find out stuff for themselves...often they [users] will ask for information because they would like to be better informed about their use of the drugs.[986]

Qualitative research studies, particularly longitudinal ones, are a very valuable addition to knowledge building in the area of drug policy. Unfortunately they also tend to be expensive and there are always problems with attrition of research 'subjects'. Nonetheless, as with any area of health policy it is essential that *all* forms of research be undertaken that is relevant to the area of investigation. It is axiomatic that quantitative data is needed to understand the dimensions of any given drug 'problem'. But such data needs to be complemented by qualitative techniques including the more 'peripheral' studies in ethnography and social research.[987]

---

985 And not only MDMA users or necessarily 'middle-class' ones. A recent research project that made excellent use of peer researchers was the survey of injecting amphetamine users conducted jointly through the auspices of Queensland Crime Commission and Queensland Health. In this project on amphetamine use in Queensland, peer researchers, most often ex-injecting users were used to administer a questionnaire to current users on their injecting use of amphetamine. It was felt that the use of such peers elicited responses that more conventional or 'professional' researchers may not have been able to achieve (see Lynch et al. 2003).

986 Dr Louisa Degenhardt, National Drug and Alcohol Research Centre, in conversation with the Drugs and Crime Prevention Committee, Sydney, 26 June 2003.

Dr Degenhardt also states that police services are not adverse to and in fact positively encourage the use of such research. By doing so they have a greater knowledge and understanding of localised drug markets and use patterns.

987 One research technique that seems to have produced some excellent results in amphetamine and other drug studies, is that of Rapid Assessment Research. This method, for example, was utilised by Vincent, Allsop and Shoobridge (1996) in their study of amphetamine users in South Australia. They describe the process as follows:

'Rapid assessment procedures consist mainly of research tools which have been adapted from anthropological investigation methods so that they can be applied within a rapid time frame, and can generate relevant information at relatively low cost. They are designed to be used in circumscribed geographical areas.

There is no single method of rapid assessment. Various combinations of research tools have been developed and utilised. These have generally included identification, examination, and analysis of existing quantitative data, "key informant" or consultant interviews, direct observation, and focus group discussions. Focused quantitative surveys, transcripts of informal conversations, personal diary entries, and other forms of qualitative and quantitative data have also been utilised. Exactly which tools are used depends on the nature and focus of the research problem, the time available for the assessment and the availability of funds... Researchers conducting rapid assessments need to be flexible in adopting techniques which are suitable to the particular situation' (Vincent, Allsop & Shoobridge 1996, p.370).

Evaluative research

Any programme or intervention that is designed or implemented should, in the view of the Committee, have an in-built requirement for evaluation. This is particularly important for harm reduction programmes and strategies. Evaluative research of both a process and outcome nature is an essential component of developing good, effective and relevant policy in this area. Moreover, in most cases funding grants to agencies who undertake drug programmes should have specific allocations to enable them to conduct such evaluations. It is a crucial aspect of determining not only what works but what doesn't work or what at least could be improved upon.

Research suggestions

It is important that any drug research agenda be implemented or at least influenced by those who have involvement with drug policy and/or practice.

During the course of this Inquiry a variety of organisations, departments and individuals have put forward some ideas for further research with regard to amphetamines and 'party drugs'. These include:

Australian Rural Centre for Addictive Behaviours (ARCAB)

- Further and disaggregated data required with regard to the incidence of drug use in rural and regional Victoria
- Better rural-specific health research, particularly conducted by people with rural backgrounds or based in rural or regional communities.[988]

Turning Point Alcohol and Drug Centre

- Better co-ordination, sharing and integration of data. Particularly with regard to police and forensic data
- Accessing new sentinel groups for research
- The relationship between amphetamine and other drugs, including alcohol
- Research into the engagement of users into treatment services
- Better balance of research between metropolitan and rural/regional centres.[989]

---

988 Submission of ARCAB to the Drugs and Crime Prevention Committee, Inquiry into Amphetamine and 'Party Drug' Use in Victoria, 7 November 2003.

989 Submission of Turning Point Alcohol and Drug Centre to the Drugs and Crime Prevention Committee, Inquiry into Amphetamine and 'Party Drug' Use in Victoria, October 2003.
The imperative need for research into rural and regional drug-related issues has already been commented upon in the context of Chapter 11 of this Report. In particular, refer to the comments and submission of ARCAB.

National Drug Research Institute – Curtin University

- More in depth social research with specific populations of users that have been identified by surveillance research as high risk. These include groups such as transport workers, party/club drug users, Aboriginal people etc.
- Studies of the use of these drugs by those who do not identify with specific subpopulations as the use of these drugs diffuses and becomes more mainstream. As the use of these drugs has changed over time there has been an overlap of their use within the dominant youth alcohol-based culture.
- Research on the diversion of prescription medication such as Ritalin and dexamphetamine for the treatment of Attention Deficit Hyperactivity Disorder among school age children. There is evidence that such tablets are traded within the school setting.
- The development and trial as demonstration projects of school based drug education interventions to reduce the harms associated with drug use for a range of drugs, including psychostimulants.
- With regards to drug use by Indigenous people there has been a call in the *NHMRC Roadmap for Aboriginal Health Research* for more intervention research, rather than epidemiological research. Consistent with this we would recommend the development of a trial of community based interventions to reduce the harm associated with psychostimulant use by Aboriginal people.[990]

Victorian Alcohol and Drug Association (VAADA)

Research is needed with regard to:

- The range of amphetamine type substances and what they contain
- The number of users who are mixing these drugs with alcohol
- Range of groups and sub populations that are using ATS
- The types of drugs being used and the environment and context they are being used in
- Pill testing research.[991]

Conclusion

The Committee believes that any strategies, interventions or policies aimed at addressing amphetamine and 'party drug' use must be based on the best available evidence and/or best practice. The following recommendations reflect the fact that up-to-date and focussed research that covers a range of quantitative and qualitative methodologies is an essential aspect of delivering effective policy outcomes in this complex area of drug use.

990 Submission of Dr Simon Lenton on behalf of the National Drug Research Institute, Curtin University, to the Drugs and Crime Prevention Committee, Inquiry into Amphetamine and 'Party Drug' Use in Victoria, October 2003.

991 Submission of VAADA to the Drugs and Crime Prevention Committee, Inquiry into Amphetamine and 'Party Drug' Use in Victoria, October 2003.

Recommendations

66. The Committee recommends that a research programme and agenda to address amphetamines and 'party drugs' be developed. This should be undertaken by the relevant agency of the Victorian Department of Human Services in association with Turning Point Alcohol and Drug Centre and other suitable research agencies.

67. The Committee recognises a substantial level of research has been undertaken in relation to amphetamine and 'party drug' use. Nonetheless, there is a noticeable absence of research that targets specific user groups, treatment issues and the effectiveness of programme delivery. The Committee therefore recommends that the research agenda outlined in Recommendation 66 should focus its priorities on the research issues which have been identified in the practice and academic literature and also reflected in the expert opinion of those who gave evidence to this Inquiry. Such issues have been highlighted in this Report.

In addition, there are a number of specific issues that the Committee has identified which form the basis of the following recommendations.

Recommendations

68. The Committee recommends that there is a need for comprehensive and timely quantitative data that, while centralised and co-ordinated, is also disaggregated at state, rural and regional and local levels. Such data should include that drawn from police, ambulance, hospital and research agencies and community agencies such as Needle and Syringe Programmes. The data will be used to inform evidence based best practice in this area.

69. The Committee recommends that such data should be made available and accessible to all tiers of government and appropriate research agencies. This is essential for any ongoing capacity by local governments in particular to address drug and alcohol issues, including those posed by psychostimulant drugs such as MDMA and amphetamines.

70. The Committee recommends that emergency hospital presentation and admissions data be disaggregated to more accurately reflect specific drug use, particularly within the rubric of amphetamines and 'party drugs'. Emergency hospital presentation and admissions data currently bundle incidences of drug overdose into the catchall 'other drug' category, unless they are primarily heroin-related or alcohol-related. This aggregation masks rather than illuminates the drug issues associated with amphetamines, 'party drugs', pharmaceuticals and some other substances.

71. The Committee recommends that ongoing research continue to be undertaken with regard to the duration and effects of the so-called 'heroin drought' and its aftermath.

72. The Committee recommends that research be undertaken into the long-term effects of the ingestion of MDMA/ecstasy including physical, psychiatric, cognitive and behavioural effects.

73. The Committee recommends that further research be undertaken into the nature and effects of 'amphetamine psychosis'.

74. The Committee recommends that in conducting research on amphetamines and 'party drugs' the complexities associated with poly-drug use need to be taken into consideration in addition to any single focus on specific drugs and/or groups of drugs.

75. The Committee recommends that research on the use, impact and diversion of prescription medication such as Ritalin/dexamphetamine for the treatment of Attention Deficit Hyperactivity Disorder among school-age children be undertaken.

76. The Committee recommends that research into the possible links between methamphetamine use and violent behaviour be further investigated.

77. The Committee recommends that further research be undertaken into effective treatment interventions, including the development of new pharmacotherapies and medications and their appropriate application. Specifically, ongoing research into possible amphetamine substitution treatments be investigated and evaluated if trialed.

78. The Committee recommends that more in-depth social research be undertaken into specific populations of users that have been identified as high risk. These may include but are not restricted to groups such as transport and other workers for whom amphetamines serve a 'functional' purpose, party/club drug users, Indigenous people, people of culturally and linguistically diverse backgrounds, homeless and street based drug users, women, gay men and lesbians.

79. The Committee acknowledges that there are many uncertainties as to why amphetamine users in particular may or may not access treatment services. The Committee recommends that further research should be undertaken to ascertain the reasons for this reluctance.

80. The Committee recommends that further research be undertaken into the difficulties faced by ambulance officers with regard to the transportation to emergency facilities and/or hospitals of people who have overdosed after having ingested amphetamines, 'party drugs' and other drugs.

81. The Committee recommends that funding be made available to enable community and local agencies such as Needle and Syringe Program outlets to undertake small-scale research to identify 'hidden' populations of amphetamine injectors and to implement appropriate strategies to reach them.

82. The Committee recommends that amphetamine and 'party drug' users should be consulted as part of any research and treatment agenda that is developed, recognising that the demography of the typical 'party drug' users is different from that of those who normally access drug treatment services.

83. The Committee recommends that all publicly funded programmes that are established to address amphetamine and 'party drugs' abuse have a requirement for evaluation to determine their effectiveness.

84. The Committee recommends the rigorous and ongoing evaluation of all publicly funded school and community based drug education programmes.

PART H: The Way Forward: Concluding Remarks

> *Albeit subject to fashion and the influence of the media icons, it seems likely that the traditional plant based drugs...will not be 'cool' and heroin and crack-cocaine will carry connotations of stigmatised and adulterated substances that would become outdated* (Klee 2001b, p.85).

This Report has not been easy to write. The topic of the Inquiry has canvassed two discrete types of drugs: amphetamines and 'party drugs'. Each of these categories contains differences in pharmacology, effects, consequences, culture and ways of addressing problems associated with the use of the drug. There are also differences within a grouping such as 'party drugs'. As has been noted throughout this report it is problematic to couple these drugs in a research document such as this.

Nonetheless, there are some commonalities that have arisen through the course of the Inquiry that can apply to both types of drug. For example, whether addressing the issue of amphetamines or 'party drugs', it is clear that focussing on one narrow target of intervention is insufficient. There must, as has been recognised in Australian drugs policy for some years, be a three-pronged attack that incorporates supply reduction, demand reduction and harm reduction. Destroying or intercepting drugs at their point of entry, for example, is necessary but not sufficient in dealing with the 'drugs menace'. Such interdiction will not of itself result in a lesser demand for drugs. As has been seen in the context of the 'heroin drought', it may simply serve to focus on a different drug of 'choice', such as amphetamines. Similarly, addressing the 'end product' of the drug's presence, that is treating a person who has become a chronic drug addict, is futile if the drugs are still crossing our borders or being 'cooked' in our backyards.

The international trend it would seem is towards an increased use in amphetamines and 'party drugs', the reasons for which are complex. Professor Hilary Klee makes the following cogent suggestions as to factors contributing to this increase:

> Four phenomena are said to have contributed to these trends: changes in social structures that lead to an emphasis on individual success and performance, a consumer society with a belief in the power of pills and an emphasis on entertainment-orientated lifestyle, the growth of industrialization, and also

> globalization. The last two facilitate the rapid spread of synthetic drugs and lead to convergence in consumption patterns across the globe (Klee 2001c, p.170).[992]

Yet, while there may be such convergence in consumption patterns, strategies to deal with illicit drug consumption vary considerably between (and sometimes within) nations. For example, one stumbling block to comprehensive international collaboration will increasingly be the opposing positions of those who subscribe to a harm minimisation philosophy compared to those who embrace a zero-tolerance stand.

In Australia, harm minimisation is an officially accepted part of national drug policy. Drug abuse is looked at as a health problem, not simply a drugs issue. The Committee endorses such as approach.

The Australian National Council on Drugs (ANCD) argues that one of the flawed aspects of current drug prevention efforts is a failure to acknowledge that substance use can be the indication of only one of a range of problem behaviours. In other words, the drug or substance is concentrated on as an 'isolated health-risk' behaviour (ANCD 2001, p.1):

> There are strong arguments for conceptualising drug misuse as one of a range of health risk behaviours, including school problems and delinquency, which have common risk and protective factors, and which share common health-and-welfare compromising outcomes, such as mental health problems, school failure, unemployment and suicidal behaviour (ANCD 2001, p.1).

Given the complexities of amphetamine and 'party drug' use and the differences between and within these classifications, it is quite clear that a 'one size fits all' approach will be inadequate to address this issue. The strategies required to prevent MDMA use among party goers will be very different to interventions needed for the chronic adult amphetamine abuser. Multifaceted strategies will therefore be required. This is particularly the case given that drug use may impact in different ways upon discrete groups in the community. As the Committee has noted, these may include Indigenous youth, young women, people from culturally and linguistically diverse backgrounds, workers in industrial settings and people with mental health problems.

The Committee has continually indicated throughout this Report that addressing amphetamine and 'party drug' abuse requires a whole of community response. Local solutions, including local partnerships, are required for local communities. Drug misuse requires interventions that range across a number of areas – policy development, training and education, legal regulation, treatment, research, media reporting, employment and recreation, and local community initiatives to name a few. *All* of these factors need to be addressed. The ANCD

992 Professor Klee has constructed a table of the factors that have both facilitated and impeded the supply and demand of amphetamines in recent years. See Appendix 35.

exhorts policymakers to learn from research experience relating to drug prevention:

> For example, be realistic about the limitations of drug education, media campaigns and law enforcement. Single, one-shot strategies are particularly ineffective. Drug abuse is a complex psychosocial issue that cannot be fixed by simple solutions (ANCD 2001, p.26).

The Committee would also concur with the following principles enunciated by the ANCD. Although they have been developed in the context of general substance use by young people, it is the Committee's belief that they are equally applicable to the specific area of amphetamine and 'party drug' use, and particularly the latter. The ANCD encourages all concerned with drug policy to:

- Adopt better practice in planning, utilising established methods such as those available in the field of health promotion. For example:
  - i Address the multiple risk and protective factors for youth drug use.
  - ii Have specific, measurable, realistic objectives.
  - iii Work at all levels of influence: the individual, the family, and the local and macro environments.
  - iv Take a long-term view – one-shot interventions are not effective.
- Acknowledge that drug use is one of a range of problem behaviours and should not be seen in isolation. Work collaboratively with others concerned with problem behaviours, including crime, suicide and educational problems, to address the shared pathways to these outcomes.
- Invest in core infrastructure. Spending on developmental health should be seen as a social investment, not just a benefit to individuals.
- Improve networks between government departments.
- Focus on the critical times in children's development.
- Monitor interventions and their outcomes to assist needs assessments and fine-tuning interventions.
- Consider the impact of all government policies and programs on the macro-environmental influences on developmental health. This needs to be done at the national, State/Territory and local government levels, and in all areas (including taxation, employment, education, urban planning, transport, justice and so on), not just the health portfolio (ANCD 2001, pp.x, xi, 27).

All the programmes, initiatives and projects which the Committee has discussed throughout this report will obviously need to be supported by adequate and ongoing funding. As such the Committee makes the following recommendations:

Recommendations

85. The Committee recommends that to address amphetamine and 'party drug' use it is imperative that adequate funding be provided for:
    a) Data collection, research and evaluation initiatives established subject to the proposed research agenda to be co-ordinated by the Department Of Human Services as outlined in Recommendation 66, p.629;
    b) Training programmes co-ordinated through the Department of Human Services;
    c) An adequate level of ongoing funding for key agencies working in the area of amphetamine and 'party drug' use, including: RaveSafe; Pt'chang Non Violence Group, Youth Substance Abuse Service; DrugInfo Clearing House (Australian Drug Foundation) and the Turning Point Alcohol and Drug Centre; and
    d) That budget allocations to drug and alcohol services take into consideration the time needed for workers to undertake professional development and keep abreast of current research developments in the area of amphetamine and 'party drugs'.
86. The Committee recommends that funding continue to be provided on a triennial basis wherever possible for appropriate community projects and programmes.
87. The Committee recommends that further funding be made available to key Needle and Syringe Program outlets in metropolitan, regional and rural settings to improve their capacity to provide primary health care and other brief interventions to current injectors.
88. The Committee recommends that funding for drug and alcohol programmes needs to acknowledge the high probability of 'changing drug use patterns and trends', such as those that occurred as a result of the so-called 'heroin drought'. It is therefore imperative that any funding for drug and alcohol programmes and initiatives, and funding arrangements, are 'flexible' enough to allow agencies to provide services and responses to emerging drug use trends.
89. The Committee recommends that the State Government's municipal 'hot spot' drug programmes continue to be funded subject to ongoing evaluation.

Summary of the Committee's position on key issues

Throughout this Report the Committee has identified a number of areas of concern that must be addressed. The remaining section of this concluding chapter contains brief summaries of the Committee's position on the key issues that have arisen from this Inquiry. It should be read in conjunction with our Recommendations located at the beginning of this Report. Reaching these positions has involved balancing and reconciling a number of competing interests and positions, all of which have strong arguments to support them.

Central to the development of the recommendations is an acknowledgement that harm minimisation forms the central platform of the Australian government's *National Drug Strategy* which is also endorsed by Victoria and all other states.

Supply reduction measures

The Committee has made a number of recommendations with regard to law and legal regulation. These have included the recommendation of new laws with regard to the amounts of amphetamine and methylamphetamine that would be sufficient to constitute various trafficking and other offences in the *Drugs, Poisons and Controlled Substances Act 1981*. The Committee has also recommended new laws with regard to the possession of precursor chemicals and apparatus in order to stem the illicit manufacture of amphetamines in Victoria. It also believes that the dangers associated with amphetamine and other drug manufacture warrant the creation of a child endangerment offence.

Clearly our police and law enforcement services, both state and federal, are at the forefront of *supply reduction* operations. In the area of amphetamine and 'party drugs' importation, manufacture and distribution, the work of law enforcement services from Customs officials to members of the state Dog Squad need to be supported and funded appropriately. In particular, the dangerous yet extremely important work of clandestine laboratory officers and illicit drug teams deserves special commendation. Yet supply reduction is not only the province of the law enforcement agencies. This Committee has written extensively of the need to have a co-operative working partnership with agencies that have a direct relationship to the drugs or components that can contribute to amphetamine manufacture in particular. These include scientific glassware manufacturers, chemical wholesalers and, most importantly, members of the pharmacy profession. The use of hitherto non-mandatory guidelines, circulars and statements produced by the Victorian Pharmacy Board in conjunction with the Pharmaceutical Society of Australia and the Pharmacy Guild to prevent the illicit diversion of pseudoephedrine products has been an encouraging step. It is one, however, that the Committee feels needs to go further. The Committee has therefore recommended that at both retail and wholesale levels guidelines covering the sale of precursors, precursor products and manufacturing apparatus should become mandatory. Moreover, the Committee believes it is not unreasonable to enact an offence making it illegal to be in the possession of a certain amount of precursor material or apparatus without lawful excuse.

When it comes to 'party drugs' in particular, regulation is required not just with regard to the drugs themselves but also the context in which they are taken. Therefore the Committee has made a number of recommendations with regard to security and health issues associated with dance clubs, rave events and associated venues.

Demand reduction measures

Education and information provision is an essential aspect of tackling problems arising from the use of these drugs from a *demand reduction* perspective. As with any area of drug use, a balance needs to be sought between providing information that may seem to encourage or condone the uptake or continuance of use and providing too little or too negative messages that may simply be ignored by the drug using populations. When it comes to the use of 'party drugs' in particular, 'just say no' messages seem to have made little headway. Innovative educational strategies that 'talk' to young people in particular, and that stress the dangers of recreational use while understanding, if not condoning, its attractions, are a necessary part of any strategy to reduce demand for these drugs. Likewise, comprehensive and age appropriate prevention strategies, particularly in schools, need to be devised based on best practice models from around Australia and overseas. Any such prevention and education strategies must at all times be culturally appropriate to the audience at which they are targeted.

Training of relevant professionals is a key aspect of demand reduction strategies. It is imperative that those in a position to affect someone who has taken or been adversely affected by drug use is able to effectively respond to that circumstance. Accordingly, the Committee has recommended that sufficient and appropriate training be given to a wide range of professionals who may come into contact with people who use amphetamines and 'party drugs', including but not restricted to medical, police, emergency services and alcohol and drug workers.

Harm reduction measures

Harm reduction works at many levels. It recognises, however unfortunately, that both licit and illicit drug use is a fact of life. This is a key aspect of the *National Drug Strategy* and one this Committee endorses. In the context of 'party drugs' it means that the venues where such drugs are taken need to take into account the fact that drug use may occur there and that appropriate safeguards are necessary to minimise the dangers to both the user and those around him or her. The protocols and recommendations of this Report with regard to harm reduction in club or rave venues are, in the opinion of this Committee, an important step in the right direction. When it comes to drugs such as methamphetamine the Committee emphatically endorses the types of harm reduction strategies already in place, particularly with regard to injecting drug use. The work of agencies such as needle and syringe exchanges and the provision of appropriate equipment to reduce the dangers associated with injecting drug use must be supported.

Treatment for those whose drug use requires intervention is also an essential aspect of any overall harm reduction strategy. The Committee has noted the lack of comprehensive and discrete treatment interventions for amphetamine users in particular. It has also noted that more research needs to be conducted on why amphetamine users are a population that seems to find it difficult to access the treatment options that are available. It encourages the excellent research work being done in Australia and Victoria, particularly that of Turning Point Alcohol and Drug Centre, to continue endeavours to explore treatment options for this particular drug.

There are other aspects of a harm reduction agenda that can not be supported. For example, the Committee believes that pill testing stations are a 'step too far'. Self-testing pill kits are particularly controversial and the Committee believes that on balance the evidence does not support their introduction as a harm reduction measure either. The Committee acknowledges that this decision will be disappointing to those who have sincerely held beliefs that such initiatives are appropriate.

Final remarks

As with most types of drug use, amphetamine and 'party drug' use needs to be addressed from many angles. One of the most important findings of the Inquiry has been that often amphetamine and 'party drugs' are merely part of a much wider 'repertoire' of licit and illicit drug use. Poly-drug use sadly seems more the norm than an aberration.

Addressing amphetamine and 'party drug' use also requires collaborative partnerships. Police, teachers, researchers, medical staff, local government and community agencies, to name a few, all have a role to play. The views and advice of user groups and former and current users should, wherever possible or relevant, inform the policies on strategies implemented as a result of the Committee's recommendations.

Finally, a constant theme throughout this Report has been that drug policy and strategy for far too long has overlooked or at least paid insufficient attention to the particular needs of rural and regional communities in Victoria. In particular, the Committee strongly exhorts authorities to meet the requirements of those who work in the alcohol, drug and allied services in the country regions of this state. The state as a whole, including Melbourne, will be the better off for such an approach.

Adopted by the Drugs and Crime Prevention Committee
Level 8
35 Spring St
Melbourne 3000

19 April 2004

Appendices

Appendix 1: List of Submissions Received

Submission Number	Name of Individual/Organisation	Date Received
1	Dr Simon Lenton, Senior Research Fellow – Curtin University of Technology	8 July 2002
2	Mr Alan Benzley	11 July 2002
3	Mr Kevin W. Walsh, Managing Director – Bio-Mediq DPC Pty Ltd	15 July 2002
4	Confidential submission	2 August 2002
5	Mr Mark Young, Community Networks Manager – Open Family Australia	5 August 2002
6	Mr David Risstrom, Councillor – City of Melbourne	5 August 2002
7	Confidential submission	6 August 2002
8	Mr Mike Hill, Executive Officer – Victorian Local Governance Association	7 August 2002
9	Mr Brendan Ball, Monash Drug and Alcohol Project – Monash City Council	7 August 2002
10	Ms Janet Farrow, Executive Director – Uniting Care Morland Hall	7 August 2002
11	Mr Andrew Paul, Chief Executive Officer – City of Greater Bendigo	7 August 2002
12	Mr Rob Skinner, Chief Executive Officer – Kingston City Council	7 August 2002
13	Mr David Murray, Chief Executive Officer – Youth Substance Abuse Service (YSAS)	7 August 2002
14	Confidential submission	7 August 2002
15	Ms Rosemary McClean, Manager, Strategic Planning – Australian Drug Foundation	7 August 2002
16	Ms Jacinta Maloney, Community Lawyer and Education Worker – St Kilda Legal Service	7 August 2002
17	Mr Graham Strathearn, Chief Executive Officer – Drug and Alcohol Services Council	8 August 2002
18	Ms Nancy Di Santo, Community Health and Safe City Planner – Hume City Council	8 August 2002
19	Ms Noelene Duff, Chief Executive Officer – City of Whitehorse	9 August 2002
20	Ms Carmel Fox, Team Leader Eastern Drug & Alcohol Service – Monash Link Community Health Service	7 August 2002

Submission Number	Name of Individual/Organisation	Date Received
21	Ms Helen Fraser, Project Worker, Drug and Health Issues – Doutta Galla Community Health Service	16 August 2002
22	Ms Michelle McDonald, Manager, Membership and Policy – YWCA Victoria	19 August 2002
23	Rev Mgr T. M. Doyle, Director of Catholic Education	23 August 2002
24	Mrs Kerrie Peters, Community Development Officer – Northern Grampians Shire Council	29 August 2002
25	Ms Gail Price, Community Development Officer – Mornington Peninsula Shire Council	28 August 2002
26	Hon. John Thwaites, MP Minister for Health, for Human Services Victoria, Drug Policy and Services Branch	28 August 2002
27	Mr John Edwards	3 July 2003
28	Ms Carol Bennett, Executive Officer – VAADA	19 August 2003
29	Mr John Perham, Moorabool Shire Council	7 Oct 2003
30	Goulburn Valley Community Health Services	7 Oct 2003
31	Mrs Susanna J Carlyon Rnd, Director – Independent Pastoral Care, Euroa	13 Oct 2003
32	Ms Susan Pascoe, Director – Catholic Education Office	9 Oct 2003
33	Ms Jenny Branton, Manager Community Services – Murrindini Shire Council	10 Oct 2003
34	Ms Alison Cran, Director, Community & Cultural Services – Shire of Yarra Ranges	13 Oct 2003
35	Professor Con Stough and Associates, Swinburne University	13 Oct 2003
36	Mr John Ryan, Chief Executive Officer – Anex	13 Oct 2003
37	Ms Angie Laussel, Manager – Macedon Ranges Shire Council	13 Oct 2003
38	Ms Kerry Thompson, Chief Executive Officer – Maribyrnong City Council	14 Oct 2003
39	Ms Jill Meade, Manager –VIVAIDS Inc	14 Oct 2003
40	Dr James Rowe, Centre for Applied Social Research – RMIT University	14 Oct 2003
41	Mr Nicholas Foa, Director, Community and Organisational Development – Maroondah City Council	3 Oct 2003
42	Ms Janet Farrow, Executive Director – Uniting Care Moreland Hall	16 Oct 2003
43	Mr Vince Keogh, Acting Director, City Assets & Services – City of Melbourne	17 Oct 2003
44	Mr Jurgen Hemmerling, A & O D Youth Outreach Worker – Open Family Australia	17 Oct 2003
45	Mr Maurice V Sheehan, Branch Director – The Pharmacy Guild of Australia	17 Oct 2003

Submission Number	Name of Individual/Organisation	Date Received
46	Ms Lydia Wilson, Chief Executive Officer – City of Yarra	20 Oct 2003
47	Ms Deb Heery, Alcohol & Other Drugs Unit – Upper Hume Community Health Service, Wodonga	21 Oct 2003
48	Mr John Parkinson, Drug Diversion Counsellor – Castlemaine District Community Health Centre	22 Oct 2003
49	Dr Ray Cleary, Chief Executive Officer – Anglicare Victoria	22 Oct 2003
50	Mr Stephen Marty, Registrar – Pharmacy Board of Victoria	23 Oct 2003
51	Mr John Iliot, Chief Executive Officer – Pharmaceutical Society of Australia (Vic)	20 Oct 2003
52	Ms Jenny Merkus, Director Social Development – Moreland City Council	24 Oct 2003
53	Mr David Murray, CEO – Youth Substance Abuse Service	27 Oct 2003
54	Ms Carol Bennett, Victorian Alcohol & Drug Association (VAADA)	27 Oct 2003
55	Confidential	27 Oct 2003
56	Ms Natalie Russell, RaveSafe Peer Education Officer – VIVAIDS	27 Oct 2003
57	Dr Simon Lenton, Senior Research Fellow – Curtin University of Technology, Perth	27 Oct 2003
58	Mr Brendan Ball, Monash Social Projects Coordinator – City of Monash	28 Oct 2003
59	Professor Margaret Hamilton, Director – Turning Point Drug and Alcohol Centre	27 Oct 2003
60	Dr David Moore, Curtin University of Technology, Perth	5 Nov 2003
61	Ms Christine Nixon APM, Chief Commissioner – Victoria Police	10 Nov 2003
62	Mr Paul McDonald, Director, Drugs Policy & Services – Dept of Human Services	11 Nov 2003
63	Dr Rodger Brough, Director – Australian Rural Centre for Addictive Behaviours (ARCAB)	7 Nov 2003
64	Mr John Paterson, State Manager – ATSIS Victorian State Office	12 Dec 2003
65	Professor Olaf H. Drummer, Victorian Institute of Forensic Medicine	6 Jan 2004
66	The Hon John Thwaites MP, Acting Premier of Victoria, Prepared by the Department of Human Services Victoria	7 Jan 2004
67	Mr Tony Parsons, Managing Director – Victoria Legal Aid	27 Jan 2004
68	Mr Ben Horan	3 Feb 2004
69	Hon. Jacinta Allan MP, Minister for Education Services	13 Feb 2004
70	Mr Edwin Lorkin, Acting Chair – Criminal Bar Association	17 Feb 2004
71	Mr Chris Dale, President – Law Institute of Victoria	24 Feb 2004

Appendix 2: Interstate Meetings and Site Visits

Meetings in Canberra – 23 & 24 June 2003

Name	Position	Organisation
Dr Toni Makkai	Director of Research	Australian Institute of Criminology
Dr Natalie Taylor	Research Analyst	Australian Institute of Criminology
Mr Chris Clark	Acting Director	Australian Crime Commission
Mr Shaun Reynolds	Team Leader – Drugs Unit	Australian Crime Commission
Mr Keith Tomlin	Federal Agent	Australian Federal Police
Mr Phil Case	Federal Agent	Australian Federal Police

Meetings in Sydney – 25 & 26 June 2003

Name	Position	Organisation
Dr John Howard	Director Clinical Services and Research	Ted Noffs Foundation
Mr Matt Stubbs	Training and Research Officer	Ted Noffs Foundation
Mr Paul Dillon	Media Liaison and Information Manager	National Drug and Alcohol Research Centre – University of New South Wales
Dr Louisa Degenhardt	Research Assistant to the Director	National Drug and Alcohol Research Centre – University of New South Wales
Dr Rebecca McKetin	Research Fellow	National Drug and Alcohol Research Centre – University of New South Wales
Ms Bronwyn Crosby	Manger of Clinical Services	St Vincent's Hospital/Alcohol and Drug Information Service
Ms Carol Stubley	Nursing Unit Manager	St Vincent's Hospital/Alcohol and Drug Information Service
Ms Lorraine Buckner Pitts	Health Education Officer/Counsellor	St Vincent's Hospital/Alcohol and Drug Information Service

Meetings in Brisbane – 27 June 2003

Name	Position	Organisation
Detective Inspector Greg Tutt	Officer in Charge, Illicit Laboratory Investigation Team	Queensland Police
Sergeant Scott Feeney	Chemical Diversion Desk Officer, State Drug Squad	Queensland Police
Detective Sergeant Jason Renwick	Illicit Laboratory Investigation Team	Queensland Police
Detective Acting Chief Supt. Graham Rynders	State Crime Operation Command	Queensland Police
Detective Superintendent Kev Robinson	State Crime Operation Command	Queensland Police
Deptective Senior Constable Fiona Hinshelwood	Sexual Crimes Investigation Unit and Project Officer – Alcohol and Drug Assisted Sexual Assault Project (ADASA)	Queensland Police
Ms Robyn Stewart	Executive Secretary, Assistant Commissioner (Crime Operations)	Queensland Police
Mr Michael Dart	Alcohol Tobacco and other Drugs Policy Advisor to the Minister	Queensland Health
Dr Kevin Lambkin	Acting Manager, Alcohol Tobacco and other Drugs Services Unit	Queensland Health
Mr Robert Kemp	Manager, Queensland Needle Availability Support Program	Queensland Health

Meetings in Western Australia – 1 & 2 October 2003

Name	Position	Organisation
Ms Carmen Acosta	Development Manager, Youth Withdrawal and Respite Service	Mission Australia
Ms Siobhan Foley	Social Worker, Yirra Youth Substance Misuse Service	Mission Australia
Ms Jen Lowe	Social Worker, Youth Withdrawal and Respite Service	Mission Australia
Prof Steve Allsop	A/g Executive Director	Drug and Alcohol Office of Western Australia
Ms Eleanor Costello	Prevention Branch	Drug and Alcohol Office of Western Australia
Mr Richard Bostwick	Director of Clinical Services, Joint Services Development Unit	Health Department of Western Australia
Detective Superintendent Jim Migro	Det. Supt In Charge, Organised Crime Division	Western Australian Police Service
Detective Senior Sergeant Roger Beer	Operations Manager for Organised Crime Investigation	Western Australian Police Service
Acting Detective Sergeant Paul Steel	Chemical Diversion Officer, Organised Crime Division	Western Australian Police Service
Senior Sergeant Gil Wilson	Acting Senior Sergeant in Charge, Alcohol and Drug Coordination Unit	Western Australian Police Service
Mr Paul Dessauer	Outreach Worker	Western Australian Substance Users Association
Dr Simon Lenton	National Drug Research Institute	Curtin University, Perth
Associate Professor Dennis Gray	National Drug Research Institute	Curtin University, Perth
Dr Richard Midford	National Drug Research Institute	Curtin University, Perth
Dr David Moore	National Drug Research Institute	Curtin University, Perth
Dr Francoise Chanteloup	National Drug Research Institute	Curtin University, Perth
Mr James Fetherston	National Drug Research Institute	Curtin University, Perth

Meetings in South Australia – 3 October 2003

Name	Position	Organisation
Mr Mal Hyde	Commissioner	South Australia Police
Ms Madeleine Woolley	Executive Director, Social Inclusion Unit	SA Department of Premier and Cabinet
Mr David Waterford	Senior Policy Officer, Drugs	SA Department of Premier and Cabinet
Mr Lindy Brinkworth	Senior Policy Officer, Drugs	SA Department of Premier and Cabinet
Mr Daniel Craker	Policy Officer, Social Inclusion Unit	SA Department of Premier and Cabinet
Professor Jason White	Director, Treatment and Rehabilitation Services	Drug and Alcohol Services Council of SA
Ms Simone Cormack	Director, Population Health Programs	Drug and Alcohol Services Council of SA
Ms Kelly Weekley	Manager, Harm Reduction	Drug and Alcohol Services Council of SA

Appendix 3: Witnesses Appearing at Public Hearings

Hearings in Melbourne – 6 October 2003

Name	Position	Organisation
Dr Rodger Brough	Director	Australian Rural Centre for Addictive Behaviours (ARCAB) and Western Region Alcohol and Drug Centre
Ms Suzan Morey	Majot Project Manager	Australian Rural Centre for Addictive Behaviours (ARCAB) and Western Region Alcohol and Drug Centre

Hearings in Melbourne – 27 October 2003

Name	Position	Organisation
Dr Chris O'Donnell	Radiologist	Frankston Hospital
Mr David Murray	Executive Officer	Youth Substance Abuse Services
Mr Rowan Fairbairn	Senior Policy Officer	Youth Substance Abuse Services
Mr Tony Palmer	Training Officer & Consultant	Youth Substance Abuse Services
Mr Steve Marty	Registrar	Pharmacy Board of Victoria
Professor Margaret Hamilton	Director	Turning Point Alcohol & Drug Centre
Dr Craig Fry	Senior Research Fellow	Turning Point Alcohol & Drug Centre
Dr Nicole Lee	Senior Clinical Psychologist	Turning Point Alcohol & Drug Centre
Ms Natalie Russell	RaveSafe Peer Education Officer	VIVAIDS
Mr Damon Brogan	Ravesafe Project	VIVAIDS
Ms Carol Bennett	Chief Executive Officer	Victorian Alcohol & Drug Association
Mr Neos Zavrou	Chairman	Victorian Alcohol & Drug Association

Hearings in Melbourne – 10 November 2003

Name	Position	Organisation
Superintendent Paul Ditchburn	Organisational Development Department	Victoria Police
Inspector Steve James	Drug and Alcohol Strategy Unit	Victoria Police
Senior Sergeant Phil Harrison	Drug and Alcohol Strategy Unit	Victoria Police
Acting Senior Sergeant Steve McGovern	Dog Squad	Victoria Police
Detective Senior Sergeant Jim O'Brien	Major Drug Investigation Division	Victoria Police
Ms Cate Quinn	Victoria Forensic Services Drug Section	Victoria Police
Mr Tim Harvey	Organiser	Transplant
Mr Garth Lategan	Organiser	SMILE Police Productions
Mr Matthew Deveson	Managing Director	ZoS Nightclub
Mr Ben Horan	First Aid and Drug Harm Reduction Officer	ZoS Nightclub
Mr Tom Walker	Owner	Seven Nightclub
Mr Josh Brooker		Individual

Hearings in Melbourne (Knox) – 11 November 2003

Name	Position	Organisation
Ms Kym Neville	Community Development Officer	Shire of Yarra Ranges
Ms Carmel Fox	Manager, Monash Link Community Health Service	Eastern Drug and Alcohol Service
Mr Graham Williams	Team Leader, AGEnDAS	Anglicare Greater Eastern Drug and Alcohol Service
Acting Supt Doug Hocking	Acting Superintendent, Knox District	Victoria Police
Snr Sgt Phil Harrison	Drug and Alcohol Strategy Unit	Victoria Police
Ms Christine Tindal	Co-ordinator, Needle and Syringe Programme	Whitehorse Community Health Centre
Mr Nick Stafford	Outreach Worker	Primary Needle and Syringe Program, Eastern Region

Hearings in Rural Victoria and Regional Areas

Benalla – 22 October 2003

Name	Position	Organisation
Inspector Steve James	Manager, Drug and Alcohol Strategy Unit	Victoria Police
Sergeant Graham Waters		Victoria Police, Benalla
Ms Deb Heery	Team Member	Alcohol & Other Drugs Upper Hume Community Health Services
Ms Elena Tauridsky	Manager	Central Hume Alcohol and Other Drugs Service
Ms Lynda Johnson	Withdrawal Nurse	Central Hume Alcohol and Other Drugs Service
Ms Rachel Meadows	Drug Diversion Worker	Central Hume Alcohol and Other Drugs Service
Pastor Daryl Marshall		Rose City Christian Life Centre
Mrs Sue Carlyon	Counsellor	Independent Pastoral Care
Mrs Mary Elder	Volunteer	Salvation Army
Mr Jurgen Hemmerling	Youth Outreach Worker	Open Family (Hume Region)
Ms Jane Campbell	Rural Manager	Odyssey House

Moe – 23 October 2003

Name	Position	Organisation
Mr Frank Coughlan	Outreach Clinician	Latrobe Community Health Service
Mr Rick Henderson	Acting Executive Officer	Central Gippsland Aboriginal Co-operative
Mr Gordon Hood	Program Co-ordinator, Bendin House	Central Gippsland Aboriginal Co-operative
Mr Laurie Marks	Juvenile Justice Program Co-ordinator	Central Gippsland Aboriginal Co-operative
Mr Huey Pepper	Youth A&D Worker	Central Gippsland Aboriginal Co-operative
Mr Steve James	Inspector, Drug and Alcohol Strategy Unit	Victoria Police
Mr Craig Gye	Senior Sergeant (Traralgon)	Victoria Police
Mr Christopher Notman	Inspector, Latrobe District	Victoria Police
Mr John Heynes	Inspector, Former Dandenong District	Victoria Police
Mr Ron Marshall	Manager, Alcohol & Drug Services	La Trobe Valley Community Health
Ms Theresa Jones	Hospital Liaison Worker	La Trobe Valley Community Health

Appendix 4: Venue Operators, Owners and Promoters who Attended the Forum

Name	Position	Organisation
Mr Tim Harvey	Organiser	Transplant
Mr Garth Lategan	Organiser	SMILE Police Productions
Mr Matthew Deveson	Managing Director	ZoS Nightclub
Mr Ben Horan	First Aid and Drug Harm Reduction Officer	ZoS Nightclub
Mr Tom Walker	Owner	Seven Nightclub

Appendix 5: List of Clubs and Events Visited

Events and Venues Attended	Date
Nightclub Visits:	14th November 2003
Sugar Suite	14th November 2003
The Croft Institute	14th November 2003
Hard Kandy	14th November 2003
ZoS	14th November 2003
Room 680	14th November 2003
Earthcore	29th November 2003

Appendix 6: Meetings with Clubbers, Ravegoers and Others and Committee Staff

Name	Position	Organisation	Date
John*	Rave and clubgoer		29th August 2003
Mr Ben Horan	Harm reduction/First aid Officer	ZoS Nightclub	25th November 2003
Bill*	Rave and clubgoer		8th December 2003
Jean*	Rave and clubgoer		8th December 2003
Angela*	Rave and clubgoer		8th December 2003
Mr Pip Darvall	Promoter	Earthcore	12th December 2003

* A pseudonym has been given to protect the anonymity of the individual

Appendix 7: Seminars and Conferences Attended

Forums and Meetings	Date
Turning Point Alcohol and Drug Centre Seminar 'Full Speed Ahead: Developments for Treatment in Amphetamine Use'	8th November 2002
4th International Conference on Drugs and Young People	26–28 May 2003
VAADA seminar 'Beyond e: exploring the impact of party drugs on current day use and culture'	23rd June 2003
Turning Point Alcohol and Drug Centre Seminar 'Work in Progress: Alcohol and Drug Research Symposium'	22nd August 2003
RaveSafe training session for Promoters, Club Owners and Workers	5th November 2003
Ethnic Communities Seminar	3rd December 2003

Appendix 8: Expert Witnesses Invited to Speak to the Committee

Name	Position	Organisation	Date
Senior Sergeant Phil Harrison	Drug and Alcohol Strategy Unit	Victoria Police	2 June 2003
Inspector Steve James	Manager, Drug and Alcohol Strategy Unit	Victoria Police	2 June 2003

Appendix 9: List of Submissions Received from Rural and Regional Victoria

Mr John Perham, Moorabool Shire Council	7 Oct 2003
Ms Merri Blair, Mobile Drugs Safety Officer – Goulburn Valley Community Health Services	7 Oct 2003
Ms Jenny Branton, Manager Community Services – Murrindindi Shire Council	10 Oct 2003
Ms Angie Laussel, Manager – Macedon Ranges Shire Council	13 Oct 2003
Mr Jurgen Hemmerling, A&OD Youth Outreach worker – Open Family Australia	17 Oct 2003
Ms Deb Heery, Alcohol & Other Drugs Unit, Upper Hume Community Health Service – Wodonga	21 Oct 2003
Mr John Parkinson, Drug Diversion Counsellor – Castlemaine District Community Health Centre	22 Oct 2003
Dr Rodger Brough, Director – Australian Rural Centre for Addictive Behaviours (ARCAB)	7 Nov 2003

Appendix 10: Drink Spiking Pamphlet

VICTORIA POLICE

CASA house
Centre Against Sexual Assault

GIPPSLAND
Centre Against Sexual Assault

Has your drink been spiked...?

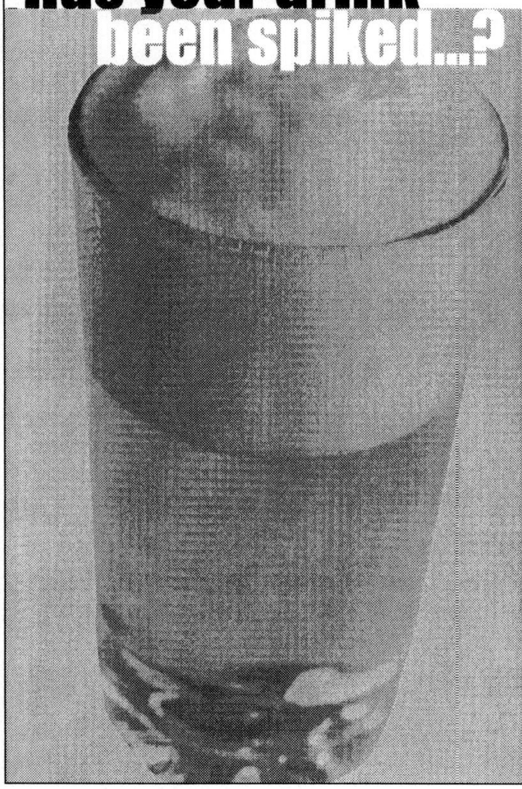

There are a number of people coming forward to Centres Against Sexual Assault (CASAs), reporting that they have been drugged and then sexually assaulted, or that their drink has been spiked. If you think this has happened to you, or someone you know, then the following information may be of interest to you.

This pamphlet has been developed by the CASAs and Victoria Police as a joint project. The aim of the project is to:

- Provide information about the options for help and support available to anyone who believes she/he may have been the victim of a sexual assault (as a result of drink spiking).
- Gather information, via an anonymous survey, about these assaults. This information may assist in two ways. Firstly, there is little known about the nature and prevalence of this type of crime in Victoria. By understanding what is happening we can ensure we are providing the best response. We can work to identify ways to prevent offences occurring. Secondly, if a specific problem is identified, police can act.

Assistance

- If you think that you have been a victim of a drug facilitated sexual assault there are options available for you to get support and assistance. This assistance may be in the form of counselling or advice on your medical and legal options, or you may decide to report the matter to police. There is more information about these options, including contact details, on the back of this pamphlet.

Drug Facilitated Sexual Assault is a Crime

- If someone gives you drugs or alcohol without your knowledge, often by simply giving drinks that are much stronger than you expect, and, as a result, you are not capable of freely consenting to sexual activity, this is an offence.
- Drug facilitated sexual assault is often a planned crime and regardless of what you may have voluntarily taken or had to drink, it is not your fault. There are laws in Victoria to protect you and services that can provide support and information about your rights and options.
- It is common for victims of drug facilitated sexual assault to have unclear, or only partial, recollections of what happened to them and as a result victims are not always confident about reporting the suspected incident to the police.

Filling out the survey: We understand you may not be able to provide all the information requested and that some of the questions may not be relevant to your circumstances. Please answer the questions to the best of your ability. If you would like to provide more information add a sheet of paper and mail it back inside the survey.

Please note that answering some of the questions presented in the survey may result in emotional distress. Should you choose to participate and find this happens to you please contact CASA House for support and information (details on rear).

Some things you should know about this survey:

- You are not required to identify yourself.
- By completing and posting this survey you are consenting to participate in this research.
- Any information you provide will be used solely for this project.
- The information will be kept for at least five years.

If you require more information about this research, please contact the Drug & Alcohol Strategy Unit, Victoria Police (9247 6725) or CASA House.

1. Your gender (circle): Female / Male
2. Age:
3. Briefly describe what has happened to you:
4. Where were you when you were drugged? (eg – offender's home, friend's house – please state the suburb/town. If it was a public venue, please provide the name/address – if known)
5. Where were you when you were assaulted? (eg own home, offender's car etc.)
6. If unconscious, where were you when you regained consciousness?
7. When did this incident occur? (eg Date/day of week / time – be as specific as possible)
8. What drug (includes alcohol) do you believe was used?

9. What makes you think it was this drug? (includes alcohol)

10. What type of drink were you having at the time you were drugged? (eg - wine, mixed drink, coffee, soft drink, cooler etc)

11. How many offenders were there?

12. Did you know the offender/s prior to the day of the assault? Circle: Yes / No.

13. Describe the primary offender.
    Age: Height:
    Build:
    Hair colour: Hair length:
    Skin colour: Gender: Male/Female
    Clothing:
    Scars/tattoos:
    Jewellery:

Other details that may help identify the offender:

14. If you wish to identify the offender (if known) please provide the following information:

Name: ____________________

Nickname: ____________________

Address: ____________________

Vehicle: ____________________

(registration/make/model/colour if possible)

15. Where did you get this form (tick box)?

☐ Community Health Centre ☐ CASA
☐ Hospital ☐ University ☐ Police Station
☐ Doctor's Office ☐ Other

Thank you - your assistance is appreciated.

Centres Against Sexual Assault

Centres Against Sexual Assault provide free and confidential services to all victims of sexual assault, including issues related to medical and legal options. There are 15 different CASAs throughout Victoria in metropolitan and regional areas. Some are listed below. If you are in a different area, contact CASA House for the details of your nearest CASA.

- CASA House (Melbourne)
  Business hours Crisis Line: (03) 9344 2210
- Gippsland CASA
  Business hours Crisis Line: (03) 5134 3922
- Afterhours Sexual Assault Crisis Line:
  Metropolitan: (03) 9349 1766
  Rural only: 1800 806 292

Victoria Police

If an urgent police response is needed, please telephone: 000

Victoria Police is responsible for investigating crimes committed in Victoria. There are specialist police units, known as Sexual Offences & Child Abuse Units (SOCA Units), that are staffed by police trained and experienced in responding to reports of sexual assault. There are 31 SOCA Units across the state and your local police station will be able to give you contact details of the nearest SOCA Unit.

- Sexual Offences & Child Abuse Units
  - Melbourne West (city) (03) 9247 5538
  - Morwell (03) 5132 2330
  - Crime Stoppers 1800 333 000

Crime Stoppers is a community based initiative which encourages members of the public to provide information (anonymously, if they wish) to the police regarding criminal activity. If you know anything about drink spiking or any other criminal activity please ring 1800 333 000.

CRIME STOPPERS 1 800 333 000

It is your choice as to whether you report this matter to police or not, however please keep in mind that it is always better from an investigation point of view to make a report as soon as possible.

Appendix 11: Injecting Drug Use

Table A: Injecting drug use: First and recent[(a)] illicit drugs injected, proportion of ever/recent injecting drug users aged 14 years and over, by sex, Australia 2001

	(Per cent)					
	First Injected[(b)]			Recently Injected[(c)]		
Drug	**Males**	**Females**	**Persons**	**Males**	**Females**	**Persons**
Heroin	30.0	31.3	30.5	18.8	30.2	22.9
Methadone	0.0	0.3	0.1	9.1	5.0	7.6
Other opiates	3.0	3.2	3.1	15.8	22.7	18.3
Amphetamines	59.8	61.2	60.3	76.4	78.3	77.1
Cocaine	2.4	1.9	2.3	11.3	18.0	13.6
Hallucinogens	0.7	0.2	0.5	3.4	0.8	2.5
Ecstasy	0.0	1.6	0.6	14.8	11.4	13.6
Steroids	4.1	0.2	2.7	5.6	4.9	5.4
Benzodiazepines	-	-	-	2.2	4.4	3.0
Other drugs	-	-	-	3.9	6.9	4.9

(a) Used in the last 12 months

(b) Answered by respondents who have ever injected

(c) Answered by respondents who have injected in the last 12 months

Source: Australian Institute of Health and Welfare (AIHW) 2002a, *National Drug Strategy Household Survey: First Results,* AIHW, Canberra, p.39.

Appendix 12: MDMA and MDEA Related Deaths in Victoria 1995–2003

Year	Case	Sex	Age	Occupation	Location	Type	BAC	Party Drug	Other Drugs
1995	1	F	25	Croupier	South Yarra	SUICIDE DRUG (HEROIN)	0	MDMA	HEROIN, METHAMPHETAMINE
1996	2	F	18	Bar Attendant	Canterbury	MVA DRIVER	0.18	MDMA	NONE
1996	3	M	25	Escort	Prahran East	DRUG	0	MDMA, MDEA	METHAMPHETAMINE
1996	4	F	32	Production Manager	Newport	MDT (Heroin)	0.09	MDMA	HEROIN
1996	5	F	29	Actress	Balwyn	DRUG	0.02	MDMA	TEMAZEPAM
1997	6	F	23	Unemployed	Kew	MDT (Heroin)	0	MDMA	HEROIN, METHAMPHETAMINE, COCAINE
1998	7	M	34	Company Director	South Yarra	MDT (Heroin)	0	MDVA	HEROIN, COCAINE
1998	8	M	26	Doctor	Collingwood	HOMICIDE	0.04	MDMA	HEROIN
1999	9	F	21	Unemployed	Hastings	HOMICIDE	0.00	MDMA	METHAMPHETAMINE, PSEUDOEPHEDRINE, DEXTROMETHORPHAN, PHOLCODIN
1999	10	M	44	Electrician	Yarraville	HOMICIDE	0.00	MDMA	CODEINE, CANNABIS
1999	11	M	20	Student	Carrum Downs	MDT (Heroin)	0.00	MDMA	MORPHINE/HEROIN
1999	12	M	22	Gardener	Malvern	MDT (Heroin)	0.09	MDMA	MORPHINE/HEROIN, CANNABIS
2900	13	F	20	Night Club Worker	Geelong	MDT (Heroin)	0	MDMA	MORPHINE/HEROIN, METHAMPHETAMINE
2000	14	M	28	Truck Driver	Hampton	MDT (Heroin)	0	MDMA	HEROIN
2000	15	M	39	Unemployed	St Kilda	MDT (Heroin)	0	MDMA	HEROIN, COCAINE, METHAMPHETAMINE
2000	16	F	33	IT Worker	Doncaster East	HOMICIDE	0	MDMA	METHAMPHETAMINE
2000	17	M	35	Unemployed	Toorak	SUICIDE GUN	0	MDMA	MORPHINE/HEROIN METHAMPHETAMINE
2000	18	M	26	Unemployed	No fixed address	MDT (Heroin)	0	MDMA	HEROIN
2001	19	M	22	Unemployed	Frankston	MVA PASSENGER	0	MDMA	METHAMPHETAMINE
2001	20	M	24	Unemployed	Emerald	SUICIDE CO	0	MDMA	METHAMPHETAMINE
2001	21	M	27	Sales Assistant	Roslyn Park, SA	MVA DRIVER	0.07	MDMA	METHAMPHETAMINE
2001	22	M	38	Manager	Mt Albert	NATURAL (INFECTION)	0	MDMA	NONE
2001	23	M	32	Police Officer	Abbotsford	MDT (Heroin)	0	MDMA	MORPHINE/HEROIN, METHAMPHETAMINE
2001	24	F	21	Sales Assistant	Carnegie	DRUG ECSTASY	0	MDMA	NONE
2001	25	M	29	Process Worker	Hampton Park	SUICIDE HANGING	0.09	MDMA	PSEUDOEPHEDRINE, CANNABIS
2001	26	M	40	Truck Driver	South Australia	SUICIDE HANGING	0	MDMA	METHAMPHETAMINE, CANNABIS
2001	27	M	23	Plasterer	St Albans	DRUG & HEART DISEASE	0	MDMA	METHAMPHETAMINE
2001	28	M	25	Sales Assistant	St Kilda	DRUG	0	MDMA	METHAMPHETAMINE
2002	29	M	33	IT Worker	Richmond	ACCIDENT HANGING	0	MDMA	NONE
2002	30	M	30	Personal Trainer	Carlton	DRUG	0	MDMA	METHAMPHETAMINE
2002	31	M	28	Unemployed	Mt Waverley	MDT (Heroin)	0	MDMA	MORPHINE/HEROIN, METHAMPHETAMINE
2002	32	M	43	Crane Operator	Port Melbourne	HOMICIDE	0	MDMA	METHAMPHETAMINE, DIAZEPAU
2002	33	M	31	Cleaner	Armadale	DRUG	0	MDMA	AMPHETAMINE, MOCCLOBEMIDE, DIAZEPAM
2003	34	M	17	Cleaner	Bayswater	MVA PASSENGER	0	MDMA	NONE
2003	35	M	30	IT Worker	Collingwood	DRUG & HEART DISEASE	0.05	MDMA	METHAMPHETAMINE
2003	36	M	20	Meat Packer	Gisborne	MVA DRIVER	0.16	MDMA	NONE
2003	37	M	23	Security Officer	Thomastown	MVA DRIVER	0	MDMA, MDEA	NONE

MVA = Motor Vehicle Accident, MDT = mixed drug toxicity, MDMA = Ecstasy, MDEA = methylenedioxyethylamphetamine, BAC = blood alcohol concentration (g%), CO = carbon monoxide

Source: Victorian Institute of Forensic Medicine, 5 January 2004

Appendix 13: Toxicological Effects of Amphetamines and Other Illicit Drugs

Table B: Toxicological effects of illicit drugs

Illicit Drug	Toxicity
Amphetamine	Vasoconstriction resulting in coronary spasm, MI, cardiomyopathy, cardiomegaly, pulmonary oedema, hypotension or hypertension, tachycardia or bradycardia, tachyarrhythmia, metabolic acidosis, seizure, intracranial haemorrhage (ICH), ischaemic stroke, rhabdomyolysis (v. high doses), hallucination, confusion, suicidal ideations.
Ecstasy and PMA	Marked hyperthermia, DIC, acute renal failure, rhabdomyolysis, arrhythmia, seizures, ICH, MI.
Gamma-Hydroxbutyric acid (GHB)	See Table D

Table C: Potential drug interactions with amphetamine

Drug	Interaction
Alcohol	Complex. Bioavailability of alcohol *slightly* increases. Amphetamine can potentially 'reverse' some of the 'euphoric' effects of alcohol.
Monoamine oxidase inhibitors (MAOI), including selegiline and Hypericum perforatum (St Johns Wort)	Accumulation of large amounts of noradrenaline in the brain and blood vessels. Amphetamines (and related compounds) release accumulated noradrenaline → massive over stimulation and hypertensive crisis. Clinical effects include neck stiffness, flushing, sweating, nausea, vomiting, increased muscle tone, intracranial bleed, arrhythmia, and cardiac arrest.
Tricyclic antidepressant (TCA)	Increase effects of amphetamine especially TCA with more serotonergic effects (e.g., clomipramine)
Chlorpromazine	Amphetamines may inhibit antipsychotic effect of chlorpromazine. Chlorpromazine may inhibit *anorectic* effect of amphetamines*
Selective Serotonin Reuptake Inhibitors (SSRIs), especially fluoxetine and paroxetine	Enhanced effects of amphetamine (↑ levels of amphetamine) ↓ metabolism of amphetamine by hepatic CYP2D6 isoenzyme. Potential serotonin syndrome.
Lithium	↓ effects of amphetamine in presence of lithium.
Dextromethorphan and L-tryptophan	Serotonergic. Possible serotonin syndrome

*Chlorpromazine can be useful in amphetamine overdose management.

Table D: Toxicology of GHB

Organ system	Toxicity
Central Nervous System (CNS)	Anaesthetic induction: Random clonic movements of face and extremities. Aggressive behaviour, combativeness Seizure-like activity (no epileptiform EEG changes) Seizures in overdose Mild toxicity: nystagmus, ataxia, sedation Severe toxicity: coma, respiratory depression, apnoea.
Cardiovascular	Bradycardia Arrhythmia (direct effect on K+ ion balance). This can occur in the presence of normal serum potassium.
Other	Reduced tissue oxygenation demands and protects cells during hypoxic and shock states Inflammatory mediator: reduced ulcer formation by indomethacin and stress Improves visual acuity in glaucoma Hypothermia (~35°C) Respiratory depression, mild respiratory acidosis.

Source of Tables B, C, D: Adapted from Kong, Fabian 2000, 'Illicit drugs: Minimising spread of a lethal cocktail', *Australian Pharmacist*, vol.19, no. 7, August, pp.419–421.

Appendix 14: Categories of Names Used to Describe MDMA Pills

PILLS	DESCRIPTIVE	PEOPLE AND ANIMALS	EFFECTS
Bayer	Amber	Dove	Magic white
Blue heart	Big white one	Super dove	Magic cube
Pellet	Blue and white	Adam & Eve	Flatliner
Purple heart	China split	Eve	Head f[**]ker
White caps	China white	Dennis the menace	Little bastard
	Dimples	EVA	Madman
	Globe	Greyhound	Shocker
	Ovals	Malcolm X	SF
	Red and black	Man united	Speed bomb
	Red and yellow	Mickey mouse	Rockets
	Smoothies	Pink panther	Flying saucer
	Squares	Robin	Bermuda triangle
	Tiddleiwink	Saddam Hussein	
		Superman	
		Wee boy	
PLACES	**FOOD AND DRINK FRUIT**	**OTHER**	
M25	Banana split	Bee bops	
New Yorker	Rhubarb and custard	Black jack	
Pink New Yorker	Strawberry	Cartoon	
Californian	Snowball	Clog	
Sunrise	Mini snowball	Diamond	
Amsterdammer	Pink snowball	Double barrel	
Milky Way	Snowman	e130	
	Disco biscuit	EA	
	Brown biscuit	Fantasy	
	White biscuit	Foreign E	
	Grey biscuit	Phase 4	
	Rusk	Pink barrel	
	Disco burger	PT	
	Coke burger	Shamrock	
	Yellow burger	Triple X	
	Love hearts	undergrounds	
	Parma violet		
	B52s		
	Blue lagoon		
	Lemon and lime		
	Maddog		
	Salt and pepper		

Source: Hammersley, Khan & Ditton 2002, *Ecstasy and the Rise of the Chemical Generation,* Routledge, London and New York, p.40.

Appendix 15: *Customs Act 1901* (Cth), Schedule Six

Table E: Schedule Six – List of scheduled and prohibited drugs, trafficable and commercial quantities

Substance quantity	Trafficable quantity (grams)	Commerc (kilograms)
ACETORPHINE	2.000	
ACETYL-ALPHA-METHYLFENTANYL	0.005	0.005
ACETYLCODEINE	2.0	
ACETYLDIHYDROCODEINE	2.0	
ACETYLMETHADOL	2.0	
ALLYLPRODINE	2.0	
ALPHACETYLMETHADOL	10.0	
ALPHAMEPRODINE	0.2	
ALPHAMETHADOL	0.2	
ALPHA-METHYLFENTANYL	0.005	0.005
ALPHA-METHYLTHIOFENTANYL	0.005	0.005
ALPHAPRODINE	25.0	
AMPHECOLORAL	2.0	
3- (2-AMINOPROPYL) INDOLE	2.0	
AMPHETAMINE	2.0	
ANILERIDINE	25.0	
BARBITURATES	50.0	
BENZETHIDINE	10.0	
BENZYLMORPHINE	5.0	
BETACETYLMETHADOL	5.0	
BETA-HYDROXYFENTANYL	0.005	0.005
BETA-HYDROXY-3-METHYLFENTANYL	0.005	0.005
BETAMEPRODINE	5.0	
BETAMETHADOL	5.0	
BETAPRODINE	5.0	
BEZITRAMIDE	5.0	
4-BROMO-2, 5-DIMETHOXYAMPHETAMINE	0.5	
BUFOTENINE	2.0	
CANNABINOIDS	2.0	
CANNABIS	100.0	100.0
CANNABIS RESIN	20.0	50.0
CHLORPHENTERMINE	2.0	
CLONITAZENE	5.0	
COCAINE	2.0	2.0
CODEINE	10.0	
CODEINE-N-OXIDE	10.0	
CODOXIME	10.0	
DESOMORPHINE	2.0	
DIAMPROMIDE	5.0	
DIETHYLPROPION	5.0	
DIETHYLTHIAMBUTENE	5.0	
N, N-DIETHYLTRYPTAMINE	2.0	
DIHYDROCODEINE	10.0	
DIHYDROMORPHINE	10.0	
DIMENOXADOL	10.0	
DIMEPHEPTANOL	10.0	
2, 5-DIMETHOXY-4-METHYLAMPHETAMINE	2.0	

Substance quantity	Trafficable quantity (grams)	Commerc (kilograms)
DIMETHYLTHIAMBUTENE	20.0	
N, N-DIMETHYLTRYPTAMINE	2.0	
DIOXAPHETYL BUTYRATE	2.0	
DIPHENOXYLATE	2.0	
DIPIPANONE	10.0	
ECGONINE	10.0	
ETHYLMETHYLTHIAMBUTENE	10.0	
ETHYLMORPHINE	2.0	
ETONITAZENE	5.0	
ETORPHINE	5.0	
ETOXERIDINE	5.0	
FENTANYL	0.005	
FURETHIDINE	1.0	
HARMALINE	2.0	
HARMINE	2.0	
HEROIN	2.0	1.5
HYDROCODONE	2.0	
HYDROMORPHINOL	2.0	
HYDROMORPHONE	2.0	
HYDROXYAMPHETAMINE	2.0	
HYDROXYPETHIDINE	5.0	
KETOBEMIDONE	2.0	
LEVORPHANOL	1.0	
LYSERGAMIDE	0.1	
LYSERGIC ACID	0.002	0.002
LYSERGIDE	0.002	0.002
MESCALINE	7.5	
METAZOCINE	7.0	
METHADONE	2.0	
METHAQUALONE	50.0	
METHORPHAN	2.0	
METHYLAMPHETAMINE	2.0	
3, 4-METHYLENEDIOXYAMPHETAMINE	0.5	
3, 4-METHYLENEDIOXYMETHAMPHETAMINE	0.50	0.50
METHYLDESORPHINE	2.0	
METHYLDIHYDROMORPHINE	2.0	
3-METHYLFENTANYL	0.005	0.005
METHYLPHENIDATE	2.0	
1-METHYL-4-PHENYL-4-PROPIONOXYPIPERIDINE (MPPP)	2.0	2.0
3-METHYLTHIOFENTANYL	0.005	0.005
METOPON	2.0	
MONOACETYLMORPHINES	2.0	
MORAMIDE	2.0	
MORPHERIDINE	2.0	
MORPHINE	2.0	1.5
MORPHINE-N-OXIDE	2.0	
MYROPHINE	20.0	
NICOCODINE	2.0	
NICODICODINE	2.0	
NICOMORPHINE	2.0	
NORACYMETHADOL	2.0	
NORCODEINE	2.0	
NORLEVORPHANOL	2.0	
NORMETHADONE	5.0	
NORMORPHINE	20.0	
NORPIPANONE	10.0	

Substance	Trafficable quantity (grams)	Commercial quantity (kilograms)
OPIUM	20.0	20.0
OXYCODONE	5.0	
OXYMORPHONE	2.0	
PARA-FLUOROFENTANYL	0.005	0.005
PENTAZOCINE	20.0	
PETHIDINE	10.0	
PHENADOXONE	10.0	
PHENAMPROMIDE	10.0	
PHENAZOCINE	1.0	
PHENDIMETRAZINE	5.0	
PHENMETRAZINE	5.0	
PHENOMORPHAN	5.0	
PHENOPERIDINE	1.0	
1-PHENYLETHYL-4-PHENYL-4-ACETOXYPIPERI-DINE (PEPAP)	2.0	2.0
PHOLCODINE	5.0	
PIMINODINE	10.0	
PIPRADROL	1.0	
PIRITRAMIDE	1.0	
PROHEPTAZINE	1.0	
PROPERIDINE	25.0	
PSILOCIN	0.1	
PSILOCYBIN	0.1	
TETRAHYDROCANNABINOLS	2.0	5.0
THEBACON	2.0	
THEBAINE	2.0	
THIOFENTANYL	0.005	0.005
TRIMEPERIDINE	10.0	

A substance ("drug analogue") which is, in relation to another substance (being a substance specified elsewhere in this Schedule, or a stereoisomer, a structural isomer (with the same constituent groups) or an alkaloid of such a substance):

(a) a stereoisomer; or
(b) a structural isomer having the same constituent groups; or
(c) an alkaloid; or
(d) a structural modification obtained in 1 or more of the following ways:
  (I) by the replacement of up to 2 carbocyclic or heterocyclic ring structures with different carbocyclic or heterocyclic ring structures;
  (ii) by the addition of hydrogen atoms to 1 or more unsaturated bonds;
  (iii) by the addition of 1 or more of the following groups, namely alkoxy, cyclic diether, acyl, acyloxy, mono-amino and dialkylamino groups with up to 6 carbon atoms in any alkyl residue; alkyl, alkenyl and alkynyl groups with up to 6 carbon atoms in the group, where the group is attached to oxygen (for example, an ester or an ether group), nitrogen, sulphur or carbon; and halogen, hydroxy, nitro and amino groups;
  (iv) by the replacement of 1 or more of the groups specified in subparagraph (iii) with another such group or groups;
  (v) by the conversion of a carboxyl or an ester group into an amide group; or
(e) otherwise an homologue, analogue, chemical derivative or substance substantially similar in chemical structure;

however obtained, except where the drug analogue is separately specified in this Schedule.

The minimum trafficable quantity of:

(a) that other substance in relation to which the substance is a drug analogue; or
(b) if there is more than 1 such other substance—that other substance having the least minimum trafficable quantity.

The minimum commercial quantity, if any, of:

(a) that other substance in relation to which the substance is a drug analogue; or
(b) if there is more than 1 such other substance— that other substance having the least minimum commercial quantity.

Appendix 16: Penalties for Drug Offences

Table F: List of penalties for drug offences, based on *Drugs, Poisons and Controlled Substances Act* 1981 (Vic)

Offence		**Penalty Section**		**Fine (penalty units: 1 unit = $100)**
Trafficking				
(1) Commercial Quantity	Indictable or summary	71(1)(a) 71(2)	25	2500
(2) Other quantity	As above	72(1)(b)	15	1000
(3) Supply of drug of dependence to a child	As above	71B	15	1000
(4) Trafficking to a child of a non-commercial quantity of a drug	As above	71(1)(ab)	20	2400
(5) Possession of substance, material, documents or equipment for trafficking in a drug of dependence	As above	71A		10
Cultivation				
(1) Not related to trafficking	As above	72(1)(a)	1	20
(2) Other	As above	72(1)(b)	15	1000
(3) Commercial quantity	As above	72(1(ab)	25	2500
Possession				
(1) Small quantity of cannabis not related to trafficking	As above	73(1)(a)		5
(2) Not related to trafficking	As above	73(1)(b)	1	30
(3) Other	As above	73(1)(c)	5	400
Use				
(1) Cannabis	Summary	75(1)	-	5
(2) Other drug	As above	75(b)	1	30
Conspiracy to:				
(1) Traffic	Indictable or summary	79(1)	As for trafficking	
(2) Cultivate	As above	79(1)	As for cultivation	
(3) Possess	As above	79(1)	As for possession	
(4) Use	Summary			
(5) Introduce drug etc.	As above			
(6) Forge etc.	As above			
(7) False representation	As above			
Introduction of a drug into the body of another	Summary	74	1	30
Forge, alter, or utter prescription	Summary	78	1	20
False representation to obtain drug, injection or prescription	Summary	78	1	20

Note: As with conspiracy, the offences of 'aid' and 'abet' carry the same maximum penalties as the substantive offence. For example, conspiracy to traffick a commercial quantity of heroin has a maximum penalty of 25 years of imprisonment and a fine of up to $250,000.

Source: Smith, G. 2002, 'Drug offences', in *The Law Handbook*, ed. K. Harper, Fitzroy, Victoria, pp.612–613.

Appendix 17: Californian Legislation Pertaining to Child Endangerment

CALIFORNIA JURY INSTRUCTION CODE

The California Jury Instruction Code [CJIC] contains the laws governing the instructions given to jurors in Californian trials. In the context of child endangerment the Code is to be read in conjunction with the California Penal Code, the Health and Safety Code and the Welfare and Institutions Code.

The most relevant sections of the CJIC are as follows:

CALIFORNIA JURY INSTRUCTION CODE

Section 9.37 *Child Abuse/Neglect/ Endangerment - Felony*

Every person who, under circumstances or conditions likely to produce great bodily harm or death, [wilfully inflicts unjustifiable physical pain or mental suffering on a child,] [or] [wilfully causes or, as a result of criminal negligence, permits a child to suffer unjustifiable physical pain or mental suffering,] [or] [has care or custody of a child and

[a] [wilfully causes or, as a result of criminal negligence, permits the child to be injured,] [or]

[b] [wilfully causes or, as a result of criminal negligence, permits the child to be placed in a situation that endangers the child's person or health.]]

is guilty of a violation of Penal Code Section 273a, subdivision (1), a crime.

The word "wilfully," as used in this instruction, means "with knowledge of the consequences" or "purposefully."

In the crime charged in the information, there must exist a union or joint operation of act or conduct and either general criminal intent or criminal negligence.

To establish general criminal intent it is not necessary that there should exist intent to violate the law. A person, who intentionally does that which the law declares to be a crime, is acting with general criminal intent, even though [he] [she] may not know that such act or conduct is unlawful.

Unjustifiable physical pain or mental suffering is the infliction of pain or suffering which is not reasonably necessary or is excessive under the circumstances.

Great bodily harm refers to significant or substantial injury and does not refer to trivial or insignificant injury.

If a child is placed in a situation likely to produce great bodily harm or death, it is not necessary that actual bodily injury occur in order to constitute the offense. However, if great bodily injury does occur, its nature and extent are to be considered in connection with all the evidence in determining whether the circumstances were likely to produce great bodily harm or death.

In order to prove this crime, each of the following elements must be proved:

[1. A person wilfully inflicted unjustifiable physical pain or mental suffering on a child;] [or]

[1. A person wilfully caused or, as a result of criminal negligence, permitted a child to suffer unjustifiable physical pain or mental suffering;] [or]

[1. A person who had care or custody of a child

[a] [wilfully caused or, as a result of criminal negligence, permitted the child to be injured;]

[or]

[b] [wilfully caused or, as a result of criminal negligence, permitted the child to be placed in a situation that endangered the child's person or health;] and

2. The person's conduct occurred under circumstances likely to produce great bodily harm or death.

Section 16.170 – *Child Abuse/Neglect/Endangerment -Misdemeanour*

Every person who:

[Wilfully inflicts unjustifiable physical pain or mental suffering on a child] [or]

[Wilfully causes or, as a result of criminal negligence, permits a child to suffer unjustifiable physical pain or mental suffering] [or]

[Has care or custody of a child and:

[a Wilfully causes or, as a result of criminal negligence, permits the child to be injured] [, or]

[b Wilfully causes or, as a result of criminal negligence, permits the child to be placed in a situation that endangers the child's person or health]]

is guilty of violation section 273a, subdivision (b) of the Penal Code, a misdemeanour.

The word "wilfully," as used in this instruction, means "with knowledge of the consequences" or "purposefully."

In the crime charged, there must exist a union or joint operation of act or conduct and either general criminal intent or criminal negligence.

To establish general criminal intent it is not necessary that there should exist intent to violate the law. When a person intentionally does that which the law declares to be a crime, [he] [she] is acting with general intent, even though [he] [she] may not know that [his] [her] may not know that [his] [her] act or conduct is unlawful.

Unjustifiable physical pain or mental suffering is the infliction or pain or suffering which, under the circumstances, is unreasonable either as to necessity or degree.

In order to prove this crime, each of the following elements must be proved:

[1. A person wilfully inflicted unjustifiable physical pain or mental suffering on a child [or]

[1. A person wilfully caused or as a result of criminal negligence permitted a child to suffer unjustifiable physical pain or mental suffering [or]

[1. A person had care or custody of a child and;

[a Wilfully caused or as a result of criminal negligence permitted the child to be injured

[or]

[b Wilfully caused or as a result of criminal negligence permitted the child to be placed in a situation that endangered the child's person or health]

CALIFORNIA HEALTH AND SAFETY CODE

Section 11379.6 *Manufacture of Controlled Substances – Penalties*

(a) except as otherwise provided by law, every person who manufactures, compounds, converts, produces, derives, processes, or prepares, either directly or indirectly by chemical extraction or independently by means of chemical synthesis, any controlled substance specified shall be punished by imprisonment in the state prison for three, five, or seven years and by a fine not exceeding fifty thousand dollars ($50,000).

(b) Except as otherwise provided by law, every person who offers to perform an act which is punishable under subdivision (a) shall be punished by imprisonment in the state prison for three, four, or five years.

(c) All fines collected pursuant to subdivision (a) shall be transferred to the State Treasury for deposit in the Clandestine Drug Lab Clean-up Account, as established by Section 5 of Chapter 1295 of the Statues of 1987. The transmission to the State Treasury shall be carried out in the same manner as fines collected for the state by the county.

Section 11379. *Additional Sentence When Children Under 16 are Present or Suffer Great Bodily Injury*

11397.7. (a) Except as provided in subdivision (b), any person convicted of a violation of subdivision (a) of Section 11379.6, or of an attempt to violate subdivision (a) of Section 11379.6, as those section[s] relate to methamphetamine or phencyclidine, when the commission or attempted commission of the crime occurs in a structure where any child under 16 years of age is present, shall, in addition and consecutive to the punishment prescribed for the felony of which he or she has been convicted, be punished by an additional term of two years in the state prison.

(b) Any person convicted of a violation of subdivision (a) of Section 11379.6 or of an attempt to violate subdivision (a) of Section 11379.6, as those section[s] relate to methamphetamine or phencyclidine, where the commission of the crime causes any child under 16 years of age to suffer great bodily injury, shall, in addition and consecutive to the punishment prescribed for the felony of which he or she has been convicted, be punished by an additional term of five years in the state prison.

(c) As used in this section, "structure" means any house, apartment building, shop, warehouse, barn, building, vessel, railroad car, cargo container, motor vehicle, housecar, trailer, trailer coach, camper, mine, floating home, or other enclosed structure capable of holding a child and manufacturing equipment.

Source: California Jury Instruction Code, California Health and Safety Code, California Penal Code.

Appendix 18: Pharmacy Board of Victoria Recommendation Regarding the Storage of Large Packs of Pseudoephedrine

Pharmacy Board
of Victoria

Large Packs of Pseudoephedrine to be Stored Out of Sight

The Pharmacy Board strongly recommends to pharmacists that they store large packs of pseudoephedrine, ie. 60's and 90's, out of sight in the dispensary or storeroom and that sale be restricted to cases where the pharmacist is fully satisfied that a genuine therapeutic need exists.

The Board has noted with concern the increasing demand for large packs of pseudoephedrine and the extraction of pseudoephedrine from these packs for the illicit manufacture of methylamphetamine.

Many pharmacists have already removed large packs from display, refused sales of large packs, not stocked large packs and notified police of the details of persons seeking large quantities. The Board commends the professional and responsible actions of these pharmacists.

People seeking large packs and/or large quantities have become more imaginative in the stories they present to pharmacists when attempting to obtain supplies. Recently a man entered a suburban pharmacy with an empty box, went directly to the Sudafed® stock and swept the entire stock from the shelf into the box before running away.

It is expected that demand for pseudoephedrine and aggressive behaviour will increase and therefore the Board believes that it is easier to refuse sales when no stock is evident.

Pseudoephedrine is indicated for the symptomatic relief of self-limiting congestive disorders. Prolonged treatment without appropriate review is not in the public interest and may in fact be harmful.

Neither the Victoria Police Drug Squad nor the Board can see any justification for the continued availability of large pack sizes and for this reason the Board has sought a change in scheduling for pseudoephedrine in packs greater than 30. It is apparent that the majority of large pack sales are for illicit use and therefore the large packs should either be discontinued or restricted to Schedule 4. This would cause little detriment to the public.

The sale of multiple packs of pseudoephedrine, including small packs, may be considered as unprofessional conduct in the same manner as other non-prescription products which are subject to abuse.

Barry L Reed
President

18 August 1999

Appendix 19: Pharmacy Board of Victoria Special Circular Number 44

PHARMACY BOARD OF VICTORIA

SPECIAL CIRCULAR No 44 **DECEMBER 1999**

Message from the President

This year has seen many activities which will have significant outcomes for the profession. The Preliminary Report of the National Competition Policy Review of Pharmacy was released on 23 November 1999 and can be viewed at www.health.gov.au/haf/pharmrev The Final Report is expected later this month and will then be considered by State and Territory Governments. It is expected that the review of the Victorian Pharmacists Act will then resume.

The future of the profession continues to rest largely in the hands of registered pharmacists - the Preliminary Report on page 27, quotes from the Consumer Health Forum submission "*Consumers go to pharmacies because they have no choice. The expert information and advice provided by pharmacists about medicines is what sets them apart from supermarkets, and it is why there are government protections such as pharmacy ownership by pharmacists...Pharmacists need to be able to show that these services are consistently provided through pharmacy to an acceptable standard, which is cost-effective for consumers and for the health system through facilitating the wise use of medicines.*"

Pharmacists who continue to believe that consumers should be supplied with any OTC medication on request, without determining the appropriateness of the medicine for the consumer, and that recipients of prescriptions should only be counselled when they request it, put the rights and privileges currently enjoyed by pharmacists in extreme jeopardy.

The Board congratulates the pharmacy organisations on the development and publication of professional practice standards and your attention is drawn to the foreword of the Board's Guidelines for Good Pharmaceutical Practice 2000. The Board has adopted the "Standards for the Provision of *Pharmacist Only* and *Pharmacy Medicines* in Community Pharmacy" published by the Pharmaceutical Society of Australia into the Guidelines and will monitor pharmacists compliance and where necessary take action in cases of non-compliance.

A Review of Drugs Poisons and Controlled Substances legislation is also being undertaken and the Board has made a joint submission with the Medical Practitioners Board of Victoria and the Dental Board of Victoria. This review will also have a major impact on the future of pharmacy practice particularly in the area of *Pharmacist Only* and *Pharmacy Medicines*.

The Board published the following statement regarding large packs of pseudoephedrine in August and I reproduce the statement here so that all pharmacists will be aware of it:

Large Packs of Pseudoephedrine to be Stored Out of Sight

The Pharmacy Board strongly recommends to pharmacists that they store large packs of pseudoephedrine, ie. 60's and 90's, out of sight in the dispensary or storeroom and that sale be restricted to cases where the pharmacist is fully satisfied that a genuine therapeutic need exists.

The Board has noted with concern the increasing demand for large packs of pseudoephedrine and the extraction of pseudoephedrine from these packs for the illicit manufacture of methylamphetamine.

Many pharmacists have already removed large packs from display, refused sales of large packs, not stocked large packs and notified police of the details of persons seeking large quantities. The Board commends the professional and responsible actions of these pharmacists.

People seeking large packs and/or large quantities have become more imaginative in the stories they present to pharmacists when attempting to obtain supplies. Recently a man entered a suburban pharmacy with an empty box, went directly to the Sudafed® stock and swept the entire stock from the shelf into the box before running away.

It is expected that demand for pseudoephedrine and aggressive behaviour will increase and therefore the Board believes that it is easier to refuse sales when no stock is evident.

Pseudoephedrine is indicated for the symptomatic relief of self-limiting congestive disorders. Prolonged treatment without appropriate review is not in the public interest and may in fact be harmful.

Neither the Victoria Police Drug Squad nor the Board can see any justification for the continued availability of large pack sizes and for this reason the Board has sought a change in scheduling for pseudoephedrine in packs greater than 30. It is apparent that the majority of large pack sales are for illicit use and therefore the large packs should either be discontinued or restricted to Schedule 4. This would cause little detriment to the public.

The sale of multiple packs of pseudoephedrine, including small packs, may be considered as unprofessional conduct in the same manner as other non-prescription products which are subject to abuse.

I congratulate the majority of pharmacists for their support and for exercising the duty of care expected of them in removing stock from sight.

Barry L Reed, President

Appendix 20: Pharmacy Board of Victoria Poster for General Public

Medicines containing pseudoephedrine

Owing to the public health problems caused by the misuse of these products,

This pharmacy reserves the right to refuse or limit the sale of medicines containing pseudoephedrine.

As recommended by

VICTORIA POLICE

Pharmacy Board of Victoria

Victoria Department of Human Services

Pharmaceutical Society of Australia (Victorian Branch) Ltd

We regret any inconvenience this measure may cause.

ISSUED AUGUST 2002

Appendix 21: Pharmacy Board of Victoria Poster for Pharmacists

To prevent the abuse of OTC solid dose pseudoephedrine-containing products:

- Keep your shelf stocks of these products to a minimum and in an area that prevents self-selection
- Store reserve stock securely and out of public view
- Other than to regular customers in exceptional circumstances, restrict sales to ONE packet
- If faced with a suspicious sale, don't put yourself or your team at risk, act discreetly, avoid confrontation and refer the sale to the Pharmacist in Charge
- Report all suspicious sales to the **Major Drug Investigation Division ☎ 9865 2618** - not your local police. If possible, provide them with a description of the suspect and a vehicle registration

Pharmacists should exercise professional judgment in the supply of S2 and S3 products in accordance with the legislation and professional practice standards. You are NOT obliged to supply these products on demand and may only do so if satisfied that the supply is consistent with the safety of the consumer.

Recommended by

VICTORIA POLICE

Pharmacy Board of Victoria

Victoria Department of Human Services

Pharmaceutical Society of Australia (Victorian Branch) Ltd

ISSUED AUGUST 2002

Appendix 22: Training Modules

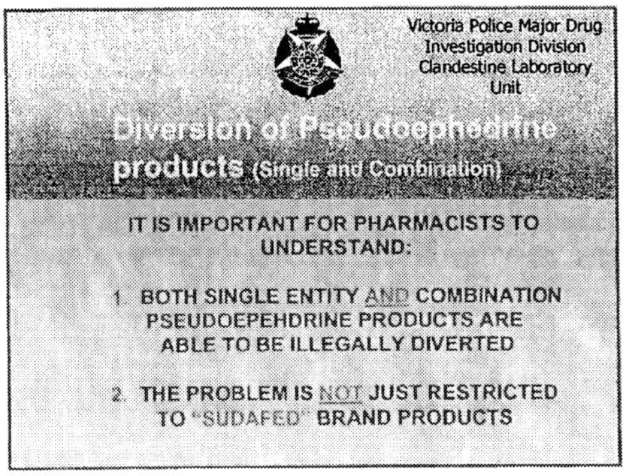
Victoria Police Major Drug
Investigation Division
Clandestine Laboratory
Unit
Diversion of Pseudoephedrine
products (Single and Combination)
IT IS IMPORTANT FOR PHARMACISTS TO UNDERSTAND:
1. BOTH SINGLE ENTITY AND COMBINATION PSEUDOEPEHDRINE PRODUCTS ARE ABLE TO BE ILLEGALLY DIVERTED
2. THE PROBLEM IS NOT JUST RESTRICTED TO "SUDAFED" BRAND PRODUCTS

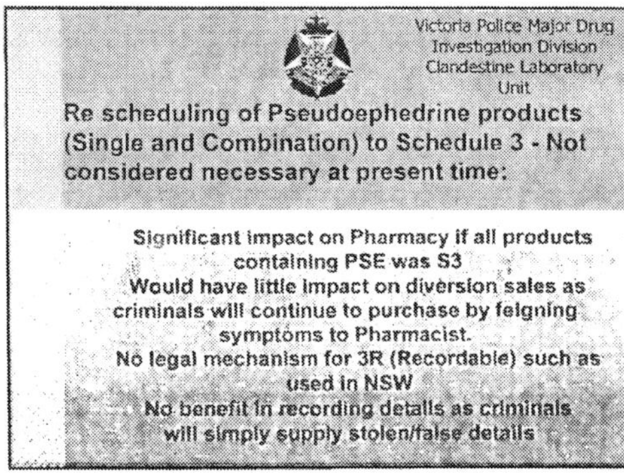

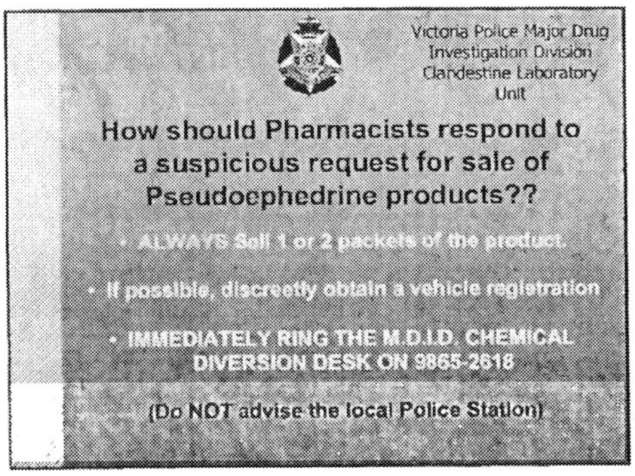

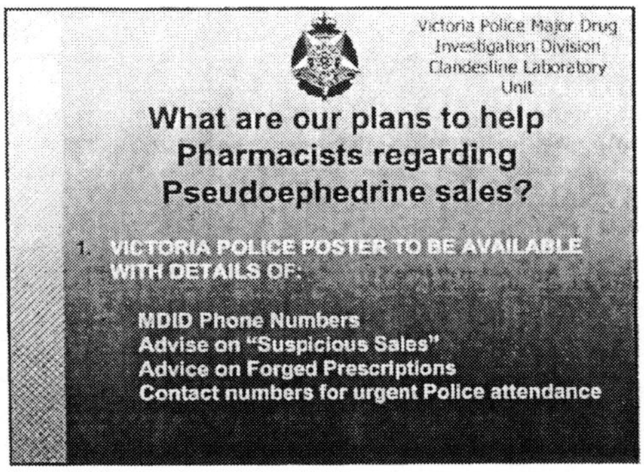
Victoria Police Major Drug
Investigation Division
Clandestine Laboratory
Unit
What are our plans to help Pharmacists regarding Pseudoephedrine sales?
1. VICTORIA POLICE POSTER TO BE AVAILABLE WITH DETAILS OF:
MDID Phone Numbers
Advise on "Suspicious Sales"
Advice on Forged Prescriptions
Contact numbers for urgent Police attendance

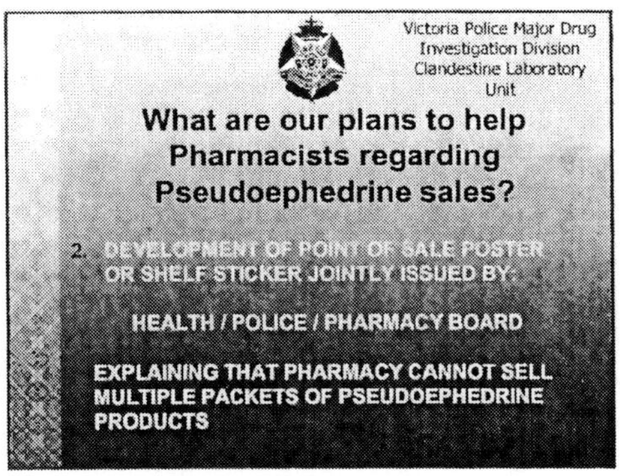

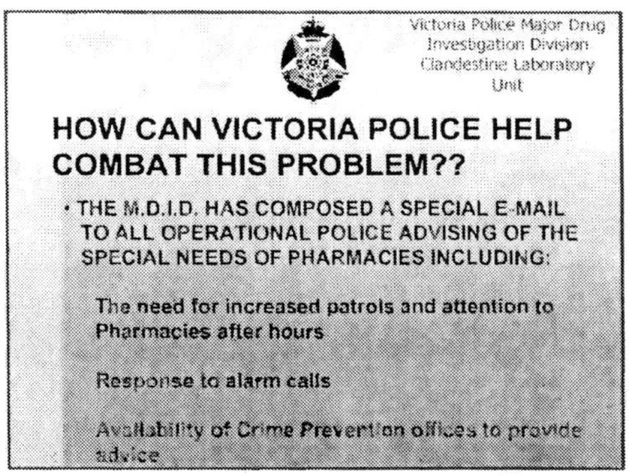

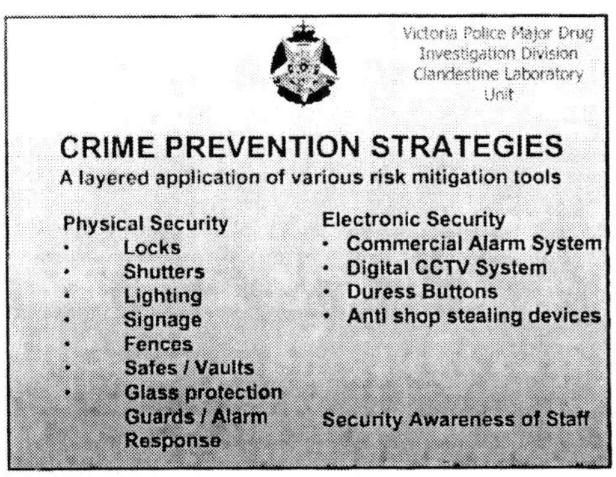
Victoria Police Major Drug
Investigation Division
Clandestine Laboratory
Unit
CRIME PREVENTION STRATEGIES
A layered application of various risk mitigation tools
Physical Security
• Locks
• Shutters
• Lighting
• Signage
• Fences
• Safes / Vaults
• Glass protection
Guards / Alarm Response
Electronic Security
• Commercial Alarm System
• Digital CCTV System
• Duress Buttons
• Anti shop stealing devices
Security Awareness of Staff

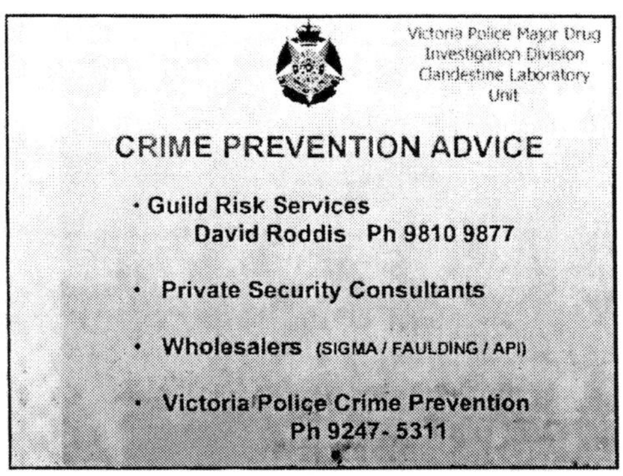
Victoria Police Major Drug
Investigation Division
Clandestine Laboratory
Unit
CRIME PREVENTION ADVICE
• Guild Risk Services
David Roddis Ph 9810 9877
• Private Security Consultants
• Wholesalers (SIGMA / FAULDING / API)
• Victoria Police Crime Prevention
Ph 9247- 5311

Source: Training Modules supplied in the submission of Pharmacy Board of Victoria to the Drugs and Crime Prevention Committee, Inquiry into Amphetamine and 'Party Drug' Use in Victoria, 23 October 2003.

Appendix 23: Suspicious Purchase of Pseudoephedrine Information Report

- Confidential -

Major Drug Investigation Division
Level 12/412 St Kilda Road
Melbourne, Victoria 3004
Tel: 03 9865 2618
Fax: 03 9865 2655

Suspicious Purchase of Pseudoephedrine Information Report

Name of Pharmacy: ____________________

Address: ____________________

Phone Number ____________________

Reporting Person: ____________________

Date of Purchase: ____________________

Time of Day: ____________________

Video Surveillance:? ☐ Is a copy available for Police:? ☐

Description of Person Making Purchase

Sex: ____________________

Ethnic Appearance: ____________________

Height (Approx): ____________________

Weight (Approx): ____________________

Hair Colour: ____________________

Hair Length: ____________________

Complexion: ____________________

Build: ____________________

Speech: ____________________

Clothing Upper Body: ____________________

Clothing Lower Body: ____________________

Distinguishing Features: ____________________

1 of 2

- Confidential -

- Confidential -

Suspicious Purchase of Pseudoephedrine Information Report (cont…)

Name given/Identification Produced? ☐ ______________________

What Type? Details: ______________________

____

____

Has this person ever been into the pharmacy:? ☐ ______________________

When and on how many occasions:?

Description of Vehicle (If Sighted)

Registration Number: ______________________

Make of Vehicle: ______________________

Model (eg. Commodore): ______________________

Type (eg. Sedan): ______________________

Colour: ______________________

Any Distinguishing Marks:

Other

Any other people sighted in car? (If 'Yes' use further information area): ☐ ______________________

Type of tablets asked for:? ______________________

What was sold:? ______________________

How many packets:? ______________________

How paid for (eg:cash/eftpos):

Any further information/comments: ______________________

____

____

____

____

Please e-mail to Natalie Bannan: nat.bannan@police.vic.gov.au
Or fax to 03 9865 2655.

2 of 2

- Confidential -

Source: Submission of Pharmacy Board of Victoria to the Drugs and Crime Prevention Committee Inquiry into Amphetamine and 'Party Drug' Use in Victoria, 23 October 2003.

Appendix 24: South Australian Guidelines for Licensees

Guidelines for Licensees

Guidelines to consider when faced with a situation where a patron has used illicit drugs.

Q. Do I need permission to call an ambulance for someone?

A. If you believe someone is in need of immediate medical assistance call an ambulance. The individual's permission is not required.

Q. What should I do if someone is reluctant, or their friend is reluctant, to receive medical assistance?

A. Remind the person that you have duty of care obligation under common law and as a licensee you are required to provide a safe environment for patrons.

Inform them of the importance of seeking immediate medical assistance for any adverse health effects related to drug use. This reduces the risk of long-term damage to the person's health or a fatal overdose. Police do not attend drug-related medical emergencies unless ambulance officers call for help or a death occurs.

Q. What should I do if someone claims to have had their drink spiked?

A. Believe them, notify management, ensure someone stays with the person, seek medical assistance and encourage the person to notify police of the incident.

Q. What are my responsibilities as a licensee under the law in relation to illicit drugs on licensed premises?

A. The Code of Practice under the *Liquor Licensing Act 1997* requires a licensee to establish and maintain appropriate practices to guard against the licensed premises being used for the purpose of illicit drug dealing. A licensee should cooperate with police in the investigation of illicit drug use.

Q. What key information should I provide to my staff in order to appropriately respond to illicit drug issues?

A. Staff should understand the legal obligations of a licensee or approved responsible person, know how to recognise illicit drugs, be vigilant and report any suspicions about illicit drug dealing in or around licensed premises. Staff should cooperate with police investigating illicit drug issues.

All staff should be aware of the premises' occupational health and safety procedures to ensure an immediate, appropriate and adequate response to any overdose that occurs in or around the licensed premises.

Q. How will authorities view my request if I ask for help to deal with illicit drug use within my premises?

A. By acknowledging the possibility of illicit drug use on or in the vicinity of premises, educating patrons and staff about the harms associated with illicit drug use and reporting illicit drug dealing to police, a licensee will be seen as taking a responsible attitude towards the safety, health and welfare of patrons and staff.

Q. What should I do if I identify someone dealing drugs on the premises?

A. A licensee or approved responsible person may bar a person who commits an offence on or adjacent to licensed premises for up to three months for a first barring. If a person is detected dealing drugs on or adjacent to licensed premises, police should be notified and the person barred.

Q. How should I deal with a patron who is violent or aggressive while under the effect of drugs?

A. To safeguard other patrons, staff and the person who is under the influence of drugs, licensees should request that police escort the person off the premises. It is important that any person suffering adverse effects from drugs is appropriately supervised to ensure they do not put themselves or others at risk of acute injury.

Source: Drug and Alcohol Services Council, South Australia, Adelaide.

Appendix 25: GHB Poster

Call 000 for an ambulance

The majority of fatal overdoses occur because people do not seek **immediate medical assistance.** Police do not attend drug-related medical emergencies unless ambulance officers call for help or a death occurs.

fantasy

GHB

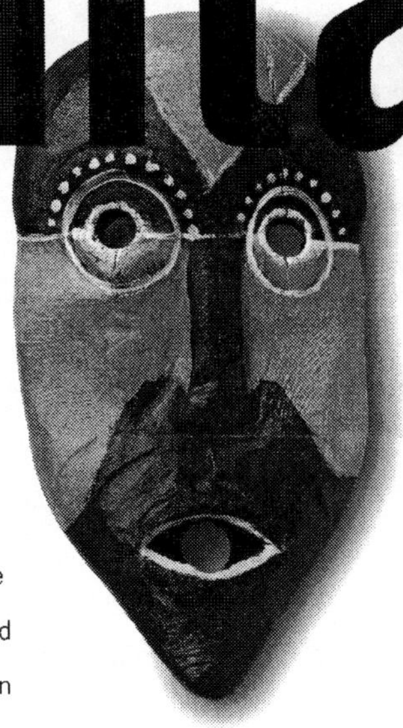

What are the effects?

- relaxation and sense of well-being
- confusion
- drowsiness
- nausea
- convulsions/seizures
- unconsciousness
- respiratory collapse

When mixed with alcohol the depressant effects of both alcohol and GHB are increased which can cause respiratory distress/overdose. These can be fatal.

How to reduce the harms

It is always safer not to use drugs, but if you do:

- Have someone who is not using look out for you.
- Always tell a friend what you are using, just in case medical assistance is required.
- Avoid poly-drug use – don't take more than one drug in a single session.
- Be aware that there is no guarantee of content with illegal drugs. Effects can be unpredictable and dangerous.
- Seek immediate medical assistance if you or a friend experience significant negative health effects.

DRUG & ALCOHOL Services Council

Government of South Australia

FOR INFORMATION ABOUT ALCOHOL AND OTHER DRUGS:
ALCOHOL & DRUG INFORMATION SERVICE
1300 13 1340 (24 HOURS)

Source: Drug and Alcohol Services Council, South Australia, Adelaide.

Appendix 26: Ready Reckoner

Illicit Drugs

IDENTIFYING ILLICIT DRUG USE AND ITS EFFECTS

	Drug Reactions	Indicators of Drug Use in or around premises	Adverse Health Effects
AMPHETAMINES			
speed, goey, whiz, uppers, point, crystal, meth, base, paste, ice	• increased pupil size • increased feelings of alertness, confidence and energy • restlessness • rapid speech • confusion • shakiness • paranoia • hallucinations • jaw clenching and teeth grinding	• a sticky, gluggy, waxy or oily form of damp powder, paste or crystal that has a yellowish or brownish hue • large translucent to white crystals or crystally course powder • injecting equipment	• blurred vision • headaches • tremor • fever • irregular heartbeat • stomach cramps • hallucinations • difficulty sleeping • psychosis • exacerbation of mental illness • injuries (potential for harm due to the drug increasing aggression) • withdrawal symptoms • occasionally collapse & convulsions • possible permanent brain damage • injecting increases the risk of blood borne viruses
BENZODIAZEPINES			
benzos, moggies, downers, sleepers, temmies, temazies, valium, diazepams, serries, pills	• lethargy • euphoria • lack of inhibition • mood swings • dizziness, confusion • slurred speech, stuttering • lack of coordination	• pill & capsules	• blurred vision • loss of short-term memory • injuries (e.g falls) • impaired thinking • stupor • withdrawal symptoms • coma
CANNABIS			
marijuana, grass, pot, ganja, mull, hash, dope, yarndi	• bloodshot eyes • loss of coordination and balance • slower reaction times • confusion, anxiety or even panic attacks • hallucinations • increased appetite • paranoia	• odour of burnt leaves • seeds • cigarette papers • pieces of foil • plastic bags	• respiratory problems • psychosis • changes in heart rate • memory problems • exacerbation of mental illness • reduced fertility • increased risk of low-birth weight babies when used during pregnancy • long term use can increase the risk of getting certain cancers • withdrawal symptoms
ECSTASY			
E, eccies, XTC, pills	• feeling of well-being • increased feelings of confidence • jaw clenching & teeth grinding • vomiting • sweating • paranoia	• tablets & capsules usually white, but many coloured with motif stamped onto one side of tablet	• severe headaches • sleep problems • nausea • dehydration • anxiety & depression • increased body temperature • brain damage
FANTASY/GHB			
grievous bodily harm (GBH), liquid ecstasy, liquid E, GHB	• extreme drowsiness • vomiting • disorientation • impaired movement and speech • shallow breathing	• a colourless, odourless, bitter or salty tasting liquid usually sold in small bottles • powder	• nausea • unconsciousness/abrupt short term coma • withdrawal symptoms
HEROIN			
hammer, H, shit, smack, horse, harry, white, scag, junk, slow, rock	• stupor • drowsiness • shallow breathing • itching • constricted pupils • vomiting	• codeine capsules • white/beige power • injecting equipment • sachets • folds/wraps of paper • spoons	• nausea • constipation • overdose • withdrawal symptoms • stop breathing • injecting increases the risk of blood borne viruses
KETAMINE			
special K, K	• vomiting • twitching • no coordination • hallucinations • heavy sedation or losing consciousness	• liquid form or powder pressed into pills by itself or mixed with other drugs and sold as ecstasy	• nausea • injuries (potential for harm due to the drug's anaesthetic properties) • exacerbation of mental illness • loss of consciousness
LSD			
trips, acid, tabs, dots, wangers	• incoherency • vomiting • seizures • dilated pupils • hallucinations	• small paper squares in various colours & designs	• nausea • 'bad trip' (severe hallucinations) • suicidal tendencies • injuries • seizures • exacerbation of mental illness

Source: Drug and Alcohol Services Council, South Australia, Adelaide.

Appendix 27: General Information Sheet for Licensees

Introduction

It is important to read these instructions before implementing the resource kit.

The purpose of this kit is to provide you, the licensee, with relevant information and realistic strategies that address illicit drug use in and around licensed premises.

Research indicates that almost 18% of the South Australian population has used illicit drugs, including cannabis, in the previous 12 months.*

People use illicit drugs in various settings, with research indicating that specific drugs, such as ecstasy, LSD and cocaine are more likely to be used at parties, restaurants and licensed premises. This is particularly concerning due to the increased health risks associated with using illicit substances with other drugs, including alcohol.

This package is designed to assist you and your patrons in preventing and reducing the harm from illicit drug use. It offers:

- comprehensive information for management and staff in identifying and responding to illicit drug use
- prevention and harm reduction information directed towards your patrons
- first aid responses in the event of an overdose within licensed premises
- responses to frequently asked questions about illicit drug use and your responsibilities as liquor licensees
- information on your responsibilities as a licensee

* Australian Institute of Health and Welfare 2002. 2001 National Drug Strategy Household Survey: State and Territory Supplement. AIHW cat. No. PHE 37. Canberra: AIHW (Drug Statistics Series No. 10).

Benefits to licensees in managing illicit drug issues within licensed premises

Improved staff and patron safety in dealing with illicit drug issues

Developing operating procedures and training staff in these procedures will reduce the risk of staff and patrons experiencing harm as a result of illicit drug use within your premises.

Reduced risk of public liability claims

Through identifying risks and developing strategies to address these risks, licensees will be more able to provide evidence of an environment that addresses their duty of care.

Increased credibility for your premises within the community

By initiating and implementing procedures that address illicit drug use within licensed premises, licensees can be seen to be making a positive contribution to the community.

Better relationships between your organisation and other key groups

Relationships with key community groups, such as the Police, Local Government and the Office of the Liquor and Gambling Commissioner, could be strengthened when your organisation is known to be caring for its patrons and community needs.

What licensees can do

- Develop operating procedures within your premises that address preventive and harm reduction strategies in order to protect the safety and health of your patrons, including guarding against the licensed premises being used for illicit drug dealing.
- Train staff on how to identify and respond to illicit drug use within your premises.
- Call for immediate ambulance assistance if a patron is suffering serious adverse health effects.
- Ensure key staff are trained in an accredited first aid program to assist patrons.
- Employ trained, licensed door and security staff – wearing name tags to be noted down if needed.
- Place the patron information contained within this kit in prominent locations throughout your premises.
- Inform glassies that unattended glasses should be collected to reduce the risk of drink spiking, and **alert patrons to this procedure.**
- Offer free unrestricted access to drinking water.
- Have adequate ventilation – turn up the air conditioner if it's getting too hot.
- Provide a chill out room for people to cool down (preferably supervised).
- Where relevant, discretely provide sharps containers to dispose of injecting equipment. These containers can be used by anyone who needs to safely dispose of injecting equipment, including the increasing number of people suffering diabetes within our community.
- Report drug offences and cooperate with police in the investigation of illicit drug dealing.

Contacts

For additional copies of the posters contained in this kit or further information about alcohol and other drugs:
Alcohol & Drug Information Service
1300 13 1340

For information about licensee responsibilities:
Office of the Liquor & Gambling Commissioner
8226 8410

To provide information about drug dealing or other illegal activity:
SA Police through Crime Stoppers
1800 333 000

Source: Drug and Alcohol Services Council, South Australia, Adelaide.

Appendix 28: Roleplays

Role Play 1

A young woman who is highly distressed approaches you freaking out and tells you that she thinks her friend has had her drink spiked. The friend is obviously intoxicated and is sprawled out on the dance floor and requires assistance.

- Inform the friend that you will call for immediate medical assistance and the police.
- Collect the beverage and put aside for the police to collect.
- Collect all unattended drinks within the premises immediately.
- Alert security of the incident and have staff monitor suspicious behaviour.

Role Play 2

A staff member finds a young man is slumped, semi-conscious in a doorway and other patrons are walking over him. His group of mates are intoxicated and refusing assistance and getting quite aggro. The staff member comes to you for assistance.

- Go with the staff member to address the situation. Inform the group that you have duty of care obligation and are required to seek immediate medical assistance for their friend.
- Check if they are conscious (shake them, call their name) – try to walk them around.
- If no response, check breathing and pulse.
- If not breathing start artificial respiration; if no pulse start CPR.
- If unconscious place in coma position.
- Call an ambulance by dialing 000.
- Stay with them.
- Ask their friends what they have taken so the ambulance officers can be informed and let them know that police do not attend drug-related medical emergencies unless ambulance officers call for help or a death occurs.

Source: Drug and Alcohol Services Council, South Australia, Adelaide.

Appendix 29: RaveSafe Audit

DATE:	EVENT:	STAFF MEMBER:

Party size (estimated numbers) **Overcrowded yes/no**	**Indoor / Outdoor / Combination**
Description of punters (age, etc) **Relaxed dress code yes/no**	**Number of male toilets________** **Number of female toilets________** **Number of disabled toilets________** **Running water in toilets cold/hot/no**
Free water for punters yes / no **if no, water price ________________** **RS strategy________________** **was enough water provided? yes/no**	**Alcohol provided at event? yes/no** **Does sound seem excessively loud? yes/no** **Secure and efficient cloakrooms yes/no** **Provide condoms, either free or vending yes/no**
Passouts for punters yes / no **Adequate ventilation/air conditioning yes/no**	**Needle/syringe facilities provided? yes/no** **RS strategy________________**
Number of exits for punters (indoor parties only)________	**Chillout space available? yes/no** **if yes, describe space________________**
First aid service provided yes/no **if yes, name of company ________________** **courteous security staff yes/no** **at least one first aider for over 500 yes/no** **basic first aid kit yes/no** **private room for treatment yes/no** **Security service provided? yes/no** **if yes, name of company________________**	**Refreshments, food and drinks available for sale? yes/no** **if yes, describe________________**
Any other services provided eg, pt'chang yes/no **if yes, name of companies________________** **clearly displayed policy about searching yes/no**	**Any health promotion, resources, posters at event?** **if yes, describe________________**
Acceptance of RaveSafe by party organisers **Poor fair good excellent** **Allow RaveSafe free access to give advice yes/no**	**Acceptance of RaveSafe by Punters** **Poor fair good excellent**

Other positive or negative harm minimisation issues relating to event/location etc
(adequate lighting outside, close to public transport, parking available, inadequate ventilation, noise etc)

Source: RaveSafe Victoria, April 2003.

Appendix 30: RaveSafe Newsletter

Want to win two tickets to War Of the Worlds 5?

We need your help! RaveSafe is keen to start holding workshops for party drug users in the lead-up to summer that are both relevant and informative. Sooooo, what issues would you like to see addressed in these FREE workshops for ravers/partygoers? If you return this section with your name and contact details, you go into the draw to win two tickets to WOW5 at Altona on 20th September at Altona.

Ps..more prizes will be given away at the workshops

Please have your say by completing this section and emailing it back to RaveSafe. (Highlight the issues you would like covered.)

Proposed workshop issues

Party drugs, their effects	*Name.........................*
Party drug interactions and mixing	*Email.........................*
Safe partying tips	*Phone........................*
The how to of pill-testing	*Preferred days/times to attend workshop.....................*
Party drugs and the law	
Dealing with an overdose	
Other.........................	
....	

WTF is GHB?

GHB (gamma hydroxybutyrate) is a naturally occurring component of human cells. It has been used as a general anaesthetic, and a treatment for insomnia and narcolepsy. It is a depressant with effects quite similar to those of alcohol, and it usually comes as an odourless liquid, slightly salty to the taste in a vial or small bottle. A similar drug 1, 4B is often sold as GHB or in place of it, and is converted to GHB in the body.

One of the major concerns with GHB is that the recreational dosage range is narrow and even small overdoses can cause temporary unrousable unconsciousness (a type of coma) and large overdoses (poisonings) can be life-threatening. The only way to know the concentration of liquid GHB is to know and trust information provided by the source. Users should be extremely careful about GHB dosages as even small overdoses can result in temporarily unrousable sleep. Effects may not peak for up to two hours, and many overdoses have occurred from people not waiting long enough before taking more.

The effects of GHB at recreational doses are physically quite similar to those of alcohol. At higher recreational doses effects can include dizziness, difficulty focusing the eyes, positive mood changes, increased appreciation of music; dancing; and talking, slurring of speech, nausea, and grogginess. At the overdose level, individuals may experience extreme grogginess (nodding in and out of consciousness) or unconsciousness, extreme dizziness and disorientation, and vomiting. During higher overdoses (poisonings), users may experience unconsciousness, convulsions, vomiting, and potentially depressed breathing. Learn more about GHB at www.erowid.org/chemicals/ghb/ghb.shtml

Safety issues

- ☺ Do not mix GHB or 1,4B with alcohol or other depressants!
- ☺ Avoid mixing GHB with other depressants such as sleep aids and opiates.
- ☺ Measure carefully!! The difference between fun and fuck-up can be less than a teaspoon's worth.
- ☺ Don't buy off random dudes in clubs.
- ☺ Always ask your source and always take less!
- ☺ Write G on your hand, in case
- ☺ Dye your GHB or 1,4B another colour to distinguish it from water
- ☺ Keep an eye on your drink at all times, as GHB may be used for drink-spiking.

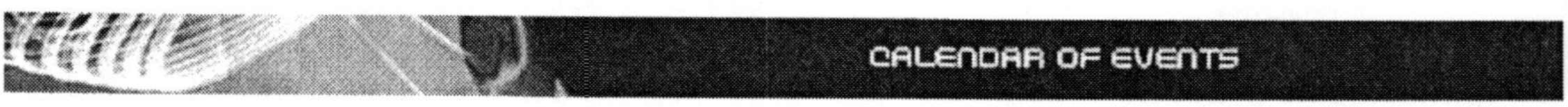

Come and see the RaveSafe crew at:

Hard Kandy – 29th August @ Dex
War Of the Worlds 5 – 20th September @ Altona
Godskitchen – 4th October @ Melbourne Park
Shrooms - 25th October - near Bendigo @ Maryborough
Earthcore – 28th November – 30th November @ Goulburn River.

At each party RaveSafe have:
Drug info and advice
Earplugs
Condoms, lube, safe sex info
Fruit
A chillout space to sit and chat if you're feeling unwell or need a break.

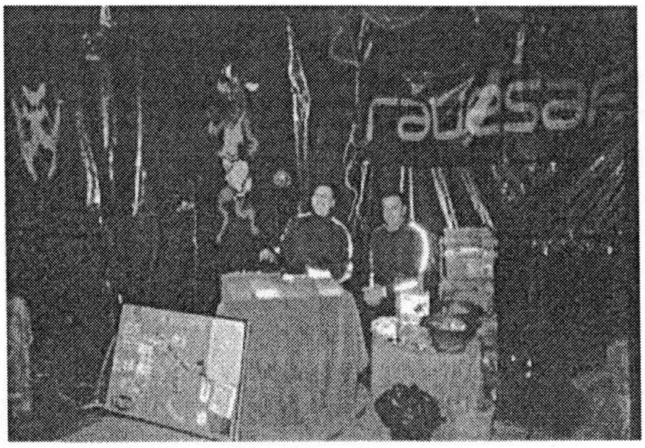

RaveSafe crew at Sonic Boom @ Lonely Planet Footscray

WARNING! WARNING!

If you are using a cough syrup called 'Robitussen" and you take MDMA the results could be fatal due to the Dextromethorrphran (DXM) in the cough syrup. A combination of these two drugs inhibits the ability of the liver to break down the MDMA and can cause heatstroke.

Each month we will keep you up-to-date with the latest possibly dodgy eccies or K-pills being sold as E's around Melbourne thanks to our friends at pillreports.com.

- Blue Safe Sex – Ketamine
- Pink Kangaroo – possibly dangerous

Learn more at:
http://www.pillreports.com/

QUESTION CORNER

Is it safe to take ecstasy 2 or more days in a row?
Taking pills three days in a row can really be just a waste of money and not good for your brain (possibly). As you need serotonin in your brain for pills to work (which takes approx 2-3 weeks to properly stock up again after dropping a pill) you may not get the ecstasy high as much on the second day you drop again. You will possibly only really get the speedy effects of the pill. There is some concern that taking pills two days in a row or more may cause some neurotoxicity in the brain.

What drugs should I avoid mixing?
GHB + Alcohol = ☠
Alcohol + K *(especially large doses)*= ☠
Benzos + alcohol or GHB or K = ☠
Speed+ Coke = blood pressure, heart strain
Alcohol + E = dehydration, kidney strain
Speed + E = heart strain, blood pressure
Antidepressants + E = can adversley interact. Take extreme caution.
Avoid *mixing GHB with anything else*
Avoid *mixing anything with high doses K*

How long do drugs stay in your system?
The following chart (taken from Erowid) gives approximate detection periods for each substance by test type. The ranges depend on amount and frequency of use, metabolic rate, body mass, age, overall health, drug tolerance, and urine pH.

SUBSTANCE	URINE	HAIR	BLOOD
Alcohol	6-24 hrs	n/a	Unknown
Amphetamine	1-4 days	up to 90 days	Unknown
Barbiturates	1-21 days	unknown	Unknown
Benzodiazepines	1-42 days	unknown	Unknown
Cannabis (single use)	48-72 hrs	up to 90 days	2-3 days
Cannabis (habitual use)	up to 12 wks	up to 90 days	2 weeks
Cocaine	4-5 days	up to 90 days	Unknown
Codeine/Morphine	2-4 days	up to 90 days	Unknown
Heroin	8 hrs	up to 90 days	Unknown
Methamphetamine	3-5 days	up to 90 days	1-3 days
PCP	3-7 days	up to 90 days	1-3 days

For more information visit: http://www.alwaystestclean.com/

SPOTLIGHT ON A SUPPORTER

There are some outstanding promoters/event organisers in Melbourne who are embracing harm reduction and supporting the work of RaveSafe. One such supporter is Richie McNeill from Hardware Corporation, who endeavours to have RaveSafe at all Hardware events. When asked why he supports RaveSafe Richie stated **'RAVESAFE is a valuable information tool to help educate and assist us in harm minimisation associated with drug use with young people. And, a lot of that goes on this day and age.'**

Come and support Hardware Corporation in collaboration with the War of the Worlds Consortium, Smile Police, the Fractured posse & Elementz Drum n' Bass arena, present on September 20th 2003, the fifth instalment of the War Of The Worlds (WOTW) at Grand sports and Entertainment complex at Altona. Don't forget that RaveSafe will also be present!

Find out more at: www.waroftheworlds.com.au

HARDWARE

HUNGRY FOR MORE?

RaveSafe is currently developing a party drugs section in the VIVAIDS Magazine 'Whack' which will be available from October/November.

If you would like to receive this magazine which will be published approximately 4 times/year then join up as a VIVAIDS member and we will send you a copy. Membership allows you to stand for the Committee of management and entitles you to voting rights at our annual general meeting, as well as a subscription to 'WHACK' Magazine.

Please forward your details back if you would to become a VIVAIDS member
Name.................................
Address..............................
State................................. postcode....................................
Ph.................................... Fax...
Email.................................

$4- students and unemployed
$15 - income earners
$30 - organisations

Why not participate in some party drug research?

Turning Point Alcohol and Drug Centre in Melbourne are conducting a study to examine trends in ecstasy and other party drug use (eg speed, crystal meth, ketamine, GHB, cocaine, LSD, etc). This study involves an interview that takes about 45-60 minutes to complete. Interviews are strictly confidential and anonymous. Please contact Jenn on (03) 8413 8417, 0413 355 890 or jenr@turningpoint.org.au for further information or to see if you are eligible for the study.

Look after your mates, and help make this e-newsletter reach more and more ravers across Melbourne by sending it on to your friends. Encourage them to send back their email address and postal details, so we can add them to our membership list. natalierussell@vivaids.org.au

Do you have a drug-related question you would like answered? Maybe you'd like some detailed info on drugs and the law, or ketamine? Whatever the problem, drop us an email and we will get onto it for you.... natalierussell@vivaids.org.au

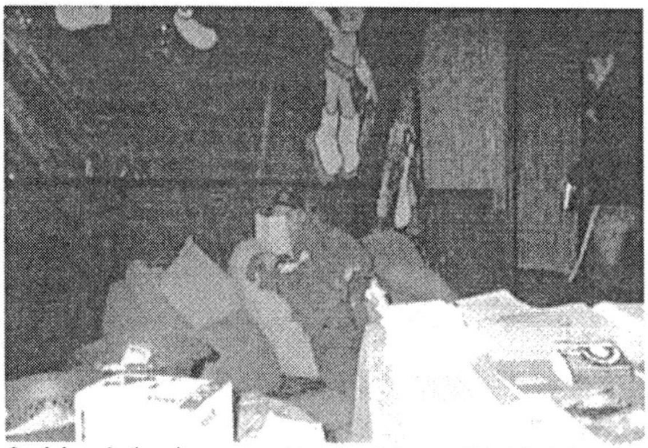

Garth from Smile police engrossed in a RaveSafe pamphlet at Sonic Boom

Outdoor Edition

With summer approaching, many partygoers are getting excited about the warm weather, and the number of outdoor events that are held in the warmer months. Goodbye to freezing our butts off in cold warehouses, and hello to sunny days and warm evenings at outdoor doofs and parties. For some, outdoor events this summer may be the first of many to come, so we thought we would dedicate this edition to safer partying at outdoor events. Bring on summer and bring on the outdoor parties!

Outdoor doofing by Hasty Bear

With spring in the air and a new season of outdoor doofs upon us, that all too familiar sound of 4/4 beats reverberating around the bush is calling you back to nature. So how do you get there? What do you wear? And how could you possibly make an al fresco party into a five star camping extravaganza?

It's all too easy to think of an outdoor doof experience like you're going to just another rave, but think again. For those of you more experienced with outdoor raves, you'll understand what I mean, you need to be a little more prepared........ I mean there is just no way you can get a pass-out and go down to the local 7-eleven and grab more chewy or chuppa-chups...... let alone water! But how big does that survival kit have to be?? That my friend depends on how long you plan to stay, what is on offer at the doof and how comfy you want to be, but for a one night gig a simple kit-out would be...

1. Water (since sometimes the water available for drinking, is... well... not so good for the stomach)
2. If you are planning to take drugs, shop in advance and don't rely on what's at the doof
3. Blankets, even in summer it can get damn cold at night, especially if there are no clouds and if you're prone to cold hands, don't forget gloves and a beanie! You loose 50-75% of your body heat through your head so a hat always comes in handy!
4. Sunglasses..... you never want to miss the morning set!!!
5. Garbage bag to take home all your rubbish (what goes in must come out!)
6. Toilet paper........ you have no idea how many times they run out!
7. Change of clothes/shoes in case you get wet or just want extra layers, and also some sort of wet weather gear
8. Fruit and nibbles for the morning, check the flyer though, they might have food available
9. Many outdoor events can mean quite a distance driving home, so try and get some sleep before you leave.

Whatever your style, make sure you read the flyer or get in touch with the organisers, they're normally pretty keen to help out if you want to know what facilities they will have on offer.

Above all look after the bush, take care of your friends and fellow ravers, and make sure we maintain a strong healthy party community!

CALENDAR OF EVENTS

Come and see the RaveSafe crew at:

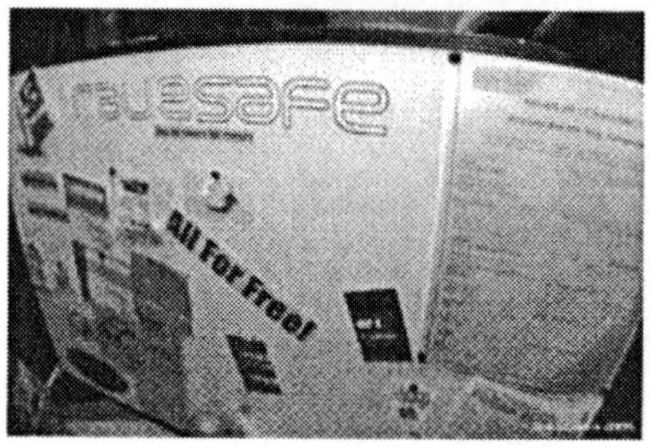

Godskitchen – 4th October @ Melbourne Park
Shrooms - 25th October - near Bendigo @ Maryborough
Earthcore – 28th November – 30th November @ Goulburn River.

At each party RaveSafe have:
Drug info and advice
Earplugs
Condoms, lube, safe sex info
Fruit
A chillout space to sit and chat if you're feeling unwell or need a break.

WARNING! WARNING!

MDMA has a potentially fatal interaction with certain antidepressants, known as MAOI's (Monoamine oxidase inhibitors.) Therefore MDMA is not recommended to anyone taking any MAOI. A Dr or pharmacist can tell you which medications fall into this category.

Each month we will keep you up-to-date with the latest possibly dodgy eccies or K-pills being sold as E's around Melbourne thanks to our friends at pillreports.com.

- Apples red/pink – ketamine
- 50 Cent/white with grey speckles – ketamine

- Blue Safe Sex Light Blue - ketamine
- Playboy white - ketamine

- Pink Kangaroo – possibly dangerous

Learn more at:
http://www.pillreports.com/

QUESTION CORNER

If I am attending events in warmer months during the day, where I will be dancing my arse off, should I drink more water than normal?
RaveSafe recommends that you stick to the guidelines of drinking 500mls water every hour if dancing and 250mls if chilling. Excess consumption of water can lead to an abnormal fluid and electrolyte balance. Sweating during MDMA use and high activity levels cause both electrolytes and water to be lost. Replacing these with water only (in large quantities) can upset the delicate balance, and hyponatremia (water intoxication) can result. One way to prevent both dehydration and hyponatremia is to drink an electrolyte drink such as Powerade, or fruit juice, rather than water. Be sure to sip drinks frequently, rather than gulping large quantities. Supplementing 250-500ml of water/ hour with 1 sports drink every 2-3 hours a good alternative if you're dancing hard. This will replenish your body's electrolytes and prevent hyponatremia (water intoxication). Also remember to take breaks from dancing and allow your body to cool down. Chill out areas are perfect for this.

....

With all the outdoor events coming up like Earthcore and Advent*jah, when a lot of driving is required, what are the laws in regards to police searching your vehicle?
The police can search you and your car at any time if they *reasonably suspect* illegal drugs, weapons or stolen goods.

FOR YOUNG PEOPLE IN TROUBLE WITH THE POLICE
... who live, work or study in ...
Fitzroy - Collingwood - Richmond - North Melbourne - East Melbourne - Brunswick - Carlton
Fitzroy Legal Service Inc. -- **ALPHALINE 9419 7427 - *EMERGENCY 24 HOURS FREE LEGAL ADVICE***
If you would like a free wallet-sized leaflet that details your rights and useful legal phone numbers please email your postal address to natalierussell@viviads.org.au and one can be sent out to you.

....

Everyone talks about pre and postloading what is it?
Preloading and postloading involves consuming certain substances in recommended amounts in order to prepare your body for the effects of MDMA. Pre/postloading is usually done during the 24-72 hour period on each side of the roll; and includes one or more of the following:
5HTP
Magnesium
Vitamin C
Alpha-lipoic Acid
Antacids
Tyrosine and DLPA

If you wish to learn more about **Pre and Postloading,** come to one of RaveSafe's **free** 'safer partying' workshops in October and November. Email natalierussell@vivaids.org.au for more info. Also visit http://www.bluelight.nu/vb/showthread.php?postid=912507#post912518

SPOTLIGHT ON A SUPPORTER

On 25th October RaveSafe will be heading off to their first outdoor event for the new season. 'Shroomz' will be an outdoor party featuring some of Melbourne's finest trance producers and DJs alongside some fantastic local talent including Sugar, Organik Magik, Aaron Smiles and many others. The whole event will be held in the lush surroundings of Victorian bush that will once again, for one weekend, become the home of giant mushrooms, madhatters, UFOs and insectoid-like alien creatures.

RaveSafe asked Warren Jackson the event organiser: **'What are you doing at Shroomz to ensure the party is safe for punters?"**

"To try and make Shroomz safer we encourage drivers to rest before they drive, check list cards are supplied by Rural Ambulance Victoria (RAV) to punters and we have provided the State Emergency Services with information on the event. We will close the site at 8pm on the 27th October 2003 thereby allowing people to rest before returning home.'

If you want to attend a party where the event organisers really care about the safety and well-being of their punters, visit http://www.shroomz.iwarp.com/ for more info. Shroomz will be held near Bendigo / Lockwood just out of kangaroo flat

HUNGRY FOR MORE?

ravesafe

Wednesday 22nd October and 12th November 2003 from 6.00pm - 9.00pm (approx), VIVAIDS, 275b Smith St Collingwood.

is holding 2 FREE Workshops specifically designed for ravers/clubbers/partygoers.

Food and drinks will be provided; all participants will receive a 'safer partying showbag' and the chance to win one of many prizes (CD vouchers, event tickets, clothing vouchers).

At no cost, and with guest speakers from Enlighten, Fitzroy Legal Service and RaveSafe, get together with your peers to discuss:

Party drugs, their effects
Safe partying tips
Party drugs and the law
Dealing with come-downs
Party drug interactions and mixing
The how to of pill-testing and pre and post loading
Dealing with an overdose

Places are very limited, so please RSVP ASAP for one of the workshops by the 10th October to Natalie on 9419 3633, or natalierussell@vivaids.org.au.

More People required to participate in Psychological Study

Project Title: Cognitive Performance and Monitoring in Dance Drug Users.

Monash University are looking for people over 18 years old:

- Who have in the past or currently use ecstasy, OR
- Who have used cannabis and/or other drugs but have not used ecstasy, OR
- Who have never used any illicit drugs
- Who would be interested in participating in a research project.

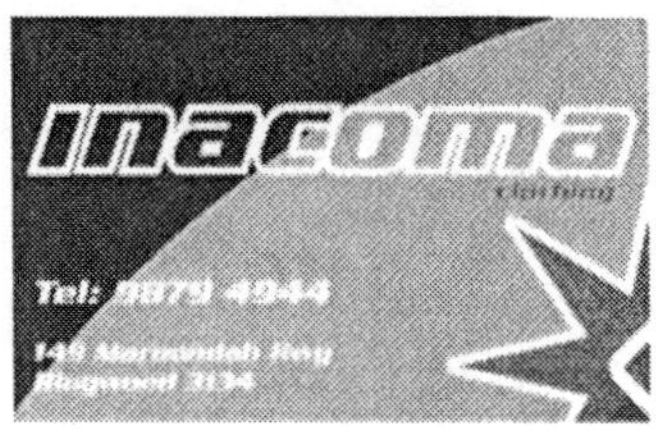

RaveSafe's groovy uniforms made by Inacoma clothing

Participants will be reimbursed for their time.
If you are interested in participating in this research, please email gillinder.bedi@med.monash.edu.au or call 9903 1149.

Don't forget to come and visit the RaveSafe tent in the foyer of the Rod Laver Arena at the Future Entertainment Event **Godskitchen** on 4th October at Melbourne Park.

You can contact RaveSafe on 9419 3633 or 0407 353 437 natalierussell@vivaids.org.au if you have any queries about safer partying or RaveSafe.

If you would like to be taken off this mailing list just send an e-mail to the address above.

Source: RaveSafe Victoria, e-news (RaveSafe email newsletter). See also www.ravesafe.com

Appendix 31: Stonnington Safe Venues Liquor Accord

Illicit Substances

Illicit Substances

Drug issues within the premises are based on a harm minimisation approach:

- **Drug dealing is not tolerated.**
- **Drug usage is not tolerated.**

	Yes	Action required
Venue has policy and procedures deterring drug dealing and drug usage.	○	______
This policy is communicated to staff and prominently displayed to customers (signage to be developed).	○	______
Any drug dealing that is detected is recorded in the incident register and full co-operation given to the Police.	○	______
Cold water is readily available.	○	______
It is preferred that a minimum of one employee, present during peak operating times holds a current accredited First-Aid Certificate.	○	______
A maintained First-Aid kit is accessible for use during trading hours.	○	______
A policy is in place to deter drink spiking and assist possible victims.	○	______

Source: Stonnington Safe Venues Liquor Accord, City of Stonnington, 2003

Appendix 32: Pill Testing Forum

myBL FORUMS SEARCH LINKS JOURNAL GALLERY CHAT PILLREPORTS ARC

www.bluelight.nu the new bluelight

You are not logged in.
To post, **register** or login:

OK

The New Bluelight > Drug Discussion > Pill Testing

(Moderated by: **Soma**)
(Users Browsing this Forum: mnrollergirl)

NEW THREAD
Subscribe to this Forum
Mark this Forum Read
Mark ALL Forums Read

Thread	Started by	Views	Replies	Last Post
Announcement: Bluelight discount for EZ-Testers + free world wide shipping	**Soma**	39	0	07-03-2004 10:46 by **Soma**
Announcement: Yet Another Research Survey (YARS) Earn $80 to $120 cash (Sydney Only)	**Johnboy**	62	0	19-02-2004 04:18 by **Johnboy**
Announcement: New Online Survey (Residents of Melbourne Australia Only)	**Johnboy**	36	0	03-02-2004 03:05 by **Johnboy**
Announcement: Do you use ice, meth, speed or base? (Sydney Australia Only)	**Johnboy**	223	0	18-12-2003 07:17 by **Johnboy**
Announcement: Attention All Media (especially the Australian media)	**Jase**	324	0	14-08-2003 11:36 by **Jase**
Instructions destroyed	**switchy85**	1	0	11-03-2004 00:32 by **switchy85**
Bank Card WTF?!	**SYSDOWN**	54	4	10-03-2004 21:55 by **Soma**
Moved: Curiois abput oxycodon	**Minx69**	-	-	07-03-2004 06:07 by **FLaGaSS**
I Just purchased my first ez test	**drgreenthumb00**	463	15	06-03-2004 11:09 by **easy e**
Ez Testers Delivered To Sydney	**Dragonsush**	35	2	03-03-2004 09:47 by **Dragonsush**
Marquis (EZ-Test) Legality in Asia	**LithiuMind**	17	1	02-03-2004 15:26 by **easy e**
Mecke and Marquis test on Speed? pills	**sasau**	50	3	29-02-2004 09:39 by **easy e**
Need Help assembling tester	**UnFuZed**	39	3	29-02-2004 04:14 by **UnFuZed**
EZ Test Affliate Program!	**easy e**	80	5	26-02-2004 14:59 by **easy e**
Mecke reagent	**robertinc**	32	2	26-02-2004 03:08 by **Soma**
Buying an Ecstacy testing kit	**EMP**	142	5	26-02-2004 02:31 by **Sleaze**
Moved: Curiois abput oxycodon	**Minx69**	-	-	07-03-2004 06:07 by **FLaGaSS**
I Just purchased my first ez test	**drgreenthumb00**	463	15	06-03-2004 11:09 by **easy e**
Ez Testers Delivered To Sydney	**Dragonsush**	35	2	03-03-2004 09:47 by **Dragonsush**
Marquis (EZ-Test) Legality in Asia	**LithiuMind**	17	1	02-03-2004 15:26 by **easy e**
Mecke and Marquis test on Speed? pills	**sasau**	50	3	29-02-2004 09:39 by **easy e**
Need Help assembling tester	**UnFuZed**	39	3	29-02-2004 04:14 by **UnFuZed**
EZ Test Affliate Program!	**easy e**	80	5	26-02-2004 14:59 by **easy e**
Mecke reagent	**robertinc**	32	2	26-02-2004 03:08 by **Soma**
Buying an Ecstacy testing kit	**EMP**	142	5	26-02-2004 02:31 by **Sleaze**
Looking to buy 1st testing kit	**JBizzle**	155	7	24-02-2004 18:00 by **Sleaze**
how to prolong life of ezy tester??	**Dragonsush**	46	1	23-02-2004 15:13 by **infinity**
Ecstasydata	**noiatrip**	135	1	23-02-2004 02:26 by **TrippieJ**
Strychnine + XTC !!??	**JohnSmith**	361	8	14-02-2004 12:46 by **Soma**
Moved: ...:-/ Help please.	**Merlyn**	-	-	12-02-2004 22:43 by **easy e**
Do these EZ test kits detect PCP?	**robertinc**	138	6	12-02-2004 18:57 by **easy e**
cocaine testing	**stz**	189	3	10-02-2004 21:47 by **easy e**
procedure in testing	**Mikkyme**	73	3	10-02-2004 08:56 by **easy e**

Showing threads 1 to 19 of 19, sorted by last post time in descending order, from last 30 days GO

Source: Pill Testing Forum www.bluelight.nu

Appendix 33: Briefing Paper by Victoria Police – Drug Testing Kits

INQUIRY INTO THE USE OF AMPHETAMINES AND 'PARTY DRUGS' IN VICTORIA
VICTORIA POLICE RESPONSE- VICTORIA POLICE RESPONSE TO DISCUSSION PAPER

VICTORIA POLICE

ATTACHMENT A

VICTORIA
FORENSIC SERVICES
CENTRE

Forensic Drive
Macleod 3085
Victoria Australia
Telephone: (61 3) 9450 3444
Facsimile: (61 3) 9459 0477

BRIEFING PAPER - DRUG TESTING KITS

Testing kits are based on colour reaction tests. Many compounds, including drugs produce a distinctive colour when reacted with various chemical reagents. The colour produced by this reaction maybe specific for the compound. However, more commonly the colour produced is not confined to a single compound, but could be produced by a number of compounds from a given class (or family) of compounds or from non-related compounds. *(In simple English the specificity of colour reactions is extremely poor and can not be relied upon for accurate identification of a particular compound).*

How do these colour tests work? In a number of cases the reaction can be correlated to particular aspects of the compounds chemical structure. However, this can not fully explain the phenomena of colour reaction, as many anomalous responses have been documented over the years.

The interpretation of these tests is also surrounded with difficulties. The most obvious being the subjectivity associated with describing the resultant colour with any true degree of accuracy – how blue is blue?? Also the consistency of reaction from one test to the next is dependent upon the many aspects present during the test (ie: the test conditions). The variation of colour seen in reference colour charts produced by the manufacturer's to explain the observed result must also be considered.

The nature of the drug presented for testing is also of significant relevance. Reference colours are usually obtained from the reaction of a drug in a particular form. This form maybe free base, acid or salt. In the case of a salt, drug compounds could exist, particularly in the illicit market place in a variety of salt forms. Since colour tests produce a reaction that has some correlation to its chemical structure it is not unexpected to see variation in results due to the differences in the drug's form.

Another aspect to consider is that these colour tests were designed to work on approximately 1mg of compound (ie: 1mg of the actual drug you wish to test). Obviously this clearly does not occur in the case of illicit testing, as only a scraping probably 1-2 mg is taken and it is unlikely if not impossible for this to contain 1mg only of the drug(s) in question.

In addition these colour tests were designed for use on single compounds. The test provides no means of separating compounds within a sample. This is of significant importance since the result is dependent on a chemical reaction between the reagent and the compound. When the reagent is presented with several compounds with which it may react and produce a colour(s) the end result colour can become unclear and misleading. Consideration must also be given when the sample is coloured (ie: green tablet) as the colour present in the sample is likely to effect the end result colour.

As you can see the process of colour testing is filled with variation and subjectivity. As a forensic tool or a field investigator tool it has value only as a simple indication test, the initial point in the process of determining the possible presence/absence of a class of drug (ie: opiates class as apposed to the compound heroin). Colour test results are never utilised to identify a drug type or provide any determination of the purity of the drug within the sample.

Information provided on the commercially available test kits indicate that they simply contain the chemical reagents which have been described for many years in scientific literature as "colour tests" (ie: Marquis (E1) and Mandelins (E2) reagent). In other words there appears to be no new chemical reagent developed by these companies. The information provided within the commercial kits, concerning the resultant colours is consistent with the available literature, which describes Marquis and Mandelins reagent. Therefore, all the above information describing the limitations of colour test (ie Marquis and Mandelins colour test) directly applies to these testing kits.

Laboratory tests have been carried out using the E1 and E2 kits. When pure standards were tested the kits responded in the manner expected, within the limitations mentioned above. When illicit street samples, containing mixtures of compounds including various drugs, were tested interpretation of the result became more complicated. As described above the test is not capable of separating the compounds.

As expected the test kits were not able to differentiate between "high" and "low" levels of drugs, between tablets containing only one drug type and tablets containing numerous drugs. No information regarding the non-drug content of the tablet could be provided by these kits.

In summary the examination of these kits demonstrates that: The kits are not able to provide clear identification of a particular drug. At best and when used under optimum conditions they provide an indication of a compound/drug class, which may be present.

- no information is provided on the non drug components which may be present in a sample
- where drug mixtures are concerned (a common occurrence in street drugs) the results become misleading
- drug levels and toxicity are not addressed at all by this testing method – *drug level (purity)and toxicity are critical issues in drug use and harm minimisation*
- interpretation of the results is extremely subjective, and the variation inherent in this testing regime is a significant limitation
- a false sense of security is bestowed upon the user which may in fact increase the risk of drug taking
- the kits themselves contain hazardous chemicals (concentrated acids) that would cause irritation, injury and damage upon contact with person (skin) or other surfaces.

Cate Quinn
Manager
Chemistry Branch

Appendix 34: Positive Benefits of Amphetamine Substitution Programmes

Table G: Positive benefits of amphetamine substitution programmes – From a review of the studies by Shearer et al. for the National Drug and Alcohol Research Centre 1999

Benefit	Author, Year
Reduced injecting behaviour	Fleming & Roberts, 1994; McBride et al., 1997; White, 1996; Pates et al., 1996; Charnaud & Griffiths, 1998
Reduced sharing of injecting equipment	McBride et al., 1997
Improved retention in treatment	McBride et al., 1997
Reduced use of illicit amphetamine	McBride et al., 1997; White, 1996; Sherman, 1990; Pates et al., 1996; Charnaud & Griffiths, 1998
Improved social functioning (reduced crime, stable housing employment)	Fleming & Roberts, 1994; Pates et al., 1996; McBride et al., 1997
Reduced cravings	Sherman, 1990

Source: National Drug and Alcohol Research Centre (NDARC) 1999, *A randomised controlled trial of the feasibility of monitoring controlled prescribing of dexamphetamine*, by J. Shearer, A. Wodak, R.P. Mattick, I van Beek, J. Lewis, W. Hall, & K. Dolan, (NDARC Technical Report No. 75), NDARC, University of New South Wales, Sydney, p.5.

Appendix 35: Factors that Facilitate and Factors that Impede the Use of Amphetamines

FACTORS THAT FACILITATE THE USE OF THE AMPHETAMINES

FACILITATING SUPPLY	FACILITATING DEMAND
Over Prescribing	Accessibility
Established dealer networks	Role models and reference groups
Poor crime control	Socially acceptable
Disparate national control policies	Reputation as controllable/harmless
Poor training of police, customs and excise	Media references to positive models
Political instability	Media coverage of positive lifestyle
Local laboratories	Low price
Ease of manufacture	Low morale, high stress
Access to precursors	Unemployment
Low price of precursors	Functional
Technical/chemical inventiveness	Need for achievement
Technical expertise	Poor understanding of effects
Poor international co-operation	Alienation of sub-cultures
Incentives for traffickers:	
Fixed costs high volume	
easy transit high profits	Few other drugs
Government preoccupation with other drugs	Other drugs dangerous/inaccessible
Poor official information base	No government strategy for prevention/education

FACTORS THAT IMPEDE THE USE OF THE AMPHETAMINES

IMPEDING SUPPLY	IMPEDING DEMAND
Risk of detection	Low accessibility
Unreliable distribution	Negative image – people, events, crime
Limited distribution networks	High price
Expert vigilant surveillance	Low purity
Punitive sanctions	Fear of additives
Community involvement	Reputation as harmful
Poor access to precursors	Dysfunctional _ mental and social
High cost of precursors	Sub-cultural preference for alternative
High production costs	Strong religious beliefs or cultural norms
High transportation costs	Highly negative media coverage
International cooperation	Community involvement
	Credible educational campaigns
	Risk of detection

Source: Klee, H. 1997c, 'Patterns of amphetamine use in seven nations: Factors affecting growth and decline', in *Amphetamine Misuse: International Perspectives on Current Trends*, ed. H. Klee, Harwood Academic Publishers, The Netherlands.

Bibliography

Ainsworth, C. 2002, 'The wrong stuff', *New Scientist*, 20 April, p.32.

Aitken, C., Kerger, M., & Crofts, N. 2000, 'Drivers who use illicit drugs: behaviour and perceived risks', *Drugs: education, prevention and policy*, vol. 7, pp.39–50.

Akram, G. & Forsyth, A.J.M. 2000, 'Speed freaks? A literature review detailing the nature and prevalence of dance drugs and driving', *International Journal of Drug Policy*, vol. 11, pp.265–277.

Albertson, T.E., Derlet, R.W. & Van Hoozen, B.E. 1999, 'Methamphetamine and the expanding complications of amphetamines', *The Western Journal of Medicine*, vol. 170, April, pp.214–218.

Alexander, B. & Tsou, J. 2001, 'Prospects for stimulant maintenance in Vancouver, Canada', *Addiction Research and Theory*, vol. 9, no. 2, pp.97–132.

Alldridge, P. 2000, *Relocating Criminal Law*, Ashgate Press, Aldershot.

Allen, B. & Tressider, J. 2003, *Of Substance*, vol. 1, no. 1, Australian National Council on Drugs, Canberra.

Allsop, S., Phillips, M. & Calogero, C. (eds) 2001, *Drugs and Work. Responding to Alcohol and Other Drug Problems in Australian Workplaces*, IP Communications Pty Ltd, East Hawthorn.

Anderson, R. & Flynn, N. 1997, 'The methamphetamine-HIV connection in Northern California', in *Amphetamine Misuse: International Perspectives on Current Trends*, ed. H. Klee, Harwood Academic Publishers, The Netherlands, pp.181–196.

Anex Bulletin, Edition 2, April 2003.

Anglin, M.D., Burke, C., Perrochet, B., Stamper, E. & Dawad-Noursi, S. 2000, 'History of the methamphetamine problem', *Journal of Psychoactive Drugs*, vol. 32, no. 2, April–June, pp.137–141.

Arnold, J. 2002, 'Drugs in clubs', *Drugs in Society*, December, pp.2–3.

Asante, J.S. 1999, 'GHB: grievous bodily harm (gamma-hydroxybutyrate)', *FBI Law Enforcement Bulletin*, vol. 68, April, pp.21–26.

Astorga, L. 2001, 'The limits of anti-drug policy in Mexico', *International Social Science Journal*, vol. 53, pp.427–434.

Australian Bureau of Criminal Intelligence (ABCI) 2002, *The Australian Illicit Drug Report 2000–2001*, Government of Australia, Canberra.

Australian Crime Commission (ACC) 2003, *Australian Illicit Drug Report 2001–2002*, Commonwealth of Australia, Canberra.

Australian Drug Foundation (ADF) 2002, 'Fact Sheet on Amphetamines', www.adf.org.au/drughit/facts/amphetamines.html

Australian Federal Police 1991, *Illicit Drugs in Australia, Situation Report 1991*, Australian Federal Police, Canberra.

Australian Institute of Health and Welfare (AIHW) 1999, *1998 National Drug Strategy Household Survey*, AIHW, Canberra.

Australian Institute of Health and Welfare (AIHW) 2001, *Statistics on Drug Use in Australia 2000*, Drug Statistics Series No. 8, (Megge Miller & Glenn Draper), AIHW Catalogue no. PHE 30, AIHW, Canberra.

Australian Institute of Health and Welfare (AIHW) 2002a, *2001 National Drug Strategy Household Survey: First Results* (Drug Statistics Series No. 9), AIHW, Canberra.

Australian Institute of Health and Welfare (AIHW) 2002b, *2001 National Drug Strategy Household Survey: State and Territory Supplement* (Drug Statistics Series No. 10), AIHW, Canberra.

Australian Institute of Health and Welfare (AIHW) 2002c, *2001 National Drug Strategy Household Survey: Detailed Findings* (Drug Statistics Series No. 11), AIHW, Canberra.

Australian Institute of Health and Welfare (AIHW) 2003, *Statistics on Drug Use in Australia 2002* (Drug Statistics Series No. 12), AIHW, Canberra.

Australian National Council on Drugs (ANCD) 2001, *National Report: Rural and Regional Alcohol and Other Drugs Consultation Forums*, Australian National Council on Drugs, September, p.5.

Backett, K. & Davidson, C. 1992, 'Rational or reasonable? Perceptions of health at stages of the lifecourse', *Health Education Journal*, vol. 51, pp.55–59.

Bagnall, D. 1997, 'Agony and ecstasy', *The Bulletin*, vol. 116, 15 April, pp.16–19.

Baker, A., Boggs, T. & Lewin, T.J. 2000, 'Characteristics of regular amphetamine users and implications for treatment', *Drug and Alcohol Review* 2001, vol. 20, pp.49–56.

Baker, A., Boggs, T. & Lewin, T.J. 2001, 'Randomised controlled trial of brief cognitive-behavioural interventions among regular users of amphetamine', *Addiction*, no. 96, pp.1279–1287.

Baker, A. & Lee, N. 2003, 'A review of psychosocial interventions for amphetamine use', *Drug and Alcohol Review*, vol. 22, pp.323–335.

Baker, A, Kay-Lambkin, F., Lee, N.K., Claire, M. & Jenner, L. 2003, *A Brief Cognitive Behavioural Intervention for Regular Amphetamine Users*, Australian Government Department of Health and Ageing, Canberra.

Battaglia, G. & Napier, T.C. 1998, 'The effects of cocaine and amphetamines on brain and brain behaviour: A conference report', *Drug and Alcohol Dependence*, vol.52, pp.41–48.

Beck, J., Harlow, D., McDonnell., Morgan, P.A., Rosenbaum, M. & Watson, L. 1989, *Exploring Ecstasy: A description of MDMA users*, Report to the National Institute on Drug Abuse, Institute for Scientific Analysis, San Francisco.

Bellis, M., Hughes, K. & Lowey, H. 2002, 'Healthy nightclubs and recreational substance use. From a harm minimisation to a healthy settings approach', *Addictive Behaviours*, vol. 27, pp.1025–1035.

Bessant, J. 1997, 'What the papers say: The media, the "underclass" and sociology', in *Youth Crime and the Media: Media Representation of and Reaction to Young People in Relation to Law and Order*, eds J. Bessant & R. Hill, National Clearinghouse for Youth Studies, Hobart, pp.22–33.

Bevan, J. & Loxley, W. 1997, The psychostimulant use and reckless or violent behaviour project: Work in progress, paper presented at the 12th Mandurah Addiction Symposium, Mandurah WA, February.

Black, J., Farrell, M. & McGuire, P. 1992, 'Ecstasy in the brain: Unproven (but cause for concern)', *Druglink*, vol.7, no. 3, pp.12–13.

Bogoras, W. 1979, 'Shamanistic performance in the inner room', in *Reader in Comparative Religion: An Anthropological Approach*, 4th edn, eds W.A. Less & E.Z. Vogt, Harper and Row, New York.

Boles, J. & Miotto, K. 2003, 'Substance abuse and violence: A review of the literature', *Aggression and Violent Behaviour*, vol. 8, no. 2, March–April, pp.155–174.

Bollinger, L. 2002, 'Recent developments regarding drug law and policy in Germany and the European Community: The evolution of drug control in Europe', *Journal of Drug Issues*, vol. 32, pp.363–378.

Boot, B., McGregor, S. & Hall, W. 2000, 'MDMA (ecstasy) neurotoxicity: Assessing and communicating the risks', *The Lancet*, vol. 355, no. 9217, pp.1818–1826.

Bourgois, P., Lettiere M. & Quesada, J. 1997, 'Social misery and the sanctions of substance abuse: Confronting HIV risk among homeless heroin addicts in San Francisco', *Social Problems*, vol. 44, no. 2, pp.155–73.

Boys, A., Lenton, S. & Norcross, K. 1997, 'Polydrug use at raves by a Western Australian sample', *Drug and Alcohol Review*, vol. 16, pp.227–234.

Boys, A., Marsden, J., Griffiths, P., Fountain, J., Stilwell, G. & Strang, J. 1999, 'Substance uses among young people: The relationship between perceived functions and intentions', *Addiction*, vol. 94, no. 7, pp.1042–1050.

Brissett, D. & Snow, R.P. 1993, 'Boredom: Where the future isn't', *Symbolic Interactionism*, vol. 16, pp.237–256.

Bronitt, S. & McSherry, B. 2001, *Principles of Criminal Law*, LBC Information Services, Sydney.

Brown, E. 2003, 'And now for my next trip', *The Australian Magazine*, 29 March, pp.10–13.

Buchanan, J. & Brown, C. 1988, 'Designer drugs': A problem in clinical toxicology', *Medical Toxicology*, vol. 3, pp.1–17.

Buckman, J., Krenske, L & Lynch, M. 2003, 'Amphetamines in Queensland Research project: Presentation to the Queensland Amphetamine Strategy Committee', Brisbane, 6 June.

Burrows D., Flaherty, B. & MacAvoy, M. (eds) 1993, *Illicit psychostimulant use in Australia*, Commonwealth Department of Housing and Community Services and Drug and Alcohol Directorate, New South Wales Health Department, Australian Government Printing Service, Canberra.

Byard, R., James, R., Gilbert, J. & Felgate, P. 1999, 'Another PMA related fatality in Adelaide', *Medical Journal of Australia*, vol. 170, 1 February, pp.139–140.

Byard, R., Rodgers, N., James, R., Kostakis, C. & Camilleri, A. 2002, 'Death and paramethoxyamphetamine – An evolving problem', *Medical Journal of Australia*, vol. 176, 20 May, p.496.

Canfield, D., Hordinsky, J., Millett, D.P., Endecott, B. & Smith, D. 2000, *Prevalence of Drugs and Alcohol in Fatal Civil Aviation Accidents between 1994 and 1998, Final Report*, Federal Aviation Administration, US Department of Transportation, Washington DC.

Cannon, A. 1999, 'Sex, drugs and sudden death (dangers of date rape drug GHB and other party drugs)', *US News and World Report*, vol. 126, 24 May, p.73.

Cantwell, B. & McBride, A. 1998, 'Self detoxification by amphetamine dependent patients: A pilot study', *Drug and Alcohol Dependence*, no. 49, pp.157–163.

Caulfield, C., Rout, M. & Anderson, P. 2004, 'Youth put lives on line to party', *Herald-Sun*, 9 March, p.3.

Centre for Addiction and Mental Health (CAMH) (Canada) 2002, *Information Bulletin: GHB (Gamma-Hydroxy-Butyrate)*, CAMH (Canada). www.camh.net/bulletins/ghb.html

Champness, S. 2000, 'Generation ecstasy', *Alive Magazine*, May, pp.48–52.

Chan Wai Leung 2003, *Who can Work Hard and Play Safe?*, Caritas Youth and Community Service, Hong Kong.

Charnaud B. & Griffiths V. 1998, 'Levels of intravenous drug misuse among clients prescribed oral dexamphetamine or oral methadone: A comparison, *Drug and Alcohol Dependence*, no. 52, pp.79–84.

Chawla, S. 1998, 'They're synthetic, They're clandestine. They can heal. They can kill', *UN Chronicle*, vol. 25, no. 2, Summer, pp.34–36.

Chesher, G. 1990a, 'Some views on Ecstasy', *Modern Medicine of Australia*, April 1990, pp.76–85.

Chesher, G. 1990b, 'Designer drugs – The 'whats' and the 'whys', *Medical Journal of Australia*, vol. 153, 6 August, pp.157–161.

Chesher, G. 1993, 'Pharmacology of the sympathomimetic psychostimulants', in *Illicit psychostimulant use in Australia*, eds D. Burrows, B. Flaherty & M. MacAvoy, Commonwealth Department of Housing and Community Services and Drug and Alcohol Directorate, New South Wales Health Department. Australian Government Printing Service, Canberra, pp.9–30.

Cho, A. & Melega, W. 2002, 'Patterns of methamphetamine use and their consequences', *Journal of Addictive Diseases*, vol. 21, no. 1, pp.21–34.

Churchill, A. 1991, 'An investigation of amphetamine dependence', in *1991 Autumn School of Studies on Alcohol and Drugs: Proceedings*, eds Ruth Godding & Greg Whelan, Department of Community Medicine, St Vincent's Hospital, Melbourne, pp.69–76.

Clark, P., Cook, P., Syed, Q., Ashton, J. & Bellis, M. 2001, *Re-emerging syphilis in the North West: Lessons from the Manchester outbreak*, Liverpool John Moores University, Liverpool.

Clinch, L. 2003, 'Victims seldom present', *Drugs in Society*, September, pp.10–11.

Cloud, J. 2001, 'Recreational pharmaceuticals: Finding new party drugs like K and ecstasy won't be easy', *Time*.

Coggans, N., Shewan, D., Henderson, M. & Davies, J.B. 1991, *National Evaluation of Drug Education in Scotland*, Institute for the Study of Drug Dependence (ISDD) Research Monograph No.4, ISDD, London.

Cohen, R.S. 1998, *The love drug: marching to the beat of ecstasy*, The Haworth Medical Press, New York.

Cole, J. 2002, 'Ecstasy tablet testing: A case of guilty until proven innocent?', in 'Letters to the Editor', *Addiction*, vol. 97, p.231.

Cole, J., Bailey, M., Sumnall, H., Wagstaff, G. & King, L. 2002, 'The content of ecstasy tablets: Implications for the study of their long term effects', *Addiction*, vol. 97, pp.1531–1536.

Collin, M. & Godfrey, J. 1997, *Altered State: The Story of Ecstasy Culture and Acid House*, Serpent's Tail, London.

Collins, D.J. & Lapsley, H.M. 1996, *The social costs of drug abuse in Australia in 1998 and 1992* (NCADA monograph No.30), Australian Government Printing Service, Canberra.

Commonwealth of Australia, House of Representatives Standing Committee on Family and Community Affairs 2003, *Road to Recovery: Report on the Inquiry into substance abuse in Australian communities*, Commonwealth of Australia, Canberra.

Commonwealth Department of Community Services and Health 1989, *Statistics on Drug Abuse in Australia*, Australian Government Printing Service, Canberra.

Commonwealth Department of Health and Family Services 1996, *National Drug Household Survey: Survey Report 1995*, Commonwealth Department of Health and Family Services, Australian Government Publishing Service, Canberra.

Commonwealth Department of Health and Aged Care (National Drug Strategy Unit) 2001, *Australian Secondary School Students' Use of Over-the-Counter and Illicit Substances in 1999*, Commonwealth Department of Health and Aged Care, Canberra.

Concar, D. 2002, 'Ecstasy on the brain', *New Scientist*, vol. 20 April, pp.26–33.

Conolly, S. 2000, *Amphetamines (Need to know)*, Heinemann Library, Oxford.

Cook, T.M. 1996, 'Cerebral oedema after ingestion of MDMA (ecstasy) and unrestricted intake of water. Letter in reply', *British Medical Journal*, vol. 313, no. 7058, 14 September, pp.689–690.

Copeland, A. & Sorensen, J.L. 2001, 'Differences between methamphetamine users and cocaine users in treatment', *Drug and Alcohol Dependence*, no. 62, pp.91–95.

Couper, F. & Logan, B. 2001, 'GHB and driving impairment', *Journal of Forensic Sciences*, vol. 46, no. 4, July, pp.919–923.

Crook, K. 2002, 'The dangers of policing drugs', *Drugs in Society*, June, pp.2–3.

Curran, H.V. & Monaghan, L. 2001, 'In and out of the K-hole: A comparison of the acute and residual effects of ketamine in frequent and infrequent ketamine users', *Addiction*, vol. 96, no. 5, pp.749–760.

Curran, H.V. & Morgan, C. 2000, 'Cognitive, dissociative and psychotogenic effects of ketamine in recreational users on the night of drug use and 3 days later', *Addiction*, vol. 95, no. 4, pp.575–590.

d'Abbs, P. & MacLean, S. 2000, *Petrol Sniffing in Aboriginal Communities: A Review of Interventions*, Cooperative Research Centre for Aboriginal and Tropical Health, Darwin.

Dalgarno, P.J. & Shewan, D. 1996, 'Illicit use of ketamine in Scotland', *Journal of Psychoactive Drugs*, vol. 28, no. 2, pp.191–196.

Darke, S. & Hall, W. 1995, 'Levels and coorelates of polydrug use among heroin users and regular amphetamine users', *Drug and Alcohol Dependency*, vol.39, pp.231–235.

Davies, J. & Ditton, J. 1990, 'The 1990s: Decade of the stimulants?', *British Journal of Addiction*, vol. 85, pp.811–813.

Deehan, A. & Saville, E. 2003, 'Recreational drug use among clubbers in the south east of England', *Findings*, no. 208, Publication of the Research, Development and Statistics Directorate, Home Office. London: Home Office, pp.1-4.

Degenhardt, L., Darke. S. & Dillon, P. 2002, 'GHB use among Australians: Characteristics, use patterns and associated harm', *Drug and Alcohol Dependence*, vol. 67, pp.89–94.

Degenhardt, L., Darke, S. & Dillon, P. 2003, 'The prevalence and correlates of gamma hydroxybutyrate (GHB) overdose among Australian users', *Addiction*, vol. 98, pp.199–204.

Degenhardt, L. & Topp, L. 2003, 'Crystal meth use among polydrug users in Sydney's dance party subculture: Characteristics, use patterns and associated harms', *International Journal of Drug Policy*, vol. 14, pp.17–24.

Denborough, M.A. & Hopkinson, K.C. 1996, 'Dantrolene and ecstasy', *Medical Journal of Australia*, vol. 166, pp.165–166.

Dennis, L. 2000, 'Fast lessons about speed', *Drugs in Society*, June, pp.12–14.

Department of Human Services and Health 1994, *Rural, Remote and Metropolitan Areas Classification*, Department of Human Services and Health, Australian Government Publishing Service, Canberra.

Department of Human Services (DHS) Victoria (Drugs Policy and Services Branch) 2001, *School Students and Drug Use: 1999 Survey of Over-the-Counter and Illicit Substances among Victorian Secondary School Students*, Department of Human Services, Melbourne.

Department of Human Services (DHS) Victoria 2004, *Drug Statistics Handbook 2003*, Department of Human Services, Victoria, Melbourne.

Derlet, R.W. & Heischober, B. 1990, 'Methamphetamine: Stimulant of the 1990s?', *Western Journal of Medicine*, vol 153, no. 6, December, pp.625–629.

Dietze, P., Laslett, A.M. & Rumbold, G. 2004, 'The epidemiology of Australian drug use', in *Drug Use in Australia: Preventing Harm*, 2nd edn, eds M. Hamilton, T. King & A. Ritter, Oxford University Press, South Melbourne, pp.33–52.

Dillon, P. 2000, 'Bopping till they drop? Drugs and the gay club scene', *Connexions*, vol. 19, no. 6, December 1999/January 2000, pp.10–11.

Dillon, P. 2001, 'The strange world of ketamine', *Connexions*, February/March, pp.11–13.

Dillon, P. & Degenhardt, L. 2001, 'Ketamine and GHB: New trends in club drug use?', *Centre Lines*, vol. 4, pp.3–4.

Dillon, P., Copeland, J. & Jansen, K. 2003, 'Patterns of use associated with non-medical ketamine use', *Drug and Alcohol Dependence*, vol. 69, pp.23–28.

Dixon, J. & Maurice, R. 2002, *Implications of Psychostimulants for Needle and Syringe Programs in New South Wales*, South Eastern Sydney Area Health Service, Sydney.

Doblin, R.A. 2002, 'A clinical plan for MDMA (ecstasy) in the treatment of post-traumatic stress disorder', *Journal of Psychoactive Drugs*, vol.34, no. 2, April–June, pp.185–194.

Donath, S. 2004, 'Women and drugs', *Drug Use in Australia: Preventing Harm*, 2nd edn, eds M. Hamilton, T. King & A. Ritter, Oxford University Press, South Melbourne, pp.102–115.

Dorn, N., Murji, K. & South, N. 1991, 'Abby, the ecstasy dealer', *Druglink*, November/December, pp.14–15.

Dornier, C.P., Simon, S.L., Rawson, R.A., Huber, A. & Ling, W. 2000, 'A comparison of injecting and non injecting methamphetamine users', *Journal of Psychoactive Drugs*, vol. 32, no. 2, April–June, pp.229–232.

Dotson, JW, Ackerman, D.L. & West, L.J. 1995, 'Ketamine abuse', *Journal of Drug Issues*, vol. 25, no. 4, pp.751–757.

Drug and Alcohol Services Council (South Australia) 2002, *Illicit Drugs and Licensed Premises Kit 2002*, Drugs and Alcohol Services Council/South Australia Police and the Office of the Liquor and Gambling Commissioner, Government of South Australia, Adelaide.

Drug and Alcohol Services Council (South Australia) 2003, *Reducing Drug Harm in the Dance Party Scene Project: Interim Progress Report*, Drug and Alcohol Services Council, Adelaide, South Australia, September.

Drug and Alcohol Services Council (South Australia) 2003, Illicit drugs and licensed premises kit: Background and update report, Internal publication.

Drug Enforcement Administration (US) (DEA) 2003, 'Fact sheet: Ketamine', at http://www.usdoj.gov/dea/concern/ketamine_factsheet.html

DrugInfo Clearinghouse 2003a, *Prevention issues for communities characterised by cultural and linguistic diversity*, Australian Drug Foundation, West Melbourne.

DrugInfo Clearinghouse 2003b, *Bilingual Information Educator (Illicit Drugs) – Facilitating drug prevention in culturally and linguistically diverse communities*, Fact Sheet No. 2.8, DrugInfo Clearinghouse, Australian Drug Foundation, West Melbourne.

Drug Policy Expert Committee (DPEC) 2000a, *Drugs: Responding to the Issues: Engaging the Community: Executive Summary and Recommendations*, Victorian Government, Melbourne.

Drug Policy Expert Committee (DPEC) 2000b, *DPEC Update*, No. 3, August, at www.dhs.vic.gov.au/phd/dpec/update3.htm

Drug Policy Expert Committee (DPEC) 2000c, *Drugs: Meeting the Challenge* (Stage Two Final Report), Drug Policy Expert Committee, Melbourne.

Drugs and Crime Prevention Committee 1998, *Harm Minimisation: Principles and Policy Frameworks* (Occasional Paper No. 1), Victorian Government Printer, Melbourne.

Drugs and Crime Prevention Committee 2002, *Inquiry into the Inhalation of Volatile Substances: Final Report,* Parliament of Victoria, Government Printer for the State of Victoria, Melbourne.

Duff, C. 2004 (in press).

Elk, C. 1996, 'MDMA (ecstasy): Useful information for health professionals involved in drug education programs', *Journal of Drug Education,* vol. 26, no. 4, pp.349–356.

Erickson, P.G., 1995, 'Harm reduction: What it is and what it is not', *Drug and Alcohol Review,* vol. 14, pp.283–285.

European Monitoring Centre for Drugs and Drug Addiction (EMCDDA) 2003, *Drugs in Focus,* September-October, Office for the Official Publications for the European Communities, Lisbon.

Farrell, M. & Marsden, J. 2002, 'Methamphetamine: Drug use and psychoses becomes a major public health issue in the Asia Pacific region', *Addiction,* vol. 97, pp.771–772.

Felgate, H., Felgate, P., James, D., Sims, N. & Vozzo, D. 1998, 'Recent Paramethoxyamphetamine deaths', *Journal of Analytical Toxicology,* vol. 22, March/April, pp.169–172.

Fitzgerald, J. 1991, 'MDMA and harm', *International Journal of Drug Policy,* vol.2, no. 4, pp.22–24.

Fleming, P. & Roberts, D. 1994, 'Is the prescription of amphetamine justified as a harm reduction measure?', *Journal of the Royal Society of Health,* June, pp.127–131.

Forsyth, A.J.M. 1995, 'Ecstasy and illegal drug design: A new concept in drug use?', *International Journal of Drug Policy,* vol. 6, no. 3, pp.103–109.

Franklin, B. 1999, 'Misleading messages: The media and social policy', in *Social Policy, the Media and Misrepresentation,* ed. B. Franklin, Routledge, London, New York.

Freese, T., Miotto, K. & Reback, C. 2002, 'The effects and consequences of selected club drugs', *Journal of Substance Abuse Treatment,* vol. 23, pp.151–156.

Frosch, D., Shoptaw, S., Huber, A., Rawson, R. & Ling, W. 1996, 'Sexual HIV risk among gay and bisexual male methamphetamine abusers', *Journal of Substance Abuse Treatment,* vol. 13, no. 6, pp.483–486.

Galloway, G., Frederick, S., Staggers, F., Gonzales, M., Stalcup, S. & Smith, D. 1997, 'Gamma-hydroxybutyrate: An emerging drug of abuse that causes physical dependence' *Addiction,* vol. 92, no. 1, pp.89–96.

Galloway, G., Newmeyer, J., Knapp, T., Stalcup, S.A. & Smith, D. 1996, 'A controlled trial of imipramine for the treatment of methamphetamine dependence', *Journal of Substance Abuse Treatment,* vol. 13, pp.453–466.

Garratt, S. 1998, *Adventures in Wonderland: A Decade in Club Culture,* Headline, London.

Gervin, M., Hughes, R., Bamford, L., Smyth, B. & Keenan, E. 2001, 'Heroin smoking by "chasing the dragon" in young opiate users in Ireland: Stability and associations with use to "come down" off "ecstasy"', *Journal of Substance Abuse Treatment,* vol. 20, pp.297–300.

Gliddon, J. 2002, 'Agony and ecstasy', *Bulletin,* 3 September, pp.14–15.

Godfrey, D. & Phillips, M. 2003, 'Driving under the influence of drugs', *Policing Issues and Practice Journal,* January, pp.16–27.

Golub, A., Johnson, B., Sifaneck, S., Chesluk, B. & Parker, H. 2001, 'Is the U.S experiencing an incipient epidemic of hallucinogen use?', *Substance Use and Misuse,* vol. 36, no. 12, pp.1699–1729.

Gore, S. 1999, 'Fatal uncertainty: Death-rate from use of ecstasy or heroin', *The Lancet,* 9 Oct, vol. 354, pp.1265–1268.

Gosling, A. 2003, 'Hong Kong's health check', *Drugs in Society,* September, pp.14–15.

Gossop, M., Marsden, J. & Stewart, D. 2000, 'Treatment outcomes of stimulant misusers: One year follow-up results from the national treatment outcome research study', *Addictive Behaviours,* vol. 25, no. 4, pp.509–522.

Gowing, L., Henry-Edwards, S., Irvine, R. & Ali, R. 2001, *Ecstasy: MDMA and other ring-substituted amphetamines,* produced for the World Health Organisation by Drugs and Alcohol Services Council (DASC) South Australia, Adelaide.

Gowing, L., Henry-Edwards, S., Irvine, R. & Ali, R. 2002, 'The health effects of ecstasy: A literature review', *Drug and Alcohol Review,* vol. 21, pp.53–63.

Gowing, L., Proudfoot, H., Henry-Edwards, S. & Teeson, M. 2001, *Evidence supporting treatment: The effectiveness of interventions for illicit drug use,* Australian National Council on Drugs (ANCD), Canberra.

Greene, S. Dargan, P., O'Connor, N., Jones, A. & Kerins, M. 2003, 'Multiple toxicity from 3,4-Methylenedioxymethamphetamine (Ecstasy)', *American Journal of Emergency Medicine,* vol. 21, no. 2, pp.121–124.

Griffin, M. 1996, 'Busting the myth about ecstasy', *Connexions,* August/September, pp.9–11.

Griffin, M. 1997, 'Not a problem!', *Connexions,* December 1996/January 1997, pp.18–20.

Grinspoon, L. & Hedblom, P. 1975, *The speed culture: Amphetamine use in America,* Harvard University Press, Cambridge.

Grob, C.S. 2000, 'Deconstructing ecstasy: The politics of MDMA research', *Addiction Research,* vol. 8, no. 6, pp.549–588.

Haire, B. 1999, 'Rising cost of party drugs', *National AIDS Bulletin*, vol. 12, no. 6, pp.17–19.

Hall, W. & Hando, J. 1993, 'Patterns of illicit psychostimulant use in Australia', in *Illicit psychostimulant use in Australia*, eds D. Burrows, B. Flaherty & M. MacAvoy, Commonwealth Department of Housing and Community Services and Drug and Alcohol Directorate, New South Wales Health Department, Australian Government Printing Service, Canberra, pp.53–70.

Hall, W. & Hando, J. 1994, 'Route of administration and adverse effects of amphetamine use among young adults in Sydney, Australia', *Drug and Alcohol Review*, vol. 13, pp.277–284.

Hall, W. & Hando, J. 1997, 'Patterns of amphetamine use in Australia', in *Amphetamine Misuse: International Perspectives on Current Trends*, ed. H. Klee, Harwood Academic Publishers, The Netherlands, pp.81–110.

Hall, W., Hando, J., Darke, S. & Ross, J. 1996, 'Psychological morbidity and route of administration among amphetamine users in Sydney, Australia', *Addiction*, vol. 91, no. 1, pp.81–87.

Hamilton, M. King, T. & Ritter, A. 2004, *Drug Use in Australia: Preventing Harm*, 2nd edn, Oxford University Press, South Melbourne.

Hammersley, R., Khan, F. & Ditton, J. 2002, *Ecstasy and the Rise of the Chemical Generation*, Routledge, London and New York.

Handley, N. 2002, 'The heroin drought: Credits and consequences', *Drugs in Society*, June, pp.14–15.

Hando, J., Topp, L. & Hall, W. 1997, 'Amphetamine-related harms and treatment preferences of regular amphetamine users in Sydney, Australia', *Drug and Alcohol Dependence*, vol. 46, pp.105–113.

Hando, J., Topp, L. & Dillon, P. 1998, 'Ecstasy use in Sydney II: Associated harms and risk taking behaviour', in *Illicit Drugs: Current Issues and Responses. Proceedings from the Eleventh National Drug and Alcohol Research Centre Annual Symposium*, eds P. Dillon, L. Topp & W. Swift, National Drug and Alcohol Research Centre, Sydney, pp.33–47.

Hansen, D., Maycock, B. & Lower, T. 2001, 'Weddings, parties, anything... a qualitative analysis of ecstasy use in Perth, Western Australia', *International Journal of Drug Policy*, vol. 12, no. 2, pp.181–199.

Hargreaves, G. 2000, 'Clandestine drug labs: Chemical time bombs', *FBI Law Enforcement Bulletin*, April, pp.1–6.

Harris, D. & Batki, S. 2000, 'Stimulant psychosis: Symptom profile and acute clinical course', *American Journal on Addictions*, vol. 9, pp.28–37.

Harvard Mental Health Letter 2001, 'GBH: Its use and misuse', March, vol. 17, no. 9, p.4.

Hawks, D. & Lenton, S. 1998. 'Harm-minimisation: A basis for decision making in drug policy?', *Risk, Decision and Policy*, vol.3, no. 2, pp.157–163.

Health Education Board of Scotland (HEBS) 2002, HEBS, *Drug education: Approaches, effectiveness and implications for delivery*, HEBS Working Paper No. 1, HEBS (online: http://www.hebs.scot.nhs.uk/ dbtw-wpd/exec/dbtwpcgi.exe)

Heckmann, W. 1997, 'The phenomenology of amphetamine use in Germany', in *Amphetamine Misuse: International Perspectives on Current Trends*, ed. H. Klee, Harwood Academic Publishers, The Netherlands, pp.237–246.

Heischober, B. & Miller, M.A. 1991, *Methamphetamine abuse in California*, (National Institute on Drug Abuse(USA) (NIDA) Research Monograph No. 115), pp.60–71.

Henderson, S. 1993, *Young women, sexuality and recreational drug use: A research and development project*, Final Report, Lifeline, Manchester.

Henry-Edwards, S. 2002, The relationship between amphetamines and violence, prepared on behalf of the National Expert Advisory Committee on Illicit Drugs, submitted to the Intergovernmental Committee on Drugs, January.

Henry-Edwards, S. & Ali, R. 2000, Amphetamine type stimulants demand reduction issues and future priorities, paper prepared for the United Nations Drug Control Program Conference on Amphetamine Type Stimulants in the East and South East Asia Region, Tokyo, Japan, 24–27 January.

Henry-Edwards, S. & Ali, R. 2003, Amphetamine type stimulants in the Asia Pacific region, Unpublished paper.

Hernandez, M., McDaniel, C.M., Costanza, C. & Hernandez, O. 1998, 'GHB induced delirium: A case report and review of the literature on gamma hydroxybutyric acid', *American Journal of Drug and Alcohol Abuse*, vol. 24, no. 1, pp.179–184.

Hinchcliff, S. 2001, 'The meaning of ecstasy use and clubbing to women in the late 1990s', *International Journal of Drug Policy*, vol. 12, pp.455–468.

Hodgins, D.C., el-Guebaly, N. & Addington, J. 1997, 'Treatment of substance abusers: single or mixed gender programs', *Addiction*, vol. 92, no. 7, pp.805–12.

Holland, J. 2001, 'The legal status of MDMA around the world', in *Ecstasy: The Complete Guide; A Comprehensive Look at the Risks and Benefits of MDMA*, ed. J Holland, Park Street Press, Rochester, Vt., pp.146–154.

Hopkins, S. 1996, 'Synthetic ecstasy: The youth culture of techno music', *Youth Studies Australia*, vol. 15, no. 2, pp.12–17.

Hopkins, W. & Frank, B. 1991, 'Street studies that work and what they show in New York City', *Journal of Addictive Diseases*, vol. 11, no. 1, pp.89–97.

Howard, J. & Arcuri A. 2003, *PALM Stats Pack 2002*, Ted Noffs Foundation, Sydney.

Howard, J., Stubbs, M. & Arcuri, A. 2004 (in prep).

Huber, A., Ling, W., Shoptaw, S., Gulati, V., Brethen, P. & Rawson, R. 1997, 'Integrating treatments for methamphetamine abuse: A psychosocial perspective', *Journal of Addictive Diseases*, vol. 16, no. 4, pp.41–50.

Hughes, R. 2000, 'Ecstasy use and dental health', *Journal of Substance Use*, vol. 5, pp.209–210.

Illicit Drug Reporting System (IDRS) 2002, *IDRS Drug Trends Bulletin*, prepared by C. Breen, L. Degenhardt & A. Roxborough, National Drug and Alcohol Research Centre, University of New South Wales, Sydney.

Ingels, M., Rangan, C., Bellezzo, J. & Clark, R. 2000, 'Coma and respiratory depression following the ingestion of GHB and its precursors: Three cases', *Journal of Emergency Medicine*, vol. 19, no. 1, pp.47–50.

Jacobs, B.A. & Miller, J. 1998, 'Crack dealing, gender and arrest avoidance', *Social Problems*, vol. 45, no. 4, pp.550–69.

Jansen, K. 1990, 'Ketamine –Can chronic use impair memory?', *International Journal of the Addictions*, vol. 25, no. 2, pp.133–139.

Jansen, K. 1993, 'Non-medical use of ketamine: Dissociative states in unprotected settings may be harmful', *British Medical Journal*, vol. 306, no. 6878, March 6, pp.601–603.

Jansen, K. 1999 'Ecstasy (MDMA) dependence', *Drug and Alcohol Dependence*, vol. 53, pp.121–124.

Jansen, K. 2001, *Ketamine: Dreams and Realities*, Multidisciplinary Association for Psychedelic Studies, Sarasota, Florida.

Jenkins, P. 1999, *Synthetic Panics: The Symbolic Politics of Designer Drugs*, New York University Press, New York and London.

Joe-Laidler, K. & Morgan, P. 1997, 'Kinship and community: The 'ice' crisis in Hawaii', in *Amphetamine Misuse: International Perspectives on Current Trends*, ed. H. Klee, Harwood Academic Publishers, The Netherlands, pp.163–179.

Johnson, D. 2001, 'Age of illicit drug initiation', *Trends and Issues in Crime and Criminal Justice*, no.201, Australian Institute of Criminology, pp. 1–6.

Jones, C. 1998, 'Why do people die from taking ecstasy?', *Journal of Substance Misuse*, vol.3, pp.95–97.

Journal of the American Medical Association 2000, 'Public health consequences among first responders to emergency events associated with illicit methamphetamine laboratories – Selected States, 1996–1999', (From the Centers for Disease Control and Prevention), *Journal of the American Medical Association*, vol. 284, December, pp.2715–2716.

Kall, K. 1997, 'Amphetamine use in Sweden', in *Amphetamine Misuse: International Perspectives on Current Trends*, ed. H. Klee, Harwood Academic Publishers, The Netherlands, pp.215–234.

Kamienicki, G., Vincent, N., Allsop, S., & Lintzeris, N. 1998, *Models of intervention and care for psychostimulant users*, (National Drug Strategy Monograph Series No 32), Commonwealth Department of Health and Family Services, Canberra.

Kaye, S. & Darke, S. 2000, 'A comparison of the harms associated with the injection of heroin and amphetamines', *Drug and Alcohol Dependence*, vol. 58, pp.189–195.

Kelsall, J., Higgs, P., Lam, T. & Crofts, N. 1999, *The Vietnamese injecting drug use and harm reduction study*, Centre for Harm Reduction, Melbourne.

Kirby, J. 1999, 'The future of criminal law', *Criminal Law Journal*, vol. 23, pp.263.

Kirn, W. 1998, 'Crank', *Time Magazine*, vol 151, no 24, 22 June, pp.24–31.

Kish, S. 2002, 'How strong is the evidence that brain serotonin neurons are damaged in human users of ecstasy?', *Pharmacology, Biochemistry and Behaviour*, vol. 71, pp.845–855.

Klee, H. 1997a, 'Amphetamine misusers in contemporary Britain: The emergence of a hidden population', in *Amphetamine Misuse: International Perspectives on Current Trends*, ed. H. Klee, Harwood Academic Publishers, The Netherlands, pp.19–34.

Klee, H. 1997b, 'A typology of amphetamine users in the United Kingdom', in *Amphetamine Misuse: International Perspectives on Current Trends*, ed. H. Klee, Harwood Academic Publishers, The Netherlands, pp.35–68.

Klee, H. 1997c, 'Patterns of amphetamine misuse in seven nations: Factors affecting growth and decline', in *Amphetamine Misuse: International Perspectives on Current Trends*, ed. H. Klee, Harwood Academic Publishers, The Netherlands, pp.291–320.

Klee, H. 1997d, 'Introduction', in *Amphetamine Misuse: International Perspectives on Current Trends*, ed. H. Klee, Harwood Academic Publishers, The Netherlands.

Klee, H. 1997e, Preliminary text in *Amphetamine Misuse: International Perspectives on Current Trends*, ed. H. Klee, Harwood Academic Publishers, The Netherlands.

Klee, H. 2001a, 'Amphetamine use: Crystal gazing into the millennium: Part one – What is driving demand?', *Journal of Substance Use*, vol. 6, pp.22–35.

Klee, H. 2001b, 'Amphetamine use: Crystal gazing into the millennium: Part two – Alternative paths', *Journal of Substance Use*, vol. 6, pp.80–95.

Klee, H. 2001c, 'Amphetamine use: Crystal gazing into the new millennium: Part three – Prospects of collaboration, containment and ultimate control', *Journal of Substance Abuse*, vol. 6, pp.158–173.

Klee, H. & Morris, J. 1994, 'Factors that lead young amphetamine misusers to seek help: Implications for drug prevention and harm reduction', *Drugs: Education, prevention and policy*, vol. 1, no. 3, pp.289–297.

Klee, H., Carnwath, T., Merill, J. & Morris J. 1995, *Amphetamine misuse and treatment: An exploration of individual and policy impediments to effective service delivery*, Centre for Social Research on Health and Substance Abuse, Manchester Metropolitan University.

Klee, H., Wright, S. & Morris, J. 1999,'Amphetamine users in treatment: Factors associated with sustained abstinence from street drugs', *Addiction Research*, vol. 7, no. 3, pp.239–265.

Klitzmann, R.L., Greenberg, J.D., Pollack, L.M. & Dolezal, C. 2002, 'MDMA (ecstasy) use, and its association with high risk behaviours, mental health, and other factors among gay/bisexual men in New York City', *Drug and Alcohol Dependence*, vol. 66, pp.115–125.

Koesters, S. Rogers, P. & Rajasingham, C. 2002, 'MDMA ('ecstasy') and other 'club drugs': The new epidemic', *Pediatric Clinics of North America*, vol. 49, no. 2, April, pp.415–433.

Kong, F. 2000, 'Illicit drugs: Minimising spread of a lethal cocktail', *Australian Pharmacist*, vol. 19, no. 7, August, pp.418–422.

Landabaso, M., Iraugi, I., Jimenez-Lerma, J., Calle, R., Sanz, J. & Gutierrez-Fraile, M. 2002, 'Ecstasy-induced psychotic disorder: Six-month follow up study', *European Addiction Research*, vol. 8, pp.133–140.

Leamon, M., Canning, R. & Benjamin, L. 2000, 'The impact of amphetamine-related disorders on community psychiatric emergency services: 1993–1997', *American Journal on Addictions*, vol. 9, pp.70–78.

Lee, J.T. 1989, 'Volatile substance abuse within a health education context', *Human Toxicology*, vol. 8, pp.331–334.

Lenton, S. 2003, 'Policy from a harm reduction perspective', *Current Opinion in Psychiatry*, vol. 16, pp.271–277.

Lenton, S., Boys, A. & Norcross, K. 1997, 'Raves, drugs and experience: Drug use by a sample of people who attend raves in Western Australia', *Addiction*, vol. 92, pp.1327–1337.

Lenton, S. & Davidson, P. 1999, 'Raves, drugs, dealing and driving: Qualitative data from a Western Australian sample', *Drug and Alcohol Review*, vol. 18, pp.153–161.

Lenton, S. & Midford, R. 1996, 'Clarifying "harm reduction"?' *Drug and Alcohol Review*, vol. 15, pp.411–413.

Lenton, S., Kerry, K., Loxley, W., Tan-Quigley, A. & Greig, R. 2000, 'Citizens who inject drugs: The "Fitpack" study', *International Journal of Drug Policy*, vol. 11, pp.285–297.

Leser, D. 1988, 'The ecstasy invasion', *The Australian Magazine*, 10 September, pp.30–36.

Lewis, L. & Ross, M.W. 1995, *A Select Body: The gay dance party subculture and the HIV/AIDS pandemic*, Cassell, London.

Ling, L. Marchant, C., Buckley, N., Prior, M. & Irvine, R. 2001, 'Poisoning with recreational drug paramethoxyamphetamine ("death")', *Medical Journal of Australia*, vol. 174, 7 May, pp.453–455.

Lintzeris, N. 1994, Exploring the relationship between psychostimulants and predatory crime, paper presented at St Vincent's Hospital Autumn School of Studies on Alcohol and Drugs, Melbourne, May. (Proceedings Papers 151-158).

Lintzeris, N. Holgate, F. & Dunlop, A. 1996, 'Addressing dependent amphetamine use: A place for prescription', *Drug and Alcohol Review*, vol. 15, pp.189–195.

Louie, R., Krouskos, D., Gonzales, M. & Crofts, N. 1998, 'Vietnamese-speaking injecting drug users in Melbourne: The need for harm reduction programs', *Australian and New Zealand Journal of Public Health*, vol. 22, no. 4, pp.481–484.

Luckman, S. 2000, 'Mapping the regulation of dance parties', in *The Beautiful and the Damned, Journal of Australian Studies*, eds J. Frow, C. Backhouse, N. Earls & G. Whitlock, no. 64, University of Queensland Press, pp.217–223.

Lumby, C. 2000, 'Anti-drugs rationale gone to pot', *The Bulletin*, no. 118, 7 March, p.47.

Lumby, C. 2003, 'The truth drug', *The Bulletin*, 4 March, p.29.

Lymb, S., Weekley, K. & Creaser, D. 2003, Reducing harm in the dance party scene in Adelaide, South Australia, to reduce drug related harm, Unpublished paper, Drugs and Alcohol Services Council, Adelaide, pp.1–7.

Lynch, M., Kemp, R., Krenske, L., Conroy, A. & Webster, J. 2003, *Patterns of Amphetamine Use: Initial findings from the Amphetamines in Queensland research project*, Crime and Misconduct Commission Queensland/Queensland Health, Brisbane.

Mabbott, N.A. & Hartley L.R. 1999, 'Patterns of stimulant drug use on Western Australian heavy transport routes', *Transportation Research*, pp.115–130.

McBride, A., Sullivan, G., Blewett, A. & Morgan, S. 1997, 'Amphetamine prescribing as a harm reduction measure: A preliminary study', *Addiction Research*, vol. 5, no. 2, pp.95–112.

McDaniel, C.H. & Miotto, K.A. 2001, 'Gamma hydroxybutyrate (GHB) and Gamma butyrolactone (GBL) withdrawal: Five case studies', *Journal of Psychoactive Drugs*, vol. 33, no. 2, April–June, pp.143–149.

Macdonald, A., Wilkins, B. & Sheldon, G. 1998, '"Clan labs" pose occupational dangers for police', *Vedette* (Journal of the Queensland Police Service), no.171, September, pp.23–25.

McElrath, K. & McEvoy, K. 1999, *Ecstasy use in Northern Ireland*, Queen's University, Belfast.

McElrath, K. & McEvoy, K. 2001, 'Heroin as evil: Ecstasy users' perceptions about heroin', *Drugs: Education, Prevention and Policy*, vol. 8, no. 2, pp.177–189.

McElrath, K. & McEvoy, K. 2002, 'Negative experiences on ecstasy: The role of drug, set and setting', *Journal of Psychoactive Drugs*, vol. 34, no. 2, April-June, pp.199–208.

McKetin, R. & Mattick R.P. 1997, 'Attention and memory in illicit amphetamine users', *Drug and Alcohol Dependence*, vol. 48, no. 3, December, pp.235–242.

McKey, J. 2000, 'Drugged and assaulted', *Connexions*, February/March, pp.21–24.

McKey, J. 2001, 'The latest trends', *Connexions*, February/March, pp.16–19.

McKoy, J. 2002, 'Getting real', *Meanjin [On Drugs 2]*, vol. 61, no. 2, pp.74–84.

Makkai, T. & McAllister, I. 1998, *Patterns of Drug Use in Australia 1985–1995*, Australian Government Printing Service, Canberra.

Malbon, B.1999, *Clubbing: Dancing, Vitality and Ecstasy*, Routledge, London and New York. Also at <ENLIGHTEN/earthcore/ravesafe/blue light>

Marsden, J., Ali, R., Adelkan, M., Perngparn, U., Liu, T., Sunga, A., Farell, M. & Monteiro, M. 2000, *WHO Multi-Site Project on Functional/Instrumental Use of Amphetamine- Type Stimulants: Study Protocol and Instrumentation*, World Health Organisation, Geneva.

Matthai, S.M., Davidson, D.C., Sills, J.A. & Alexandrou, D. 1996, 'Cerebral oedema after ingestion of MDMA (ecstasy) and unrestricted intake of water', *British Medical Journal*, vol. 312, no. 7042, p.1359.

Mattick, R.P. & Darke, S. 1995, 'Drug replacement treatments: Is amphetamine substitution a horse of a different colour?', *Drug and Alcohol Review*, vol. 14, pp.389–394.

Mayrhauser, C. von, Brecht, M. & Anglin, M.D. 2002, 'Use ecology and drug use motivations of methamphetamine users admitted to substance abuse treatment facilities in Los Angeles: An emerging profile', *Journal of Addictive Diseases*, vol. 21, no. 1, pp.45–60.

Measham, F., Aldridge, J. & Parker, H. 2001, *Dancing on Drugs: Risk, Health and Hedonism in the British Club Scene*, Free Association Books, London.

Measham, F., Newcombe, R. & Parker, H. 1994, 'The normalisation of recreational drug use amongst young people in North West England', *BJS*, vol. 45, no. 2, June, pp.287–312.

Melechi, A. 1993, 'The ecstasy of disappearance', in *Rave Off: Politics and Disappearance in Contemporary Youth Culture*, ed. S. Redhead, Avebury, Aldershot, pp.29–40.

Messenger, M. 1998, 'Is decriminalisation of drugs the answer?', *Police News*, vol. 78, no. 10, October, pp.36–38.

Midford, R., McBride, N. & Farringdon, F. 1999, 'Drug education: The need for an evidence based approach', *Centrelines*, A quarterly newsletter from the National Centre for Drug & Alcohol Research, vol. 33, pp.4–7.

Midford, R., McBride, N. & Munro, G. 1998, 'Harm reduction in school drug education: Developing an Australian approach', *Drug and Alcohol Review*, vol.17, pp.317–328.

Miller, M. 1997, 'History and epidemiology of amphetamine abuse in the United States', in *Amphetamine Misuse: International Perspectives on Current Trends*, ed. H. Klee, Harwood Academic Publishers, The Netherlands, pp.113–133.

Ministerial Council on Drug Strategy (MCDS) 1998, *National Drug Strategic Framework 1998–99 to 2002–03. Building Partnerships: A way to reduce the harm caused by drugs in our community*, Canberra.

Moore, D. 1990, 'Anthropological reflections on youth drug research in Australia: What we don't know and how we should find out', *Drug and Alcohol Review*, vol. 9, pp.333–342.

Moore, D. 1992, *Recreational Drug Use, with Particular Reference to Amphetamines, Ecstasy and LSD, Amongst a Social Network of Young People in Perth, Western Australia*, National Centre for Research into the Prevention of Drug Abuse, Curtin University of Technology, Perth.

Moore, D. 1993, '"Speeding, ecking and tripping": Ethnographic notes from a small world of psychostimulant use', in *Illicit Psychostimulant Use in Australia*, eds D. Burrows, B. Flaherty & M. MacAvoy, Commonwealth Department of Housing and Community Services and Drug and Alcohol Directorate, New South Wales Health Department. Australian Government Printing Service, Canberra, pp.71–90.

Moore, D. 1995, 'Raves and the bohemian search for self and the community: A contribution to the anthropology at public events', *Anthropological Forum*, vol. 7, no. 2, pp.193–214.

Moore, D. 2002a, 'Opening up the cul-de-sac of youth drug studies: A contribution to the construction of some alternative truths', *Contemporary Drug Problems*, vol. 9, Spring, pp.13–63.

Moore, D. 2002b, 'Ethnography and the Australian drug field: Emaciation, appropriation and multidisciplinary myopia', *International Journal of Drug Policy*, no. 13, pp.271–284.

Moreland Hall 2003, *The Big Book on Party Drugs*, by John Hartley, for Uniting Care Moreland Hall, Education and Training Unit, Moreland Hall, Moreland, Victoria.

Morgan, M.J. 1999, 'Memory deficits associated with recreational use of ecstasy (MDMA)', *Psychopharmacology*, vol. 141, pp. 30–36.

Morgan, P. & Beck, J. 1997, 'Hidden contexts of methamphetamine use in the United States', in *Amphetamine Misuse: International Perspectives on Current Trends,* ed. H. Klee, Harwood Academic Publishers, The Netherlands, pp.135–162.

Moriarty, K. 2001, 'The ecstasy lucky dip', *Drugs in Society,* June, pp.8–9.

Mundy J. 2001, 'Methamphetamines: A growing epidemic?', *Connexions,* April/May 2, pp.2–6.

Murnane, A., Smith, A., Crompton, L., Snow, P. & Munro, G. 2000, *Beyond Perceptions: A report on alcohol and other drug use among gay, lesbian, bisexual and queer communities in Victoria,* The ALSO Foundation, Centre for Youth Drug Studies, Vic Health, Melbourne.

Myles, J. 1997, 'Treatment for amphetamine use in the United Kingdom', in *Amphetamine Misuse: International Perspectives on Current Trends,* ed. H. Klee, Harwood Academic Publishers, The Netherlands, pp.69–80.

National Drug and Alcohol Research Centre (NDARC) 1997, *The Illicit Drug Reporting System (IDRS) Trial: Final Report,* by J. Hando, S. O'Brien, S. Darke, L. Maher & W. Hall, (NDARC Monograph No. 31), NDARC, University of New South Wales, Sydney.

National Drug and Alcohol Research Centre (NDARC) 1998, *Ecstasy Use in Australia,* by L. Topp, J. Hando, L. Degenhardt, P. Dillon, A. Roche & N. Solowij, (NDARC Monograph No. 39), NDARC, University of New South Wales, Sydney.

National Drug and Alcohol Research Centre (NDARC) 1999, *A randomised controlled trial of the feasibility of monitoring controlled prescribing of dexamphetamine,* by J. Shearer, A. Wodak, R.P. Mattick, I van Beek, J. Lewis, W. Hall, & K. Dolan, (NDARC Technical Report No. 75), NDARC, University of New South Wales, Sydney.

National Drug and Alcohol Research Centre (NDARC) 2001a, *SA Party Drug Trends: Findings from the Illicit Drug Reporting System (IDRS) Party Drugs Model,* by M. Longo, R. Humeniuk, L. Topp, C. McGregor, R. Cooke, R. Ali & S. Shimamoto, (NDARC Technical Report No. 115), NDARC, University of New South Wales, Sydney.

National Drug and Alcohol Research Centre (NDARC) 2001, 'Structural determinants of youth drug use', by Catherine Spooner, W. Hall & M. Lynskey, *ANCD Research Paper,* National Drug and Alcohol Research Centre, UNSW, Sydney.

National Drug and Alcohol Research Centre (NDARC) 2002a, *Victorian Drug Trends 2001: Findings from the Illicit Drug Reporting System (IDRS),* by C. Fry & P. Miller, (NDARC Technical Report No. 129), NDARC, University of New South Wales, Sydney.

National Drug and Alcohol Research Centre (NDARC) 2002b, *Australian Drug Trends 2001: Findings of the Illicit Drug Reporting System (IDRS)*, by L. Topp, S. Kaye, R. Bruno, M. Longo, P. Williams, B. O'Reilly, C. Fry, G. Rose, S. & Darke, (NDARC Monograph No. 48), NDARC, University of New South Wales, Sydney.

National Drug and Alcohol Research Centre (NDARC) 2002c, *SA Party Drug Trends: Findings from the Illicit Drug Reporting System (IDRS) Party Drugs Model*, by M. Longo, R. Humeniuk, P. Christie, L. Topp & R. Ali, (NDARC Technical Report No. 131, NDARC, University of New South Wales, Sydney.

National Drug and Alcohol Research Centre (NDARC) 2002d, *New South Wales Party Drug Trends 2001: Findings from the Illicit Drug Reporting System (IDRS) Party Drugs Module*, by L. Topp, C. Breen, S. Kaye & S. Darke (NDARC Technical Report No. 136, NDARC, University of New South Wales, Sydney.

National Drug and Alcohol Research Centre (NDARC) 2002e, *Queensland Drug Trends 2001: Findings from the Illicit Drug Reporting System (IDRS) Party Drugs Module*, by G. Rose & J. Najman (NDARC Technical Report No. 132, NDARC, University of New South Wales, Sydney.

National Drug and Alcohol Research Centre (NDARC) 2003a, 'Fact Sheet –Amphetamines', http://ndarc.med.unsw.edu.au/ndarc.nsf

National Drug and Alcohol Research Centre (NDARC) 2003b, *Australian Drug Trends 2002: Findings from the Illicit Drug Reporting System* (IDRS), by C. Breen, I. Degenhardt, A. Roxburg, R. Bruno, A. Duquemin, A. Fetherston, J. Fischer, R. Jenjinson, S. Kinner, M. Longo & C. Rushforth (NDARC Monograph No 50), NDARC.

National Drug and Alcohol Research Centre (NDARC) 2003c, *Victorian Drug Trends 2002: Findings from the Illicit Drug Reporting System*, by C. Breen, I. Degenhardt, A. Roxburg, R. Bruno, A. Duquemin, A. Fetherston, J. Fischer, R. Jenjinson, S. Kinner, M. Longo & C. Rushforth (NDARC Technical report No. 145), NDARC.

National Expert Advisory Committee on Alcohol (NEACA) 2000b, *Alcohol in Australia: Issues and Strategies*, AGPS, Canberra. www.health.gov.au/pubhlth/strateg/drugs/alcohol.pdf

National Institute on Drug Abuse (USA) (NIDA) 1998, *Research Report – Methamphetamine Abuse and Addiction*, National Institutes of Health Research Report Series, NIH Publication Number 98-4210, April, pp.1–7.

National Rural Health Alliance (NRHA) & Department of Health and Ageing 1999, *Rural, Regional and Remote Australians: An Overview of the People, their Health and Health Services*, NRHA & Department of Health and Ageing, p.28.

Neale, J. 2001, 'Driving on recreational drugs: A qualitative investigation of experiences from behind the wheel', *Drugs education, prevention and policy*, vol. 8, no. 4, pp.315–325.

Nencini, P. 2002, 'The shaman and the rave party: Social pharmacology of ecstasy', *Substance Use and Misuse*, vol. 37, nos. 8–10, pp. 923–939.

Newcombe, R. 1992, *The Use of Ecstasy and Dance Drugs at Rave Parties and Nightclubs*, 3D, Liverpool.

Nicholson, K.L. & Balster, R.L. 2001, 'GHB: A new and novel drug of abuse', *Drug and Alcohol Dependence*, vol. 63, no. 1, pp.1–22.

Nolan, R. 1998, 'Transcendence, communality and resistance in rave culture: An observation of youth at a Townsville rave', *Northern Radius*, vol. 5, no. 1, April, pp.7–8.

Norberry, J. 1997, *Illicit Drugs, their Use and the Law in Australia*, Background Paper Number 12, Parliamentary Library of Australia, Canberra.

Nutting, A., Lee, N.K., Jenner, L. & & Davies, J. (forthcoming), The prevalence of mental health disorders among clients in substance use treatment.

O'Donovan, E. 1992, 'Amphetamine: The new drug problem?', *Connexions*, vol. 12, no. 6, Nov/Dec, pp.2–8.

Oetting, E., Deffenbacher, J., Taylor, M., Luther, N., Beauvais, F. & Edwards, R. 2000, 'Methamphetamine use by high school students: Recent trends, gender and ethnicity differences, and the use of other drugs', *Journal of Child and Adolescent Substance Abuse*, vol. 10, no. 1, pp.33–50.

O'Neill, J.1996, 'E equals jail, Prozac equals euphoria', *The Independent Monthly*, July, pp.26–31.

Ovenden, C. & Loxley, W. 1996, 'Bingeing on psychostimulants in Australia: Do we know what it means (And does it matter)?', *Addiction Research*, vol. 4, no. 1, pp.33–43.

Parr, M.J.A., Low, H.M. & Botterill, P. 1997, 'Hyponatraemia and death after "ecstasy" ingestion', *Medical Journal of Australia*, vol. 166, no. 3, February, pp.136–137.

Parrott, A.C., Lees, A., Garnham, N.J., Jones, M. & Wesnes, K. 1998, 'Cognitive performance in recreational users of MDMA/ecstasy: Evidence for memory deficits', *Journal of Psychopharmacology*, vol 12, pp.79–83.

Parrott, A.C., Sisk, E. & Turner, J.J.D. 2000, 'Psychobiological problems in heavy "ecstasy" (MDMA) polydrug users', *Drug and Alcohol Dependence*, vol. 60, no. 1, pp.105–110.

Patterson, I. & Pegg, S. 1999, 'Nothing to do', *Youth Studies Australia*, vol. 18, no. 2, pp.24–29.

Paul, J.P., Stall, R. & Davis, F. 1993, 'Sexual risk for HIV transmission among gay and bisexual men in substance abuse treatment', *AIDS Education and Prevention*, vol. 5, no. 1, pp.11–24.

Pedersen, W. & Skrondal, A. 1999, 'Ecstasy and new patterns of drug use: A normal population study', *Addiction*, vol. 94, no. 11, pp.1695–1706.

Pennell S. 1999, *Meth matters: A report from 5 cities*, National Institute of Justice Report, Washington DC, US Department of Justice.

Pentney, A.R. 2001, An exploration of the history and controversies surrounding MDMA and MDA', *Journal of Psychoactive Drugs*, vol. 33, no. 3, July-September, pp.213–221.

Pharmacy Board of Victoria 2001, *Special Circular*, No. 48, November.

Pharmacy Board of Victoria 2002, *Special Circular*, No. 50, November.

Pharmacy Board of Victoria, 2003, *Circular*, No. 52, October.

Pietschmann, T. 1997, 'Economic forces driving manufacture, trafficking and consumption of amphetamine-type stimulants', in *Amphetamine Misuse: International Perspectives on Current Trends*, ed. H. Klee, Harwood Academic Publishers, The Netherlands, pp.275–290.

Queensland Department of Health and Research and Prevention Unit 2003, *Experiences and Views of Amphetamine Users in Queensland, Questionnaire*, Queensland Department of Health and Research and Prevention Unit, Queensland Crime and Misconduct Commission, Queensland Government Printer.

Queensland Government 1999, *Beyond a Quick Fix: Queensland Drug Strategic Framework 1999/2000 to 2003/2004*, Queensland Government Printer, Brisbane.

Ramsey, J., Butcher, M., Murphy, M., Lee, T., Johnston, A. & Holt, D. 2001, 'A new method to monitor drugs at dance venues', *BMJ*, vol. 323, September, p.603.

Rawson, R., Gonzales, R & Brethen, P. 2002, 'Treatment of methamphetamine disorders: An update', *Journal of Substance Abuse Treatment*, vol. 23, pp.145–150.

Rawson, R., Huber, A., Brethen, P., Obert, J., Gulati, V., Shoptaw, S. & Ling W. 2002, 'Status of methamphetamine users 2–5 years after outpatient treatment', *Journal of Addictive Diseases*, vol. 21, no. 1, pp.107–119.

Reback, C. & Grella, C. 1999, 'HIV risk behaviours of gay and bisexual male methamphetamine users contacted through street outreach', *Journal of Drug Issues*, vol. 29, no. 1, pp.155–166.

Redfearn, P.J, Agrawal, N. & Mair, L.H. 1998, 'An association between the regular use of 3,4 methylenedioxy-methamphetamine (ecstasy) and excessive wear of the teeth', *Addiction*, vol. 93, no. 5, pp.745–748.

Reeves, J. & Duda, R. 2003, 'GHB/GBL intoxication and withdrawal: A review and case presentation, *Addictive Disorders and their Treatment*', vol. 2, no. 1, pp.25–28.

Reid, G. 2003, 'Drugs in a multicultural community', *DrugInfo Clearinghouse Newsletter*, vol. 2, no. 2, November, Australian Drug Foundation, West Melbourne.

Reid, G., Higgs, P., Beyer, L. & Crofts, N. 2002, 'Vulnerability among Vietnamese illicit drug users in Australia: Challenges for change', *International Journal of Drug Policy*, vol. 13, pp.127–136.

Reynolds, S. 1998, *Energy Flash: A Journey through Rave Music and Dance Culture*, Macmillan, London.

Richards, J.R., Bretz, S.W., Johnson, E.B., Turnipseed, S.D., Brofeldt, B.T. & Derlet, R.W. 1999, 'Methamphetamine abuse and emergency department utilisation', *The Western Journal of Medicine*, vol. 170, April, pp.198–202.

Ricuarte, G.A & McCann U.D. 1992, 'Neurotoxic amphetamine analogues: Effects in monkeys and implications for humans', *Annals of the New York Academy of Sciences*, no. 648, pp.371–82.

Ricaurte, G.A., Yuan, J. & McCann U.D. 2000, '3,4-methylenedioxymethamphetamine ('Ecstasy') induced neurotoxicity: Studies in animals', *Neuropsychobiology*, vol. 42, pp.5–10.

Ricaurte, G.A., De Lanney, L.E., Irwin, I. & Langston, J.W. 1988, 'Toxic effects of MDMA on central serotonergic neurons in the primate: Importance of route and frequency of drug administration', *Brain Res*, no.446, pp.165–168.

Ricuarte, G.A., Finnegan, K.T., Irwin, I. & Langston, J.W. 1990, 'Aminergic metabolites in cerebrospinal fluid of humans previously exposed to MDMA: Preliminary observations', *Annals of the New York Academy of Sciences*, no. 600, pp.699–708.

Ricaurte, G.A., Markowska, A.L., Wenk, G.L., Hatzdimitrou, G., Wlos, J. & Olton, D. 1993, '3,4-methylenedioxymethamphetamine, serotonin and memory', *Journal of Pharmacological and Experimental Therapeutics*, vol. 266, pp.1097–1105.

Riedlinger, T.J. & Riedlinger, J.E. 1994, 'Psychedelic and entactogenic drugs in the treatment of depression', *Journal of Psychoactive Drugs*, vol. 26, no. 1, pp.41–55.

Roddis, D. 2000, 'Pharmacy crime watch', *Security Australia*, vol. 20, no. 9, p.31.

Rosenbaum, M. 2002, 'Ecstasy: America's new reefer madness?', *Journal of Psychoactive Drugs*, vol. 34, no. 2, April–June, pp.1–9.

Rosenbaum, M., Morgan, P. & Beck, J. 1989, 'Ethnographic notes on ecstasy use among professionals', *International Journal on Drug Policy*, vol. 1, no. 2, pp.16–19.

Rowland, B., Toumbourou, J. & Stevens, C. 2003, 'Preventing drug related harm in communities characterised by cultural and linguistic diversity', *DrugInfo Clearinghouse, Prevention research evaluation report*, no. 8, November, Australian Drug Foundation, West Melbourne.

Ryan, D. & Keen, P. 2001, 'The party faithful', *Users' News* (NSW Users and Aids Association), no. 34, Summer, pp.4–5. First published in *Wanted*, Australian Federation of Aids Organisations, 1999.

Ryder, D., Salmon, S. & Walker, N. 2001, *Drug Use and Drug-Related Harm: A Delicate Balance*, IP Communications, Melbourne.

Safe, M. & Sager, M. 1990, 'Ice', *The Australian Magazine*, 26-27 May, pp.8-14.

Sanguineti, V.R., Angelo, A. & Frank, M.R. 1997, 'GHB: A home brew', *American Journal of Drug and Alcohol Abuse*, vol. 23, no. 4, November, pp.637–643.

Saunders, N. 1998, 'How the media report ecstasy', *Journal of Substance Misuse*, vol. 3, pp.98–100.

Schifano, F., Di Furia, L., Forza, G., Minicuci, N. & Bricolo, R. 1998, 'MDMA (ecstasy) consumption in the context of polydrug abuse: A report on 150 patients', *Drug and Alcohol Dependence*, vol. 52, pp.85–90.

Schlosser, E. 2002, *Fast Food Nation*, Penguin Books, London.

Semple, S., Patterson, T. & Grant I. 2002, 'Motivations associated with methamphetamine use among HIV+ men who have sex with men', *Journal of Substance Abuse Treatment*, vol. 22, pp.149–156.

Shannon, M. 2002, *Drugs in Australia: Ecstasy*, Binara Publishing, Carlton, Victoria.

Shapiro, H. 1989, 'MDMA in perspective: The speed trip', *Drugslink*, March/April, pp.14–15.

Sheldon, G. 1997, 'The Illicit Laboratory Investigation Task Force', *Queensland Police Union Journal*, August, pp.15–19.

Sherlock, K., Hay, A., Wolff, K. & Conner, M. 1999, 'Validating the consumption of MDMA in an examination of the behavioural effects of 'ecstasy' amongst recreational users', *Addiction Research*, vol. 7, no. 1, pp.47–62.

Shewan, D., Dalgarno, P. & Reith, G. 2000, 'Perceived risk and risk reduction among ecstasy users: The role of drug, set and setting', *International Journal On Drug Policy*, vol. 10, pp.431–453.

Shoptaw, S., Reback, C. & Freese, T. 2002, 'Patient characteristics, HIV serostatus, and risk behaviours among gay and bisexual males seeking treatment for methamphetamine abuse and dependence in Los Angeles', *Journal of Addictive Diseases*, vol. 21, no. 1, pp.91–105.

Sim, T., Simon, S., Dornier, C., Richardson, K., Rawson, R. & Ling, W. 2002, 'Cognitive deficits among methamphetamine users with attention deficit hyperactivity disorder symptomatology', *Journal of Addictive Diseases*, vol. 21, no. 1, pp.75–89.

Simon, N.G. & Mattick, R.P. 2002, 'The impact of regular ecstasy use on memory function', *Addiction*, vol. 97, no. 12, December, pp.1523–1529.

Simon, S., Dornier, C., Carnell, J., Brethen, P., Rawson, R. & Ling, M.D. 2000, 'Cognitive impairment in individuals currently using methamphetamine', *American Journal on Addictions*, vol. 9, pp.222–231.

Simon, S., Dornier, C., Sim, T., Richardson, K., Rawson, R., and Ling, W. 2002, 'Cognitive performance of current methamphetamine and cocaine abusers', *Journal of Addictive Diseases*, vol. 21, no. 1, pp.61–74.

Single, E., 1995, 'Defining harm reduction', *Drug and Alcohol Review*, vol. 14, pp.287–290.

Siokou, C. 2002, 'Seeking the vibe', *Youth Studies Australia*, vol. 21, no.1, pp.11–18.

Slaughter, L. 2000, 'Involvement of drugs in sexual assault', *Journal of Reproductive Medicine* , vol. 45, pp.425–430.

Smith, D., Wesson, D.R., Buxton, M.E., Seymour, R.B., Ross, S., Bishop, M.P. & Zerkin, E. 1982, *PCP: Problems and Prevention*, Kendall/Hunt Publishing Company, Iowa.

Smith, G. 2002, 'Drug offences in Fitzroy Legal Service', in *The Law Handbook*, ed. K. Harper, Fitzroy, Victoria, pp.603–621.

Smith, N. & Temple, W. 2000, 'Date rape drugs', *Australian Pharmacist*, vol. 19, no. 6, July, p.357.

Solowij, N. 1993, 'Ecstasy (3,4-methylenedioxymethamphetamine)', *Current Opinion in Psychiatry*, vol. 6, pp.411–415.

Solowij, N., Hall, W. & Lee, N. 1992, 'Recreational MDMA use in Sydney: A profile of Ecstasy users and their experiences with the drug', *British Journal of Addiction*, vol. 87, pp.1161–1172.

South Australian Drugs Summit Communique 2002a, Issues Papers and Final Recommendations for Plenary Discussion, June 24-June 28, Drug and Alcohol Services Council, Department of Human Services, South Australia, Adelaide.

South Australian Drugs Summit Issues Paper 2002b, *Health Maintenance and Treatment*, Drug and Alcohol Services Council, Department of Human Services, South Australia, Adelaide.

South Australian Drugs Summit 2003, *Tackling Drugs: Government Responses, Further Initiatives*, Government of South Australia/Social Inclusion Initiative, Adelaide.

Stas, T. 2001, 'Crackdown on drugs: Strike Force Sibret', *Police Service Weekly*, vol. 13, no. 44, 5 November, pp.4–5.

Steel, P. (Detective First Class Constable, WA Police Service & Churchill Fellow) 2003, *Report* (the Steel Report), Winston Churchill Memorial Trust of Australia.

Strang, J. & Farrell, M., 1992, 'Harm-minimisation for drug misusers: When second best may be best first', *British Medical Journal*, vol. 304, no.6835, pp.1127–1129.

Strang, J., Ruben, S. & Farrell, M. 1994, 'Prescribing heroin and other injectable drugs', in *Heroin Addiction and Drug Policy: The British System*, eds J. Strang & M. Gossop, Oxford University Press, Oxford.

Suwaki, H., Fukui, S. & Konuma, K. 1997, 'Methamphetamine abuse in Japan', in *Amphetamine Misuse: International Perspectives on Current Trends*, ed. H. Klee, Harwood Academic Publishers, The Netherlands, pp.199–214.

Sweet, M.1997, 'A drug called E', *Sydney Morning Herald* (Spectrum Section), 6 December, pp.6–12.

Swift, W. & Copeland, J. 1998, 'Treatment needs of women with alcohol and other drug problems: Findings of an Australian National Survey', *Addiction*, vol. 91, no. 8, pp.1141–50.

Tancer, M. & Johanson, C. 2001, 'The subjective effects of MDMA and *m*CPP in moderate MDMA users', *Drug and Alcohol Dependence*, vol. 65, pp.97–101.

Teece, M. & Makkai, T. 2000, 'Print media reporting on drugs and crime 1995–1998', *Trends & Issues in Crime and Criminal Justice*, no. 158, pp.1–6.

Ter Bogt, T., Engels, R., Hibbel, B., Van Wel, F. & Verhagen, S. 2002, 'Dancestasy: Dance and MDMA use in Dutch youth culture', *Contemporary Drug Problems*, vol. 29, Spring, pp.157–181.

Thomas, G., Bonner, S. & Gascoigne, A. 1997, 'Coma induced by abuse of hydroxybutyrate (GBH or liquid ecstasy): A case report', *British Medical Journal*, vol. 314, no. 35, 4 January, pp.1–4.

Thornton, M. 1991, 'Feminism and the contradiction of law reform', *International Journal of the Sociology of Law*, vol. 19, pp.453–474.

Thornton, M. (ed.) 1995, *Public and Private: Feminist Legal Debates*, Oxford University Press, Melbourne.

Thornton, S. 1994, 'Moral panic, the media and British rave culture', in *Microphone Fiends: Youth Music And Youth Culture*, eds A. Ross & T. Rose, Routledge, London, pp.177–192.

Thwaites, J., Minister for Health, Victoria Government 2002, *Warnings on Overdoses from 'Fantasy' Party Drug*, media release, 25 July.

'Timeline of a PMA death' 2001, *Drugs in Society*, June, p.9.

Topp L. 2001, 'The use of Methamphetamine in Australia', *Centre Lines*, Newsletter of the National Centre for Drug and Alcohol Research, February, pp.3–4.

Topp, L. & Darke, S. 1997, 'The applicability of the dependence syndrome to amphetamine', *Drug and Alcohol Dependence*, vol. 48, pp.113–118.

Topp, L, Hando, J. & Dillon, P. 1999, 'Sexual behaviour of ecstasy users in Sydney, Australia', *Culture, Health and Sexuality,* vol. 1, no. 2, pp.147–159.

Tossmann, P., Boldt, S. & Tensil, M. 2001, 'The use of drugs within the techno-party scene in European metropolitan cities', *European Addiction Research,* no. 7, pp.2–23.

Traub, S., Hoffmann, R. & Nelson, L. 2002, 'The "ecstasy" hangover: Hyponatremia due to 3,4-Methylenedioxymethamphetamine', *Journal Of Urban Health: New York Academy of Medicine,* vol. 79, no. 4, December, pp.549–555.

Turnbull, M. 1993, 'Developing amphetamine related strategies within a harm reduction framework', *International Journal of Drug Policy,* vol. 4, no. 2, pp.98–103.

Turning Point Drug and Alcohol Centre 2001, *A study of the impact of the heroin 'drought' in Melbourne: Results of the Drug Availability Monitoring Project (DAMP),* by P. Miller, C. Fry & P. Dietze, Turning Point Drug and Alcohol Centre, Melbourne.

Turning Point Alcohol and Drug Centre 2003, 'Discussion Paper No. 8: Alcohol and drug service delivery in rural and regional Victoria', by Ron Tiffen & Lynda Berends, *Service System Review,* Turning Point Alcohol and Drug Centre, Melbourne.

United Nations Drug Control Programme (UNDCP) 1996, *Amphetamine-type stimulants: A global review,* United Nations International Drug Control Programme, (UNCDP Technical Series Number 3), Vienna.

United Nations Office on Drugs and Crime (UNODC) 2003, *Global Illicit Drug Trends,* UNODC, New York.

Vaiva, G., Boss, V., Bailly, D., Thomas, P., Lestavel, P. & Goudemand, M. 2001, 'An "accidental" acute psychosis with ecstasy use', *Journal of Psychoactive Drugs,* vol. 33, no. 1, pp.95–98.

van de Wijngaart, G., Braam, R., de Bruin D., Fris, M., Maalste N. & Verbraeck, H. (199) 'Ecstasy use at large scale dance events in the Netherlands', *Journal of Drug Issues,* vol. 29, pp.679–702.

Van Laar, M. & Spruit, I. 1997, 'Use and abuse of amphetamine in the Netherlands', in *Amphetamine Misuse: International Perspectives on Current Trends,* ed. H. Klee, Harwood Academic Publishers, The Netherlands, pp.247–272.

Vastag, B. 2001, 'Ecstasy experts want realistic messages', *Journal of the American Medical Association,* vol. 286, no. 7, pp.777–779.

Vincent, N., Allsop, S. & Shoobridge, J. 1996, *Responding to Hazardous and Harmful Use of Amphetamines,* Proceedings of the Reshaping the Future: Drugs and Young People Conference, Australian Drug Foundation, Canberra, pp.369–383.

Vincent, N., Allsop, S. & Shoobridge, J. 1997, *Responding to the Hazardous and Harmful use of Amphetamines Final Report (Phase 1)*, Commonwealth Department of Health and Family Services (Drugs of Dependence Branch), Canberra.

Vincent, N., Shoobridge, J., Ask, A., Allsop, S. & Ali, R. 1999, 'Characteristics of amphetamine users seeking help and treatment in Adelaide, South Australia', *Drug and Alcohol Review*, no. 18, pp.63–73.

Von Sydow, K., Lieb, R., Pfister, H., Hofler, M. & Wittchen, H. 2002, 'Use, abuse and dependence of ecstasy and related drugs in adolescents and young adults – A transient phenomenon? Results from a longitudinal community study', *Drug and Alcohol Dependence*, vol. 66, pp.147–159.

Vuori, E., Henry, J., Ojanpera, I., Nieminen, R., Savolainen, T., Wahlsten, P. & Jantii, M. 2003, 'Death following ingestion of MDMA (ecstasy) and moclobemide', *Addiction*, vol. 98, pp.365–368.

Wardlaw, G. 1993, 'Supply reduction (law enforcement strategies pertaining to illicit use of psychostimulants)', in *Illicit psychostimulant use in Australia*, eds D. Burrows, B. Flaherty & M. MacAvoy, Commonwealth Department of Housing and Community Services and Drug and Alcohol Directorate, New South Wales Health Department, Australian Government Printing Service, Canberra, pp.91–104.

Wareing, M., Fisk, J.E. & Murphy, P.N. 2000, 'Working memory deficits in current and previous users of MDMA ('ecstasy')', *British Journal of Psychology*, vol. 91, no. 2, pp.181–188.

Webb, M.B. 1998, '"E" is for... emerging drug policy issue', *Social Policy Journal of New Zealand*, no. 10, June, pp.86–100.

Webb, T. 2003, 'Ecstasy and the law: The past, present and the future of MDMA's legal regulation in the Australian Capital Territory', *Australian Law Students' Association Academic Journal*, Australian Law Students' Association Inc, pp.80–129.

Weierter, S. & Lynch, M. 2002, *Drug Use and Crime: Findings from the DUMA Survey*, Crime and Misconduct Commission, Queensland, Research and Issues Paper Series, Number 3, June, pp.1–6.

Wermuth, L. 2000, 'Methamphetamine use: Hazards and social influences', *Journal of Drug Education*, vol. 30, no. 4, pp.423–433.

Western Australia Chamber of Mines and Energy 1996, *Alcohol and Drugs in the workplace: Issues, trends and practices*, WA Chamber of Mines and Energy, Perth.

White, J., Bochner, F. & Irvine, R. 1997, 'The agony of "ecstasy": How can we avoid more "ecstasy" related deaths?', *Medical Journal of Australia*, vol. 166, pp.117–118.

White, J., Irvine, R. & Bochner, F. 1996 *Toxic Effects of MDMA*, a report commissioned by the Commonwealth Department of Human Services, Canberra.

White, J. & Ryan, C.F. 1996, 'Pharmacological properties of ketamine', *Drug and Alcohol Review*, vol. 15, no. 2, pp.145–155.

White, R. 2000, 'Dexamphetamine substitution in the treatment of amphetamine abuse: An initial investigation', *Addiction*, vol. 95, no. 2, pp.229–238.

Wickes, W. 1993a, 'Medical aspects of psychostimulant use', in *Illicit psychostimulant use in Australia*, eds D. Burrows, B. Flaherty & M. MacAvoy, Commonwealth Department of Housing and Community Services and Drug and Alcohol Directorate, New South Wales Health Department, Australian Government Printing Service, Canberra, pp.31–52.

Wickes, W. 1993b, *Amphetamines and other psychostimulants: A guide to the management of users*, Australian Government Publishing Service, Canberra.

Wilkins, B. 1996, 'Cerebral oedema after MDMA (ecstasy) and unrestricted water intake: Hypnatraemia must be treated with low water input', *British Medical Journal*, vol. 313, no. 7058, September, pp.689–690.

Wilkins, C. 2002, 'Designer amphetamines in New Zealand: Policy challenges and initiatives', *Social Policy Journal of New Zealand*, December, pp.14–28.

Williams, L. & Parker, H. 2001, 'Alcohol, cannabis, ecstasy and cocaine: Drugs of reasoned choice amongst young adult recreational drug users in England', *International Journal of Drug Policy*, vol. 12, pp.397–413.

Williams, P. 2001, 'Illicit drug use in regional Australia, 1988–1998', in *Trends & Issues in Crime and Criminal Justice*, No.192, Australian Institute of Criminology, Canberra, February, p.8.

Williamson, S., Gossop, M., Powis, B., Griffiths, P., Fountain, J. & Strang, J. 1997, 'Adverse effects of stimulant drugs in a community sample of drug users', *Drug and Alcohol Dependence*, vol. 44, pp.87–94.

Winstock, A., Griffiths, P. & Stewart, D. 2001, 'Drugs and the dance music scene: A survey of current drug use patterns among a sample of dance music enthusiasts in the UK', *Drug and Alcohol Dependence*, vol. 64, pp.9–17.

Winstock, A., Wolff, K. & Ramsey, J. 2001, 'Ecstasy pill testing: Harm minimization gone too far?' *Addiction*, vol. 96, pp.1139–1148.

Wodak, A. 1996, 'What are the real risks of ecstasy?', *Modern Medicine of Australia*, June, p.155.

Wodak, A, 2001, 'Editorial: Developing a medical response to psychostimulants', *Addiction Research and Theory*, vol. 9, no. 2, pp.93–96.

Wood, C. 1998a, 'Speed: A matter of treatment', *Connexions*, vol. 17, no. 6, December 1997/January, pp.19–22.

Wood, C. 1998b, 'Raving about the mix', *Connexions*, vol. 18, no. 1, February/March, pp.17–19.

Wray, J. 2000, 'Psychopysiological aspects of methamphetamine abuse', *Journal of Addictions Nursing*, vol. 12, no. 3/4, pp.143–147.

Wright, S. & Klee, H. 1999, 'A profile of amphetamine users who present to treatment services and do not return', *Drugs: Education, prevention and policy*, vol. 6, no. 2, pp.227–239.

Wright, S., Klee, H. & Reid, P. 1999, 'Attitudes of amphetamine users towards treatment services', *Drugs: Education, prevention and policy*, vol. 6, no. 1, pp.71–86.

Yacoubian, G.S. 2001, 'The global proliferation of ecstasy', *International Journal of Comparative Criminology*, vol. 1, no. 1, pp.127–136.

Youth Studies Australia 2002, 'Ecstasy update', *Youth Studies Australia*, vol. 21, no.1, p.15.

Yui, K., Goto, K., Ikemoto, S. & Ishiguro, T. 2000, 'Stress induced spontaneous recurrence of methamphetamine psychosis: The relation between stressful experiences and sensitivity to stress', *Drug and Alcohol Dependence*, vol. 58, pp.67–75.

Zakzanis, K. & Young, D. 2001, Memory impairment in abstinent MDMA ('Ecstasy') users: A longitudinal investigation. *Neurology*, vol. 56, pp.966–969.

Zinberg, N.E. 1979, 'Social interactions, drug use, and drug research', in *Substance abuse: Clinical problems and perspectives*, eds J.H. Lowinson & P. Ruiz, Williams and Wilkins, Baltimore, pp.91–108.

Zinberg, N.E. 1984, *Drug, set and setting: The basis for controlled intoxicant use*, Yale University Press, New Haven.

Zule, W. & Desmond, D. 1999, 'An ethnographic comparison of HIV risk behaviours among heroin and methamphetamine injectors', *American Journal of Drug and Alcohol Abuse*, vol. 25, no. 1, pp.1–22.

Minority Report

Pursuant to Section 34(2) of the Parliamentary Committees Act 2003

We:

Hon Robin Cooper M.L.A. (Deputy Chairman)

Mr Kim Wells M.L.A.

submit this minority report in response to the Inquiry into Amphetamines and 'Party Drug' Use in Victoria.

We are not satisfied that the Bracks Government has permitted Victoria Police to provide a submission that is a true and accurate reflection of the Police position on this important issue.

We are of that view because of a Government directive issued by the Secretary of the Department of Premier and Cabinet (DPC), Mr Terry Moran, which prevents all Government Departments from directly making submissions to Joint Parliamentary Committees of the Victorian Parliament. That directive instructs Departments to first provide their submissions to their Minister for vetting and approval, before then sending it to the DPC for further vetting and approval.

In issuing that directive Mr Moran claimed that he was simply following a precedent established by the Kennett Government. His claim is incorrect as the previous Government's protocols were based on Victorian Government departments making submissions to Federal Government Parliamentary committees or Parliamentary committees of other states or territories, not to committees of the Victorian Parliament.

What has particularly disturbed us is that the Moran directive included Victoria Police. Such a stance is clearly contrary to many statements made by the Police Minister, Mr Haermeyer, both inside and outside of Parliament, that all operational matters are the total responsibility of the Police Commissioner. We support that commitment by the Minister to the "separation of powers doctrine" in regard to Victoria Police, but it now seems that his commitment is rhetoric rather than real.

Political intervention by the Government in the response by Victoria Police to the Committee, and the specific issues of the separation of powers doctrine and the independence of the Police, was raised as a matter of real concern in an email of 27 October 2003 to the office of the Chief Commissioner by Superintendent Paul Ditchburn, Manager of the Legal and Corporate Policy Division of Victoria Police.

An additional confirmation of the level of political control being applied by the State Government can be seen in a Victoria Police memorandum of 7 November 2003 which states that "approval" by the Minister's Chief of Staff, Mr Rob McDonald, had been given for a Police officer to attend a meeting of the Committee at Knox on 11 November 2003. It is our view that approval, or otherwise, for a Police officer to attend a meeting of the Committee should rest solely with the Chief Commissioner.

It is now clear that Victoria Police was directed by the Government not to appear before the Drugs and Crime Prevention Committee on 27 October 2003 because the Government did not approve of the contents of their submission. In a document dated 30 October 2003, written by Superintendent Ditchburn that was released to Mr Wells under the FOI Act it is stated, "A hearing to the (D&CP) committee for Monday 27 October 2003 was cancelled due to non-receipt of DPC approval under the guidelines. A heavily censored version may now proceed". That statement by Superintendent Ditchburn must call into question the content of the submission that the Committee eventually received.

The "Inquiry into Amphetamine and 'Party Drug' Use in Victoria" Discussion Paper was released to the public in September 2003. Victoria Police used this discussion paper as the basis of its submission.

We became concerned about the Police submission after Mr Wells received a telephone call from a Police member stating that, "you are not going to receive the full story".

After receiving a copy of the submission we noted that while it addressed most of the issues relating to Police operational roles, two crucial issues were omitted.

Firstly, there was no reference to the question, "what level of policing should exist in and around rave parties and associated venues?"

Secondly, there was no reference to the question, "to what extent is addressing the importation and distribution of amphetamines and 'party drugs' (not manufactured locally) a resource problem at Commonwealth and State levels?"

Members of Victoria Police eventually attended a Public Hearing on 10 November 2003 where questions relating to the accuracy and frankness of their written submission were directed to the leader of the group, Superintendent Ditchburn.

Mr Cooper asked Superintendent Ditchburn whether the Victoria Police submission had been changed in any way from its original submission. Superintendent Ditchburn stated that it had not.

Mr Wells then asked Superintendent Ditchburn why certain answers had been removed from the 'draft' response which had been prepared.

The Chair then stated that Superintendent Ditchburn had already answered questions regarding the original submission however the original submission refers to the finished product prepared by Victoria Police. This is significantly different to the question put by Mr Wells which referred to the draft responses.

Mr Wells then repeated the question by asking, "Whose decision was it to pull certain answers out of your draft responses?"

Members of Victoria Police were not given the chance to answer this question. A Government Member answered the question on behalf of Victoria Police by stating that, "I believe there were no answers taken from responses".

Mr Cooper then correctly pointed out that there were two separate issues which remained unresolved.

One issue related to the draft response and the second issue to the official submission provided to the Committee.

This vital point raised by Mr Cooper was ruled out of order by the Chair and Victoria Police were not required to answer.

Mr Wells then rephrased his question. In referring to the official response to the Committee, Mr Wells asked why two vital answers were removed from the official response in regards to resourcing.

Superintendent Ditchburn replied that Victoria Police did not answer all the questions and propositions that were in the discussion paper. He went on to state that they "selected some key ones. There were certainly none removed in that respect".

We are aware that Victoria Police did not answer all of the questions in the discussion paper because some issues did not affect Victoria Police, however, the second part of his comment, "key ones were selected and certainly none were removed in that respect", neatly avoided the question.

We are concerned that the draft document was formulated in such a way, with only the so-called "key" issues being selected, so as to not embarrass the Bracks Government in regards to the resourcing of Victoria Police.

Mr Wells then asked the same question in another way by referring to the Victoria Police Annual Report 2002-03 stating that there was a target of 600,000 hours allocated for illegal drug activity investigation, however the number of actual hours of policing that was achieved came to only 400,000 hours. He pursued that matter because of his belief that the shortfall of 200,000 hours policing work on illegal drug activity would be a major concern to the Victoria Police.

Superintendent Ditchburn answered by stating that there was no particular reason why specific questions were not answered.

When Mr Wells further asked, "So is the issue of resourcing not a main concern of Victoria Police?" Superintendent Ditchburn was not given the opportunity by the Chair to respond.

The issue of amphetamine and 'party drug' use in Victoria is extremely serious and should be well above the petty concerns of a Government or a Minister thinking they may be seen in a bad light. Political interference in the way Victoria Police deals with this Committee, or other Parliamentary committees, and the censoring of its submission for this particular Inquiry, is reprehensible.

The general community, rightly, wants to better understand the issue itself, and to be assured that those who are charged with the responsibility of dealing with the problem are doing everything within their power to eliminate, or at the least minimise, the damage that is caused by these illicit drugs.

In light of the concerns that we have, which are outlined in this minority report, we regret to say that we have serious doubts about whether that assurance to the community can be honestly provided.

Minority Report

Pursuant to Section 34(2) of the Parliamentary Committees Act 2003

I: Dr Bill Sykes M.L.A., submit this minority report in response to the Inquiry into Amphetamine and 'Party Drug' Use in Victoria.

I wish to register my concern about political interference with a formal submission of to the Inquiry into Amphetamine and 'Party Drug' Use in Victoria.

I believe that the submission from Victoria Police, to this Inquiry (dated 10 November 2003) was subject to interference. This submission had the potential to provide a source of extremely pertinent information on this issue which impacts on the lives of so many young (and not so young people) and their families.

In expressing this concern I confirm my support for the Report itself. The Report explores a wide range of issues, establishes a number of key principles and makes a series of recommendations. These recommendations will assist in reducing demand and restricting supply of illicit drugs and will also minimise the harm they cause.